Orthopaedic and trauma nursing

An evidence-based approach to musculoskeletal care

Orthopaedic and trauma nursing

An evidence-based approach to musculoskeletal care

EDITED BY

Sonya Clarke and Julie Santy-Tomlinson

WILEY Blackwell

This edition first published 2014 © 2014 by John Wiley & Sons, Ltd

Registered Office
John Wiley & Sons, Ltd, The Atrium, Southern Gate, Chichester, West Sussex, PO19 8SQ, UK

Editorial Offices
9600 Garsington Road, Oxford, OX4 2DQ, UK
The Atrium, Southern Gate, Chichester, West Sussex, PO19 8SQ, UK
111 River Street, Hoboken, NJ 07030-5774, USA

For details of our global editorial offices, for customer services and for information about how to apply for permission to reuse the copyright material in this book please see our website at www.wiley.com/wiley-blackwell

Library of Congress Cataloging-in-Publication Data

Orthopaedic and trauma nursing (Clarke)
Orthopaedic and trauma nursing : an evidence-based approach to musculoskeletal care /
edited by Sonya Clarke and Julie Santy-Tomlinson.
p. ; cm.
Includes bibliographical references and index.
ISBN 978-1-118-43885-5 (paper)
I. Clarke, Sonya, editor. II. Santy-Tomlinson, Julie, 1961– editor. III. Title.
[DNLM: 1. Orthopedic Nursing–methods. 2. Evidence-Based Nursing. 3. Musculoskeletal System–injuries. 4. Wounds and Injuries–nursing. WY 157.6]
RD753
616.7'0231–dc23

2014013802

A catalogue record for this book is available from the British Library.

Wiley also publishes its books in a variety of electronic formats. Some content that appears in print may not be available in electronic books.

Cover image: ©iStock/Raycat
Cover design by Meaden Creative

Set in 8.5/12pt Meridien by SPi Publisher Services, Pondicherry, India
Printed and bound in Malaysia by Vivar Printing Sdn Bhd

1 2014

Contents

Contributors

Thelma Begley, Assistant Professor in Children's Nursing, School of Nursing and Midwifery, Trinity College Dublin, MSc (Nursing), Bachelor Nursing Studies (Hons), Higher Diploma in Nursing Studies (Children's Nursing) & (Nurse Education), Orthopaedic Nursing Certificate, RGN, RCN, RNT

Thelma, a nurse for over 20 years, holds qualifications in both adult and child nursing. Her clinical experience includes adult, children and young people's medical and surgical nursing and in particular children's orthopaedic nursing. She has significant teaching experience in the development and delivery of undergraduate and postgraduate nursing programmes with specialist expertise in children's and orthopaedic nursing. Thelma's conference presentations and publications are related to these areas of interest. She is module leader on undergraduate, postgraduate and MSc Children's Nursing programmes and is Course Coordinator for the Higher Diploma in Children's Nursing in Trinity College.

Vanessa Blair, Staff Nurse, Belfast Health and Social Care Trust, Northern Ireland

Vanessa is an Australian-born and trained Registered Nurse, currently residing and working in Northern Ireland. Vanessa has gained experience across multiple nursing disciplines in what has been a varied career. She is currently developing specialist knowledge in orthopaedics and her experience of working in different nursing jurisdictions has provided her a platform for academic commentary on nursing best practice in orthopaedics. With a primary nursing degree at the University of New England, Australia, Vanessa has since completed a Certificate in Orthopaedics at Queen's University, Belfast. Vanessa has had one publication and is an examiner for orthopaedic and trauma OSCE's at Queen's University Belfast.

Sonya Clarke (*Editor*), Senior Lecturer (Education), Discipline Lead for Children's Nursing and Pathway Coordinator for continuing orthopaedic and trauma education programmes, School of Nursing & Midwifery, Queen's University Belfast (QUB), Northern Ireland. MSc, PGCE (Higher education), PgCert (Pain management), BSc (Hons) Specialist Practitioner in Orthopaedic Nursing, RCN, RGN

Sonya's career reflects adult and children's nursing within orthopaedic and fracture trauma, with an additional 15 years' clinical experience acquired as a Marie Curie nurse within palliative care. In 1988 Sonya commenced her RGN training and, through an appreciation of paediatrics, completed a Diploma in Children's Nursing in 1996. A Lecturer Practitioner position between QUB and a regional orthopaedic hospital encouraged the transition into full time higher education in 2003. Teaching both undergraduate and continuing education Sonya became Discipline Lead for Children's Nursing in 2012. Her academic portfolio incorporates a second role of 'pathway coordinator' where she actively develops, manages and delivers education to RN's practising within orthopaedic and trauma across the life span.

Scholarly activity reflects both specialist areas with an edited book published in 2012 on planning care for children. Annual publications include peer reviewed national and international journals, plus reviewer and editorial roles. Joint student publications motivate and challenge students with conference presentations ongoing nationally and internationally. This co-editor is currently registered on a taught Doctorate programme of study in Education (EdD) at QUB and a national forum member of RCN Society of Orthopaedic and Trauma Nursing (SOTN).

Alison Collins, Tissue Viability Nurse Belfast Health and Social Care Trust RGN (Royal Victoria Hospital, Belfast), BSc (Hons). District Nursing qualification Certificate in Orthopaedic Nursing, Post Grad Dip in Wound Healing and Tissue Repair, MSc.

Alison is an experienced nurse of more than 20 years; she currently holds a specialist nursing post within the largest Health and Social care Trust within Northern Ireland.

Peter Davis MBE Cert.Ed, BEd (Hons), RGN, DN, ONC, MA, Associate Professor (retired), part time lecturer University of Nottingham, Emeritus Editor International Journal of Orthopaedic and Trauma Nursing.

During the late 1980s, Peter held posts in pre- and post-basic nursing education with a specific remit for orthopaedic nurse education. In 1989 he gained a master's degree in nursing and education. In 1994 his first book, as editor and contributor, was published 'Nursing the Orthopaedic Patient'. From 1992 to 1994 he was chair of the RCN Society of Orthopaedic and Trauma Nursing and has spent several years as a committee member. He was founding editor of the Journal of Orthopaedic Nursing and now Emeritus Editor of the new International Journal of Orthopaedic & Trauma Nursing. He has presented numerous papers at national and international conferences. A personal philosophy of practice being primary to theory has kept him close to nursing care throughout his career and ensures an emphasis on research utilisation and evidence-based practice. In 2000 Her Majesty Queen Elizabeth II conferred on him the honour of Member of the Order of the British Empire (MBE) for services to orthopaedic nursing.

Mary Drozd, Senior Lecturer/Advanced Practitioner University of Wolverhampton MSc, BSc, RGN

Mary is a Senior Lecturer and pathway leader for the post-qualifying orthopaedic and trauma practitioner course plus course leader for the Return to Nursing Programme and also teaches on the post-qualifying mentorship courses. She is currently involved in the development of a new Master's in Nursing (Advanced Practice) course. Mary was elected onto the Royal College of Nursing (RCN) Society of Orthopaedic and Trauma Nursing (SOTN) Forum in 2009. She has led on the revision of the RCN Orthopaedic and Trauma Practitioner Competences which were published in September 2012. Alongside this she has contributed on behalf of the RCN at the National Institute for Health and Care Excellence on technology appraisals related to orthopaedic and trauma nursing plus co-chairing the Scientific Committee for SOTN. She has presented plenary, concurrent and workshop sessions at international conferences and has published papers related to orthopaedic and trauma nursing as well as nurse education. Mary is currently studying for a Doctorate.

Dr Jeannie Donnelly, Lead Nurse Tissue Viability, Belfast Health & Social Care Trust, and part-time teacher in the Faculty of Life and Health Sciences at Queens's University Belfast, PhD, BSc, RGN, ONC

Jeannie has a wealth of experience and knowledge as a clinical nurse specialist and educator. She currently has a dual role as practitioner and academic that best places her within post-registration education to teach and supervise RNs plus practice as a lead clinician in Northern Ireland.

Dr Sandra Flynn, Consultant Nurse Elective Orthopaedics, Countess of Chester NHS Foundation Trust, Chester, RN

Sandra Flynn currently holds the post of Nurse Consultant in Elective Orthopaedics at the Countess of Chester NHS Foundation Trust. Her clinical focus is mainly upper limb work which includes hand surgery, nurse-led clinics, performing nerve conduction studies and providing treatment for patients with bone and joint infections. As a nurse consultant Sandra is responsible for service development, education and training and research. She currently mentors and is responsible for the professional development of senior surgical specialist nurses within the Trust. Her recent PhD thesis at the University of Chester was entitled 'Perceptions of Care and Caring: An Orthopaedic Perspective.' Sandra is currently a committee member on the RCN SOTN forum.

Sinead Hahessy, RGN, BA, MA (Soc. Sc) is a Lecturer and Postgraduate Programme Director in Orthopaedic Nursing in the School of Nursing & Midwifery at the National University of Ireland, Galway.

Sinead has 14 years' experience as a lecturer in nurse education. Her clinical nursing career includes experience in orthopaedics, gerontology, emergency and theatre nursing. With a postgraduate background in sociology she has contributed to the professional and educational development of undergraduate and post-graduate nursing in Ireland through involvement in curriculum design and teaching. Her teaching and research interests are in orthopaedic/theatre nursing, professional development and clinical governance within the context of higher education in Ireland and qualitative research methods. She is currently undertaking a PhD in Education & Health Sciences at the University of Limerick, exploring the academic identity of nurse lecturers.

Fiona Heaney, Development Co-ordinator Orthopaedics, Clinical Facilitator/Practice RGN, MHSc (Nursing/Education), PG Diploma (Nursing Studies/ Orthopaedics), PG Diploma (Clinical Teaching), Galway

Fiona has worked in orthopaedics for over 13 years. Her main interest and experience is in the area of orthopaedic trauma, but also within orthopaedic rehabilitative and elective units. Currently she works as Clinical Facilitator/Practice Development Co-ordinator for the specialty of orthopaedics in Galway University Hospitals in Ireland. Fiona has an interest in developing practice and clinical education, and works closely with the National University of Ireland Galway in the development and delivery of the postgraduate diploma in orthopaedic nursing studies. Fiona is also interested in developing orthopaedic nursing nationally and is involved in the co-ordination of national orthopaedic nursing conferences, and has recently taken over as chairperson for the Irish Orthopaedic Nurses Section.

Karen Hertz, Advanced Practitioner, MSc, BSc, DPSN, RGN

Karen spent the last 30 years working in adult nursing. Post-qualification she practiced exclusively within orthopaedic nursing in a variety of positions in direct clinical practice. For the last eight years she has assumed the role of Advanced Practitioner in a busy trauma unit focusing on the development of care for older patients. She has a particular interest in patients with fragility fractures and specifically hip fracture care. Additional activity includes development of NICE Guidance for hip fractures and an active role in developing orthopaedic nursing. Karen is a current committee member of RCN national Society of Orthopaedic and Trauma Nursing forum.

Professor Rebecca Jester, RN, PhD

Rebecca qualified as a registered nurse in 1985 following completion of her pre-registration orthopaedic nursing certificate and then her registered general nurse training. She has worked as a staff nurse, sister and ward manager in a variety of trauma and orthopaedic settings since qualifying. She was awarded her PhD in Health Sciences from the University of Birmingham in 2001 and a personal professorship in orthopaedic nursing by Keele University in 2008. She has worked across the interface of education, research and practice since 1995 and currently is the Head of Department of adult nursing and midwifery at London South Bank University and also works part-time as an Advanced Nurse Practitioner in Orthopaedics at Dudley Group of Hospitals.

Julia Judd, Advanced Nurse Practitioner, University Hospital, Southampton, MSc, RSCN, RGN, ENB 219

Julia is an Advanced Nurse Practitioner in Children's Orthopaedics at the University Hospital Southampton, UK. She completed her joint training as a RSCN and RGN at Queen Mary's Hospital for Children in Carshalton and her orthopaedic training at Lord Mayor Treloar Hospital in Alton. Julia has jointly convened and chaired twelve national paediatric orthopaedic conferences based in Southampton and regularly presents at national and international conferences. She was instrumental in establishing the RCN Children and Young People's Orthopaedic and Trauma Community in 1998, and is current treasurer. Julia has published extensively, both articles and book contributions, and is a reviewer for the International Journal of Orthopaedic Nursing. She is actively involved with a number of different national and international research projects, specifically focusing on developmental dysplasia of the hip, Perthes disease, clubfoot and the orthopaedic manifestations of vitamin D deficiency. Her professional objective is to continue to promote the specialty of paediatric orthopaedic nursing.

Dr Mark Limb, Senior University Teacher, the University of Sheffield School of Nursing and Midwifery, Sheffield, England, PhD, BSc(Hons), ENB 219, RGN

Mark qualified as an adult nurse in 1988 and spent the first few years of his career in an orthopaedic and trauma setting. Since 1992 he has been in the field of education and has taught orthopaedic nursing to both pre- and post-registration student nurses. He has previously undertaken research into the psychological impact of limb reconstruction procedures but now focuses much of his time leading on educational quality and standards at school, faculty and university level as well as acting as leader for the pre-registration programme delivered within the school. He still remains committed to the delivery of education for orthopaedic nurses and maintains leadership of units with an orthoapedic trauma focus.

Dr Brian Lucas, Lead Nurse Practice, QUE Kings Lynn NHS Foundation Trust, RN, PhD

Brian has over 20 years experience in orthopaedic and trauma nursing as both a practitioner and educator. He is Chair of the RCN SOTN, an editorial board member of the International Journal of Orthopaedic and Trauma Nursing and has written a number of articles and book chapters on aspects of orthopaedic nursing. He was the nurse member on the NICE Guideline Development Group for the updating of the osteoarthritis guidelines. His current role as Lead Nurse Practice and Innovation at The Queen Elizabeth Hospital King's Lynn NHS Foundation Trust, Norfolk, involves ensuring that staff trust-wide have the skills and knowledge to deliver quality care and that nursing is organised in ways that maximise patient benefit.

Lorna Liggett, (Retired) Former Discipline Lead for Children's Nursing (Queen's University Belfast), BSc, RSCN

Lorna, a passionate and innovative nurse educator for over 40 years, is now retired. Her final position was within nurse education as the Discipline Lead for undergraduate children's nursing at Queen's University, Belfast. She co-edited the 2012 Wiley Blackwell text 'Planning Care for Children', prior to contributing to a forthcoming RCN book, 'Nurses' Voices From the Northern Ireland Troubles.'

Dr Carolyn Mackintosh-Franklin, University of Hull

Carolyn is a registered nurse with many years' experience in pain management, as a pioneering Clinical Nurse Specialist and educationalist. Her most recent work focuses on educating nurses and other health care professionals to develop greater understanding of the nature of pain, so that assessment and management can be improved for all pain sufferers. This includes the development of both undergraduate and postgraduate educational programmes, as well as contributions to pre-registration nurse education. Carolyn's own area of research focuses on health care staff and their attitudes towards people experiencing pain. There is considerable evidence that improvements in pain management have been slow to occur, with many people experiencing unnecessary and prolonged suffering as a result of both poor assessment and inadequate pain management. The attitudes of health care staff are likely to be a significant factor underpinning this failure to improve care, and current research indicates that individuals' own priorities and values play a key role in determining the standards of pain assessment and management of pain that sufferers receive.

Rosemary Masterson, Nurse Tutor, Cappagh National Orthopaedic Hospital, Dublin, RGN, ONC ENB 219, BNS, MSc in Nursing

Rosemary undertook her general training in the north-west of Ireland before completing the ENB 219 certificate in Orthopaedic Nursing at the Royal National Orthopaedic Hospital in Stanmore, London. She worked in both orthopaedic elective and trauma settings in Ireland and London. Rosemary undertook her Bachelor of Nursing Studies degree at University College Dublin and, in conjunction with the RCN and University of Manchester, completed a Masters in Nursing. She currently works in Cappagh National Orthopaedic Hospital, Dublin as a nurse tutor.

Sinead McDonald, Fracture Outcomes and Research Manager Royal Victoria Hospital, Belfast Health and Social Care Trust, RGN, Certificate in Fracture Trauma.

Sinead a registered Nurse since 1990, with 23 years' experience in Trauma and Orthopaedics. Her current position is Fracture Outcomes and Research Manager in the Royal Victoria Hospital since 2004. This involves the management of a regional database which holds data on all fractures in Northern Ireland under the supervision of Sinead, with special focus on hip fracture for the purpose of audit and research, contributing to the National Hip Fracture Database. The data Sinead provides and analyses using SPSS is recognised for its data completeness and accuracy and as a rich source of quality data used extensively by orthopaedic management, performance management and service improvement. She is also responsible for teaching trauma research and audit for both nursing and medical staff and the supervision of all in-house auditing.

Pamela Moore, Sister in Fracture Clinic, Royal Victoria Hospital Belfast, PgCert Specialist Practitioner in Orthopaedic Nursing, BSc Hons, RGN

Pamela has many years of experience in both managerial and 'hands on' roles within a busy dedicated fracture clinic/unit. She is passionate about orthopaedic and fracture trauma care and values ongoing nurse education. Pamela is a frequent specialist lecturer on the orthopaedic and fracture trauma programmes and OSCE examiner at Queen's University, Belfast.

Lynne Newtown-Triggs, MA, RGN, Pre Assessment Sister, Bedford Hospital NHS Trust

Lynne currently works as a Pre Assessment Nurse Manager at a district general hospital with her main focus being the orthopaedic specialty. She qualified as an RGN in 1984 and has since worked in both elective and trauma environments as a ward sister and specialist nurse. She completed the ENB 219 at the RJAH Orthopaedic Hospital in 1987 and has since completed a BA (Hons) degree in nursing studies and an MA in Healthcare Ethics.

Donna Poole, Lecturer and joint Unit Co-ordinator BSc Professional Nursing Practice (Spinal Cord Injury), MA in Practice Education (currently studying), PgCert in Practice Education, Certificate in video streaming technology and education, Certificate in Spinal Cord Injuries, Certificate in Continence Management, Diploma Applied Science (Nursing), RGN

Donna, a registered nurse for 25 years, has experience in spinal cord injury nursing, rehabilitation, community and domiciliary care and case management. Her current position is lead nurse for education in a specialist neuromusculoskeletal NHS Trust. Prior to this post Donna facilitated and coordinated the rehabilitation and discharge of spinal cord injured persons in the London Spinal Cord Injury Centre. She graduated in Sydney, Australia in 1987, with a Diploma in Applied Science (Nursing). Following this she completed her certificate in spinal cord injury nursing and after working in two spinal units, she worked in remote communities of Australia as a registered nurse and as manager of a home and community care project. Director of Nursing of a district nursing service, teaching and presenting on care of the spinal cord injured person statewide and community nursing with a continence focus followed, then teaching the Diploma in Nursing (pre-enrolment). In all of these posts Donna has utilised and shared her knowledge of care of the spinal cord injured person to promote awareness and knowledge of spinal cord injury and to lead and motivate those caring for people with spinal cord injury. In her current post she also teaches and part coordinates BSc Professional Nursing Practice (spinal cord injury) for London South Bank University. Member of MASCIP, ISCoS, various contributions for guidelines and research in the field; 'Enhancing the Emotional Dimensions of Nursing Care in Spinal Cord Injury', an action research project in collaboration with LSBU (2005–ongoing), contributor to publication Huntleigh/SIA (2009) 'Moving and Handling Guidelines.'

Hannagh Pugh, Orthopaedic Trauma CNS, University College Hospital, London

Hannah trained 'up north' before coming to London as an RN and has worked in a variety of orthopaedic positions including a sister's post at a major trauma centre and as a specialist nurse for limb reconstruction. She is now an orthopaedic CNS at The Princess Grace Hospital. A frequent presenter at both national and international events and author on various orthopaedic topics, Hannah is also a committee member of the RCN Society of Orthopaedic and Trauma Nursing, is secretary of The London Orthopaedic Nurses Group and is on the editorial committee for the international Journal of Orthopaedic and Trauma Nursing.

Pauline Robertson Lecturer and joint Unit Co-ordinator, BSc Professional Nursing Practice (Spinal Cord Injury), London South Bank University and Spinal Outreach Practitioner London Spinal Cord Injury Centre, Royal National Orthopaedic Hospital; PgCert in Practice Education, qualified moving and handling trainer, MA in Practice Education (ongoing), RGN

Pauline has worked in nursing for the last 26 years and in spinal cord injury (SCI) for the last 22 plus having worked overseas to develop a SCIC with a British wheelchair charity and relief work for agencies that treat people with SCI through conflict or natural disaster. Pauline currently works clinically as an Acute SCI Outreach Practitioner helping to support newly injured patients and helped develop many new innovations such as a new national database to register all new SCI patients to enable research and audit throughout the patient's journey. Teaching commitments mainly consist of post-registration for adult nurses, usually on the topic of SCI and how it relates to that specialty and regularly supports the Spinal Injuries Association.

Jean Rogers, Practice Education Facilitator for Stockport NHS Foundation Trust, Stockport, RGN, BSc (Hons), MSc, ONC, Cert. Ed(Fe)

Jean qualified as an RGN in 1988 from Salford NHS Foundation Trust. She has worked in a number of areas including elective orthopaedics, acute trauma and ENT, rheumatology and endocrinology, acute medicine and acute rehabilitation. She undertook the orthopaedic course at the Robert Jones and Agnes Hunt Orthopaedic Hospital in 1991 where she was in the last group to undertake the twelve-month course and in her spare time completed a certificate in higher education. Following this Jean held the posts of senior staff nurse, junior sister and lecturer/practitioner and completed a BSc (Hons) in nursing practice. She is co-author of the Oxford University Press 'Handbook of Orthopaedic and Trauma Nursing' as well as numerous articles. She is chair of the Northwest Orthopaedic and Trauma Forum, chair of RCN Cheshire East and sits on the North West Regional Board and is a staff governor. Her main interests lie in Orthopaedics, nurse education and the politics of nursing and she takes an active role in these areas being a member of the orthopaedic forum, the practice educator's special interest group and the RCN Education Forum. Jean is currently undertaking a PhD in Health and Social Care at the University of Salford. Jean's current post is as practice education facilitator for Stockport NHS Foundation Trust where she believes that she has the best of both worlds educating the nurses of the future in the practice setting.

Julie Santy-Tomlinson *(Editor)*, Senior Lecturer University of Hull, BSc, MSc, RGN, ENB 219

Julie trained as a nurse at St Mary's Hospital Paddington, London in the early 1980s. She has always been an orthopaedic nurse at heart and took up various clinical posts as staff nurse, ward sister and practice development nurse in a variety of orthopaedic units in London, South Africa, Cambridge, Shropshire and Hull in the 1980s and early 1990s. She undertook the ENB 219 certificate in Orthopaedic Nursing at the Robert Jones and Agnes Hunt Orthopaedic Hospital, Oswestry in 1986/7. In 1996 Julie moved to her first post in nursing education at the University of Bradford where she taught and managed various modules concerning evidence-based practice, orthopaedic and trauma nursing, older people and wound management and tissue viability until moving to the University of Hull where she has worked since 2002. She is currently a Senior Lecturer and University Teaching Fellow there. Her PhD considers the diagnosis of infection in external fixator pin site wounds. The study was supported by a nursing research scholarship from the Smith and Nephew Foundation. Involvement with the Royal College of Nursing Society of Orthopaedic and Trauma Nursing for the past 20 years (for some of that period as a committee member) enabled Julie to develop world-wide networks with orthopaedic and trauma nurses which she has maintained and developed over the last decade. Julie speaks regularly at international conferences on numerous topics relevant to orthopaedic and trauma nursing. She has also published widely on a variety of issues. She became co-editor of the International Journal of Orthopaedic and Trauma Nursing (formerly the Journal of Orthopaedic Nursing) in 2009.

Helen Stradling, Macmillan Advanced Nurse Practitioner Sarcoma, Nuffield Orthopaedic Centre, Oxford University Hospitals NHS Trust, Oxford

I qualified from the University of Birmingham in 1998. From there I took up the post of staff nurse at the Nuffield Orthopaedic Centre in Oxford. It was here that I was able to mix my passion for orthopaedics and oncology as the sarcoma patients were nursed on the ward. During the first few years on the ward I began to increase my knowledge relating to sarcoma and undertook study in both oncology and orthopaedics. In 2004 the Nuffield Orthopaedic Centre became one of seven national centres for the care of bone sarcoma and it was at this point that I was successful in my application for the role of Macmillan Specialist Nurse for musculoskeletal oncology. Over the last seven years this role has grown and I have been able to implement changes for the benefit of all sarcoma patients treated in Oxford. We now offer a 'one stop shop' for diagnostics; all patients are nursed in the same ward area by nurses with oncology and orthopaedic experience, and follow-up is now nurse-led. The service took over the care of the bone sarcoma patients previously treated in Bristol in 2007 which has again increased our referral numbers.

I was awarded the Nursing Times Cancer Nurse Leader of the Year award in 2010 in recognition of all the work which had been put into improving the pathway for sarcoma patients and their families in Oxford. I became the first Chair of the National Sarcoma Forum in September 2011 and this is now a forum in which things are being taken forward by professionals in order to continue to improve the care of sarcoma patients in the UK.

Anna Timms, Limb Reconstruction Clinical Nurse Specialist, Royal National Orthopaedic Hospital, Stanmore, RGN, BSc Psychology, ONC

Anna qualified from the Queen Elizabeth School of Nursing, Birmingham in 1994. Since then she has specialised within the fields of rheumatology and orthopaedics. Working within the trauma environment at the Royal London Hospital she became a Limb Reconstruction Nurse Specialist in 2005, leaving to become a member of the team at the Royal National Orthopaedic Hospital in 2012. She has authored articles and presented both nationally and internationally in the field of limb reconstruction.

Elizabeth Wright, Advanced Nurse Practitioner, University Hospital, Southampton, RGN, RSCN, MSc Advanced Clinical Practice

Liz commenced her nursing career in 1984. She trained at the Hammersmith Hospital, London and then gained experience in general paediatric and neonatal intensive care nursing. She entered the specialist field of orthopaedic paediatric nursing in 1990. She was Sister of a paediatric orthopaedic ward for six years, then a Nurse Specialist until she commenced her current post of Advanced Nurse Practitioner, completing her MSc in Advanced Nurse Practice in 2004. Her professional objective is to raise the awareness of the unique speciality of paediatric orthopaedics. She strives to achieve this by having jointly convened and chaired several national paediatric orthopaedic conferences based in Southampton, as well as having established and chaired the RCN Children and Young Peoples Orthopaedic and Trauma Group in 1998. She continues to be actively involved in this group and is the current treasurer. Liz participates in the RCN Society of Orthopaedic and Trauma Nursing (SOTN); being a member of various SOTN work panels and is a part of the SOTN Scientific Committee. She has published several times on the subject of paediatric orthopaedics.

Beverly Wellington, MSc Advanced Practice, BSc (Hons) Nursing Studies, PgCert TLHE, RGN, ONC, Dip CN, Certificate in Cognitive Behavioural Therapy, Certificate in Counselling Skills, Professional Certificate in Management

Beverley has many years of experience in orthopaedic nursing, having worked in Ward Manager roles in both trauma and elective areas before becoming a Clinical Nurse Specialist covering both of those areas. She later moved into the specialised area of brachial plexus injuries and since 2004 has been working with the Scottish National Brachial Plexus Injury Service as a Clinical Nurse Specialist based at the New Victoria Hospital, Glasgow, Scotland. She has a dual role and also works as Programme Leader and Lecturer for a Graduate Certificate in Orthopaedic Care programme at the University of the West of Scotland. Beverley regularly presents papers at national and international conferences and has written for both book and journal publications. She has worked on projects for both national and international collaborations including guideline development, care pathways, ementoring and orthopaedic nursing competencies. Her other interests include partnership working for several years with Malawi and she has made regular visits to the country and facilitates ongoing projects.

Elaine Wylie, Nurse Specialist, Southern Health and Social Care Trust, Northern Ireland, RGN, BSc (Hons), PgDip Specialist Practice Registration Rheumatology

Elaine has worked in rheumatology for 23 years and the last 13 as a Nurse Specialist. She is currently based at Craigavon Area Hospital, where her clinical responsibilities include nurse-led review, joint injections and biologic therapy clinics, as well as running a telephone helpline service. She is involved in service development locally and has mentored rheumatology nurses in Jesi, Italy to extend their role and service. Her specific interests in rheumatology are inflammatory arthritis, patient and family education and support, and staff training and development. She is currently developing her skills in musculoskeletal ultrasound. Elaine teaches on both rheumatology and orthopaedic specialist courses at Queen's University Belfast and the University of Ulster. She has a keen interest in research and audit and has presented a variety of papers locally, nationally and internationally.

Foreword

To many nurses orthopaedics is like Marmite (a brown, sticky, edible spread made from yeast extract, commonly eaten in the UK and known for its strong salty taste), you either love it or hate it! How anyone does not want to be involved in a form of nursing that can actually make such a huge difference to the patient is beyond me, but that's the nature of care. With their saws and screws, plates and nails the orthopaedic surgeon can often rebuild the skeleton, the muscles, the ligaments and tendons so that function is restored. However, that's not the end of the journey as many of us know. It is the specialist knowledge of the nurse, the physiotherapist, the occupational therapist and the rest of the specialist team that cares, advises and encourages the patient in the pre/post-surgery phases, or following injury. Here much of the restorative accountability lies with the orthopaedic practitioner.

We have come a long way since Jean-Andre Venel who established the first orthopaedic institute in 1780 and Dame Agnes Hunt, whose meeting with orthopaedic surgeon Robert Jones in 1903 was to see her embark on journey that would develop into the origins of orthopaedic nursing in the UK. Nursing practice has seen many changes since the turn of the 20th century. Long gone are the 'Nightingale' wards with rows of patients, legs aloft in traction. Gone are the days where patients would be pushed out on their beds to specially constructed verandas for fresh air. Now efforts are squarely focused on early rehabilitation, mobilisation, complication prevention, education and safe discharge. Of course, evidence-based practice and the unique contribution of the orthopaedic practitioner ensures all this is possible.

I have had the privilege of working with many of the contributors to this book through being the co-editor of the International Journal of Orthopaedic and Trauma Nursing. I can vouch for their energy and enthusiasm around the subject area and know that the co-editors of this book would have had 'all on' reigning in the team to get this book complete. However, you occasionally hit on a winning formula, a group of people that just work, people who share a vision and passion that drive a project forward. This is one such case. Here is the culmination of all that energy which has produced an inspired book to aid those who want to learn more about the nature of orthopaedic care.

If you have looked on the shelves for a new orthopaedic nursing book you will know that they are few and far between. The evolution of this book is an important step in taking orthopaedic care forward. No matter where in the world you care for your patients you will find this book essential for current evidenced-based orthopaedic care. It captures so many of the changes that now drive orthopaedic care around the globe by drawing on expertise and clinical innovations that often form the basis of articles found in the International Journal of Orthopaedic and Trauma Nursing. Drawing on experience from both practice and education the editors have bound together so many topic areas, making them relevant to current practice. Chapters range from pure anatomy and physiology to the place of research in orthopaedic care and from musculoskeletal injuries to the needs of the child with specific orthopaedic issues; all capturing relevant and up to date orthopaedic astuteness. There is something for everyone and little is missing.

My vision for this book is that it will not sit on a shelf in a library somewhere, occasionally used as reference material, but will find its way onto wards and departments where it can be used and applied by practitioners delivering care. If you're looking to improve your patients' experience of orthopaedic care, no matter what continent of the world you work in, this book can be the catalyst for that change.

I'm sure this will become a key text for many orthopaedic practitioners whilst finding its way onto the reading lists of orthopaedic courses globally. If you are looking for an orthopaedic book linking theory to practice whilst focusing on evidence-based care of the orthopaedic patient this is a must-have read – for your team or to add to your own collection.

Bryan Smith
University of Nottingham, UK and former
Co-Editor International Journal of Orthopaedic
and Trauma Nursing

Preface

Orthopaedic and trauma care are highly specialised aspects of health care focused on the person with musculoskeletal problems, injury and following orthopaedic surgery. Such care is delivered across the lifespan from birth to death and in a wide range of community and hospital settings. The skills required for effective, evidence-based practice must be developed through a regard for the knowledge and evidence base for practice coupled with development of competence and expertise. This branch of care shares generic skills but encompasses specialist skills like no other. The aim of this book is to provide practitioners working in orthopaedic and musculoskeletal trauma settings with the evidence, guidance and knowledge required to develop their skills and underpin effective practice.

The title of this book reflects the focus on the practice of musculoskeletal care as well as signifies a specific focus on the evidence base for that practice. The editors and contributors have not tried to achieve the impossible in providing information about all of the available knowledge on a given topic, but offer building blocks for extending knowledge and understanding the issues that drive safe, effective practice. The book provides relevant information about key theory and summaries of the evidence base underpinning all the main aspects of orthopaedic and trauma practice. This approach will enable the practitioner to easily gain an understanding of the existing evidence base for their practice. This will ensure that the book is relevant for those studying for a degree as well as for those clinicians practicing in developing and advanced orthopaedic and trauma practitioner roles. Evidence is rarely out of date, but sometimes superseded. One danger with this approach in this book, therefore, is that the evidence base is likely to move on as time progresses, so it is important that the practitioner is also encouraged to seek more up to date evidence through knowledge of how to access and appraise it.

Because the focus of this text is on evidence based practice, each chapter is supported by summaries, or digests, of the available evidence as well as reference to relevant and seminal research. Guidance for this practice is based on this evidence. This will enable the practitioner to focus on the evidence essential for modern practice. Whilst much of the focus of the book is on the care of the adult it also includes sections focusing specifically on children and young people and on older people with orthopaedic conditions, following surgical intervention and after injury.

Although the title of the book reflects a focus on nursing care of the orthopaedic and trauma patient, it also aims to provide a wealth of useful and thought provoking information for other practitioners working in the orthopaedic and trauma setting. Equally, the book is aimed at practitioners beyond the shores of the United Kingdom where the editors are based.

Part one of the book provides an overview of the key issues that relate to orthopaedic and trauma nursing practice. It considers the theory underpinning orthopaedic care and places it in context with the history and development of practice in the musculoskeletal care environment. An important aspect of this is a discussion of how the evidence base for orthopaedic and trauma practice has developed and how the reader might develop skills in seeking out and evaluating evidence. There is also an overview of how professional and practice development, based on theoretical knowledge and evidence, can lead to ensuring and developing competence and effective practice. Integral to this introductory section is an overview of the musculoskeletal system that will enable to the practitioner to underpin a knowledge of relevant anatomy and physiology to the other sections of the book. Rehabilitation begins at the patient's very first contact with health care services and the central concepts within, and practice of, rehabilitative care are also considered.

Part two of the book focuses on six specific aspects of practice which, although generic, take on a specific specialist focus in the musculoskeletal care setting. Consideration of general and specialist assessment of the patient, casting, traction and external fixation, prevention and management of complications and patient safety, nutrition and hydration, pain assessment and management and wound management and tissue viability are considered specifically within the context of orthopaedic and trauma care. These aspects of care, along with the key principles discussed in the previous section, need to be applied to the practice advice provided in the remainder of the book.

Part three of the book considers the care of the patient with musculoskeletal conditions not attributed to trauma, but to degeneration of the bones, joints and soft tissue with a specific focus on arthropathies such as osteoarthritis. The section considers the management of these conditions with a specific focus on elective surgery which constitutes much of the need for orthopaedic care in the non-emergency setting.

Part four of the book provides an overview of the principles and practice of care of the patient following musculoskeletal trauma and injury. It begins with a discussion of the principles of trauma care, providing the practitioner with important knowledge to underpin safe and effective trauma care practice both in the emergency situation and subsequently. This is followed by specific consideration of the principles of fracture management and care and then by specific consideration of fractures in the older person with a focus on fragility fracture. This if followed by an overview of the care of the person with spinal cord injury aimed specifically at practitioners who provide that care in the general hospital setting. Finally there is a brief overview of the knowledge required to care for the patient with soft tissue and nerve injury including brachial plexus injuries.

Part five of the book provides an overview of key concepts and fundamental issues that relate to the neonate, infant, child and young person. The material is specific to this client group and values the expertise of children's nursing relating to skeletal growth and development, family-centred care, safeguarding/non-accidental injury and pain management. This is followed by key information relating to the assessment and management of common children's musculoskeletal conditions that the practitioner may come across in everyday practice. A review of fracture healing, diagnosis and classification then follows before the complexities of diagnosing and treating children's fractures considering the immature and developing skeleton are then discussed along with the principles of conservative and surgical treatment.

We hope that the readers of this book will use the text as a general reference source for maintaining and developing their knowledge, but that they will also extend that knowledge by accessing the further reading and seeking new material that is relevant to their own learning needs through online and traditional sources of information. We hope that this will help to ensure that orthopaedic and trauma practice will become increasingly safe, effective and evidence-based.

Sonya Clarke and Julie Santy-Tomlinson
Belfast and Hull

PART I

Key issues in orthopaedic and musculoskeletal trauma nursing

CHAPTER 1

An introduction to orthopaedic and trauma care

Julie Santy-Tomlinson[1] and Sonya Clarke[2]

[1] *University of Hull, Hull, UK*

[2] *Queen's University Belfast, Belfast, UK*

Introduction

The aim of this chapter is to provide an introduction to orthopaedic and trauma nursing and the care of the orthopaedic and musculoskeletal trauma patient. The focus is on the diversity of the individuals in need of that care and the culture, settings, theory and contexts in which that care takes place. Orthopaedic and trauma nursing is a discrete but diverse specialty focused on the care of the patient with musculoskeletal problems. These problems are related to either disease or injury of the bones, joints, muscle and soft tissues which are central to human movement. Orthopaedic and trauma practitioners must develop knowledge and skills in order to provide expert specialist care based on diverse, highly specific and specialised patient needs. One of the defining features of orthopaedic care is that it is provided across the life span from birth through to death and in every care setting.

Historical perspectives

In an early textbook, Mary Powell (1951) wrote of the general principles of orthopaedic nursing, which embodied the principles of rest balanced with movement and exercise, treatment of the patient as a whole, optimum positioning for joints using splinting and traction, relief of pain and the provision of the best conditions for recovery and healing. This encompassed pre-operative and post-surgical care, trauma care and rehabilitation. With a focus on the nurse–patient relationship and team work, many parallels can be drawn with orthopaedic and trauma nursing today. The book was based on her many experiences up to that time of inter- and post-war orthopaedic care and what she had learnt from the teachings of Dame Agnes Hunt. Although care must have been provided to patients with musculoskeletal conditions and injuries in earlier times, it is often said that orthopaedic nursing's history – particularly in the UK – began with Dame Agnes Hunt in Shropshire, England in the early decades of the 20th century. Widely associated with the early development of orthopaedic nursing, Agnes Hunt took an approach to the care of individuals with musculoskeletal problems and disability that focused on the importance of rest, fresh air and good nutrition in ensuring the proper development and recovery of diseased, injured and deformed bone, joints and soft tissue. Many common musculoskeletal diseases of that time such as tuberculosis and poliomyelitis were largely eradicated in developed countries during the twentieth century and this has resulted in important and far reaching change in the priorities for orthopaedic and trauma care since that time. Even so, this history remains pertinent to the way in which care is provided today.

The early literature relating to musculoskeletal care focused on the practice of many weeks and months of enforced rest, while the current focus is on early mobilisation and avoiding inactivity. Although much is very different in the second decade of the 21st century, there are some principles of early 20th century care that remain relevant – in particular the need for what Mary Powell (1951) would have called an 'orthopaedic conscience' (which she later renamed the 'orthopaedic

Orthopaedic and Trauma Nursing: An Evidence-based Approach to Musculoskeletal Care, First Edition. Edited by Sonya Clarke and Julie Santy-Tomlinson.

eye') – a special 'sense' or consciousness of how movement, position, posture and comfort is central to both the assessment and care of the orthopaedic patient in modern health care. This is largely based on the practitioner's experience of working with patients. This is reflected in the way in which skilled and experienced orthopaedic and trauma practitioners are able, for example, to recognise nursing needs by instinctively observing the way in which people move or hold themselves. Skilled orthopaedic practitioners, for example, understand how gentle and minimal repositioning of a limb or supporting it with a pillow can improve comfort and support healing and recovery. Such observation and subsequent intervention still demonstrate how nurses make judgments about the needs of patients and formulate decisions about care based on clinical information derived from a variety of sources including, but not exclusively, evidence (Thompson and Dowding 2002).

As a specific entity, orthopaedic nursing has parallels with the development of orthopaedic and trauma surgery and famous surgeons such as Hugh Owen Thomas and Robert Jones. Their efforts led to the inception of orthopaedic surgery in the 1940s as part of the development of the National Health Service (NHS) in the United Kingdom as well as the development of orthopaedic and trauma services around the world. Even so, orthopaedic care has been provided for as long as the musculoskeletal system has been prone to disease and injury, although this previously took place under the auspices of bone setters, barber surgeons and other 'informal' carers. Trauma nursing is most often evident in nursing stories from war such as those surrounding the Crimean War and the role played by both Florence Nightingale and Mary Seacole. The care of patients sustaining musculoskeletal trauma has often made strides forward during times of conflict, war, great societal change and disaster whilst the development of elective surgery has been driven by a desire to improve lives by, for example, ameliorating the pain and disability of osteoarthritis and other chronic conditions.

At the beginning of the 20th century a number of specialist orthopaedic hospitals sprang up in the UK. This led to the rapid creation of a network of centres, often in rural or suburban locations, focused on the specialist care of patients and the education of practitioners in the principles and specifics of musculoskeletal care. These organisations also became early developers of the evidence base for orthopaedic care. As services have become more centralised, a number of these hospitals have closed and been integrated into acute urban hospital centres. Those remaining specialist hospitals continue to develop the specialist knowledge for musculoskeletal care alongside emergency departments and acute, outpatient and community units.

As the 20th century progressed musculoskeletal care began to evolve into two related entities – those of elective care and of musculoskeletal trauma care. Elective orthopaedic surgery involves procedures that are planned in advance and are designed to treat or manage known conditions which are causing pain and/or disability. This often includes surgery for arthropathies such as osteo- and rheumatoid arthritis and might also involve surgery to further manage the effects of trauma once initial recovery and healing has taken place. This might include surgery to correct deformity or the removal of 'metal work.' Patients with arthropathies such as rheumatoid arthritis are often cared for in specialist centres where the focus is on medical management and rehabilitation rather than on surgery. These patients might, however, be referred for elective surgery when this is thought to be of potential benefit.

Trauma care, on the other hand, is unplanned and involves the management, care and rehabilitation of patients who have suffered injury following a specific event such as a fall, road traffic accident, sporting injury or other mechanism of injury. All structures in the human body are prone to injury and trauma care, therefore, takes place in a variety of settings including the emergency department, intensive care unit and neurosurgical setting as well as the orthopaedic trauma unit. Orthopaedic trauma care is focused specifically on trauma to the musculoskeletal system whilst taking into account the need to include other aspects of trauma management as necessary. The focus in this book is specifically, therefore, on those aspects of trauma care which involve the musculoskeletal system. Often orthopaedic nurses are specialists in one or the other of elective or trauma orthopaedics but many have skills in both areas.

The nature of orthopaedic and musculoskeletal trauma nursing

The orthopaedic practitioner has a unique role, with associated skills and knowledge. Nursing theory applied to orthopaedic and musculoskeletal trauma nursing comes both from general sources relating to nursing and healthcare as a whole, and from specialist sources. The theory which underpins practice is often based on an in-depth knowledge of anatomy and physiology of the musculoskeletal system and of those physical and psychosocial factors which affect musculoskeletal health and well-being and recovery from injury and surgery.

The nature of orthopaedic nursing and associated practice has been a matter of some discussion over many years. Work has focused on its status as a discrete specialty and the specific nursing actions which make it distinct from other nursing specialisms and from 'generic' nursing. This has highlighted the importance of specialist skills and the need for specific education for orthopaedic and trauma nursing. One example of this is the assessment skills needed to recognise a very specific set of potential complications of orthopaedic surgery, conditions and injuries (see Chapter 9 for further detail) that are not part of the generic skills required of nurses and other practitioners. See Box 1.1 for further detail of the present state of inquiry into the specialist nature of orthopaedic nursing.

Box 1.1 Evidence Digest: The nature of orthopaedic nursing

An early study by Love (1995) attempted to clarify and discriminate between orthopaedic and general nursing using a questionnaire survey of orthopaedic nurses that asked which nursing activities were highly orthopaedic nursing functions and which were not. There were a range of activities deemed to be 'unique' to orthopedic nursing including 'elevation of limbs to prevent swelling' and 'removal of splintage if ischaemia is threatening safety of a limb'.

More recently a number of researchers (Santy 2001, Drozd *et al.*, 2007) have used qualitative approaches to research such as grounded theory to explore the nature of orthopaedic and trauma nursing and examine the detail of what specific interventions practitioners undertake with orthopaedic patients. Work by Judd (2010) has undertaken similar inquiry into issues related to working with children with orthopaedic problems.

This work is a foundation on which theory, education and practice frameworks can be developed to ensure that musculoskeletal care can be increasingly effective in the future and enable practitioners to articulate their specialist role and value. The studies collectively demonstrate that there are many specialist interventions which focus on supporting mobility, managing and caring for the patient with orthopaedic devices such as splints, traction, casts and external fixators and caring for the patient following specific surgical procedures and injuries as well as preventing and recognising the complications of those interventions. The studies also highlight how specialist skills are developed and used alongside the generic interventions and actions considered to be fundamental aspects of nursing as a whole. The studies can be used as evidence to help ensure that the skills, knowledge and attitudes required for effective orthopaedic and trauma nursing practice are maintained. The findings, therefore, ensure that the specialty of orthopaedic care is protected from erosion and that patients are cared for by practitioners who are competent in providing that care in all its forms.

Mobility and function

The focus on the musculoskeletal system and its function in facilitating movement and mobility is an inherent aspect of orthopaedic care. Mobility, movement and function are concepts, therefore, which have long been argued to be central to orthopaedic nursing (Davis 1994, Love 1995, Balcombe *et al.*, 1991). Even so, the concept of mobility itself has been difficult to define and work which considered this is described in more detail in an evidence summary in Box 1.2, in which Ouellet and Rush (1992, 1996, 1998) and Rush and Ouellet (1998) have begun to highlight the complex and essential nature of mobility and its link with immobility as well as the care needs these present. Davis (1994) also emphasised the centrality of mobility for patients with musculoskeletal problems within the physical, psychological and social domains of care. Key to this discussion is an acknowledgement that movement is an essential aspect of human health and wellbeing. It also acknowledges that both musculoskeletal problems and the resulting nursing interventions can lead to immobility and that such immobility or restricted mobility leads to consequences which include serious complications.

The centrality of mobility in orthopaedic and trauma nursing practice has led to one proposed model for orthopaedic nursing (Balcombe *et al.*, 1991, Davis 1994) which holds mobility at its core. Even so, orthopaedic nursing has tended to continue to use generic nursing models applied to the care of the adult or child. Nursing models ideally aim to illustrate the theory of nursing practice to enable the practitioner to organise and prioritise effective and safe patient care. The 'nursing process,' developed by Orlando

Box 1.2 Evidence digest: Mobility as a concept for orthopaedic care

The work of Ouellet and Rush in the 1990s has done much to illuminate the centrality of mobility in caring for patients with musculoskeletal problems. Even though the work has largely been conducted in older people's care settings, the findings have direct relevance to orthopaedic and trauma nursing.

A group of papers report on a series of studies which aimed to explore the concept of mobility and its relationship to nursing practice. The researchers used a 'concept development' approach (as is often the case with work which aims to clarify and develop a concept for use in practice) which began with an in-depth exploration and analysis of the literature relating to mobility. This first phase identified, using literature from the health and social sciences, a limited view of mobility in nursing with a focus on immobility and impaired physical mobility without much provided in the way of direction for nursing (Ouellet and Rush 1992).

The second phase of the work (Ouellet and Rush 1996) employed a qualitative approach to explore the concepts identified in the literature by conducting a series of interviews with nurses and analysing the data using content analysis. The interviews showed that the practical approaches and experience of the nurses supported the findings of the literature, but that there was a need to explore this in more detail with patients across different client groups. Hence, in a second phase of data collection (Rush and Ouellet 1998), thematic content analysis of semi-structured interviews with elderly clients was used to explore the concept of mobility in more detail. Patient descriptions resulted in the emergence of three interrelated dimensions of mobility: physical, cognitive and social. From the patients' descriptions of mobility six qualities emerged: *ease and freedom of movement, independence, automaticity, purposefulness, self-environmental awareness* and *continuity*.

The authors moved on to use this work to develop a proposed conceptual model of mobility (Ouellet and Rush 1998) which is broken down into six components: *Mobility capacity, forces, perceptions, actuation in all dimensions, patterns and consequences*. These components can have direct relevance to the role of the orthopaedic practitioner in directing assessment and interventions which assess and improve mobility capacity. This takes account of the forces involved in mobilisation for patients with specific conditions, allowing for the patient and carer perceptions of their own mobility, how people actually mobilise and the results of both mobilisation and the care provided.

(1961), provides a logical, structured approach that directs the practitioner's critical thinking in a dynamic manner. It encourages the nurse to balance scientific evidence, personal interpretation and judgement when delivering patient/family-centred care. This is supported by models of nursing and philosophies of care that help to define the care role and guide practice (Corkin *et al.*, 2012). The nursing process presents as a four stage procedure to: assess (often extended to 'nursing diagnosis'), plan, implement and evaluate care. Nursing diagnosis involves a professional judgement based on holistic assessment. Figure 1.1 not only identifies the four components, but reinforces its cyclical nature. A variety of models and frameworks have been developed on the basis of the nursing process to plan care.

Influential work by Fawcett (1995) encouraged many nursing models to incorporate four key components:

- the person
- their environment
- health
- nursing.

Commonly adopted nursing models in orthopaedic and trauma care settings include the Roper, Logan and Tierney's (2000) model of nursing care (particularly in use in the UK, originally published in 1980, and subsequently revised) based upon activities of living, Orem's self-care model (2001) and Roy's Adaptation model (1984). Such models of care have value for the orthopaedic and trauma patient as a way of ensuring that care is provided within a philosophy that ensures that specific individual needs are met. A joint approach is sometimes adopted, especially when planning care for children; for example by combining Casey's partnership model (1988) and Roper, Logan and Tierney's (2000) model of care. The first is the founding model of family-centred care and the latter encompasses the 12 activities of daily living and life continuum along with consideration of dependence/ independence. In combination they produce a comprehensive approach to planning of care. Recently, nursing models have been overshadowed by a focus on evidence-based practice, but they continue to play an important part in providing a holistic theoretical foundation for nursing that has the potential to enhance

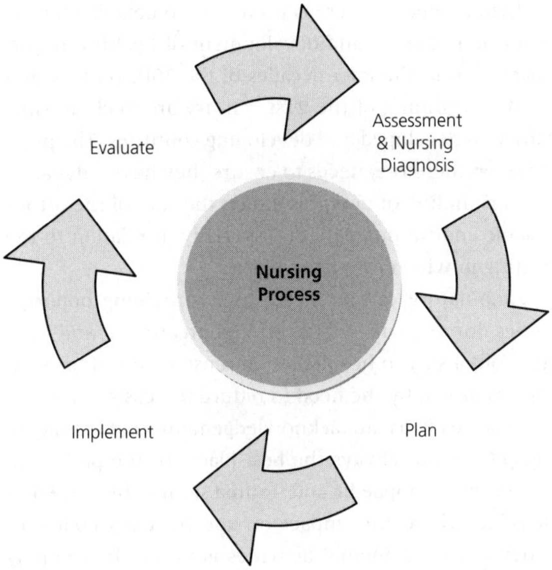

Figure 1.1 The nursing process

practice (McCrae 2012) within orthopaedic and trauma care. Even so, orthopaedic and trauma nursing perhaps has yet to embrace nursing models fully.

Public health and musculoskeletal conditions and injury

Public health focuses on the health and wellbeing of individuals from a societal perspective. It is synonymous with the prevention of disease and ill health through public action. The public health agenda applied to orthopaedic and trauma care is complex. It is mainly focused on skeletal health but this, in itself, is a multi-faceted issue and necessarily involves consideration of numerous factors which affect musculoskeletal health such as:

- bone development in the child and young adult
- bone health – including, specifically, vitamin D deficiency, osteoporosis, rickets and osteomalacia
- exercise and musculoskeletal fitness
- diet, nutrition and obesity
- life style factors and risk taking behaviours
- accidental injury and its prevention – e.g. road traffic, work place and sports injuries
- ageing.

Musculoskeletal conditions and injuries can affect any member of society and there are few personal, social and cultural boundaries. Human anatomy evolves slowly, but injury can be a result of immediate changes in the weather and other natural conditions as well as societal variations such as diverse and migrating cultures amongst countries. This is apparent, for example, in the reported increase in tuberculosis in immigrant communities in part due to the migration of Asian families (WHO 2012) to other parts of the world. Other issues include changes in population dynamics with an increasingly ageing population leading to an upsurge in fragility fractures. For the adolescent and young adult there is a heightened rate of injury due to 'risk taking' behaviour. The epidemiology of orthopaedic-related conditions alters as the pathophysiology of disease processes and the treatment options continue to evolve as a result of emerging technology, research evidence and the ongoing drive for safe, cost-effective care.

Recent renewed concerns about vitamin D deficiency illustrate the changing nature of the public health agenda and musculoskeletal care. Deficiency is associated with rickets, fractures and musculoskeletal symptoms and studies suggest a worrying link with deformity and generalised bone and muscle pain (Judd 2013). Such deficiency is attributed to an increasingly multiethnic population, poor diet and lifestyle choices made by families. Previously a condition linked with poverty, the recent recurrence of rickets in the UK, for example, is linked to changes in the lifestyle of children which has resulted in them spending less time playing out of doors, reducing their exposure to the sunlight that is important for vitamin D and calcium synthesis.

The diverse orthopaedic patient

The vast age range of the orthopaedic trauma patient means that there are a number of conditions and injuries which are more common in different age groups. Age groups carry different risk factors for musculoskeletal problems; these are outlined in Table 1.1. Changes occur as the musculoskeletal system develops, grows and deteriorates and as humans age. Many orthopaedic conditions and fracture trauma injuries are related to changing musculoskeletal structure. Normal and abnormal changes occur in utero, at birth, childhood, adulthood and from old age to death. Intrinsic factors affecting this include abnormal musculoskeletal development such as developmental dysplasia of the hip (DDH), scoliosis and osteogenseis imperfecta with which there are considerable

Table 1.1 Age groups In relation to orthopaedic problems

Age group	Examples often specific to age group
Familial/hereditary	Paget's Osteogenesis imperfecta
Congenital	DDH Talipes
Post natal and pre-walking	Birth injuries
Early childhood	Rickets and osteomalacia Non-accidental injury Accidental injury
Mid to late childhood	Juvenile chronic arthritis Perthes' disease
Young person/ adolescence	Slipped upper femoral epiphysis Osgood-Schlatter disease
Early adulthood	Injuries resulting from high energy trauma Sports injuries Rheumatoid arthritis Ankylosing spondylitis
Middle and late adulthood	Work related injury Back pain
Later life/older age	Injuries resulting from low energy trauma Fragility fractures Osteoporosis Degenerative joint conditions

variations in treatment and outcome. Other conditions are often age-related such as osteoporosis and osteoarthritis which are associated with intrinsic factors such as increasing age. Such variations can hopefully be reduced as a result of national guidance and globally relevant initiatives such as those published by the World Health Organization (WHO). Extrinsic factors include the risk-taking of the young person/adolescent leading road traffic trauma alongside accidental and non-accidental injury in vulnerable children and adults. In spite of political and economic development in most parts of the world, social status and environmental conditions continue to impact on musculoskeletal health problems due to issues such as low income and poor education leading to poor diet.

The care journey in different settings

In many of the chapters in this book we see that the care journey takes place against a background of changing health services and political priorities as well as individual needs. There is no reason to believe that the enormous change and development of health care services seen in the later decades of the 20th century and at the beginning of the 21st century are likely to slow down in developed and developing countries. The practitioner, therefore, needs to ensure they have a dynamic understanding of how this affects the care of the orthopaedic and trauma patient, especially in relation to the setting in which care takes place.

Ambulatory care is increasingly providing opportunities for patients to be offered treatment and care without a stay in hospital or, at most, a very short stay. This is driven by the need to reduce the costs of healthcare as well as an acknowledgement that an acute hospital is not always the best place for the patient to be. In the orthopaedic and trauma setting this is seen as feasible where the impact on the patient's ability to carry out fundamental activities is minor. It is important to bear in mind, however, that non-admission to or early discharge from hospital can be both anxiety provoking and uncomfortable for patients and their families and there is a need to provide support that ensures that specialist orthopaedic advice and services are accessible remotely from the hospital. In particular, services need to ensure that patients recovering at a distance from an acute hospital setting in their own homes are afforded support and a care package which includes fundamental elements such as effective pain relief, good nutrition, support for rehabilitation, access to advice and support and all of those things the patient needs to reach both their recovery and rehabilitation potential as well as maintain their safety. Such services can be complex and difficult to coordinate. One of the difficulties in providing adequate support in the patient's home can be funding and purchasing mismatches between the acute hospital and community services, which may be quite separate entities depending on the structure and funding of the health care system. Family support for care in the home is also becoming increasingly challenging as the role and employment of family members change.

For more than a quarter of a century there has been a strong focus on reducing lengths of stay and moving from hospital-based to community-based care. This focus is driven by the need to stretch limited resources while maintaining the quality of care. While this shift has long been an important aim for health care managers and policy makers, the reality has been more problematic and this change is taking place slowly.

Musculoskeletal conditions, injuries and surgery are problems which take time to resolve and may leave the individual of any age with varying degrees of temporary or permanent disability which require careful support and rehabilitation. Within this drive is a danger that patients are being discharged from hospital with residual nursing needs and there is a consequent need to develop care practice at the boundaries of the care settings. The development of technology is offering new opportunities for monitoring and supporting patients in their homes, especially in rural and remote settings, but in many areas this has yet to be applied to the orthopaedic patient. Meanwhile orthopaedic and trauma practitioners need to develop skills in providing care and support from a distance and the use of communication technology is likely to increase as this aim becomes more relevant in the future.

Ethical and legal aspects of orthopaedic and trauma care

Practitioners are increasingly required to consider the complex nature of ethical issues which affect the orthopaedic and trauma patient. As with all other branches of nursing, there are both specialised and general issues that affect the specific patient group and the orthopaedic practitioner needs a deep working understanding of these.

Much of the discussion about ethical issues in all aspects of nursing is related to the nature and quality of care. Nursing care is often seen as being synonymous with holistic patient-centred approaches which are non-judgmental and include the demonstration of attitudes and behaviours that are sensitive to the needs of patients and carers and respect individuality and choice (McSherry *et al.*, 2012). This is especially important when orthopaedic and trauma care takes place in highly pressurised environments in which it is possible to lose sight of patient-centred priorities. Effective education of orthopaedic practitioners, insightful and transformational leadership and the development of a strong patient priority-centred evidence base are central to this. Within this is the need to develop practitioners not only with the right knowledge, skills and attitudes but with a passion for working with patients with very specific and significant needs related to their musculoskeletal problem.

The provision of quality care within a framework which values and respects dignity is a constant source of discussion in all health care settings. This is particularly important in maintaining their own safety when the patient is a vulnerable child or older adult or other individual with impairment. As people with learning disabilities live longer they are more likely to require care in orthopaedic settings. Mental health problems such as debilitating depression frequently affect care and recovery. There remains a need for the practitioner to develop the skills to care for orthopaedic patients with a wide variety of needs which make them vulnerable. The 'safeguarding' from harm of both children and vulnerable adults is becoming an increasing priority and must be central to all care provided.

In any health care setting, informed consent to all procedures and activities is an important part of care along with consideration of the mental capacity of the patient. Orthopaedic interventions carry with them significant risks. Understanding how to assess the capacity of an individual to make decisions about their care is an important part of informed consent – as is the ability to ensure that patients, carers and families understand the risks of the decisions they are being asked to make. Practitioners must adhere to Acts of Parliament in their own country which provide a statutory framework to empower and protect people of all ages who may lack capacity to make their own decisions.

There is a danger that orthopaedic practitioners assume that 'do not resuscitate' orders and 'living wills' do not relate to the orthopaedic/trauma patient group except in the oncology setting. This can perhaps be traced to the specialty's focus on 'healing and recovery.' However, as caring develops in the coming decades it is likely that there will be a greater focus on end of life issues and practitioners must be aware of national guidance and legislation that requires them to be aware of best practice in both decision making and communication. One example of this is in the discussion regarding the need to consider palliative care for frail older patients with major orthopaedic injuries. Research increasingly shows that some conditions are life-limiting. One example is hip fracture which often occurs in very frail elderly patients and may need to instigate a sensitive discussion about the need to implement end of life care (Murray *et al.*, 2012). Decisions and discussions about such matters may not have been, but will need to be, part of the orthopaedic practitioners' skills set as the quality of end of life care reaches a more prominent place in all settings.

Summary

This chapter has examined the nature of orthopaedic and trauma nursing and the main issues which drive its development including public health, political, practical and legal and ethical agendas. It has highlighted the diverse needs of the orthopaedic patient along the entire age continuum and in the variety of settings in which care takes place. It acknowledges that modern health care is complicated and has many drivers and that this leads to numerous complex ethical issues with which the practitioner must engage. It is hoped that these principles can be successfully applied to the material contained within the remainder of this book.

Recommended further reading

Judd, J. (2010) Defining expertise in paediatric orthopaedic nursing. *International Journal of Orthopaedic and Trauma Nursing*, **14**(3), 159–168.

McSherry, W., McSherry, R. & Watson, R. (2012) *Care in Nursing. Principles, Values and Skills*. Oxford University Press, Oxford.

Santy, J. (2001) An investigation of the reality of nursing work with orthopaedic patients. *Journal of Orthopaedic Nursing*, **5**(1), 22–29.

Sellman, D. (2011) *What Makes a Good Nurse?* Jessica Kingsley, London.

References

Balcombe, K. Davis, P. and Lim, E. (1991) A nursing model for orthopaedics. *Nursing Standard*, **5**(49), 26–28.

Casey, A. (1988) A Partnership With Child and Family. *Senior Nurse*, **8**(4), 8–9.

Corkin, D., Clarke, S. and Liggett, L. (Eds) (2012) *Care Planning in Children and Young People's Nursing*. Wiley-Blackwell, Oxford.

Davis, P.S. (1994) *Nursing the Orthopaedic Patient*. Churchill Livingstone, Edinburgh.

Drozd, M., Jester, R. and Santy, J. (2007) The inherent components of the orthopaedic nursing role: an exploratory study. *Journal of Orthopaedic Nursing*, **11**(1), 43–52.

Fawcett, J. (1995) *Analysis and Evaluation of Conceptual Models of Nursing*, 3rd edn. F.A. Davis Company, Philadelphia.

Judd, J. (2010) Defining expertise in paediatric orthopaedic nursing. *International Journal of Orthopaedic and Trauma Nursing*, **14**(3), 159–168.

Judd, J. (2013) Rickets in the 21st-century: a review of low vitamin D and its management. *International Journal of Orthopaedic and Trauma Nursing*, **17**(4), 199–208.

Love, C. (1995) Orthopaedic nursing: a study of its specialty status. *Nursing Standard*, **9**(44), 36–40.

Ouellet, L.L. and Rush, K.L. (1992) A synthesis of selected literature on mobility: A basis for studying impaired mobility. *International Journal of Nursing Knowledge*, **3**(2), 72–80.

Ouellet, L.L. and Rush, K.L. (1996) A study of nurses' perceptions of client mobility. *Western Journal of Nursing Research*, **18**(5), 565–579.

Ouellet, L.L. and Rush, K.L. (1998) Conceptual Module of Client Mobility. *Journal of Orthopaedic Nursing*, **2**(3), 132–135.

McCrae, N. (2012) Wither Nursing Models? The value of nursing theory in the context of evidence-based practice and multidisciplinary health care. *Journal of Advanced Nursing*, **68**(1), 222–229.

McSherry, W., McSherry, R. and Watson, R. (2012) *Care in Nursing. Principles, Values and Skills*. Oxford University Press, Oxford.

Murray, I.R., Biant, L.C., Clement, N.C. and Murray, S.A. (2012) Should a hip fracture in a frail older person be a trigger for assessment of palliative care needs? *Supportive and Palliative Care*, **1**(1), 3–4.

Orem, D.E. (2001) *Nursing: Concepts of Practice*, 6th edn. Mosby, London.

Orlando, I.J. (1961) *The Dynamic Nurse-patient Relationship: Function, Process and Principles*. G.P. Putnam's Sons, New York.

Powell, M. (1951) *Orthopaedic Nursing*. E. & S. Livingstone, Edinburgh.

Roper, N., Logan, W.W. and Tierney, A.J. (2000) *The Roper-Logan-Tierney Model of Nursing: Based on Activities of Living*. Elsevier Health Sciences, Edinburgh.

Roy, C. (1984) *Introduction to Nursing: An Adaptation Model*, 2nd edn. Prentice Hall, Englewood Cliffs, NJ.

Rush, K.L. and Ouellet, L.L. (1998) An analysis of elderly clients' views of mobility. *Western Journal of Nursing Research*, **20**(3), 295–311.

Santy, J. (2001) An investigation of the reality of nursing work with orthopaedic patients. *Journal of Orthopaedic Nursing*, **5**(1), 22–29.

Thompson, C. Dowding, D. (Eds) (2002) *Clinical Decision Making and Judgement in Nursing*. Churchill Livingstone, Edinburgh.

World Health Organization (WHO) (2012) *Global Tuberculosis Report 2012: Executive Summary*. Available at: http://www.who.int/tb/publications/global_report/en/ (accessed: 14 April 2013).

CHAPTER 2

The knowledge and evidence base for practice

Peter Davis MBE[1] and Mark Limb[2]

[1] *Newark, Nottinghamshire, UK*

[2] *School of Nursing and Midwifery, University of Sheffield, UK*

Introduction

The aim of this chapter is to enable the orthopaedic practitioner to appraise evidence related to daily care decisions in a sound and unbiased manner and then apply the findings and evaluate the care outcomes. Hunt (1938) gives a very insightful view of her experience in developing orthopaedic nursing and the impact of social and political factors she had to face. Since this publication there have been many books written to help both student and qualified orthopaedic practitioners (Powell 1986, Footner 1987, Davis 1994, Maher *et al.*, 2002, Kneale and Davis 2005) along with journals and individual papers. Over time, there has developed a rich and varied body of knowledge. Content has gradually moved away from descriptions of what should be done to patients to a more considered view of patient care based on current evidence and more of a focus on how to engage with the patient.

There have been a number of influences on the development of nursing knowledge. The Briggs report in 1972 (Committee on Nursing) suggested that nursing should become a research-based profession and there has been much written about how and why this is necessary, the impact it has on patient care and the view of nursing by other professions. Care up to this point had often been based upon what had traditionally been delivered under the authority of senior staff. Whilst this may have been based on years of experience there was no real assurance that the care delivered was the best possible or was even effective. Policies and education began to respond to this but, over subsequent decades, it had been noted that the uptake of research by nurses had been sporadic and sometimes limited. Hunt (1981) identified that research was still not really finding its way into practice a decade after the report was published. Another decade later Closs and Cheater (1994) felt that research had started to permeate the culture of nursing, although they did not think it was a clearly embedded concept. Nearly thirty years later Batteson (1999) felt that many practices were still based on local circumstance rather than research.

There appears to have been a number of driving forces for the need to use research in practice over the years since 1972 and these have been propelled by both economic and educational factors. Clarke (1999) looks at this in terms of efficiency and effectiveness in clinical decision making and Gerrish and Clayton (1998) add the concern for quality improvement and cost consciousness. Particular attention was paid to effectiveness by the NHS executive (1998) as they began to ask that clinical decisions should be based on the best possible evidence of effectiveness. This often results in the generation and application of clinical guidelines. But effectiveness is not the only criteria by which to judge new knowledge and evidence: feasibility, appropriateness and meaningfulness, particularly for the patient, are also important.

Effectiveness and economics may not have been the only driving force. French (1998) noted that as data were collected regarding practice on computer databases, there were geographical variations in care and this may not have been what is most effective, but what individual practitioners had traditionally done or wanted to do. This, according to Hicks and Hennessey (1997), brings in the notion of accountability as care cannot be delivered based upon opinion and/or authority; it needs some form of justification. This has

Orthopaedic and Trauma Nursing: An Evidence-based Approach to Musculoskeletal Care, First Edition. Edited by Sonya Clarke and Julie Santy-Tomlinson.

also led to a number of organisations such as Cochrane, Joanna Briggs and NICE (National Institute for Clinical Excellence) developing a number of resources and databases for both practice and teaching purposes.

There was also the encouragement of research utilisation, and Horsely *et al.* (1978) examined the complex organisational functions that range from problem identification to the implementation of an innovation. Many research texts were then published looking at how to undertake and critique research including chapters on change management. However, research can be used in more than one way and may not just be about innovation and change in practice. Estabrooks (1998) identified that it can be used as action research when directly applied to practice with change and evaluation taking place as part of the research. However, it can also be used conceptually to enlighten understanding and persuasively to change the views of others. As Bircumshaw (1990) suggests, research can be used in other ways without the need to directly implement it.

Evidence-based practice

Until recently there has been little mention of evidence-based practice and more of a focus on research and its utilisation. This can be regarded as a problem as there is a tendency to use these terms interchangeably. Whilst evidence-based practice may encompass research utilisation, evidence is more than the findings of research and, as pointed out by McKenna and Cutcliffe (1999), the absence of research does not mean that evidence-based decisions cannot be made.

The most frequently cited definition of evidence-based practice is that of Sacket *et al.* (1996) and focusses on ensuring that current best evidence should be used in making decisions about medical care. They identify the best evidence as systematic research but note that individual clinical expertise needs to be integrated with this. This does not, however, help us to understand what would happen in the absence of research or consider the patient in the decision making process. Ryecroft-Malone *et al.* (2004) provide a more encompassing definition and incorporate the need to look at the impact of research, the effectiveness of expert knowledge and the need to integrate patients' experiences into decision making. See Figure 2.1

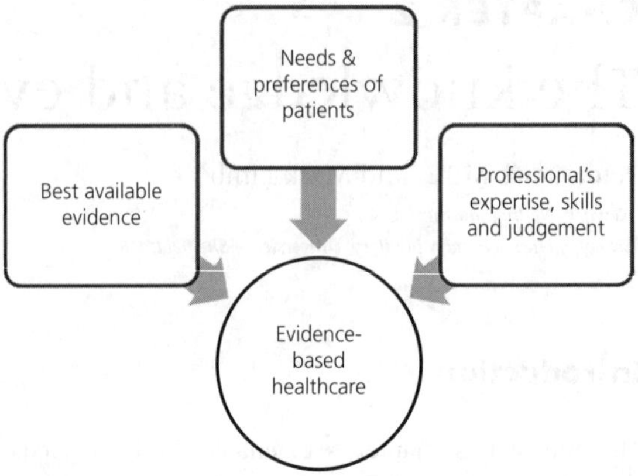

Figure 2.1 Elements of evidence-based healthcare

Ingersoll *et al.*'s (2000) definition brings in the nursing context and notes that it is more about theory-derived research-based information, about care delivery to groups and individuals and, most importantly, is considerate of individual needs and preferences. This definition does not imply that primary research is the only form of evidence and it includes the patient in decisions reflecting the increased levels of health related knowledge of patients and the view that 'medicine knows best' is quickly being eroded by the 'expert' patient.

Nurses must embrace this issue from their own professional perspective as well as differentiate their professional roles and responsibilities. Whilst evidence-based care is becoming a priority in health care, Banning (2005) found that nurses were not able to differentiate very well between evidence-based medicine and evidence-based practice. Whilst nurses take on more advanced roles that often merge with the boundaries of other disciplines, the development of knowledge and understanding must continue to build on their professional knowledge.

More recent research into evidence-based practice tends to move away from how it is defined and considers how it works in practice. This is important in relation to the changing roles of the nurse in modern health care. Some may argue that, up to now, there is little indication that evidence-based practice works. Gerrish *et al.* (2011), for example, examined how nurses in advanced roles act as 'knowledge brokers' for clinical nurses, thus enabling them to use evidence effectively. Whilst nurses may be working in complex and advanced roles, they can develop and use knowledge and skills that facilitate the use of evidence by others who are less experienced. Thus evidence is combined with expertise in helping others deliver care.

There are two main misperceptions within EBP. The first is the assumption that research has been carried out on the particular clinical issue or problem of interest. This is often not the case. For example, if a search is conducted for evidence to support the premise that early mobilisation in orthopaedic patients is beneficial, very little if any original research will be found. The second assumption is that all published research is of good quality. The appraisal process often shows research to be poorly constructed and conducted, and therefore cannot be trusted for implementation. Santy and Temple (2004) identify in their critical review of skeletal pin site care that only two pieces of evidence were found that were of sufficient quality to be trusted and used to direct nursing care.

Evidence-based practice has three components (Aveyard 2010). Firstly, the evidence about the feasibility, appropriateness, meaningfulness and effectiveness of health care practices is sought. Secondly, the quality of that evidence is assessed and appraised. Finally, the evidence should be applied to the context in which it is relevant. An example of the entire process, from setting the question to implementing findings, is provided in a review of pre-operative exercise in knee replacement surgery (Lucas 2004).

Hierarchies of evidence

There is a good deal of debate about what is best evidence and nurses need to be able to navigate this complex, evolving web of information. When deciding what evidence is best a number of authors have made some attempt to apply categories to help clarify what may be the most rigorous. Bircumshaw (1990) suggests a fairly simplistic hierarchy to help the reader understand the relationship between research and practice, tying the availability of research into the responsibility of the nurse. This model places the emphasis on the primacy of empirical research, as do the hierarchies of Fawcett (1984) and Davis (1990). This should not be seen as too much of a problem as different research designs may be regarded as more valid and reliable than others. However, other models are much more encompassing than this and encapsulate a broader range of evidence types ranging from personal and peer experience to meta-analyses and systematic reviews. A succinct overview of these may be as follows:

- quantitative research
- qualitative research
- expert opinion
- personal experience.

This is not too far removed from Carper's (1978) classification of nursing knowledge that identified four levels that were evident in nursing practice at the time:

- empirical
- aesthetic
- ethical
- personal.

Empirical research appears to have great pre-eminence in these hierarchies and Griffiths (2002) feels that this may be because questions about issues such as effectiveness and efficiency are best addressed by such methods, particularly the randomised controlled trial (RCT). Quantitative research may not, however, be able to solve all problems. Mulhall (1998) points out that there are 'untidy' aspects of caring that need to be examined such as emotion and feeling. Decision-making around these may not be best served by the RCT. McCormack (2004) suggests that qualitative research is an important element of practice but, because of perceived problems relating to reliability and validity, it is placed lower in the hierarchies. Howard and Davis (2002) describe and explain the relatively weak position of qualitative research in orthopaedics and suggest a new approach they label as 'diagnostic research'. Evidence has to be selected on the basis of the problem being addressed and, with this in mind, Naish (1997) feels that the levels of evidence should be regarded as more elastic and without one having privilege over another. Quantitative research may identify a clinical problem but qualitative research may set it in context.

Mantzoukas (2007) suggests we abandon the hierarchy altogether as this often serves to impede the implementation of evidence-based practice. An alternative offered is reflection on practice in order to make decisions relating to care. To do this a good deal of clinical experience is required and, at the same time as there is a growing body of evidence in nursing, there is also a growing body of experience that has been gained by individual practitioners. Gerrish and Clayton (2004) found that experience was frequently used as a source of evidence. Intuition and experience in expert practice is important as the development of quality services cannot be delayed by lack of research findings (Ellis 2000) and intuition uses the untapped resource of tacit knowledge (Meerabeau 1992). This complicates matters; on the one hand evidence-based practice tends to under-emphasise intuition and experiential knowledge and stresses the examination of clinical research, whilst on the other hand it can never replace individual expertise (Rolfe 1999).

Finding and dealing with the evidence

Having examined the meaning of evidence-based practice it is useful to consider the skills required for delivering this effectively. These can be categorised under two broad areas:

- specific
- general.

Specific skills include being able to find, filter and extract relevant information (Bryar *et al.*, 2003) as well as being able to appraise the evidence (Hek 2000), decide on its quality and its relevance to their practice. Information technology and development of critical reading skills are essential.

More general research appreciation skills are necessary to be able to understand some of the complex evidence that may need to be appraised prior to application in practice. The practitioner may also need to mentor and teach others about the nature of the evidence and its relationship to and potential impact on practice. Practitioners have to be able to extract evidence that is relevant and be able to recognise the different range of approaches that can inform practice. Finally, there is a need for good management and time management skills and to be able to create an appropriate culture for evidence-based practice to work effectively (Mulhall 1998).

Asking a question and developing your knowledge

Having looked at some of the issues around research and evidence, we now must look at how you can start to develop your own knowledge base relevant to orthopaedic or trauma practice. The ability to think critically in solving a health care problem is of essence to the process of EBP. Jones-Devitt and Smith (2007, p. 7) define critical thinking as:

> Making sense of the world through a process of questioning the questions, challenging assumptions, recognising that bodies of knowledge can be chaotic and evolving; ultimately with the aim of continually improving thinking.

Lipe and Beasley (2004) warn of two main pitfalls in problem solving; firstly, the failure to clearly identify the real problem and secondly, the failure to eliminate preconceived ideas in identification of solutions. For example, with respect to surgical wound care the orthopaedic nurse may consider the fundamental question to be what type of dressing to use and search for evidence on whether to use honey, gel, occlusive, transparent or silver dressings. However, the first question should be do we need to dress the wound? Once this is answered the question of dressing type can then be addressed if necessary.

Below is a step-by-step method by which you can start to do this. It does not have to lead to a full research project and be undertaken for educational purposes; you can do it just to improve patient care.

1. Choose a subject area or set a question and discuss this with your managers and peers. Think about an area of expertise that you want to consolidate or develop. Maybe there's something in your clinical area that makes you and others just stop and question why? Or could this be done in a better way? This first stage is probably the most important as without a clear search question the end result will be weak, inconclusive or unusable.
2. Start to look for information and identify the articles that pertain to your chosen area. Make notes of:
   - the databases that you searched
   - the key words that you used for your search and how you refined them
   - if you undertook any incremental searching (looking at the reference list at the back of published articles)
   - conversations with others who have a particular specialist interest in the area you have chosen.

   All the above are ways of accessing existing sources of knowledge but each will have its own issues for consideration:
   - Databases may be selective in the information that they hold or may contain so much information that it is difficult to decide what is important. You may have to limit to local holdings for financial reasons but this limits the scope of your knowledge development as well. Don't limit your search to primary research only as evidence/knowledge is much wider than this, but do try to make sure the information you collect is peer-reviewed in order to ensure its credibility. Key words can be difficult

to determine and define so it is important to ensure that you have been very specific in the choice of subject. Again, it is useful to discuss this with managers and peers in order to ensure that you have the correct words for the correct focus.

- Incremental searching (looking at the reference lists on articles that you already have) is useful, particularly when the databases do not appear to be yielding very much. However, if you have an article from 2005 all the additional articles you get from this will pre-date it and may be considered too old to use.
- Asking specialist/advanced nurses for information is also very useful and may yield some articles that you had not thought of or may be finding difficult to obtain. However, because of their specialist focus, you may find that the article selection is biased.

While each method may have its limitations, if you identify material from a wider range of sources it is likely that you will end up with a pertinent dataset for use in the development of your knowledge base.

3 Once you have collected all the articles, read through them and identify from this the ones that you will select for consideration. You need to justify how you narrowed the articles down by setting inclusion and exclusion criteria. Once you have decided which are relevant, obtain a copy of each.

4 Start to acquaint yourself with the articles that you have identified. Get a feel for the area. Identify those that are primary research and those that are literature reviews, editorials, professional opinion etc.

5 Start to summarise the research articles using 'research evidence summaries' (see Table 2.1) and the other articles using 'literature evidence summaries' (see Table 2.2). You may want to design your own format if you find these too restrictive.

Table 2.1 Research summary

Reference	Make a note of the full reference here so that you have a lasting record of it	
Themes/key words	Under what theme/key word can the work be summarised?	
Principal findings	What are the main findings of the research?	
Ethics	Is there evidence that the research project was subject to ethical scrutiny? Are there any obvious problems to note?	
Sample	Has the population under study been described?	
	What type of sample was drawn from the population?	
	How many were selected for the study and what was the response rate?	
	How many dropped out of the study/what was the attrition rate?	
	How might the above affect the **generalisability (external validity)** of the study?	
Design	**Quantitative**	**Qualitative**
	RCT	Grounded theory
	Experiment	Phenomenology
	Quasi-experiment	Ethnography
	Correlational	
	Survey	
	Try to ascertain if the study is retrospective or prospective	
	In terms of hierarchies of evidence is the design used trustworthy?	
Data collection	Identify the ways data have been collected. Some studies may use more than one method. Some examples are as follows: interviews, observations, care records, clinical data, scales, questionnaires	
	How valid/reliable is the method utilised?	
Data analysis	**Quantitative**	**Qualitative**
	What is/are the name(s) of the test(s) used?	How have the data been dealt with?
	Are these parametric or non-parametric?	How **trustworthy** do you feel this is?
	What is the level of significance?	
Clinical significance	Have the researchers looked at the clinical as opposed to the statistical significance of the findings?	

6 Once you have completed all the summaries, have a look through and see if you can identify any themes. For example; if you are looking at pre-operative fasting you may find that some of the articles are about fasting times whilst others may look at the outcomes associated with fasting times. Separate these and then put each of the articles on a matrix for each theme. Matrices for the research articles and other literature can be found in Tables 2.3 and 2.4 respectively.

7 Once you have identified all the different approaches taken in the research articles and inserted them into the matrix start reading around the research methods that have been utilised by the authors. Justham (2007) suggests a simple check list of questions that will get you started. The Critical Appraisal Skills Programme (2013) and the Joanna Briggs Institute (2013) web sites provide more in-depth appraisal tools. Access research methods texts from the library to help you to understand the methods discussed in the papers.

8 For the other articles it is useful to identify what type of evidence they represent (professional opinion, group consensus etc.) and their position relative to research in a hierarchy of evidence.

Table 2.2 Literature summary

Reference	Make a note of the full reference here so that you have a lasting record of it
Summary	What are the main points being made by the author(s)?
Themes/ Key words	Under what theme/key word can the work be summarised?
Article type	Is the article type any of the following? Opinion editorial Group consensus Conference proceedings Review **In terms of hierarchies of evidence what is the position of this material relative to research?**
Clinical relevance	Of what clinical relevance is the article?

Table 2.3 Research matrix

Author/ Date/ Source	Summary of findings	Ethics	Sample type/size	Design	Data Collection	Tests/Analysis	Discussion/ clinical relevance

Models of application

Having gone some way to develop your knowledge base what do you do with it now? There seem to be three major models by which evidence may be applied in the clinical setting:

Table 2.4 Literature matrix

Author/date/ source	Article type	Summary of points for comment	Clinical reflections

- linear
- multi-dimensional
- partnership.

The linear models indicate that there is some logical process occurring that has a beginning and an end starting with some form of problem assessment and ending with some form of evaluation and including the need to select and review evidence, develop policy, implement change and evaluate services/ outcomes (Hewitt-Taylor 2002, Gerrish and Clayton 2004). Kitson *et al.* (1999) and Fitzgerald (2003) regard these models as problematic in the complex health care systems in which they are supposed to work.

Kitson *et al.* (1998) therefore propose a multi-dimensional model that identifies factors contributing to the successful implementation of evidence-based practice as a function of three factors:

- the type of evidence available
- the context in which the evidence is being applied
- the level of facilitation available.

This goes some way to explaining the complexities that nurses face, as does the partnership model described by Ross *et al.* (2001) who identify the value of the collaborative efforts of a number of individuals within the organisation.

A criticism of these models is that, in trying to move away from the linear models they lack the logicality that is often required for the purposes of accountability. However, we should look at all these models as being a partial representation of the reality of practice and see the "implementation" noted in the latter two models described as the logical processes of the former linear models. If we merge all these models we get the overall picture that there is some linear process occurring and that this is affected by the evidence, the context, the facilitator and the collaborative efforts of all involved. Davis (2004) exemplifies this in his critical discourse on venous thromboembolism prevention in orthopaedic health care practice. The discussion concentrates on three related elements: clinical practice improvement itself, the evidence base and aspects of change.

Context and collaboration may be particularly important in the field of orthopaedics and trauma because of the multi-professional nature of the speciality as Field (1987) identifies the different roles of the professionals:

- Doctor = Curative
- Physiotherapist = Restorative
- Nurse = Evaluative.

Each member of the team will have a different role but will need common knowledge to function effectively. Therefore, it makes sense to make sure that all are involved if there is to be any development in evidence-based practice as this may involve multiple adoption decisions.

In summary, an approach that develops knowledge and understanding to use in an evidence-based practice approach has six elements:

- search for evidence
- appraise evidence
- summarise evidence
- utilise
- embed
- evaluate the impact.

At its simplest, EBP is about good practice and improving the quality of health care (Baker 2010). Practitioners must continue to strive to generate and identify new knowledge for practice and apply it only after casting a critical orthopaedic nursing eye over it. We must listen to patient stories or narratives as they can be powerful and enlightening directors of decisions about care (Davis 2007). We must also listen to our own hearts and instincts and utilise evidence in a caring and empathetic manner.

Recommended further reading

Aveyard, H. (2010) *Doing a Literature Review in Health and Social Care*, 2nd edn. Open University Press, Maidenhead.
Aveyard, H. and Sharp, P. (2013) *A Beginner's Guide to Evidence Based Practice in Health and Social Care*, 2nd edn. Open University Press, Maidenhead.
Bowling, A. (2009) *Research Methods in Health*, 3rd edn. Open University Press, Maidenhead.
Gerrish, K. and Lacey, A. (2010) *The Research Process in Nursing*, 6th edn. Wiley Blackwell, Oxford.
Jones-Devitt, S. and Smith, L. (2007) *Critical Thinking in Health and Social Care*. Sage, London.

References

Aveyard, H. (2010) *Doing a Literature Review in Health and Social Care*, 2nd edn. Open University Press, Maidenhead.
Baker, J. (2010) *Evidence-based Practice for Nurses*. Sage, London.

Banning, M. (2005) Conceptions of evidence, evidence-based medicine, evidence-based practice and their use in nursing: independent nurse prescribers' views. *Journal of Clinical Nursing*, **14**(4), 411–417.

Batteson, L. (1999) Health visiting and clinical benchmarking. *Primary Health Care*, **9**(9), 10, 12, 14.

Bircumshaw, D. (1990) The utilization of research findings in clinical nursing practice. *Journal of Advanced Nursing*, **15**, 1272–1280.

Bryar, R., Closs, S.J., Baum, G. *et al.* (2003) The Yorkshire BARRIERS project: diagnostic analysis of barriers to research utilisation. *International Journal of Nursing Studies*, **40**(1), 73–84.

Carper, B.A. (1978) Fundamental Patterns of Knowing in Nursing. *Advances in Nursing Science*, **1**(1), 13–24.

Clarke, J. (1999) Evidence-based practice: a retrograde step? The importance of pluralism in evidence generation for the practice of health care. *Journal of Clinical Nursing*, **8**, 89–94.

Closs, S. and F. Cheater (1994) Utilization of nursing research: culture, interest and support. *Journal of Advanced Nursing*, **19**, 762–773.

Critical Appraisal Skills Programme (2013) Available at: http://www.casp-uk.net/ (accessed March 2013).

Committee on Nursing (1972) *Report of the Committee of Nursing*, Briggs Report, Cmnd 5115. HMSO, London.

Davis, B. (1990) Research-based teaching. *Nursing Standard*, **4**(48), 38–40.

Davis, P.S. (1994) *Nursing the Orthopaedic Patient*. Churchill-Livingstone, Edinburgh.

Davis, P. (2004) A critical exploration of practice improvement in orthopaedic nursing with reference to venous thromboembolism. *Journal of Orthopaedic Nursing*, **8**, 208–214.

Davis, P. (2007) Listening to patient stories. *Journal of Orthopaedic Nursing*, **11**(1), 1.

Ellis, J. (2000) Sharing the evidence: clinical practice benchmarking to improve continuously the quality of care. *Journal of Advanced Nursing*, **21**(1), 215–225.

Estabrooks, C. A. (1998) Will evidence-based nursing practice make practice perfect? *Canadian Journal of Nursing Research*, **30**(1), 15–36.

Fawcett, J. (1984) Another look at utilization of nursing research. *The Journal of Nursing Scholarship*, **16**(2), 59–62.

Field, P. A. (1987) The impact of nursing theory on the clinical decision making process. *Journal of Advanced Nursing*, **12**, 563–571.

Fitzgerald, L., Ferlie, E. and Hawkins, C. (2003) Innovation in healthcare: How does credible evidence influence professionals? *Health and Social Care in the Community*, **11**(3), 219–228.

Footner, A. (1987) *Orthopaedic Nursing*. Balliere-Tindall, London.

French, B. (1998) Developing the skills required for evidence-based practice. *Nurse Education Today*, **18**, 46–51.

Gerrish, K., Nolan, M., Todd, A., Kirschbaum, M. and Guillaume, L. (2011) Factors influencing advanced practice nurses' ability to promote evidence-based Practice among frontline nurses. *Worldviews on Evidence-Based Nursing*, **9**(1), 30–39.

Gerrish, K. and J. Clayton (1998) Improving clinical effectiveness through an evidence-based approach: Meeting the challenge for nursing in the United Kingdom. *Nursing Administration Quarterly*, **22**(4), 55–65.

Griffiths, P. (2002) Evidence informing practice: Introducing the mini review. *British Journal of Community Nursing*, **7**(1), 38-40.

Hek, G. (2000) Evidence-based practice: finding the evidence. *Journal of Community Nursing*, **14**(11), 19–22.

Hewitt-Taylor, J. (2002) Evidence-based practice. *Nursing Standard*, **17**(14-15), 47–52.

Hicks, C. and Hennessy, D. (1997) Mixed messages in nursing research: their contribution to the persisting hiatus between evidence and practice. *Journal of Advanced Nursing*, **25**, 595–601.

Horsley, J. A., Crane, J. and Bingle, J.D. (1978) Research utilization as an organizational process. *Journal of Nursing Administration*, (July), **4–6**.

Howard, D. and Davis, P. (2002) The use of qualitative research methodology in orthopaedics – tell it as it is. *Journal of Orthopaedic Nursing*, **6**, 135–139.

Hunt, A. (1938) *This is My Life*. Blackie, London.

Hunt, J. (1981) Indicators for nursing practice: The use of research findings. *Journal of Advanced Nursing*, **6**, 189–194.

Ingersoll, G., E. McIntosh, and Williams, M. (2000) Nurse-sensitive outcomes of advanced practice. *Journal of Advanced Nursing*, **32**(5), 1272–1281.

Joanna Briggs Institute (2013) Available at: http://www.joannabriggs.edu.au/ (accessed March 2013).

Jones-Devitt, S. and Smith, L. (2007) *Critical Thinking in Health and Social Care*. Sage, London.

Justham, D. (2007) Finding and evaluating an article. *Journal of Orthopaedic Nursing*, **11**, 60–65.

Kitson, A., Harvey, G. and McCormack, B. (1998) Enabling the implementation of evidence-based practice: a conceptual framework. *Quality in Health Care*, **7**, 149–158.

Kneale, J.D. and Davis, P.S. (2005) *Orthopaedic and Trauma Nursing*. Churchill Livingstone, Edinburgh.

Lipe, S.K. and Beasley, S. (2004) *Critical Thinking in Nursing*. Lipincott Williams and Wilkins, Philadelphia.

Lucas, B. (2004) Does a pre-operative exercise programme improve mobility and function post total knee replacement: a mini-review. *Journal of Orthopaedic Nursing*, **8**, 25–33.

Maher, A.B., Salmond, S.W. and Pellino, T. (2002) *Orthopaedic Nursing*. Saunders, Philadelphia.

Mantzoukas, S. (2007) The evidence-based practice ideologies. *Nursing Philosophy*, **8**(4), 244–255.

McCormack, B. (2004) Commentary on fortuitous phenomena: On complexity, pragmatic randomised controlled trials, and knowledge for evidence-based practice by Carl Thompson. *Worldviews on Evidence-Based Practice (First Quarter)*, **18–19**.

McKenna, H. and Cutcliffe, J. (1999) Evidence-based practice demolishing some myths. *Nursing Standard*, **14**(6), 39–42.

Meerabeau, L. (1992) Tacit nursing knowledge: an untapped resource or a methodological headache? *Journal of Advanced Nursing*, **17**(1), 108–112.

Mulhall, A. (1998) Nursing, research, and the evidence. *Evidence-Based Nursing*, **1**(1), 4–6.

Naish, J. (1997) So where's the evidence? *Nursing Times*, **93**(12), 64–66.

NHS Executive (1998) *Information for Health: an Information Strategy for the Modern NHS 1998–2005*. DoH, London.

Powell, M. (1986) *Orthopaedic Nursing and Rehabilitation*. Churchill Livingstone, Edinburgh.

Rolfe, G. (1999) Insufficient evidence: the problems of evidence-based nursing. *Nurse Education Today*, **19**, 433–442.

Ross, F., McLaren, S., Relfeirn, S. and Warwick, C. (2001) Partnerships for changing practice: Lessons from the South Thames Evidence-Based Practice Project (STEP). *Nursing Times Research*, **6**(5), 817–828.

Rycroft-Malone, J., and Stetler C. (2004) Commentary of evidence, research, knowledge: a call for conceptual clarity. *Worldviews on Evidence-Based Nursing*, **1**(2), 98–101.

Sackett, D., Rosenberg, W., Muir Gray, J., Haynes, R.B. and Richardson, W.S. (1996) Evidence based medicine: what it is and what it isn't. *British Medical Journal*, **312**, 71–72.

Santy, J., Temple, J. (2004) A critical review of two research papers on skeletal pin site care. *Journal of Orthopaedic Nursing*, **8**, 132–135.

CHAPTER 3

Professional development, competence and education

Mary Drozd[1] and Sinead Hahessy[2]

[1] *University of Wolverhampton, Walsall, West Midlands, UK*
[2] *National University of Ireland, Galway, Ireland*

Introduction

The aim of this chapter is to discuss ongoing or continuing professional development (CPD) for orthopaedic and trauma nurses. Nursing is a constantly changing profession and continuing professional development is a compulsory part of being a professional. Keeping up to date with best practice and research and acquiring new skills helps to facilitate an effective contribution to patient care. Patients have a right to expect, at the very least, a practitioner who is competent in their sphere of practice. One existing competency framework (Royal College of Nursing 2012) will be discussed along with specialist orthopaedic and trauma nurse education, mentorship in orthopaedic and trauma nursing practice and the role of reflection in continuing professional development.

Professional development

Continuing professional development (CPD) can be defined as *'the systematic maintenance, improvement and broadening of knowledge and skills, and the development of personal qualities necessary for the execution of professional, managerial and technical duties throughout one's working life'* (Tomlinson 1993, p. 231) and is at the heart of professional development (Hawkins and Smith 2008). Activities to promote professional development can take the form of both informal and formal activity and can help the practitioner to move beyond prescribed parameters of practice and develop expertise.

Professional regulation is the hallmark of professions and ensures that standards are met and that practice is maintained and developed (Munro 2008). In many countries regulatory bodies require practitioners to meet specific standards for both practice and education. The purpose is to link professional development and the maintenance of competence to protect the public through safe practice. Nurses have a specific professional responsibility to engage with CPD (O'Shea 2008) and employers recognise that their most valuable resource is their staff, but it is often learning and development opportunities that are sacrificed in financially constrained environments. Barriers to professional development often include financial issues, employment demands, work schedules, anxiety, the learning climate, support for learning, lack of job satisfaction (Cooley 2008), individual motivation and lack of financial support from employers (Lawton and Wimpenney 2003).

The employer has an important role in facilitating and encouraging CPD and in investing in staff to ensure that professional learning occurs in the workplace alongside development of the organisation (Gopee 2002). They expect individuals to contribute to their own learning and that of others because of the perceived benefit to the individual and team's professional growth, future employability and ability to perform their current role effectively. Modernisation agendas for health services include the development of a culture of learning that enables staff to progress and develop. CPD is often an obligatory element of this that values evidence of personal development and this is achieved in various ways.

Literature detailing the relevance of CPD emerged in the 1980s and is mainly UK orientated (e.g. Charles 1982, Brown 1988, Hunt 1991). It focused on

Orthopaedic and Trauma Nursing: An Evidence-based Approach to Musculoskeletal Care, First Edition. Edited by Sonya Clarke and Julie Santy-Tomlinson.

Box 3.1 Evidence digest: printed educational materials – effects on professional practice and healthcare outcomes

Printed educational materials widely use passive dissemination strategies to improve the quality of clinical practice and patient outcomes. Traditionally they are presented in paper formats such as monographs, publication in peer-reviewed journals and clinical guidelines. A review by Giguère *et al.* (2012) includes 45 studies: 14 RCTs and 31 ITS studies that evaluated the impact of printed educational materials (PEMs) on healthcare professionals' practice or patient outcomes, or both. Almost all the included studies (44/45) compared the effectiveness of PEM to no intervention. One single study compared paper-based PEM to the same document delivered on CD-ROM. Based on seven RCTs and 54 outcomes, the median absolute risk difference in categorical practice outcomes was 0.02 when PEMs were compared to no intervention (range from 0 to +0.11). Based on three RCTs and eight outcomes, the median improvement in standardised mean difference for continuous profession practice outcomes was 0.13 when PEMs were compared to no intervention (range from -0.16 to +0.36). Only two RCTs and two ITS studies reported patient outcomes. In addition, they re-analysed 54 outcomes from 25 ITS studies, using time series regression and observed a statistically significant improvement in level or in slope in 27 outcomes. From the ITS studies, the authors calculated improvements in professional practice outcomes across studies after PEM dissemination (standardised median change in level = 1.69). From the data gathered, they could not comment on which PEM characteristic influenced their effectiveness.

The results of this review suggest that when used alone and compared to no intervention, PEMs may have a small beneficial effect on professional practice outcomes. There is insufficient information to reliably estimate the effect of PEMs on patient outcomes and clinical significance of the observed effect sizes is not known. The effectiveness of PEMs compared to other interventions, or of PEMs as part of a multifaceted intervention, is uncertain.

philosophical debates, underpinning frameworks, the relevance of continuing education and the challenges associated with implementation. Barriball *et al.* (1992) noted a lack of empirical data analysing nurses' perceptions of their continuing education needs. Further debates focused on what constituted an effective continuing professional education (CPE) system (Nolan *et al.*, 1995) or the tensions between the 'luxury or necessity' of the endeavour (Perry 1995). Nonetheless, CPE has developed at an accelerated pace. The pioneers of educational change embraced the pursuit of 'new' knowledge through various curricular and pedagogical approaches. Concepts central to the professionalisation debate such as pursuing the accumulation of a distinct body of knowledge through research activity and reflective practice have emerged. CPE in orthopaedic and trauma nursing strives to promote the specialist nature of knowledge and the majority of postgraduate/post-qualifying programmes are designed to address this. The 'artistic' forms of nursing knowledge such as intuition and experience are increasingly being accepted as valid forms of knowledge.

The current focus of CPD has now moved to evaluating the impact of post-registration programmes from the perspectives of the student and the impact learning has on clinical practice and patient outcomes, although there is a paucity of research in relation to the latter. A review of the CPD literature (Hegarty *et al.*, 2008) concludes that patient outcomes are neglected in 61 studies and they advise that future research endeavours should aim to include patient outcomes. Gijbels *et al.*'s (2010) systematic review focused on the student perspective and concluded that nurses welcomed the effects that CPD has on professional and career trajectories. There is little research that has addressed the impact of orthopaedic and trauma CPD from either the student perspective or measurement of patient outcomes as a consequence of CPD (See box 3.1 for a general example).

Mentors

Literature from a wide range of disciplines refers to the use of mentoring to assist career development. This is practiced differently in particular locations, settings and healthcare professions. Mentors are crucial in facilitating the development of other practitioners as they assist the next generation in developing skills and knowledge. They must have a sound evidence-based knowledge and skill base along with an understanding of how individuals learn and grow professionally in order to be able to nurture practitioner development (Gray 2011). At the point of socialisation to the orthopaedic and trauma environment the mentor can help to instill values associated with life-long learning and professional development in the specialty by relating a 'sense of partnership' (Ali and Panther 2008) in which the student or practitioner feels assimilated into the clinical setting.

Mentors provide a spectrum of learning and supportive behaviours such as challenging and being a critical friend, being a role model, helping to build networks and develop resourcefulness, simply being there to listen, helping people work out what they want to achieve and planning how they will bring change about (Clutterbuck 2004). Price (2004) suggests that a mentor will be in a position to shape other nurses' understanding of practice and practice wisdom for years to come. The specialist knowledge and skills such as postoperative orthopaedic care, the prevention and recognition of complications or the application of traction are best learned in the practice setting. Great responsibility for this is placed on mentors even though resources are finite and mentors must juggle the delivery of care with their teaching and supportive roles (Price 2004). No other role in nursing has such power to shape other nurses' practice and knowledge and nothing can be more important than passing on clinical skills and knowledge to others while caring for patients and their families (Price 2004). A system of mentorship is essential in enabling the less experienced practitioner to be supported in specialist knowledge and skill development and such a mentor should aim to provide leadership in developing learning (Gopee 2011).

Competence

Competence has become a defining feature of practice-based professions (Bradshaw 2000). Axley (2008, p. 217) argued that *"there is no officially agreed upon theoretical or operational definition of competency among nurses, educators, employers, regulating bodies, government and patients"* and that the attributes of 'competency' are multi-faceted and context-dependent, which can lead to confusion. Aspects of competence most frequently cited are:

(a) knowledge (information, teaching, training)
(b) actions (ability, skill)
(c) professional standards (criteria, requirements, qualification)
(d) internal regulation (accountability, attitude, autonomy)
(e) dynamic state (ongoing change, consistent improvement).

Competence is not fixed or static but part of the development of expertise and an intrinsic aspect of professional practice (Eraut 1994). It is concerned not only with skill acquisition and application but also with the development of knowledge to support assessment and decision-making (Proctor-Childs 2011). Other professional qualities such as attitude, motives, personal insight, interpretative ability, maturity and self-assessment should be included (Axley 2008).

It is essential that decision making is examined (Hagbaghery *et al.*, 2004) and understood by orthopaedic and trauma nurses to ensure critical analysis is applied to the decision making process, as this enhances competency development. Patients with orthopaedic or traumatic conditions or injuries require specialist knowledge and skills which develop over time, and via various strategies that will be discussed later. Benner (1984) highlights that a nurse who was expert in coronary care found it difficult to perform even at the competent level on an intermediate care surgical unit, supporting clinical specialisation and a structure of clinical preceptors or mentors to teach the beginning nurse or the experienced nurse who transfers to a new unit.

Orthopaedic and trauma practitioner competences

Contemporary healthcare requires efficiency and competence. The Royal College of Nursing (RCN) Society of Orthopaedic and Trauma Nurses (SOTN) in the UK has recently provided an example of specialist competences for orthopaedic and trauma practitioners (RCN SOTN 2012). The benefit of a competency framework is that it provides a foundation on which to develop and evaluate safe and effective practitioners. The framework aims to provide a solid foundation to optimise evidence-based practice and provide safe and competent care.

Orthopaedic and trauma practitioner competences highlight the specialist nature of orthopaedic and trauma practice and provide clarity for organisations regarding what they can expect from orthopaedic and trauma practitioners. They can also be used as benchmarks for organisations to use in recruitment, selection, development, appraisal and individual performance management as well as contribute to the CPD of practitioners. The specialist orthopaedic and trauma practitioner domains within the RCN (2012) framework include the following:

Partner/guide

The partnership between the patient and the health care professional highlights the unique role in guiding the patient through their journey in orthopaedic and trauma health care. Supporting the patient and ensuring they are at the centre of their care is essential, as is working in partnership with the patient's family/informal carers along with liaison and collaboration with all members of the multi-professional team (MPT) to ensure seamless, holistic care.

Comfort enhancer

Comfort is a concept which is fundamental to the care of the orthopaedic/trauma patient. It is a complex human experience which can be interpreted in different ways. It is closely related to the experience of pain, especially for patients who have received an assault to musculoskeletal tissue (Cohen 2009). The comfort of orthopaedic/trauma patients is central to good health-care outcomes. This aspect of care may become more complex for the patient depending on the nature of their condition, injury or surgery. Musculoskeletal instability and movement can result in significant pain and discomfort. Competence in providing essential care within this context is therefore central to high quality care and highlights the need for that care to be provided in a specialist setting where practitioners possess the requisite specialist competence (Santy *et al.*, 2005, Drozd *et al.*, 2007).

Risk manager

One of the most central aspects of orthopaedic and trauma practice is the fact that orthopaedic and trauma surgery and injuries may carry with them a high risk of complications. The range of complications varies from those which are common to all situations where there is immobility and /or an assault to body tissues. However, there are a number of complications which are specific to trauma and orthopaedic patients such as compartment syndrome, fat embolism, osteomyelitis, neurovascular impairment, venous thromboembolism (VTE) and complex regional pain syndrome. It is the nature of these complications which requires highly specialised care.

Technician

The highly technical aspects of orthopaedic and trauma practice require knowledge, understanding and skill in managing, for example, specialised devices and equipment which are used to either treat orthopaedic conditions and injuries or to protect patients from complications. The practitioner needs to be competent in managing such treatment modalities which are highly specialised and carry their own risk of complications (linked to the risk management domain). Some practitioners develop enhanced expertise in specific aspects. For example, while many practitioners care for patients with casts, additional expertise is required for the application of casts. In turn, these highly skilled and educated practitioners require focused, in-depth training and education. Appropriate education, training and development of practitioners is essential in ensuring that the right level of practitioner, with the requisite knowledge, understanding and skills are caring for orthopaedic and trauma patients. Maintaining the currency of such specialist skills is imperative for safe and effective care. For example, the use of traction for adults is now used less extensively and such competences may require regular updating.

Although these domains relate directly to UK practice, there is scope for transferability internationally with work ongoing by the International Collaboration of Orthopaedic Nurses (ICON) to produce international related competences.

There are various strategies for achieving ongoing professional development within orthopaedic and trauma nursing, such as:

- self-study by engaging with current evidence-based material (see Chapter 2)
- seeking learning opportunities in the workplace
- supervised practice by experienced mentors
- case studies
- viva voce
- observed structured clinical examinations (OSCE)
- oral and/or written reflections about care
- critical incident analysis
- reflecting on practice
- self and peer assessments
- formal appraisals with line managers
- in-house courses and study programmes
- accredited university progammes
- learning through electronic means such as online applications and other mobile media with instant access to evidence-based information
- professional portfolios containing evidence of learning and development.

Learning can also occur through personal experience, for example, from personal family experiences that can be transferred to the work context (Munro 2008). There should be a forum for discussion of clinical practice in which nursing knowledge is coherently charted and explored (Benner 1984). Careful record keeping and sharing of paradigm cases are important strategies for documenting the significance of nursing practice. Teaching rounds/master classes by expert nurses open vistas to other nurses while recognising the value of expertise and its importance in transmitting wisdom and judgment.

Reflection

An essential aspect of professional development is to undertake structured, facilitated reflection as a central component of CPD (Cowan *et al.*, 2007, Kim 2007) in order to explore practice and competence, although CPD does not guarantee competence. Lillyman (2011) believes that reflection is a strategy that helps the practitioner to link evidence-based theory with current practice. Alongside this, reflective learning involves actively thinking about and learning from experience. Moloney and Hahessy (2006, p. 50) state that:

> "for educational development to happen the reflective nurse must see knowledge attainment as part of a developmental cycle where new knowledge is mixed with existing knowledge and practice, in order for a change in practice to occur."

This is in accordance with Schon's (1987) notion of integrating formal and espoused theory to develop personal knowledge.

The majority of reflective models suggest three main stages including awareness, critical analysis and the development of new perspectives (Freshwater 2008). Effective reflection requires a supportive and reflective culture and is a process that all individuals can use to develop professionally and maintain professional accreditation as part of their involvement in daily care delivery (Lillyman 2011). Learning can change attitudes as well as outdated practices and is often stimulating and rewarding, but can also be associated with a degree of discomfort as existing knowledge is tested and attitudes challenged (Pross 2005).

Education

Pre-registration nurse education and training programmes may cover limited aspects of orthopaedic and trauma nursing and it can be wrongly subsumed under the surgical nursing specialty without the recognition of it as a separate specialism. Orthopaedic and trauma practitioners require specific, specialist knowledge and skills at different levels of practice (Clarke 2003, Santy *et al.*, 2005, RCN 2005, Lucas 2006, Flynn and Whitehead 2006, Drozd *et al.*, 2007, RCN 2012). An assumption is often made that postqualifying/graduate nurses who undertake further academic courses relating to orthopaedic and trauma nursing will have an appreciation of basic anatomy and physiology of the musculoskeletal system. This is often unsubstantiated and basic anatomy and physiology needs to be revisited early in postqualifying orthopaedic and trauma nursing courses in order to build upon this underpinning basic knowledge.

One way that nurses can achieve personal and professional growth is by learning through formal defined education programmes (Munro 2008) at postgraduate levels, but learning can also be non-accredited workplace learning. It is vital that the evidence of this ongoing learning and development is documented by practitioners. Further education can lead to opportunities for advancing role development but there is a lack of standardisation of orthopaedic and trauma nursing education in many countries.

Summary

It is essential that practitioners are enabled to provide the highest quality of effective orthopaedic and trauma patient care and professional development should be an ongoing and integrated activity. Practitioners must recognise and seize opportunities for professional development. Ongoing learning and role development is essential for the dramatic changes practitioners are experiencing but educators also have a significant responsibility to maintain links with the clinical environment to ensure that they remain cognisant of clinical developments along with appropriate pedagogical approaches. Meskell *et al.* (2009, p. 789) have argued that:

> "lecturers must demonstrate a value for the practice component of the role and the maintenance of clinical credibility appears to be crucial in order to address the theory-practice divide and preserve the right to continue teaching nurses."

Various strategies for accessing ongoing professional development have been discussed along with active engagement in reflection and the consistent support and challenge from current mentors in practice. Excellence in orthopaedic and trauma nursing practice is the aim of CPD. Registered nurses have a code of conduct and statutory requirements for maintaining registration that necessitate CPD. Other practitioners in orthopaedic and trauma settings must also keep updated and continue to develop both personally and professionally.

Orthopaedic and trauma nursing will continue to evolve and encouragement is needed to pursue lines of inquiry and raise research questions from clinical knowledge and practice for the benefit of patients. It is clear that further research is required into the effects and outcomes of CPD on patient care in clinical practice as currently there is a dearth of evidence.

Recommended further reading

Gopee, N. (2011) *Mentoring and Supervision in Healthcare*, 2nd edn. Sage, London.

McIntosh, A., Gidman, J. and Mason-Whitehead, E. (eds) (2011) *Key Concepts in Healthcare Education*. Sage, London.

RCN Society of Orthopaedic and Trauma Nurses (SOTN) (2012) Orthopaedic and Trauma Practitioner Competences. RCN, London. Available at: http://www.rcn.org.uk/__data/assets/pdf_file/0010/476047/004316.pdf (accessed 14 October 2013).

References

Ali, P.A. and Panther, W. (2008) Professional development and the role of mentorship. *Nursing Standard*, **22**(42), 35–39.

Axley, L. (2008) Competency: a concept analysis. *Nursing Forum*, **43**(4), 214–222.

Bradshaw, A. (2000) Competence and British nursing: a view from history. *Journal of Clinical Nursing*, **9**, 321–329.

Barribal, K.L., While, A.E. and Norman, I.J. (1992) Continuing professional education for registered nurses: a review of the literature. *Journal of Advanced Nursing*, **17**, 1129–1140.

Benner, P. (1984) *From Novice to Expert. Excellence and Power in Clinical Nursing Practice*. Prentice Hall, New Jersey.

Brown, L.A. (1988) Maintaining professional practice – is continuing education a cure or merely a tonic. *Nurse Education Today*, **8**, 251–257.

Charles, M. (1982) Continuing education in Nursing: Whose responsibility? *Nurse Education Today*, **2**, 5–11.

Clarke, S. (2003) A definitional analysis of specialist practice in orthopaedic nursing. *Journal of Orthopaedic Nursing*, **7**(2), 82–86.

Clutterbuck, D. (2004) *Everyone Needs a Mentor*. Chartered Institute of Personnel and Development, London.

Cohen, S. (2009) Orthopaedic patient's perceptions of using a bed pan. *Journal of Orthopaedic Nursing*, **13**(2), 78–84.

Cooley, M.C. (2008) Nurses' motivations for studying third level post-registration programmes and the effects of studying on their personal and work lives. *Nurse Education Today*, **28**(5), 588–594.

Cowan, D. Wilson-Barnett, J. and Norman, I. (2007) A European survey of general nurses' self assessment of competence. *Nurse Education Today*, **27**(5), 452–458.

Drozd, M., Jester, R. and Santy, J. (2007) The inherent components of the orthopaedic nursing role: an exploratory study, *Journal of Orthopaedic Nursing*, **11**(1), 43–52.

Eraut, M. (1994) *Developing Professional Knowledge and Competence*. The Falmer Press, London.

Flynn, S. and Whitehead, E. (2006) An exploration of issues related to nurse led clinics. *Journal of Orthopaedic Nursing*, **10**(2), 86–94.

Freshwater, D, Taylor, B.J. and Sherwood, G. (2008) *International Textbook of Reflective Practice in Nursing*. Wiley Blackwell, Oxford.

Giguère, A., Légaré, F., Grimshaw, J. *et al.* (2012) Printed educational materials: effects on professional practice and healthcare outcomes. *Cochrane Database of Systematic Reviews* **10** (Art. No.: CD004398). DOI: 10.1002/14651858.CD004398.pub3.

Gijbels, H., O' Connell, R., Dalton-O'Connor, C. and O'Donovan, M. (2010) A systematic review evaluating the impact of post registration nursing and midwifery education on practice. *Nurse Education in Practice*, **10**(1), 64–69.

Gopee, N. (2002) Human and social capital as facilitators of lifelong learning in nursing. *Nurse Education Today*, **22**(8), 608–616.

Gopee, N. (2011) *Mentoring and Supervision in Healthcare*, 2nd edn. Sage, London.

Gray, M. (2011) Mentorship, in *Key Concepts in Healthcare Education* (eds A. McIntosh, J. Gidman, and E. Mason-Whitehead), Sage, London, pp. 117–123.

Hagbaghery, M.A., Salsali, M. and Ahmadi, F. (2004) The factors facilitating and inhibiting effective clinical decision making in nursing: a qualitative study. *Biomed Central Open Access*. Available at: http://www.biomedcentral.com/1472-6955/3/2 (accessed 26 November 2012).

Hawkins, P. and Smith, N. (2008) *Coaching, Mentoring and Organisational Consultancy, Supervision and Development*. Open University Press, Maidenhead.

Hegarty, J., Mc Carthy, G., O 'Sullivan, D. and Lehane, B. (2008) A review of nursing and midwifery education research in the Republic of Ireland. *Nurse Education Today*, **28**, 720–736.

Hunt, S. (1991) Continuing education for midwives – a woman's right. *Midwives Chronicle and Nursing Notes* (January), **6–7**.

Kim, K. (2007) Clinical competence among senior nursing students after their preceptorship experiences. *Journal of Professional Nursing*, **23**(6), 369–375.

Lawton, S. and Wimpenny, P. (2003) Continuing professional development: a review. *Nursing Standard*, **17**(24), 41–45.

Lillyman, S. (2011) Reflection, in *Key Concepts in Healthcare Education* (eds A. McIntosh, J. Gidman, and E. Mason-Whitehead), Sage, London, pp. 156–161.

Lucas, B. (2006) Judgment and decision making in advanced orthopaedic nursing practice in relation to chronic knee pain. *Journal of Orthopaedic Nursing*, **10**(4), 206–216.

Meskell, P., Murphy, K. and Shaw, D. (2009) The clinical role of lecturers in nursing in Ireland: Perceptions from key stakeholder groups in nurse education on the role. *Nurse Education Today*, **29**, 784–790.

Moloney, J. and Hahessy, S. (2006) Using reflection in everyday orthopaedic nursing practice. *Journal of Orthopaedic Nursing*, **10**, 49–55.

Munro, K.M. (2008) Continuing professional development and the charity paradigm: interrelated individual, collective and organisational issues about professional development. *Nurse Education Today*, **28**(8), 953–961.

Nolan, M., Owens, R.G., Nolan, J. (1995) Continuing professional education: Identifying the characteristics of an effective system. *Journal of Advanced Nursing*, **21**, 551–560.

O'Shea, Y. (2008) *Nursing and Midwifery in Ireland. A Strategy for Professional Development in a Changing Health Service*. Blackhall Publishing, Dublin.

Perry, L. (1995) Continuing professional education: Luxury or necessity? *Journal of Advanced Nursing*, **21**, 766–771.

Price, B. (2004) Mentoring: the key to clinical learning. *Nursing Standard*, **18**(52), suppl.1–2.

Proctor-Childs, T. (2011) Clinical competence, in *Key Concepts in Healthcare Education* (eds A. McIntosh, J. Gidman, and E. Mason-Whitehead), Sage, London, pp. 17–22.

Pross E. (2005) International nursing students: a phenomenological perspective. *Nurse Education Today*, **25**, 627–633.

Royal College of Nursing (RCN) (2005) *Competencies: An Integrated Career and Competency Framework for Orthopaedic and Trauma Nursing*. RCN, London.

RCN Society of Orthopaedic and Trauma Nurses (SOTN) (2012) *Orthopaedic and Trauma Practitioner Competences*. RCN, London. Available at: http://www.rcn.org.uk/__data/assets/pdf_file/0010/476047/004316.pdf (accessed 14 October 2013).

Santy, J., Rogers, J., Davis, P. *et al.* (2005) A competency framework for orthopaedic and trauma nursing. *Journal of Orthopaedic Nursing*, **9**(2), 81–86.

Schon, D. A. (1987) *Educating the Reflective Practitioner*. Temple Smith, London.

Tomlinson, H. (1993) *Developing professionals. Education*, **182**(13), 231.

CHAPTER 4

The musculoskeletal system and human movement

Lynne Newton-Triggs[1] and Jean Rogers[2]

[1] *Bedford Hospital, Bedford, UK*

[2] *Stepping Hill Hospital, Stockport, UK*

Introduction

The aim of this chapter is to provide an overview of musculoskeletal structure and function while relating it to human movement. Structure and function are linked and it is impossible to discuss one without the other. It is essential that orthopaedic and trauma practitioners know and understand the terms used to describe anatomical positions and the structures involved in musculoskeletal conditions, injuries and surgery to facilitate safe, high quality care. It is also essential to provide a common language which is effective in interdisciplinary communication as this ensures practitioners can explain specific conditions, injuries, surgery and treatment to other staff, patients and relatives to enable them to engage in their care.

Anatomical positioning

The human body is described as being in anatomical position when the body is upright with the head facing forward, hands at the side facing forward with the thumbs pointing away from the body and the feet hip-width apart with the feet and toes pointing forward (Figure 4.1). This position is known universally. When referring to the right and left of the body it is the right and left of the person who is the subject of discussion (e.g. the patient) not the left and right of the observer.

The skeleton has two distinct sections: The axial skeleton consists of the skull bones, inner ear, ribs, vertebrae and sternum. It provides structural support, attachment points for ligaments and muscles and protection for the brain, spinal cord and major organs of the chest. The appendicular skeleton consists of the pectoral girdle and the upper limbs, pelvic girdle and lower limbs that make movement possible and protect the organs of the pelvis.

Human movement is described in three dimensions (or planes) which divide the human body (Figure 4.2)

- The sagittal (vertical/median) plane – lies vertically through the body dividing it into left and right parts.
- The coronal (frontal) plane – lies vertically through the body dividing it into anterior and posterior parts.
- The transverse (horizontal) plane – lies horizontally through the body dividing it into superior and inferior parts.

Anatomical terminology and movement

Anatomical directions and terminology assists practitioners to use a systematic approach to describing and orientating the human body. Box 4.1 gives the most commonly used terms.

Movement can be described in a variety of ways depending on where and how the movement occurs. Types of movement are often described in pairs describing opposite movements (See Box 4.2).

Orthopaedic and Trauma Nursing: An Evidence-based Approach to Musculoskeletal Care, First Edition. Edited by Sonya Clarke and Julie Santy-Tomlinson.

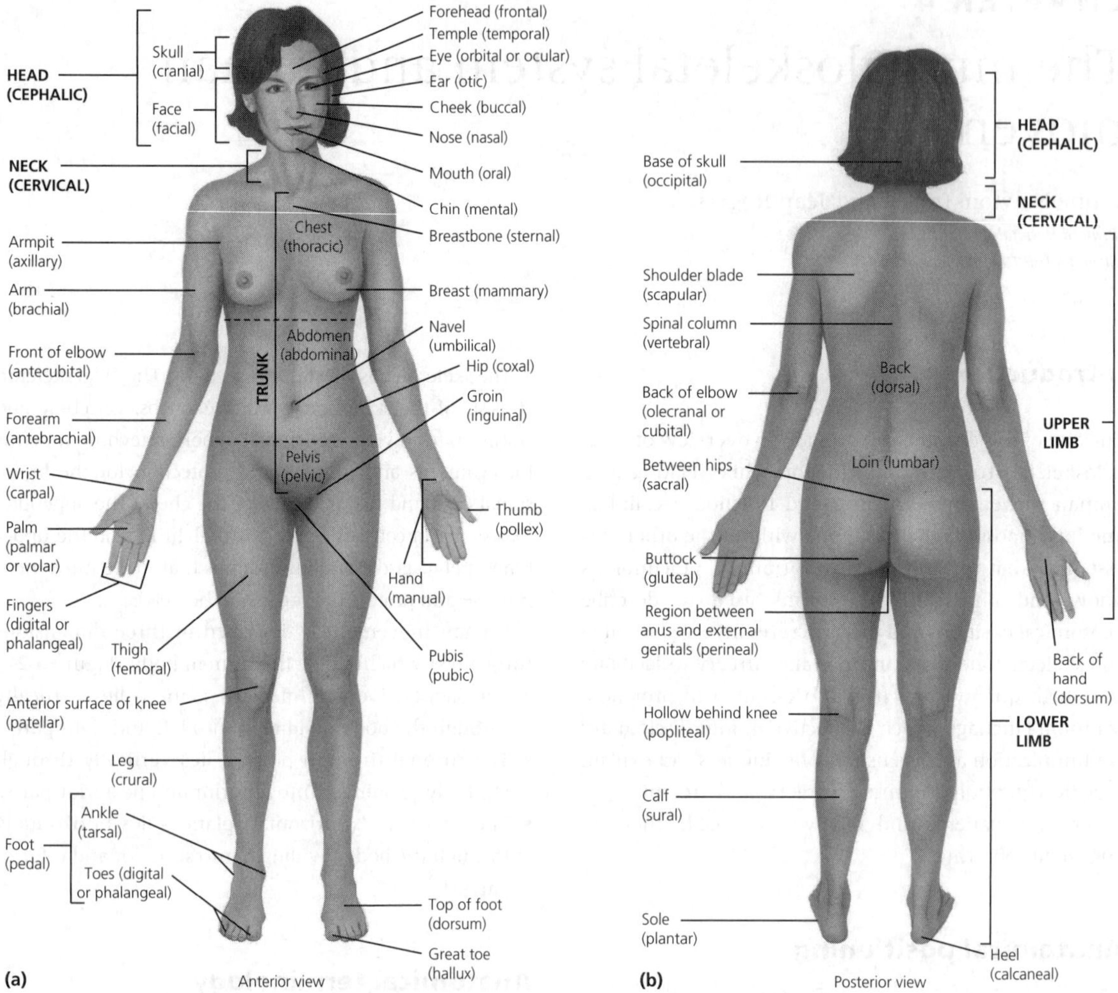

Figure 4.1 Anatomical position. Tortora, G.J. and Derrickson, B.H. *Essentials of Anatomy and Physiology*. 2013, Wiley. This material is reproduced with permission of John Wiley & Sons, Inc.

The skeleton

The skeleton is made of bone, cartilage and ligaments. These structures work in unison to allow movement. The skeleton is strong, light and flexible, representing about 20% of the total body weight, half of which is water. At birth there are over 300 bones, some of which fuse later. Adults have approximately 206, varying slightly between individuals depending on small bone fusion during growth.

Bones are classified in many ways. Their shape and structure are governed by genetic, metabolic and mechanical factors (see Table 4.1).

Bone physiology

Bone is a highly vascular tissue containing intercellular substance surrounding widely separated cells. This dynamic tissue is continuously remodelled and features four characteristic types of cells (see Table 4.2).

Bone is made up mainly of collagen and mineral salts; principally calcium phosphate and some calcium carbonate with small amounts of magnesium hydroxide, fluoride and sulphate. These salts are deposited in a framework of collagen fibres which then calcify. Bone is not completely solid, with some spaces between its hard

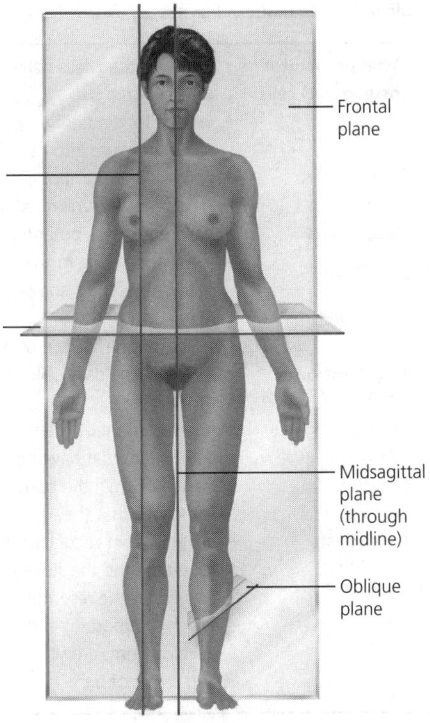

Figure 4.2 Planes of the body. Tortora, G.J. and Derrickson, B.H. *Essentials of Anatomy and Physiology*. 2013, Wiley. This material is reproduced with permission of John Wiley & Sons, Inc.

Box 4.1 Common anatomical terms

- **Anterior/ventral** – towards the front of the body
- **Deep** – away from the surface of the body
- **Distal** – away from the body
- **Inferior/caudal** – away from the head or towards the lower part of the body
- **Lateral** – away from the midline of the body
- **Medial** – towards the midline of the body
- **Midline** – the centre line of the body when it is in the anatomical position
- **Posterior/dorsal** – means towards the back of the body
- **Proximal** – closer to the trunk
- **Superficial** – close to the surface of the body
- **Superior/cranial/cephalic** – towards the head or upper part of the body
- **Valgus** – deviated away from the midline
- **Varus** – deviated towards the midline.

Box 4.2 Terminology for describing movement

- **Flexion** – bending movement; the angle of a joint is decreased
- **Extension** – straightening movement; the angle of the joint is increased
- **Pronation** – rotation of the arm; the hand faces away from the anatomical position to face backwards
- **Supination** – rotation of the arm so the hand faces forwards
- **Abduction** – movement of the limb away from the midline
- **Adduction** – movement of the limb towards the midline
- **Inversion** – movement of the foot and ankle, leaving the sole of the foot facing towards the midline
- **Eversion** – movement of the foot and ankle, leaving the sole of the foot facing away from the midline
- **Plantar flexion** – the toes are pushed down away from the body
- **Dorsiflexion** – the toes are pushed up towards the body
- **Rotation** – rotation of a joint along the horizontal axis of the bone laterally or medially
- **Protraction** – movement forward in the transverse plane e.g. biting the upper lip with the lower teeth.
- **Retraction** – movement backwards in the transverse plane e.g. moving the teeth back into position
- **Elevation** – motion of the limb upwards e.g. shrugging the shoulders
- **Depression** – motion of the limb downwards e.g. opening the jaw

One term does not relate to a pair and is unique to the movement of the thumb:

- **Opposition** – moving of the thumb to the fingers or the palm for grasping objects.

components, providing channels for blood vessels and a lighter structure. Bone tissue can be categorised into compact or cancellous (spongy) depending on the size and distribution of the spaces.

Compact bone surrounds cancellous bone and is thicker in the diaphysis (shaft) than the epiphyses (ends). It provides support and protection and helps long bones resist the stress of weight bearing. Adult compact bone has a concentric ring structure with blood vessels and nerves traversing it from the periosteum through Volkmann's canals that connect with the blood vessels and nerves of the medullary cavity and the central Haversian canals. The Haversian canals run longitudinally through the bone and are surrounded by rings of hard

Box 4.3 Functions of the skeleton

- **Support** – framework for support of the body and maintaining its shape
- **Movement** – muscles, bones and joints provide the principal mechanics for movement, all coordinated by the nervous system
- **Protection** – encases and protects vital organs
- **Blood cell production** – haematopoietic stem cells (HSCs) in the medulla of the bone (bone marrow) give rise to all of the different mature blood cell types and tissues; this is a vital process in the body
- **Storage** – the matrix of bone stores calcium and the bone marrow stores iron
- **Endocrine regulation** – bone cells release the hormone osteocalcin, which contributes to the regulation of blood sugar and fat deposition.

Table 4.1 Bone classifications

Bone	Examples	Features
Long bones	Femur, tibia, humerus	Tubular in shape with a central shaft **(diaphysis)** which contains bone marrow Two extremities **(epiphyses)** Completely covered (except for joint surfaces) in **periosteum** The epiphyses contain **epiphyseal cartilage/plates** near each end of the bone. These are active in growth and ossify when growth is completed in early adulthood
Short bones	Found in the wrist and ankle (carpals and tarsals)	Cuboid in shape No shaft Hard outer shell of compact bone Spongy (cancellous) bone in the centre
Flat bones	Cranium, scapula, pelvis and ribs	Hard compact bone outer casing with a soft cancellous bone centre Usually curved
Irregular bones	Bones of the face, vertebrae	Do not fit in other categories
Sesamoid bones	Patella, distal portion of first and second metacarpals, pisiform, first metatarsal	Embedded in tendons

Table 4.2 Bone tissue cell types

Osteoprogenitor (osteogenic) cells	• un-specialised cells derived from mesenchyme • with mitotic potential and the ability to differentiate into osteoblasts • within the periosteum, endosteum, Haversian and Volkman's canals
Osteoblasts	• have no mitotic potential • involved in bone formation by secreting organic compounds and mineral salts • found on the surface of bone
Osteocytes	• maintain the daily cellular activities of bone • have no mitotic potential and are osteoblasts that have become trapped within the bony intercellular substance that they have laid down
Osteoclasts	• develop from circulating monocytes • found around the surfaces of bone • function is the resorption of bone which is important in the development, growth, maintenance and repair of bone.

calcified bone – concentric lamellae between which are spaces called lacunae which contain osteocytes. Canaliculi radiate in all directions from the lacunae, forming an intricate network providing numerous routes for nutrients to reach the osteocytes and for the removal of waste. Each central canal with the surrounding lamellae, lacunae, osteocytes and canaliculi is known as a Haversian system or osteon (see Figure 4.3).

Cancellous (spongy) bone consists of an irregular latticework of thin plates of bone called trabeculae within which lie lacunae containing osteocytes. The spaces between the trabeculae of some bones are filled with red marrow (responsible for red cell production). Blood vessels from the periosteum penetrate through to the cancellous bone.

Bone growth and development

The process of bone formation, 'ossification', begins in the embryo in which the 'skeleton' at this time is composed of fibrous membranes and hyaline cartilage shaped like bones and providing the medium for ossification. Ossification occurs in two ways:

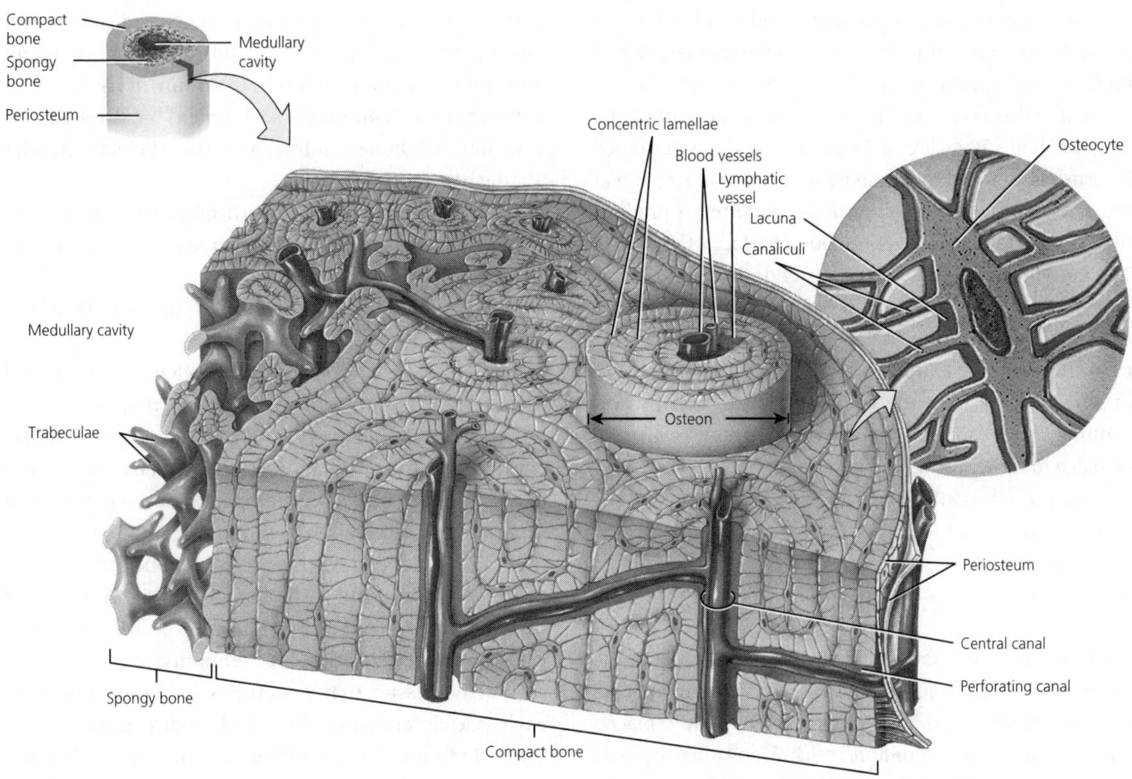

Figure 4.3 Haversian system (osteon). Tortora, G.J. and Derrickson, B.H. *Essentials of Anatomy and Physiology*. 2013, Wiley. This material is reproduced with permission of John Wiley & Sons, Inc.

Intramembranous ossification – osteoblasts cluster in a fibrous membrane forming a centre of ossification and secrete intercellular substances partly composed of collagenous fibres which form a framework around which calcium salts are deposited (calcification). When the cluster of osteoblasts is completely surrounded by the calcified matrix, it is called a trabecula (plural trabeculae). Trabeculae radiate out from each centre of ossification into a framework. The original connective tissue becomes the periosteum and the ossified area becomes cancellous (spongy) bone with a covering of compact bone. Bone is continuously destroyed and reformed until it reaches its final adult size and shape.

Endochondral ossification – the replacement of cartilage by bone. Most bones of the body are formed by this process. Early on in embryonic development a cartilage template of the future bone is laid down and covered by a membrane – the 'perichondrium'. Midway along the shaft a blood vessel penetrates the perichondrium, stimulating osteoprogenitor cells within the perichondrium to enlarge and become osteoblasts. These cells then form osteocytes which form a periosteal collar of compact bone around the middle of the diaphysis of the cartilage model. This then forms the membranous covering of bone known as the periosteum. At the primary centre of ossification, chondrocytes hypertrophy and the matrix becomes mineralised and spaces in the shaft of the bone join together forming the medullary cavity which then fills with bone marrow. Secondary centres of ossification form at the extremities of long bones in the epiphyses and lay down spongy bone. One secondary ossification centre develops in the proximal epiphysis soon after birth and the other centre develops in the distal epiphysis during a child's second year. After the two secondary ossification centres have formed, bone tissue completely replaces the cartilage except in two regions: cartilage continues to cover the articular surfaces of the epiphyses as 'articular cartilage' as well as in the region between the epiphysis and diaphysis (the 'epiphyseal plate') where lengthwise growth of bone continues into early adulthood.

Bones continue to grow in length and width following birth. Appositional growth is the growth in diameter of bone by the formation of new bone on the surface of existing bone. This occurs at the same time as growth in the length of bone. Bone lining the marrow cavity is destroyed by osteoclasts allowing the cavity to increase in size and at the same time osteoblasts from the periosteum produce new compact bone to cover the outer surface of the bone. The growth in length is known as endochondral growth which takes place in the epiphyseal plates until their ossification. The cartilage in the epiphysis is replaced by bone from the shaft side and this is matched by the production of new cartilage from the epiphyseal plate. This process continues until early adulthood when hormones cause the cartilage in the epiphyseal plate to ossify.

Bone growth is influenced by:

- nutrition
- sunlight
- hormones
- exercise.

Bone is constantly remodelling and re-appropriating its matrix and minerals along lines of mechanical stress allowing worn or damaged bone to be removed and replaced with new tissue. Bone also stores calcium and phosphorous. There is a delicate homeostasis maintained between the action of osteoclasts removing calcium and collagen from the bone and osteoblasts depositing calcium and collagen. If too much tissue or calcium is removed, the bones become weakened and break easily, leading to osteoporosis.

There are a number of other hormones involved in the metabolism of bone:

- Vitamin D (calcitriol) – regulates calcium and phosphorous levels and the mineralisation of bone.
- Calcitonin – inhibits the action of osteoclasts thus inhibiting the removal of calcium from bone.
- Parathyroid hormone – increases the number and activity of the osteoclasts which release calcium and phosphate from bones into blood.
- Oestrogens – inhibit the activity of osteoclasts, protecting the bones from excessive bone turnover.
- Human growth hormone – responsible for the general growth of bones at the epiphyseal plates.

Skeletal muscle

Skeletal muscle appears striated (striped) and has the fastest contraction rate under voluntary control of all muscles. It is controlled by the central and autonomic nervous system and provides force and power for movement. Muscles contract and relax to bring about movement and perform three main functions:

1 movement (voluntary and reflex) – through the actions of bones, joints and the skeletal muscles attached to the bones
2 maintenance of posture – through the contraction of muscles to support the body in a stationary position
3 heat production – contraction produces most of the body's heat.

Skeletal muscles are composed of collections of striated muscle fibres and some connective tissues such as blood vessels and nerves. Deep fascia is a dense connective tissue that lines the body wall and extremities as well as holding muscles together and separating them into functioning groups. The entire muscle is wrapped with a fibrous connective tissue called the epimysium. Bundles of muscle fibres called fasciculi are covered by fibrous connective tissue known as perimysium and endomysium – fibrous connective tissue that penetrates into the interior of each fascicle and surrounds and separates the muscle fibres. Individual muscle fibres are long and cylindrical structures with multiple nuclei and their length and width varies depending on the function and purpose of each muscle. Each muscle fibre contains thousands of microscopic contractile units known as myofibrils that bring about contraction following electrical stimulation in a complex process of sliding filaments within the myofibrils.

Muscles are named according to their shape, location, or a combination of both and according to function e.g. flexion, extension, or rotation.

Skeletal muscle attachment

Skeletal muscles produce movement by exerting force on tendons which in turn pull on bones. When a muscle contracts it draws one articulating bone towards the other. The attachment of a muscle tendon to the stationary bone is called the origin. The attachment of the other muscle tendon to the moveable bone is known as the **insertion**. Levers are created by the bones and joints. Tendons attach muscles to the bone and act on the skeleton by contracting and shortening or relaxing to allow two bones to move closer or move away.

Ligaments, tendons and cartilage

Ligaments, tendons and cartilage connect bones, joints and muscles and guide and protect movement that has been initiated by muscles.

Ligaments and tendons are formed from regularly arranged dense connective tissue with strong parallel fibres that attach muscles to bone. Aponeoroses are the flattened sheet-like tendons which connect muscle to bone or muscle to muscle. Large fibrous sacs known as bursae protect some tendons such as those at the hip, knee and elbow. Ligament elasticity allows stretch. They stabilise the joint to ensure movement remains within its normal planes.

Dense irregular connective tissue forms cartilage. Fibres are arranged irregularly, allowing them to endure more stress than ligaments and tendons. There is no blood or nerve supply and minimal ability for healing. There are two types of cartilage that relate to the skeletal system:

- hyaline cartilage – the most abundant type found at joints over the ends of the long bones as 'articular cartilage'. It provides flexibility and support, absorbs shock and reduces friction.
- fibrocartilage – allows greater resistance to compression and tension due to its fibrous structure. It can be found at the symphysis pubis, the intervertebral discs between vertebrae and the menisci of the knee.

Neurovascular supply

Bone has a rich nerve and blood supply, supplying the nutrients for bone growth and muscle contraction and supporting biofeedback systems.

Bone has a rich blood supply from which it acquires nutrients required for growth, remodelling and repair. Large nutrient arteries enter bones through holes known as nutrient foramen into the diaphysis of the bone and then divide into the proximal and distal branches and supply the head of the bone. Blood vessels and capillaries divide from the nutrient artery and enter the central/Haversian canals to supply the compact bone. Perforating canals within the compact bone allow entry of the capillaries into the cancellous bone, supplying the nutrients required for bone cell and bone marrow activity. The central canal of long bones and central area of flat bones contain red marrow (haematopoietic tissue) which is responsible for the production of red blood cells.

Nerves are prolific throughout bone, allowing communication with the central nervous system and providing feedback as well as being responsible for some of the pain felt when there is bone disease or injury. Blood vessels and nerves run side by side and are most prolific in the ends of long bones where they provide autonomic feedback/proprioception from the joints.

Joints

Bones are held together at joints by flexible connective tissue where all movement takes place. The structure of the joint determines how it functions. Some joints permit no movement, whilst others permit slight or considerable movement. The structural classification of joints is based on whether there is a synovial cavity and the type of connective tissue that binds the bones together. Structurally joints are classified as:

- **Fibrous Joints** – lack a synovial cavity and the articulating bones fit very closely together. There is little or no movement. There are three types:
  - Suture – between the bones of the skull. The bones are united by a thin layer of dense fibrous connective tissue. The irregular structure of sutures gives added strength and decreases the chance of fracture. Some sutures present during growth are replaced by bone in the adult and these are called synostoses.
  - Syndesmosis – is a fibrous joint where the fibrous connective tissue is present in a greater amount than in a suture but the fit between the bones is not quite as tight. The fibrous connective tissue forms an interosseous membrane or ligament. The syndesmosis is slightly moveable because the bones are separated more than in a suture and some flexibility is permitted by the interosseous membrane e.g. the talofibular joint.
  - Gomphosis – a type of fibrous joint where a cone-shaped peg fits into a socket e.g. the articulation of the roots of teeth with the sockets.
- **Cartilagenous Joints** – have no synovial cavity and articulating bones are tightly connected by cartilage, allowing little or no movement. There are two types:
  - Synchondrosis – the connecting tissue is hyaline cartilage. The commonest type is the epiphyseal plate found between the epiphysis and diaphysis of a

growing bone. The joint is eventually replaced by bone when growth ceases – synostosis e.g. the joint between the first rib and the sternum.

  - Symphysis – a cartilaginous joint in which the connecting material is a broad flat disc of fibrocartilage e.g. between the bodies of the vertebrae and the symphysis pubis. These joints are slightly moveable – amphiarthrotic.

- **Synovial Joints** – the most common joints have a space known as the synovial cavity between the articulating bones and are freely moveable. Synovial joints have five main features:
  - Joint cavity – the space between articulating bones which provides the space for movement.
  - Articular cartilage – covers the surfaces of the articulating bones and is formed of hyaline cartilage. Prevents friction and absorbs shock.
  - Articular capsule – synovial joints are surrounded by a sleeve-like structure enclosing the synovial cavity and uniting the articulating bones. It is composed of two layers – the fibrous capsule and the synovial membrane. The fibrous capsule consists of dense connective tissue and is attached to the periosteum at a variable distance from the edge of the articular cartilage. The flexibility of the fibrous capsule allows for movement at the joint while its tensile strength resists dislocation.
  - Synovial membrane – the inner layer of the articular capsule and covers all surfaces of the joint not already covered by articular cartilage. It is composed of loose connective tissue and secretes synovial fluid.
  - Synovial fluid – secreted by the synovial membrane, fills the joint cavity, lubricates the joint, provides nourishment for the articular cartilage, reduces friction, supplies nutrients and removes metabolic wastes from the cells of the articular cartilage. Synovial fluid contains phagocytic cells that remove microbes and debris from wear and tear in the joint.

  Synovial joints are further classified by their movement and the structures of the articulating bones:

- Hinge joint – the convex surface of one bone fits into the concave surface of another bone. The movement is in a single plane and is similar to that of a hinged door e.g. hinge joints are the knee, elbow and interphalangeal joints where the movement allowed is flexion and extension.
- Ball and Socket Joint – a ball-like surface of one bone fitted into a cuplike depression of another bone, allowing movement in three planes: flexion/extension, abduction/adduction and rotation/circumduction e.g. the shoulder joint and hip joint. The stability of the joint depends on how deep the socket is and the fit of the ball within the socket.
- Plane joint (gliding) – the articulating surfaces glide against each other in one plane only and are usually flat, allowing only limited movement e.g. the joints between the carpal bones, tarsal bones and the sternum and clavicle.
- Pivot joint – the conical surface of one bone articulates within a ring formed partly by another bone and a ligament, allowing rotation e.g. the joint between the atlas and axis allowing rotation of the head.
- Condyloid joint – an oval shaped condyle of one bone fits into an elliptical cavity of another bone, allowing side to side and back and forth movements and allowing flexion/extension, abduction/adduction and circumduction e.g. the joint at the wrist between the radius and carpals.
- Saddle joint – the articular surface of one bone is saddle shaped and the other articular surface is shaped like a rider sitting in the saddle – a modified condyloid joint with freer movement. Movements are side to side and back and forth e.g. the joint between the trapezium and the metacarpal of the thumb. Figure 4.4 illustrates the different types of synovial joints.

The cranium (the skull)

The bony skeleton of the head (cranium) supports the structure of the face and forms a cavity for the brain. It is thin, light and solid and is usually described via the eight bones that make it up (Table 4.3), sometimes referred to as the neurocranium. The inner surfaces attach to membranes that position and stabilise the brain, blood vessels and nerves. The outer surfaces act as an attachment for muscles so the head can move in various ways.

The cranium is proportionally more developed at birth and grows more quickly during the first years of life than the rest of the skeleton. To allow flexion so

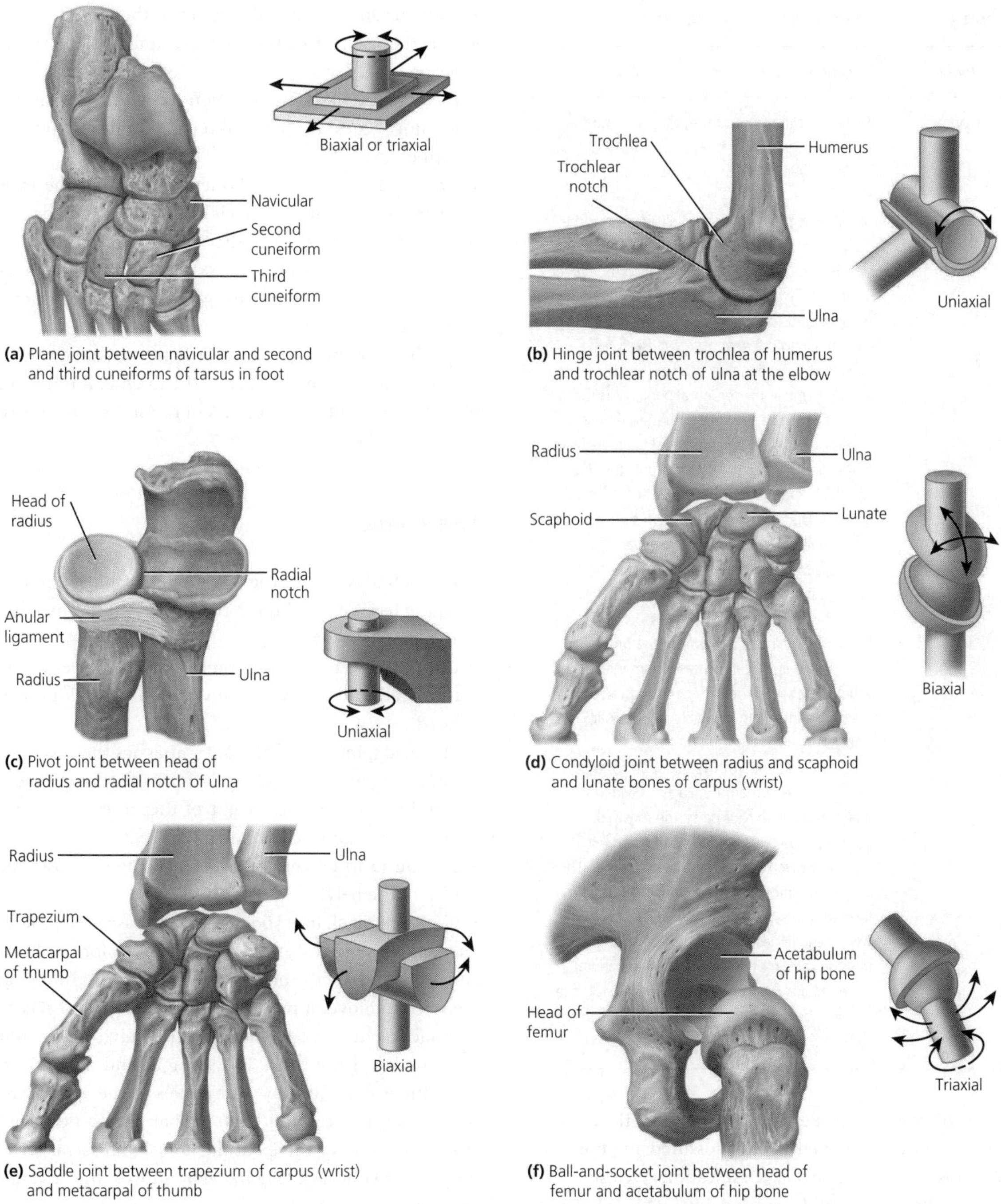

Figure 4.4 Types of synovial joint. Tortora, G.J. and Derrickson, B.H. *Essentials of Anatomy and Physiology*. 2013, Wiley. This material is reproduced with permission of John Wiley & Sons, Inc.

Table 4.3 The function of the bones of the skull

Bones	Function
Frontal	Situated at the front of the head forming the forehead, the roof of the eye sockets and nasal cavity as well as the base of the anterior of the skull.
Occipital	Situated at the rear of the skull just above the nape of the neck. It has a hole at the base which is the channel of the spinal cord between skull and the spinal column. The occipital bone is connected to the top two vertebrae (atlas and axis) allowing the head to move freely.
Sphenoid	A wing shaped bone situated at the base of the skull in front of the temporal bones. It is the only bone that articulates with the other seven bones of the skull. It spans the skull laterally and helps form the base of the cranium, the sides of the skull, and the floors and sides of the eye sockets. The central body has two sinuses within it which lie side by side and are separated by a bony septum that projects downward into the nasal cavity, and channels for the optic nerve and other nerves.
Ethmoid	Separates the nasal cavity from the brain. It is spongy and light, can be easily damaged and is situated between the eye sockets at the roof of the nose. The external walls contain small sinuses.
Temporal x 2	Found on each side of the skull and form part of the sides and the base. Each is divided anatomically into four parts: the mastoid, petrous, squamous, and tympanic parts. It is closely involved in the anatomy of the ear. They also form a projection from the cheekbone to the eye (the zygoma).
Parietal x 2	Two of the largest bones of the skull and form the sides and roof. In the front each parietal bone adjoins the frontal bone; in the back, the occipital bone; and below, the temporal and sphenoid bones.

that childbirth can take place, the bones of the cranium at birth are connected by non-ossified membranous regions (fontanelles). Ossification closes the fontanelles by a child's second birthday. Where the bones meet they become connected to each other by immobile solid fibrous articulations called cranial sutures.

The cranium has four main functions:

- protection of the brain
- contains and supports the eyes and the face
- fixes the distance between the eyes to allow stereoscopic vision
- the ears are fixed into position to help the brain use auditory cues to judge direction and distance of sounds.

There are fourteen facial bones which hold the eyes in place and form the facial features. The face is sometimes referred to as the splanchnocranium and makes the cranium into the skull. These bones meet with the cranial bones to give each face unique individual form.

The hyoid bone is one further bone – it stands alone and is located in the neck below the tongue. It is held in place by ligaments and muscles of the styloid process of the temporal bone.

The spine

The vertebral column, (the 'backbone' or spine) extends from the base of the skull to the pelvis and has five distinct regions:

- Cervical spine (7 vertebrae) – the neck, supports the head and allows for nodding and shaking the head
- Thoracic spine (12 vertebrae) – attaches the ribs
- Lumbar spine (5 vertebrae) – forms the lower back, carrying most of the weight of the upper body and providing a stable centre of gravity
- Sacrum (5 fused vertebrae) – makes up the posterior wall of the pelvis
- Coccyx (4 small fused bones) – at the base of the spine.

The spine provides strong flexible support for the head and body and keeps the trunk straight whilst allowing the torso to move. It protects the spinal cord and acts as an attachment point for the ribs, the pelvic girdle and the muscles of the back. The strength and mobility of the spine is enhanced by four curves of the spine, two concave at the cervical and lumbar levels (lordosis/lordoses) and two convex at the dorsal and sacral areas (kyphosis/kyphoses). Figure 4.5 shows the overall structure of the spine.

The main functions of the spine are:

- protection of the spinal cord and nerve roots
- supports and balances the body in an upright position with the help of surrounding muscles and ligaments

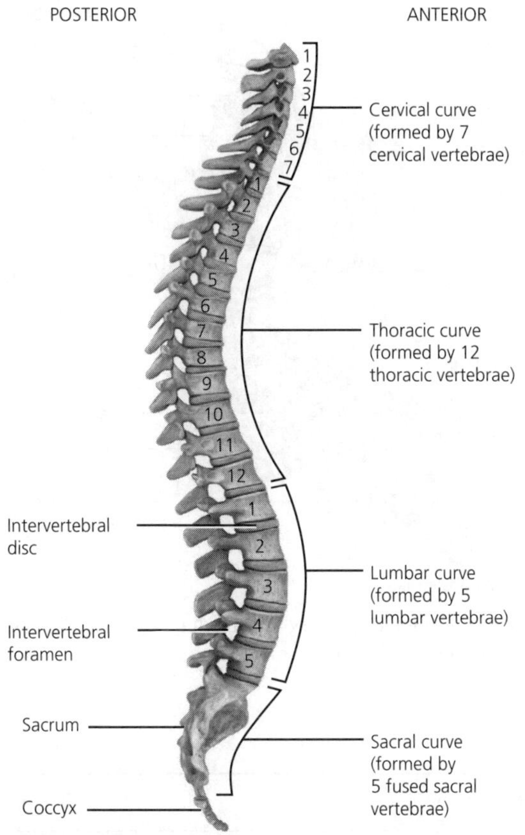

Figure 4.5 The spine. Tortora, G.J. and Derrickson, B.H. *Essentials of Anatomy and Physiology*. 2013, Wiley. This material is reproduced with permission of John Wiley & Sons, Inc.

- attachment for the ribs, pelvic girdle, muscles, ligaments and tendons
- mobility of the vertebrae and the intervertebral discs allow mobility in the trunk of the body.

The vertebrae

The vertebrae are named by using the initial of the area concerned i.e. C = cervical, D (or T) = dorsal (or thoracic) etc. and the number according to the vertebra's position in the spine i.e. C3 is the third cervical vertebra. Figure 4.6 illustrates the structure of a typical vertebra. The basic structure is the same at all levels and consists of:

- A vertebral body which is the thickest and loadbearing part of the vertebrae. Rough surfaces provide excellent adhesion for the intervertebral discs. It also contains two foramina that allow blood vessels to pass through.
- A vertebral arch – composed of two thick projections (vertebral pedicles) and two flat sections of bone (vertebral laminae) and completed by the vertebral body. This forms the vertebral foramen that encloses the spinal cord. Once the vertebrae are stacked on each other the vertebral foramen form the vertebral canal. The stacked pedicles create a gap on each side, each allowing for the passage of a spinal nerve.
- Seven processes commence from the vertebral arch – two transverse, four articular and one spinous process. The four articular processes are covered in hyaline cartilage and articulate with the vertebrae above and below.

The vertebrae are different depending on the level of the spine they correspond to (see Table 4.4); however, two vertebrae are unique – C1 and C2.

- C1 (atlas) – supports the head and is a ring of bone with two transverse processes and has articular facets on its upper side that are concave and articulate with the occipital condyles allowing the head to move up and down. On the lower surfaces it articulates with the second vertebra.
- C2 (the axis) – has a characteristic protrusion on the upper surface known as the dens. This serves as a pivot for the rotation of the atlas and the head allowing it to rotate from side to side.

Soft tissues of the spine

Intervertebral discs have two functions:

- to attach the vertebrae to one another
- to absorb and dampen shock to the spine.

All the vertebrae are separated by the intervertebral discs except for C1 and C2 and the coccyx. These are made of varying thickness of cartilage – the thickest in the lumbar vertebrae which take the most stress.

The annulus fibrosus of the disc is a strong outer structure made up of concentric sheets of collagen fibres connected to the vertebral end plates. This encloses the nucleus pulposus. The nucleus pulposus contains a gel-like matter full of water that resists compression; the amount of water in the nucleus

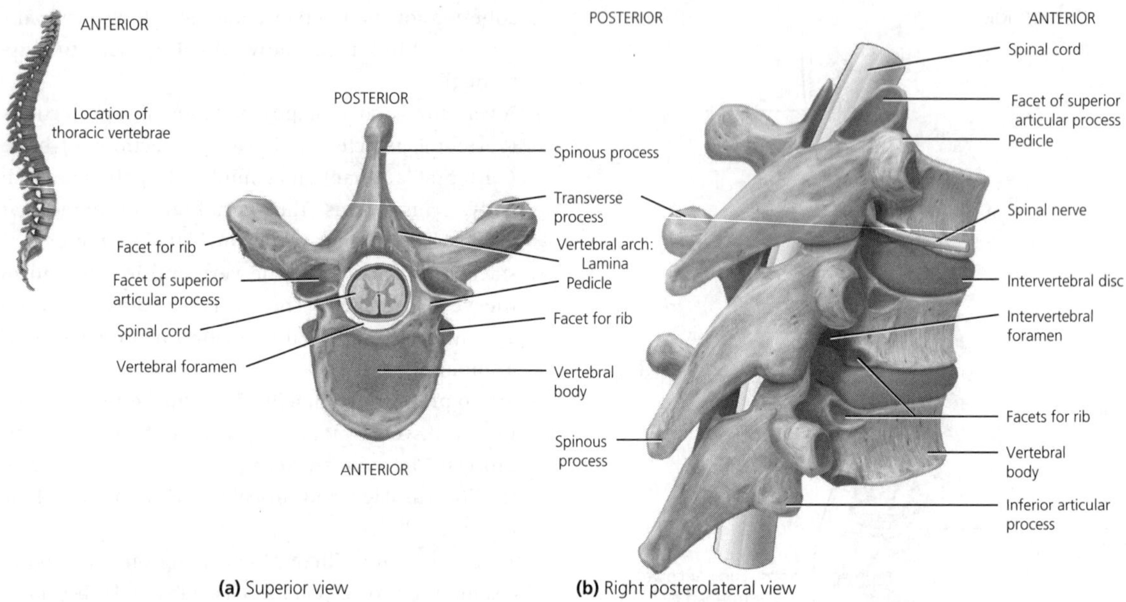

Figure 4.6 Structure of a typical vertebrae (illustrated by a thoracic vertebra). Tortora, G.J. and Derrickson, B.H. *Essentials of Anatomy and Physiology*. 2013, Wiley. This material is reproduced with permission of John Wiley & Sons, Inc.

Table 4.4 The characteristics of vertebrae

Vertebral position	Size and structure	Characteristics
Cervical (C1–C7)	Smaller than other vertebrae but with wider arches	• form the bony structure of the neck – includes C1 and C2 • three foramina – one vertebral which accommodates the spinal cord and two transverse which allow the vertebral artery to pass through with its corresponding vein and nerve.
Thoracic (T1–T12)	Large and robust except for T11, T12, T1 and T2 they have longer transverse processes.	• at the back of the thoracic cavity and articulate with the ribs.
Lumbar (L1–L5)	Largest and most robust vertebrae with short thick processes.	• carry most of the body weight and support the lower back.
Sacrum	5 fused vertebrae	• forms a triangle and part of the posterior wall of the pelvic cavity • it is wider in women than in men.
Coccyx	4 fused vertebrae	• forms a smaller triangle and the posterior portion of the bones of the pelvis • connected to the sacrum.

varies throughout the day depending on activity (see Figure 4.7).

The ligaments of the spine (listed in Table 4.5) connect bone to bone and are fibrous connective tissues made up of densely packed collagen fibres. These help to provide structural stability and a natural brace along with the tendons and muscles which help to protect the spine from injury. There are two primary ligament systems in the spine. The intrasegmental system includes the ligamentum flavum, interspinous and intertransverse ligaments. This holds many vertebrae together. The intersegmental system includes the anterior and posterior longitudinal ligaments, and the supraspinous ligaments.

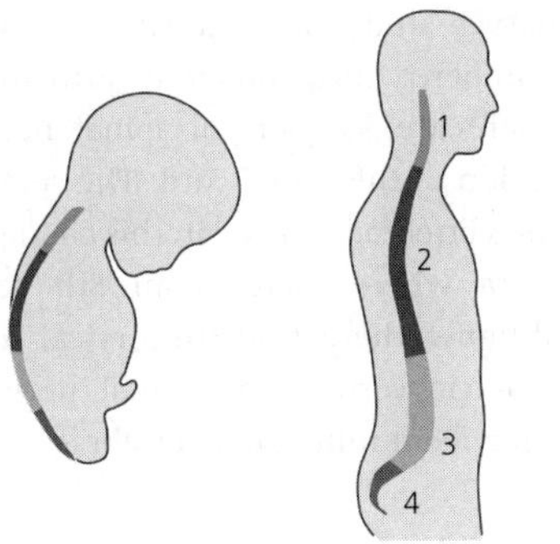

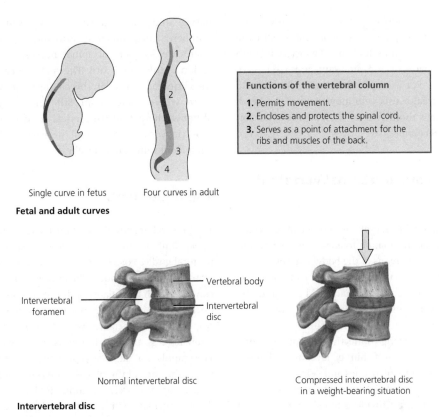

Functions of the vertebral column

1. Permits movement.
2. Encloses and protects the spinal cord.
3. Serves as a point of attachment for the ribs and muscles of the back.

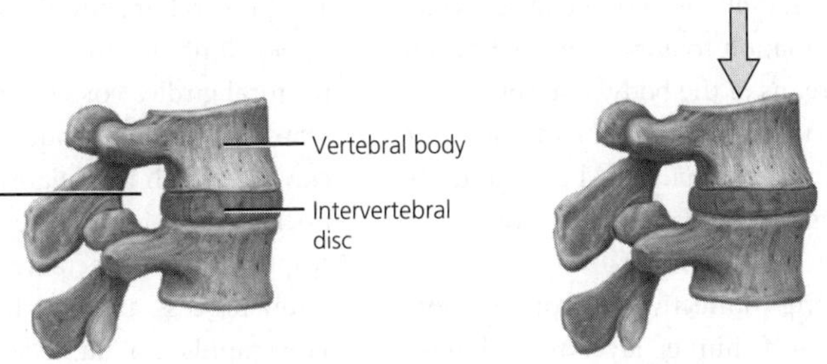

Figure 4.7 Intervertebral discs. Tortora, G.J. and Derrickson, B.H. *Essentials of Anatomy and Physiology*. 2013, Wiley. This material is reproduced with permission of John Wiley & Sons, Inc.

Table 4.5 The ligaments of the spine

Ligament Name	System	Description
Anterior longitudinal ligament	Intersegmental system	• One of the primary spine stabilisers and runs the entire length of the spine from the base of the skull to the sacrum. • Connects the front (anterior) of the vertebral body to the front of the annulus fibrosis.
Posterior longitudinal ligament	Intersegmental system	• Another primary spine stabiliser and runs the entire length of the spine from the base of the skull to the sacrum. • Connects the back (posterior) of the vertebral body to the back of the annulus fibrosus.
Supraspinous ligament	Intrasegmental system	• Attaches the tip of each spinous process to the next one.
Interspinous ligament	Intrasegmental system	• A thin ligament. • Attaches to the ligamentum flavum that runs deep into the spinal column.
Ligamentum flavum	Intrasegmental system	• The strongest ligament. • Runs from the base of the skull to the pelvis, in front of and between the lamina, and in front of the facet joint capsules. • Protects the spinal cord and nerves.

The primary function of the complex muscle and tendon system of the spine is to support and stabilise the structure. Specific muscles are associated with movement of parts of the anatomy and have very important roles. For example, the sternocleidomastoid muscle (neck area) assists with movement of the head, while the spinalis thoracis is associated with extension of the vertebral column.

The spinal cord and spinal/vertebral nerves

The spinal cord consists of millions of nerve fibres which transmit electrical information to and from the brain to the limbs, trunk and organs of the body. The spinal cord descends through the vertebral foramen of each vertebra down to the cauda equina. The brain and the spinal cord are surrounded by the meninges which have three distinct layers:

- the dura mater – strong connective grey outer layer
- the arachnoid mater – a thinner layer resembling a loosely woven fabric of arteries and veins
- the pia mater – a delicate inner layer of highly vascular membrane providing blood to the neural structures.

The space between the arachnoid mater and pia mater (subarachnoid space) is filled with cerebrospinal fluid (CSF) – a clear fluid found in the ventricles, spinal canal and spinal cord that is secreted from a vascular part of the ventricles in the brain, the choroid plexus. This acts as a shock absorber to protect against injury and contains different electrolytes, proteins and glucose.

The communication system from the spinal cord is via spinal nerves which link to the peripheral nervous system which branch off and pass out from the cord through the foramen of the vertebra. Figure 4.8 shows the spinal cord and spinal nerves. There are four main groups of spinal nerves, which exit different levels of the spinal cord:

- cervical nerves – supply movement and feeling to the arms, neck and upper trunk and control breathing
- thoracic nerves – supply the trunk and abdomen
- lumbar and sacral nerves – supply the legs, bladder, bowel and sexual organs.

The spinal nerves carry information to and from different levels (segments) in the spinal cord. Both the nerves and the segments in the spinal cord are numbered in a similar way to the vertebrae e.g. T3. There are 31 pairs of spinal nerves, in the cervical region of the spinal cord. The spinal nerves exit above the vertebrae. However, this changes below the C7 vertebra where there is an 8th cervical spinal nerve although there is no 8th cervical vertebra. From the 1st thoracic vertebra all spinal nerves exit below their equivalent numbered vertebrae.

The upper limb

The pectoral or shoulder girdle attaches the bones of the upper limb to the axial skeleton. Each of the two pectoral girdles consists of a clavicle (collar bone) and a scapula (shoulder blade). The anterior component is the clavicle which articulates with the sternum at the sternoclavicular joint. The posterior component is the scapula which articulates with the clavicle at the acromion process and the humerus at the glenoid cavity. The scapula is a flat, triangular bone which lies over the ribs at the back of the rib cage and is held within a complex group of muscle attachments. The pectoral girdles do not articulate with the vertebral column.

The clavicle (collarbone) is a long slender bone with a double curve that lies horizontally in the superior anterior part of the thorax. The medial end articulates with the sternum at the sternoclavicular joint and the lateral end articulates with the acromion of the scapula at the acromioclavicular joint. The clavicle transmits forces from the upper limb to the trunk of the body.

The Scapula (shoulder blade) is a large triangular flat bone which sits posteriorly over the thoracic cage between the levels of the second and seventh rib. A sharp spine runs diagonally across the posterior surface and ends at a flattened projection known as the acromion which articulates with the clavicle at the acromioclavicular joint and can easily be felt as the high point of the shoulder. Below the acromion, the glenoid cavity articulates with the humerus to form the shoulder joint. Figure 4.9 shows the right upper limb.

The ball and socket joint of the **shoulder (glenohumeral joint)** is freely moveable in many directions but is relatively unstable because the glenoid cavity is very shallow. The rim is slightly deepened by cartilage but has little effect on the stability of the joint.

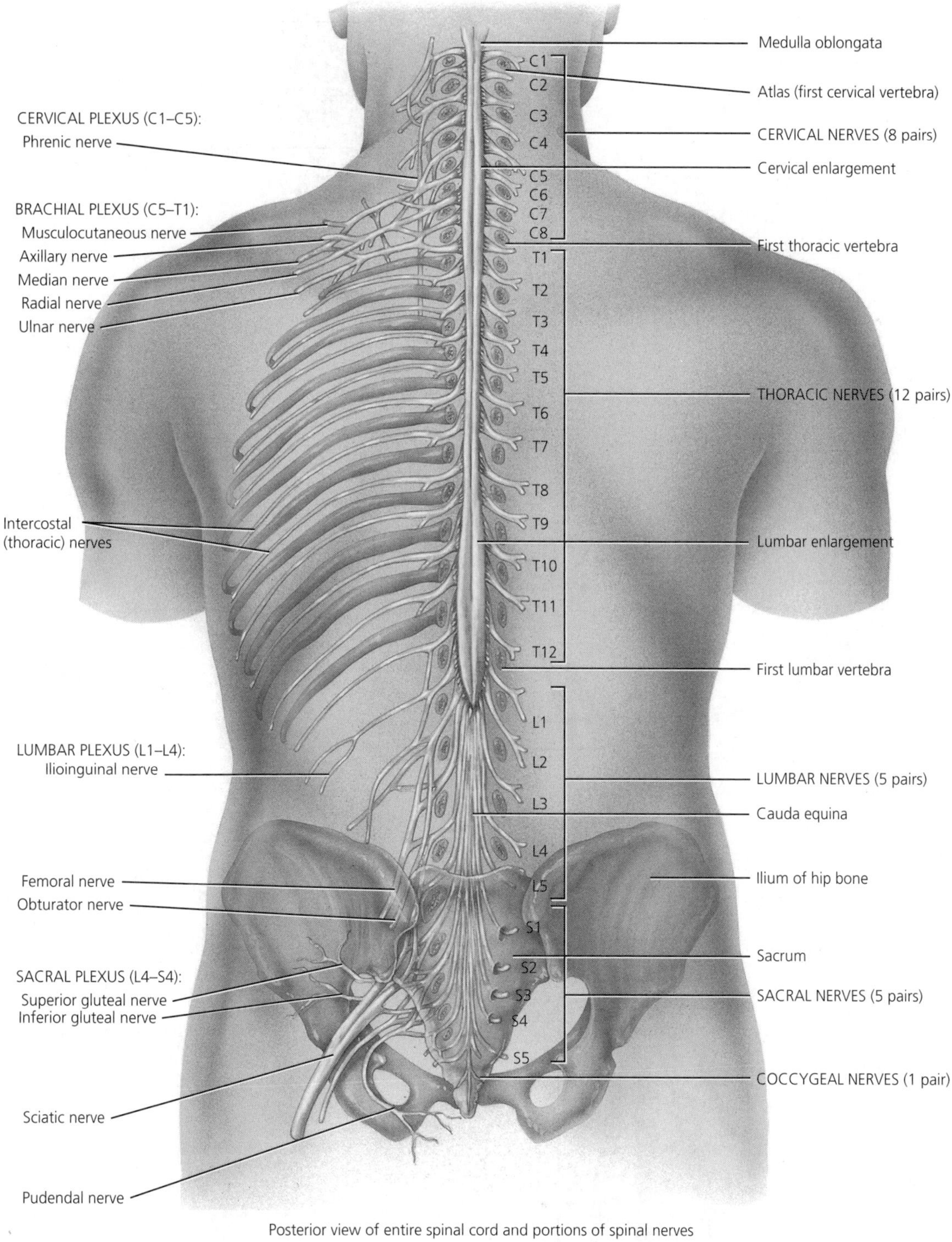

Posterior view of entire spinal cord and portions of spinal nerves

Figure 4.8 Spinal cord and spinal nerves. Tortora, G.J. and Derrickson, B.H. *Essentials of Anatomy and Physiology*. 2013, Wiley. This material is reproduced with permission of John Wiley & Sons, Inc.

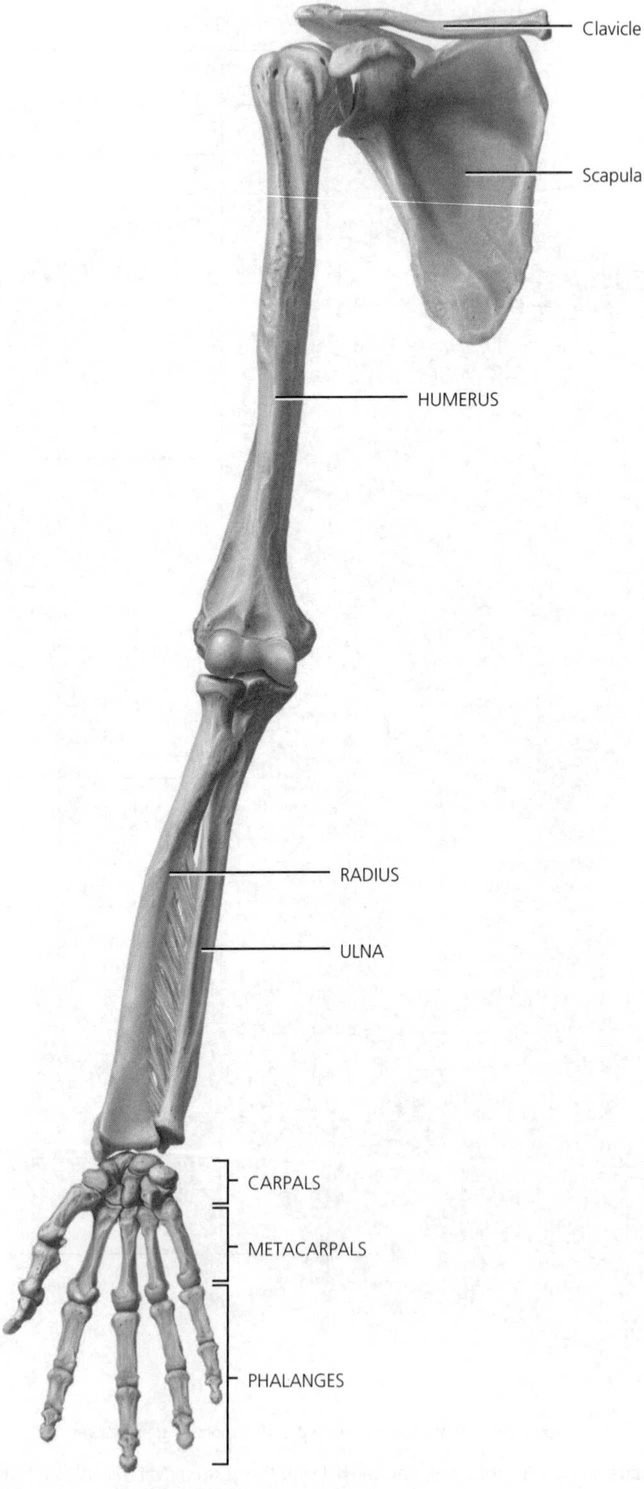

Figure 4.9 Right upper limb. Kuntzman, A.J. and Tortora, G.J. *Anatomy and physiology for the manual therapies*. 2010, Wiley. This material is reproduced with permission of John Wiley & Sons, Inc.

A number of ligaments and tendons help to secure the humeral head in the joint cavity along with the series of four tendons (subscapularis, supraspinatus, infraspinatus and teres minor) which make up the rotator cuff.

The humerus is the longest and largest bone of the upper limb. The proximal end consists of a head that articulates with the glenoid cavity. It has an anatomical neck just distal to the head. The neck of the humerus is a constricted area just distal to the greater and lesser tubercles and is liable to fracture. The shaft of the humerus is cylindrical but gradually becomes flattened and triangular at its distal end.

The elbow is a synovial hinge joint which allows flexion and extension and is important to the flexibility and function of the upper limb. Supination and pronation of the forearm take place at the proximal radioulnar joint contained within the elbow joint capsule. The distal end of the humerus articulates with the proximal end of the ulna and radius. At the distal end of the humerus:

- The capitulum is a rounded knob that articulates with the head of the radius.
- The radial fossa is a depression which receives the head of the radius when the elbow is flexed.
- The trochlea is the surface that articulates with the ulna.
- An anterior depression known as the coronoid fossa receives the ulna head when the forearm is flexed.
- The olecranon fossa is a posterior depression that receives the olecranon of the ulna when the elbow is extended.

Most of the muscles of the forearm are attached to the distal end of the humerus at the medial and lateral epicondyles and the ulnar nerve lies on the posterior surface of the medial epicondyle.

The radius is the lateral bone of the forearm situated on the thumb side and the ulna is the medial bone of the forearm situated on the little finger side. The head of the radius articulates with the capitulum of the humerus and the radial notch of the ulna. The shaft of the radius widens at its distal end and articulates with two of the wrist bones – lunate and scaphoid. At the proximal end of the ulna the olecranon process forms the point of the elbow. The elbow is stabilised by ligaments which prevent rotation and provide stability and strength.

The wrist and hand are capable of very fine, flexible movements. The wrist consists of eight small bones – the carpals, in two transverse rows with four bones in each row, united by ligaments. The proximal row of carpal bones (from lateral to medial) are the scaphoid, lunate, triquetrum and pisiform. The distal row (from lateral to medial) are the trapezium, trapezoid, capitate and hamate. A passageway on the palmar side of the carpal bones known as the carpal tunnel provides a conduit through which the median nerve and flexor tendons of the hand pass. The nerve supply to the arm and hand, with specific reference to the brachial plexus is considered in some detail in Chapter 20.

The metacarpals which form the palm of the hand each consist of a proximal base which articulates with the distal row of carpal bones, a shaft and a distal head which articulate with the proximal phalanges of the fingers. The metacarpal bones are numbered 1 to 5. The phalanges are the bones of the fingers and there are 14 in each hand – 2 in the pollex (thumb) and 3 in each of the remaining four fingers. A single bone of the finger is referred to as a phalanx. The articulations between the metacarpal bones and the phalanges are referred to as the metacarpophalangeal (MCP) joints which flex and extend the fingers and thumb. The two joints in the fingers are known as the interphalangeal joints – the joint closest to the MCP joint is referred to as the proximal interphalangeal joint (PIP) and the joint near the end of the finger is called the distal interphalangeal joint (DIP). The thumb has only one interphalangeal joint.

The pelvis

The pelvis is a bowl-shaped ring of bones that transmits weight from the spine through the legs. Its two (right and left) innominate bones are made up of three bones – the ilium, ischium and pubis – which fuse together at puberty. The pelvic girdle consists of the innominate bones connected at the pubic symphysis anteriorly and the sacrum posteriorly at the sacroiliac joint to form the highly stable but immobile pelvic ring (see Figure 4.10). The pelvic cavity contains the reproductive organs, bladder and rectum. The female pelvis is wider and shallower than the male to facilitate childbirth. The functions of the pelvis are summarised in Box 4.4

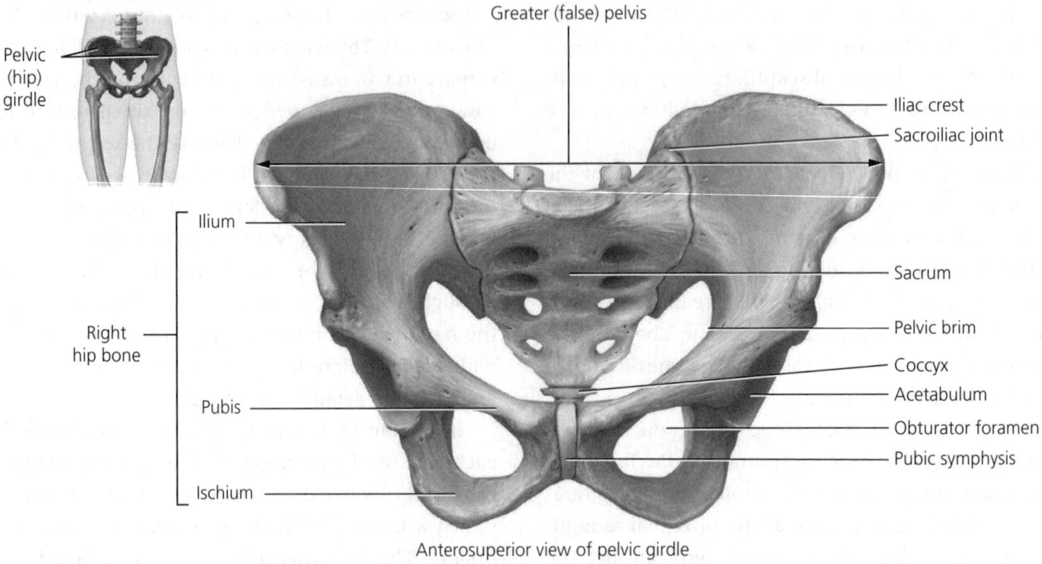

Figure 4.10 The female pelvis – anterior view. Tortora, G.J. and Derrickson, B.H. *Essentials of Anatomy and Physiology*. 2013, Wiley. This material is reproduced with permission of John Wiley & Sons, Inc.

Box 4.4 Functions of the pelvis

Weight bearing – bears the weight of the upper body in sitting and standing
Transfer – transfers weight from the axial skeleton to the appendicular skeleton in standing and walking
Attachments – provides attachments for and withstands the forces of the muscles used for posture and movement
Protection – contains and protects the pelvic and abdominopelvic viscera.

The lower limb

The lower limbs are composed of 60 bones (see Figures 4.11 and 4.12). Each limb includes the femur, patella, tibia, fibula, tarsals, metatarsals and phalanges.

The ball and socket arrangement of the hip joint allows flexion/extension, adduction/abduction and medial/lateral rotation and is central to the transfer of weight from the trunk and upper body to the legs. The proximal end, or head, of the femur articulates with the acetabulum of the innominate bone. The neck of the femur is a constricted region distal to the head. The greater and lesser trochanters are projections that serve as points for the attachment of some of the thigh and buttock muscles. The joint is supported by a series of strong muscles and ligaments with a main nerve supply from the femoral and obturator nerves formed from the lumbar plexus. The main blood supply comes from the femoral artery.

The femur is the longest and heaviest bone of the body and distally articulates with the tibia at the knee joint. The diaphysis of the femur has a rough vertical ridge on its posterior surface which serves as the attachment for several thigh muscles. The distal end of the femur expands and includes the medial and lateral condyles.

The knee is the largest joint. It is a hinge joint allowing flexion and extension supported by a complex system of ligaments and made up of three joints: the lateral and medial femorotibial and the patellofemoral. The two femorotibial joints are articulations between the lateral and medial condyles of the femur and the tibial condyles, separated by the intercondylar eminence. The patella is a small triangular sesamoid bone that sits in the quadriceps tendon anterior to the knee joint and provides protection to the knee joint during kneeling and glides over the distal femur during flexion and

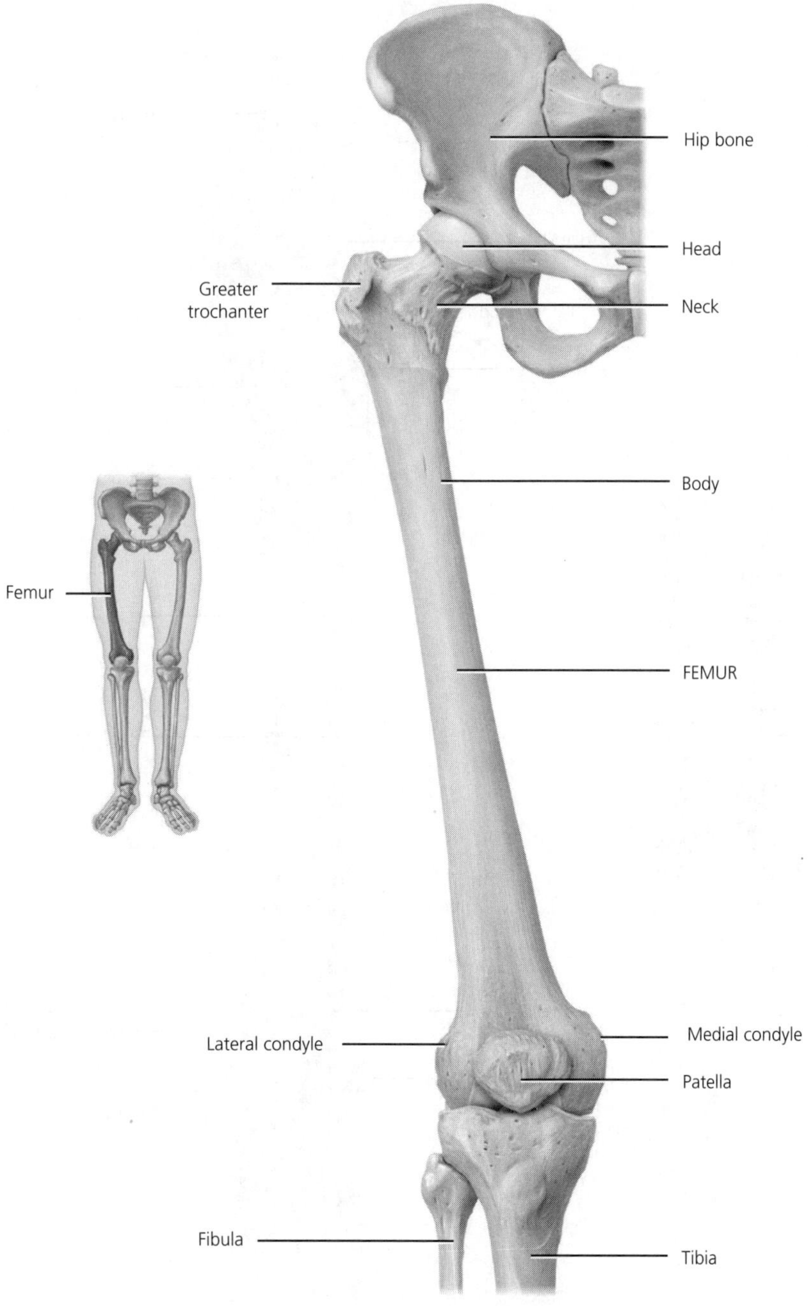

Figure 4.11 Lower limb – hip to knee. Tortora, G.J. and Derrickson, B.H. *Essentials of Anatomy and Physiology*. 2013, Wiley. This material is reproduced with permission of John Wiley & Sons, Inc.

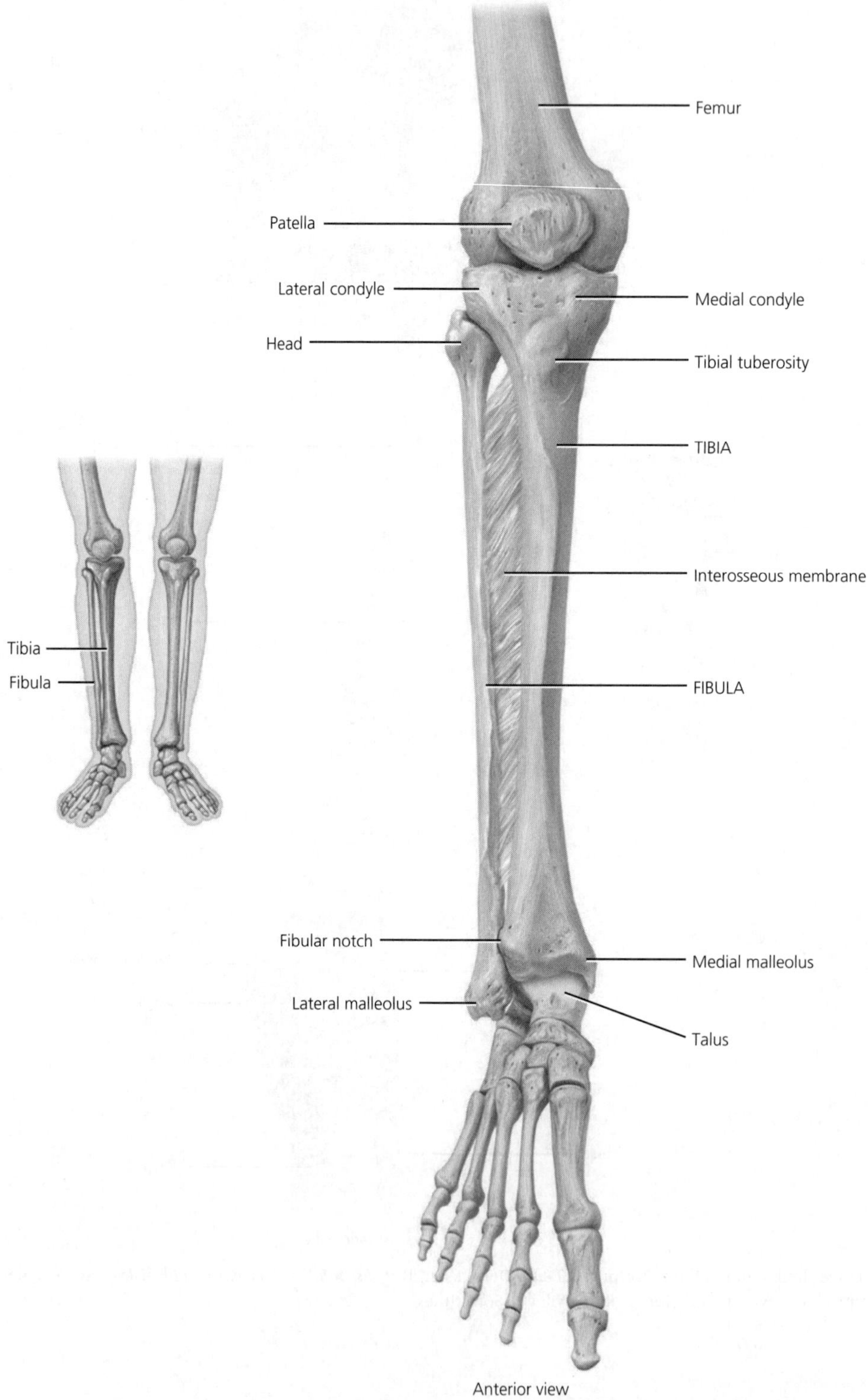

Figure 4.12 Lower limb – knee to foot. Tortora, G.J. and Derrickson, B.H. *Essentials of Anatomy and Physiology*. 2013, Wiley. This material is reproduced with permission of John Wiley & Sons, Inc.

extension of the knee forming the patellofemoral joint. Stability is provided by the ligaments, cartilages and tendons of the joint, particularly the cruciate ligaments in the centre of the knee, but these are vulnerable to injury under excessive rotational forces. Two cartilage shock absorbers, the menisci, sit on the medial and lateral tibial condyles. The medial and lateral collateral ligaments lie external to the joint capsule and attach the medial and lateral femoral condyles to the medial tibial condyle and the head of the fibula laterally to prevent rotation.

There are 28 bones in the foot and ankle allowing adaptation to various surfaces, providing balance, mobility and weight bearing stability and shock absorbency. The ankle joint is the articulation between the distal ends of the tibia and fibula and the talus bone. During walking the talus initially bears the entire weight of the body and half of that weight is then transferred to the calcaneus. The remaining weight is transmitted to the other tarsal bones – cuboid, navicular and three cuneiform bones. The talus and calcaneum are located at the posterior part of the foot and the rest of the tarsal bones are located anteriorly. The cuneiform bone and cuboid bone articulate with the metatarsals. There are five metatarsals each consisting of a proximal base, shaft and distal head. Distally the metatarsals articulate with the proximal row of phalanges which consist of a proximal base, middle shaft, and distal head. The hallux (big toe) has two large heavy phalanges while the other four toes each have three phalanges – proximal, middle and distal. The bones of the foot are arranged in two arches which enable the foot to support and distribute weight. The arches of the foot are maintained by the bones, ligaments and tendons of the foot; these are not rigid, but yield when weight is applied and spring back when the weight is released.

Tendons and ligaments are vital to the foot for flexibility and movement and the muscles of the foot work in partnership with those of the lower leg. There are many **nerves** within the foot which permit sensation, particularly feeling the surface when walking.

Conclusion

A fundamental guide to musculoskeletal anatomy and physiology has been provided in this chapter. It is recognised, however, that considerable further detailed knowledge is required to support expert and effective practice. This can be gained from attention to further reading. This should include a deeper review of muscle anatomy and physiology than it has been possible to include here.

Anatomy and physiology act as part of the diverse evidence base that underpins musculoskeletal care. Practitioners cannot understand what has gone wrong with a system and meet patients' needs if they do not know how it works when it is undamaged. To understand musculoskeletal diseases and disorders and the care and treatment associated with these health problems, the practitioner must have, as a priority, an in-depth working knowledge of the anatomy and physiology of the musculoskeletal system along with a general knowledge of other systems. Orthopaedic and trauma care covers the full span of life and most people will access some form of orthopaedic and trauma service in their lifetime A knowledge of anatomy and physiology is essential in facilitating prompt assessment and treatment as well as providing the tools for post-injury education of the patient.

Suggested further reading

Kuntzman, A.J. and Tortora, G.J. (2010) *Anatomy and Physiology for the Manual Therapies.* : John Wiley & Sons, Inc., New Jersey.

Palastanga, N. and Soames, R.W. (2012) *Anatomy and Human Movement: Structure and Function* 6th edn. Churchill Livingstone, Edinburgh.

References

Kuntzman, A.J. and Tortora, G.J. (2010) *Anatomy and Physiology for the Manual Therapies.* John Wiley & Sons, Inc., New Jersey.

Tortora, G.J. and Derrickson, B.H. (2013) *Essentials of Anatomy and Physiology.* John Wiley & Sons, Inc., New Jersey.

CHAPTER 5

The team approach and nursing roles in orthopaedic and musculoskeletal trauma care

Sandra Flynn[1] and Brian Lucas[2]

[1] *Countess of Chester Hospital, Chester, UK*

[2] *Queen Elizabeth Hospital, Kings Lynn, UK*

Introduction

The aim of this chapter is to introduce the notion of multi-disciplinary team working and the disciplines that make up the team within orthopaedic and trauma care. The term 'multi-disciplinary' is used to describe the collaborative work of the various health professional groups (Finn *et al.*, 2010) who are drawn together to use their knowledge and skills towards a common patient goal (Solheim *et al.*, 2007). The multi-disciplinary approach can facilitate positive outcomes, helping to ensure that the needs of the patient, family or carer are fully met. Healthcare professionals assume responsibility for promoting and restoring health, preventing illness and relieving suffering. Clinical expertise that is based on sound clinical knowledge, employing discretionary judgement, understanding illness and its trajectory and appreciating the varied human response to illness is central to professional healthcare practice. The ability to take care of patients well requires healthcare professionals who can project an open and warm presence that allows them to connect with each patient in a personalised way (Paulson 2004).

The team and importance of a multidisciplinary approach

The complexity of chronic conditions and the expanding development in medical care and treatment options available has led to the need for effective and efficient health care teams (Wiecha and Pollard 2004) and a multi-disciplinary approach to the provision of care and rehabilitation. The orthopaedic multi-disciplinary team comprises a group of individuals who are committed to a shared purpose in the best care of the patient with musculoskeletal conditions or injuries, shared performance goals, skills which overlap and complementary expertise. A common approach and focus on teamwork consists of several key dimensions relating to team coordination including effective communication, shared knowledge, problem solving and mutual respect (Gittell *et al.*, 2000). It is important for orthopaedic and trauma practitioners to understand and engage the varied roles of the multi-disciplinary team so that they complement each other and work together to deliver a high quality service and provision of care for a diverse patient population. In addition to promoting better outcomes for patients, research has demonstrated that multidisciplinary collaborative working affords opportunties to enhance skills and knowledge, provide informal education and promote a culture of respect and understanding amongst healthcare professionals (Tzenalis and Sotiriadou 2010).

The role of the multi-disciplinary team includes:

- assessment
- treatment/management of conditions
- education/advocacy
- referral/collaboration
- research and clinical audit.

Musculoskeletal pathways of care differ from patient to patient and the number of healthcare professionals involved in an individual pathway of care will vary

Orthopaedic and Trauma Nursing: An Evidence-based Approach to Musculoskeletal Care, First Edition. Edited by Sonya Clarke and Julie Santy-Tomlinson.

according to the complexity of their needs (Jester *et al.*, 2011). Care needs to be client-centred and a team approach helps to ensure services are delivered in partnership with the patient and their family/carer.

Team roles

Optimal management and care of patients with musculoskeletal conditions requires the expertise of specialists from different disciplines. Collectively the multi-disciplinary team provides a holistic, seamless service over the full continuum of care. The individual practitioners who have roles within the musculoskeletal multi-disciplinary team are discussed in the following section, but it is acknowledged that teams may vary according to sub-specialty and locality and that not all roles may be represented.

The nursing role in orthopaedic and trauma care

Nursing roles within the specialty of trauma and orthopaedics are diverse and found in a variety of settings within secondary care. Nursing areas of practice include, but are not limited to, adult and paediatric orthopaedic units, trauma units, outpatient departments, day surgery centres, operating theatres, accident and emergency departments and rehabilitation units. Nursing staff provide an important link within the team, working with the patient and other health care professionals to develop, plan, implement, coordinate and evaluate plans of care. Nursing roles include:

- Health Care Assistant/Assistant Practitioner
- Registered Nurse
- Ward/Unit/Department Manager
- Matron
- Pre-assessment Nurse
- Clinical Nurse Specialist
- Nurse Practitioner
- Trauma Co-ordinator
- Surgical Care Practitioner
- Consultant Nurse.

The notions of 'advanced' and 'specialist' practice/practitioner encompass a number of job tiles and roles within the specialty of trauma and orthopaedic nursing. Each role is multifaceted and exhibits contrasting quantities of clinical activity, education, management, leadership, collaboration and research, depending upon the individual job profile and client/service requirements. Advanced level nursing is concerned with a higher level of clinical practice, regardless of specialist area or role, which is beyond that of first level registration (DoH 2010) and is continually evolving while remaining firmly rooted in the provision of direct care or clinical work with patients, families and populations. The main activities of advanced roles lie within four domains:

- clinical
- leadership and collaborative practice
- practice development and quality improvement
- continuing professional development, education and training.

In 2000 the role of Nurse Consultant was established in the UK with the following aim (DoH 1999):

> (…help to provide better outcomes for patients by improving services and quality, to strengthen leadership and to provide a new career opportunity to help retain expert nurses…)

The nurse consultant provides highly specialised professional advice, consultancy, clinical expertise and leadership to patients, carers and colleagues in collaboration with medical, nursing and allied health professional colleagues. The nurse consultant develops and delivers highly specialised care using advanced skills and competencies. An essential component of the role in musculoskeletal care is to initiate research in the field of orthopaedic and trauma nursing to ensure evidence-based practice is embedded in all aspects of care and treatment. The role is structured around four core functions:

- expert clinical practice
- education, training and development
- professional leadership and consultancy
- practice and service development, research and evaluation.

In the *National Curriculum Framework for Surgical Care Practitioners* (DoH 2006) a surgical care practitioner is defined as:

> (A non-medical practitioner, working in clinical practice as a member of the extended surgical team, who performs surgical intervention, pre-operative and post-operative care under the direction and supervision of a consultant surgeon.)

The role of the Surgical Care Practitioner (SCP) is varied and the practitioner works under the supervision of a consultant surgeon or senior member of the surgical team. Responsibilities include:

- pre-operative assessment and physical examination
- assisting with preparation of patients for surgery
- assisting with surgical procedures in the operating theatre under the supervision and direction of the operating surgeon
- being first or second assistant at operations
- ordering of pre and post-operative investigations as part of the multi-professional team
- post-operative care e.g. wound assessment.

Patients requiring orthopaedic or trauma care need skilled nursing intervention throughout their pathway of care from initial diagnosis through to long-term follow-up. This may be provided by one practitioner across the entire pathway or through different nurses working in specific roles, such as in pre-operative assessment, ward care or post-operative and post-discharge review. Each has its own merits and drawbacks (Lucas 2002a). For clarity the pathway elements and the potential nursing roles within them will be described separately.

Elective Care

Diagnosis

Some orthopaedic nurse practitioners are involved in the initial diagnosis of an orthopaedic condition in primary or secondary care and in developing, with the patient, a treatment plan. This can include adding the patient's name to the waiting list for surgery if appropriate (Lucas 2006). To do this they require advanced assessment and decision making skills and a good working relationship with orthopaedic surgeons (Judd 2005, Lucas 2006).

Preparation of patients for surgery

Patients waiting for surgery have complex needs and a multifactorial assessment/education, taking into account physical and psychosocial needs, should be undertaken (Lucas *et al.*, 2013). With shorter waiting times for surgery, due to initiatives that reduce the pathway from initial consultation to definitive treatment, it is important that patients are well prepared for surgery. Within joint replacement/arthroplasty services there has been the development of information classes which support this education. The nursing role within this may include education about the procedure, hospital stay and post-operative recovery, as well as the collecting of patient assessment data such as Patient Reported Outcome Measures (PROMs). In order to maximize the learning experience for patients, nurses who lead such classes need knowledge of educational principles (Hartley *et al.*, 2012). Orthopaedic nurses may also carry out the pre-operative assessment of patients to ensure they are fit for anaesthesia and surgery, although this may also be seen as the role of an anaesthetic nurse practitioner. Box 5.1 examines the evidence base for nurse-led preoperative assessment. For some day case surgery the nurse practitioner may carry out a procedure such as carpal tunnel release following appropriate education and training (Newey *et al.*, 2006).

Inpatient stay

The nursing role within the inpatient stay spans from the fundamental care from a nurse on an orthopaedic ward, to the nurse practitioner whose role encompasses many aspects of traditional junior doctor roles such as prescribing and discharging patients. All of these require suitable skills and competencies (see Chapter 3). Nurses are also central to the implementation of enhanced recovery programmes, with criteria-based discharge by nurses and an emphasis on 'normality' with drips/drains removed as soon as possible (Wainwright and Middleton 2010) (see Chapter 14).

Post-hospital care

After discharge following elective orthopaedic surgery patients may have information needs, and nurses can provide telephone advice (Hodgins *et al.*, 2008). Early supported discharge schemes with nursing involvement have proved to be cost-effective and popular with patients (Hill *et al.*, 2000). A Cochrane Review concluded that there is high patient satisfaction with such schemes although the evidence is inconclusive on cost savings and readmission rates (Shepperd *et al.*, 2009). Nurse practitioners may review patients in the outpatient setting for physical care such as wound dressings/suture removal or to monitor recovery from surgery. Such follow-up may be short-term, with patients being discharged after 4–6 weeks or, in the case of joint replacement, for long periods or, even, life (Flynn 2005).

Box 5.1 Evidence Digest: Nurse-led preoperative assessment (Craig 2005)

This review by Craig (2005) was led by the question: "Does nurse-led pre-operative assessment reduce the cancellation rate of elective surgical in-patient procedures: a systematic review of the research literature". The review assessed whether pre-assessment by a nurse reduces the number of elective surgical operations that are cancelled on the day of surgery. The evidence was weak and it was uncertain that pre-assessment reduced cancellations.

RCTs, prospective and retrospective cohort studies of nurse-led POA carried out prior to hospital admission were included. Some patients in one study were seen following their out-patient appointment. In two studies the nurses' decisions on all assessed patients were checked by a doctor; in one study only assessments judged by the nurse to be of concern were checked by a doctor; and in one study the independence of the nurses' decisions was unclear. The types of surgery in the included studies were total hip or knee replacement, urology and general surgical procedures. Studies that reported surgical cancellation rates were eligible for inclusion. The review reported on cancellation rates on admission for surgery or on the day of surgery.

Review criteria included the clarity of the study question, prospective or retrospective design, similarity between exposed and control groups, follow-up and the measure and size of effect. Sample size calculation was also recorded. The author did not state how the validity assessment was performed. Four cohort studies were included. The total number of participants was 3,667. One study was retrospective; it was unclear whether the other three studies were prospective or retrospective regarding data collection. In one study there were no cancellations for reasons that could have been foreseen at POA among 59 patients assessed by a nurse specialist or among the control group of 52 patients seen by a doctor. In the largest study, eight (0.4%) of 2,762 patients were cancelled on admission for reasons that could have been resolved at the POA. The comparative rate of cancellation for the Health Trust was 10.9%. However, it was uncertain that nurse-led POA was solely responsible for the lower rate of cancellations in the study population, owing to other differences between the ward investigated and the rest of the Trust. In another study there were eight cancellations out of 314 patients who had attended the POA clinic over a period of two years, compared with 12 out of 162 in the control year before the POA clinic was established. Cancellation due to POA failure could not be ascertained with certainty because the reasons for cancellation were not specified. The fourth study reported two cancellations (1.1%) for preventable reasons out of 179 patients who underwent POA, compared with 10 (5.9%) of 175 patients in the control group ($p<0.05$). This corresponded to a 46% absolute reduction in the risk of cancellation (number-needed-to-treat 22).The authors concluded that it was uncertain that POA reduced the rate of adult elective surgery cancellations.

Centre for Reviews and Dissemination commentary

"The review addressed a clear question. However, the search could have missed relevant studies not indexed on the databases searched. Furthermore, possible publication bias, which the author acknowledged, could mean that studies with favourable results were more likely to be included. The derivation of the search strategy was reported in sufficient detail to allow an independent assessment of its sensitivity to identify relevant studies, including international literature (should readers query why studies conducted outside the UK and studies published in languages other than English were not identified). The review appeared to have been conducted by a single author and no methods to minimise reviewer bias or errors in the study selection, data extraction or validity assessment processes were reported. Appropriate aspects of study quality were assessed systematically. The description of the individual study characteristics was thorough. The narrative synthesis was appropriate and study quality was taken into account in the interpretation of the findings. On the basis of the evidence reviewed, the author's conclusion is appropriate."

Trauma care

The orthopaedic and trauma nursing role in trauma care varies depending on the severity of injury and the nature of the treatment required.

Minor orthopaedic trauma not requiring admission

For patients with injuries such as a Colles fracture, care is usually entirely within the outpatient setting. The role of the orthopaedic trauma nurse is multifaceted. In some clinics nurse practitioners are involved in diagnosing the injury, requesting and interpreting X-rays and undertaking the appropriate treatment such as cast application (Wardman 2002). They may also review patients after initial treatment and discharge them to primary care. Fragility Fracture Nurses may ensure that those with fragility fractures are referred to osteoporosis screening services if appropriate or run a fragility fracture service (Clunie and Stephenson 2008) (see Chapter 18).

Major orthopaedic trauma requiring inpatient admission

Nurse practitioners within trauma services fast-track patients from the emergency department (ED) to an inpatient trauma unit, particularly patients such as those with a hip fracture. Such practitioners can often prescribe intravenous fluids and order and interpret X-rays. Trauma Coordinator roles have also developed in many units and involve ensuring the patient undergoes appropriate timely admission procedures, is prepared for surgery and that patient transfer to and from surgery is well coordinated. Some also assist during surgery or help in pain control through such initiatives as femoral nerve block (Randall *et al.*, 2008). Post-operatively the nursing role encompasses the acute recovery of patients and may also include nurse practitioner roles such as nurse initiated discharge (Webster *et al.*, 2011). After discharge the nurse in the trauma pathway may have a similar role to that described in the elective pathway; a point of contact/advice for patients and involvement in the post-operative follow-up of patients. This may include specialist roles with specific groups of patients requiring long-term follow-up such as those with external fixators which includes care of the device as well as psychological care of the patients through self-management and nurse-led support groups (Dheensa and Thomas 2012). Box 5.2 examines the value of multidisciplinary rehabilitation programmes.

Box 5.2 Evidence Digest Cochrane Review: Multidisciplinary rehabilitation programmes following joint replacement at the hip and knee in chronic arthropathy (Khan *et al.*, 2009). Reproduced with permission from The Cochrane Collaboration

Khan *et al.* (2009) assessed the effectiveness of multidisciplinary rehabilitation programmes on activity and participation following joint replacement surgery in adults. The evidence revealed that the included trials were of low quality and long-term effects of early rehabilitation were not investigated.

Review questions

- Does organised multidisciplinary rehabilitation achieve better outcomes than the absence of such services following hip or knee joint replacement?
- Which programme models are effective and in which setting?
- Which participants benefit most?
- Which specific outcomes are influenced?
- Does the intensity of multidisciplinary rehabilitation lead to greater gain?
- Are cost benefits demonstrable?

RCTs were included if they applied multidisciplinary rehabilitation following hip/knee joint replacement surgery and compared a given intervention with a controlled condition. Quality appraisal of individual studies was performed using the three Jadad *et al.* (1996) criteria: randomisation, double blinding and description of withdrawals. An additional criterion was employed to give an overall assessment of quality as recommended by the Cochrane Collaboration (Higgins 2006). Best evidence synthesis was performed using qualitative analysis.

Five trials were included, participants totaled 619. Two studies involved in-patient rehabilitation and three home-based settings. Pooling of data was impractical due to study design variance and types of outcomes employed. The authors reported that for inpatient settings early implementation of clinical and rehabilitation pathways helped accomplish functional milestones, reduced length of stay, lowered post-operative complications and reduced cost within the first four months. Home-based multidisciplinary care enhanced functional ability and quality of life.

Author's conclusions

Some evidence to suggest that early multidisciplinary rehabilitation improves activity level and patient participation. Little consideration is given to optimal intensity, frequency and effects of rehabilitation programmes and associated social costs over time. The methodological and scientific rigor of clinical trials in this field requires improvement.

Centre for Reviews and Dissemination commentary

The diverse nature of trials in this review presented a challenge with the assimilation of available evidence. The authors acknowledge possibility of:

- selection bias from the literature search
- publication bias
- reference bias in respect of the included published studies.

The authors acknowledge adopting a low inclusion threshold for studies but argue the approach was necessary to ensure that best evidence was presented and to acknowledge the limited evidence resulting from these 'poorer' studies.

Medical roles in orthopaedic and trauma care

Orthopaedic Surgeons and supporting medical staff are concerned with all aspects of heath care relating to the patient requiring elective orthopaedic and orthopaedic trauma care be it conservative or surgical. Medical, physical and rehabilitative methods as well as surgery are employed in order to provide the most appropriate treatment. Surgery may be indicated when it is the best option for restoring function following injury or disease of bones, joint and related soft tissues. Medical staff work closely with the multi-disciplinary team, playing an important role in diagnosis and decision making and in prescribing and delivering musculoskeletal treatment and care.

Allied Health Professional roles

Allied Health Professionals are other clinical staff uniquely placed to provide a wide range of specific services that include diagnostic, therapeutic and direct patient care. They work closely with other health care professionals to ensure an integrated and coordinated service to patients and service users (DoH 2010). Within the specialty of orthopaedics and musculoskeletal trauma in many countries, allied healthcare professionals include:

- Physiotherapists
- Occupational Therapists
- Diagnostic Radiologists
- Orthotists
- Prosthetists
- Dieticians.

Physiotherapists in musculoskeletal care are concerned with identifying, maximising and maintaining movement and the functional ability and potential of the patient by focusing on health promotion, disease or injury prevention as well as treatment and rehabilitation (Atkinson *et al.*, 2005). The role of the physiotherapist has evolved considerably in recent years along with a range of skills in assessment, diagnosis and management. The emergence of the role of the extended scope physiotherapist (ESP) has enabled the treatment of patients where appropriate with many ESPs qualified to request radiological and pathological investigations, interpret results, prescribe medications and refer to other services (Lowe and Prior 2008).

Occupational therapy plays a fundamental role in recovery and rehabilitation, working with the orthopaedic multi-disciplinary team to meet treatment goals. The role of the occupational therapist (OT) in musculoskeletal care is to perform a thorough assessment that facilitates an individual's discharge aiming to assist the patient to live and work as independently as possible (Mooney and Ireson 2009). Physical strength and stamina, proper movement and ability can be affected following musculoskeletal disease or injury and subsequent treatment and OTs work with individuals to promote maximum functional ability so that activities of daily living can be maintained. The occupational therapist will obtain information about the patient's lifestyle abilities prior to injury, illness or surgery to develop a plan of care which will assist the patient in adjusting to their current physical condition. There may be a need for the individual to learn new skills or adapt the way in which they live and/or work to address disability such as where joint and limb function has been impaired. This is achieved by assisting patients to overcome and manage limitations resulting from their conditions.

Musculoskeletal radiology is concerned with the diagnostic imaging and diagnosis of the skeleton and associated soft tissue. Imaging includes X-rays, computed tomography (CT), ultrasound and MRI. Radiologists are health care professionals who are experts in obtaining and interpreting medical images. They work with other clinicians by reporting findings of examinations and tests and confer with referring medical staff to recommend further examinations or treatments.

Orthotics and prosthetics are applied physical disciplines that use assessment, diagnosis and management of the body as a whole to address neuromuscular and structural skeletal problems by providing orthotic appliances and prostheses including artificial limbs. The orthotist and prosthetist liaise directly with members of the multi-disciplinary orthopaedic team to achieve maximum function, prevent further disability and facilitate improved body image and play an important role in advising on the rehabilitation of patients with physical challenges and disabilities (Lusardi *et al.*, 2012). Orthoses, usually a brace, splint or special footwear, are designed to provide one or more of the following:

- relieve pressure on a diseased joint or stress in a bone weakened by disease or injury
- correct or prevent physical deformity
- stabilise a joint or several joints

- improve mobility
- protect the joint from further injury.

An orthotic prescription is formulated by a member of the multi-disciplinary team and the orthotist will assess the patient's needs, take measurements, design and then fit and adjust the orthosis. This can be an ongoing process for many patients but more so for children and young people due to their growing and changing immature skeletal frame. An essential part of the role is to educate the individual and/or carer in the fitting and using of the device.

The prosthetist provides artificial replacements for individuals who have lost or were born without all or part of a limb and may face disability. The prosthetist will design and select the most suitable prosthesis from a range of components with the aim of enabling the individual to lead a normal life.

Dietitians are clinicians who apply expert knowledge of nutrition to support individuals in understanding and applying the principles of healthy eating and maximising nutrition throughout their lifespan. They assess patients' nutritional needs, developing and implementing nutrition programs thus contributing to health promotion and illness prevention strategies (Webster-Gandy *et al.*, 2011).

Additional supporting team members

Additional members of the health care team that are central to patient care include

- Pharmacists – health care professionals who are experts in medicines and how they work and are concerned with the safe and effective use of medication. Their role encompasses an understanding of the biochemical mechanisms of action of drugs, the way medicines are selected and supplied, therapeutic roles, side effects, potential drug interactions and monitoring. Pharmacists are directly involved in patient care and use their expertise to work collaboratively within the team. The overall aim is to ensure patient safety and improve the quality of all medicine related practices (Price 2012).
- Operating Department Practitioners (ODPs) – an integral part of the operating department multi-professional team, helping to ensure effective and safe peri-operative care. This incorporates the anaesthetic, surgical and recovery stages of the patient pathway in orthopaedic and trauma care (see Chapter 14).
- Social worker – collaborates with the multi-disciplinary team on discharge planning to ensure that patients' needs are met in order that they may be discharged from hospital in a safe and timely fashion. They connect patients and families to appropriate resources and support in the community (Beder 2006).
- Clinical psychologist – assists in the assessment of the mental health needs of the patient. They form part of the healthcare team where patients require assistance through periods of emotional adjustment, information and where there is a need to establish health-inducing behaviour (Beinart *et al.*, 2009).
- Multi-faith workers – the provision of spiritual care is an important consideration and a multi-disciplinary responsibility. Spiritual care encompasses emotional, psychological, social and pastoral support, together with a requirement to meet the religious needs of the patient.

Nurse-led services

The nursing roles described earlier can be part of a traditional consultant-led service or there may be an identified need for a nurse-led service. For example, a nurse-led service for patients requiring joint replacement may have a nurse practitioner assessing referrals from general practitioners, providing pre-operative education, reviewing the patient as an inpatient and providing post-discharge follow-up (Lucas 2002a). Before such services can be established, the case for them has to be made. One method of ensuring that all issues are identified is the ESSENCE model, devised through discussion with extended scope practitioners within the Royal College of Nursing's Society of Orthopaedic and Trauma Nursing in the UK (see Figure 5.1).

Establish the need/case

A first step is to understand and identify what the drivers for the new service are and what benefits it might bring. These can be local, such as the length of time patients are waiting for a particular service (Judd 2009, Murray 2011) or national initiatives/guidance such as the Best Practice Tariff for hip fractures (see Chapter 18). Those who may benefit are patients (reduced waiting times), commissioners of care (more cost-effective care for larger numbers of patients), nursing itself (the opportunity to develop new skills and

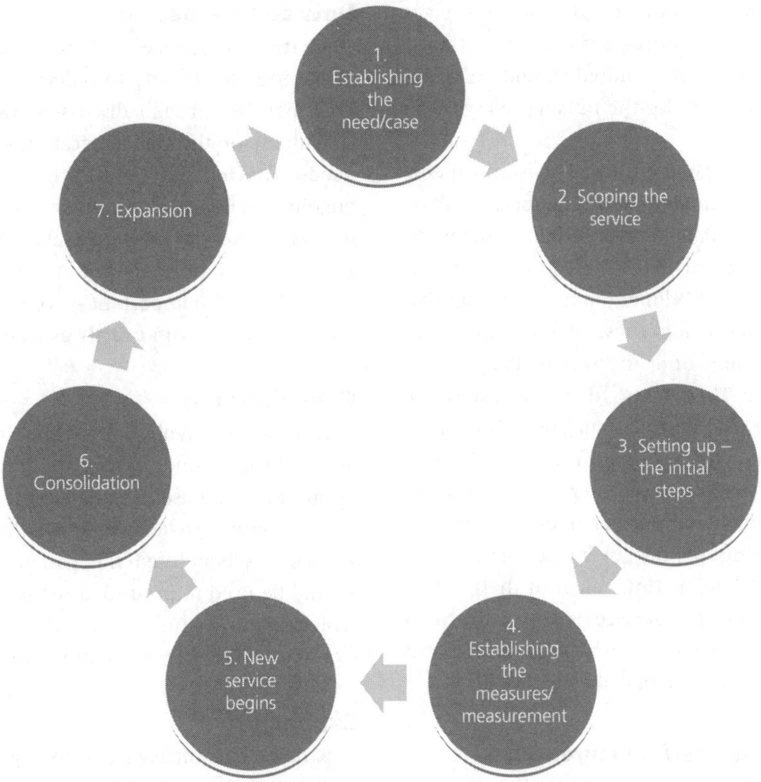

Figure 5.1 The essence model of nurse-led services

knowledge) and the hospital/health care organisation (increased revenue and patient satisfaction). Local champions for change and potential barriers should be considered. This can be through process mapping the current patient journey to identify issues and problems. A written business case can then be devised, which establishes why the nurse-led service is required and what benefits it will bring.

Scoping the service

It should be clear what patient group or groups will be included in the nurse-led service, how they will be referred to the service and how the service links with other existing services. It is advisable to begin with well-defined conditions or patient groups such as simple fractures or post-operative care (Wardman 2002, Judd 2009). Scoping should also include determining whether there is an existing service within your organisation which has similar attributes (nurse-led, protocol driven) and from which learning can take place. External scoping can identify whether a similar service is already functioning elsewhere and this can be found from the literature, conference presentations or professional organisations.

Setting up – the initial steps

Once the case has been accepted for the nurse-led clinic or service, the planning of how it will work in practice can begin in earnest. It will take time to set up well, especially if the development is taking place alongside existing workloads (Lucas 2002b). The service will need to have clear governance arrangements with protocols and procedures setting out the scope of nursing practice (Judd 2009). Issues such as how patients will access the service might be difficult to resolve due to contracting arrangements (Clunie and Stephenson 2008). The nurse should have control over the length of appointments and the numbers booked onto clinics, so that this does not become unmanageable. The education and training required to carry out the roles within the services should also be established and included in the protocols for the clinics or service (Murray 2011). Such training/

education may be provided by external providers such as universities or in-house by orthopaedic surgeons (Lucas 2006, Judd 2009). The skills required should be recognised in the job description for the nursing roles within the service.

The establishment of good governance arrangements will also mean that the nurses within the service will be covered by vicarious liability from their employers. There are many practical issues to consider such as facilities (office space, a clinic room, administrative support, clinical support) and these may be difficult to obtain in the beginning until the service has 'proved itself' (Judd 2009). The ability to access diagnostic services may be crucial, such as magnetic resonance imaging for patients with back pain (Murray 2011). A risk analysis of the proposed service should be undertaken to identify and answer questions such as what happens during periods of nurse planned or unplanned leave (sickness). Time taken in these initial steps will ensure that the service is more likely to succeed, but some questions cannot be identified and answered until the service actually begins.

Establishing measures/measurements

The rationale for the service outlined in the 'establish the need/case' stage indicates what needs to be measured. Considering what data are already being collected that may help establish the value of the new service, such as length of stay or readmission rates, is advisable. Other potential measures could be the safety of the nurse practitioner in carrying out an extended role (Murray 2011), admission avoidance (telephone follow-up), patient outcomes such as pain reduction, number of patients seen, mortality, financial savings and patient satisfaction (Judd 2009, Murray 2011). These measures might be collected over time, as reports on services often have short follow-up only (Flynn and Whitehead 2006) and need to be measures that stakeholders in the service value – for example commissioners may want to see financial savings, such as less GP consultations and less prescribed analgesia (Murray 2011). Once the measures have been identified the use of audit should be considered in the design of measurement tools. If national databases are available for inputting data then it is advisable to use these (Clunie and Stephenson 2008). Good evidence is crucial if the case for continuation or further development of the nurse-led service is to be made.

New service begins

Once the new service or clinic begins it is important to create the opportunity to reflect on how it is working. This may be through discussion with an orthopaedic consultant or through clinical supervision. The nurse needs sufficient support during the early days and ongoing feedback about their own performance and that of the service. It is advisable to start small with a small number of patients until clinical skills develop. Flexibility is also important – even well planned clinics/services may not run exactly as planned (Judd 2009).

Consolidation

Consolidation involves knowing how the service is doing through undertaking the audit already decided upon. It may be useful to repeat the process map of the patient journey to determine whether the implemented service has benefitted the patients. This information should be used to produce a report on the early results which should be presented within the organisation, for example to the Management Board.

Expansion

Expansion encompasses developing nursing knowledge and the service itself. The nurse-led service should be celebrated and publicised within the organisation, externally at conferences and by publication, and visits from others should be encouraged. In these ways the service will become well-known and others can learn from its successes and challenges. Expansion of the service itself may also be considered, this may be expanding the range of patients seen (Wardman 2002) and/or the number of nurses involved in the service (Murray 2011). Such expansion requires returning to the 'establishing the need' stage of the ESSENCE model.

Conclusion

There are a variety of multi-faceted roles within orthopaedic and trauma care that complement the role of the nurse in providing effective, coordinated care for the patient. Each practitioner has a set of complementary skills and their roles are equally important but may be required in different parts of the patient journey. The last few decades have seen significant developments in the flexibility and extension of roles which has aimed to more effectively meet patient and service needs. The evidence base for these roles is currently in its infancy.

Recommended further reading

Cox, C., Hill, M. and Lack, V. (eds) (2011) *Advanced Practice in Healthcare: Skills for Nurses and Allied Health Professionals*. Routledge, London.

McGee, P. (Ed.) (2009) *Advanced Practice in Nursing and the Allied Health Professions*, 3rd edn. Wiley Blackwell, Oxford.

Wainwright, T. and Middleton, R. (2010) An orthopaedic enhanced recovery pathway. *Current Anaesthesia and Critical Care*, **21**(3), 114–120.

References

Atkinson, K., Coutts, F.J. and Hassenkamp, A. (2005) *Physiotherapy in Orthopaedics: A Problem-Solving Approach*. Churchill Livingstone, London.

Beinart, H., Kennedy, P. and Llewelyn, S. (2009) *Clinical Psychology in Practice*. Blackwell, Oxford.

Beder, J. (2006). *Hospital Social Work: The Interface of Medicine and Caring*. Routledge, New York.

Clunie, G. and Stephenson, S. (2008) Implementing and running a fracture liaison service: An integrated clinical service providing a comprehensive bone health assessment at the point of fracture management. *Journal of Orthopaedic Nursing*, **12**(3–4), 159–165.

Craig, S.E. (2005) Does nurse-led pre-operative assessment reduce the cancellation rate of elective surgical in-patient procedures: a systematic review of the research literature (structured abstract). *Cochrane Database of Abstracts of Reviews of Effects 2012* Issue 3. Available at: http://onlinelibrary.wiley.com/o/cochrane/cldare/articles/DARE-12006005095/frame.html Centre for Reviews and Dissemination (accessed 1 September 2012).

Department of Health (DoH) (1999) *Nurse, Midwife and Health Visitor Consultants. Establishing posts and Making Appointments*. Health Service Circular. DoH, London.

Department of Health (DoH) (2006) *The National Curriculum Framework for Surgical Care Practitioners*. DoH, London.

Department of Health (DoH) (2010) *Advanced Level Nursing: A Position Statement*. DoH, London.

Dheensa, S. and Thomas, S. (2012) Investigating the relationship between coping, quality of life and depression/anxiety in patients with external fixation devices. *International Journal of Orthopaedic and Trauma Nursing*, **16**(1), 30–38.

Finn, R., Learmonth, M. and Reedy, P. (2010) Some unintended effects of teamwork in healthcare. *Social Science and Medicine*, **70**(8), 1148–1154.

Flynn, S. (2005) Nursing effectiveness: An evaluation of patient satisfaction with a nurse-led orthopaedic joint replacement review clinic. *Journal of Orthopaedic Nursing*, **9**(3), 156–165.

Flynn, S.D. and Whitehead, E. (2006) An exploration of issues related to nurse-led clinics. *Journal of Orthopaedic Nursing*, **10**(2), 86–94.

Gittell, J.H., Fairfield, K.M., Bierbaum, B., Head, W. and Jackson R. (2000) Impact of relational co-ordination on quality of care, post-operative pain and functioning and length of stay: a nine hospital study of surgical patients. *Medical Care*, **38**(8), 807–819.

Hartley, M., Neubrander, J. and Repede, E. (2012) Evidence-based spine preoperative education. *International Journal of Orthopaedic and Trauma Nursing*, **16**(2), 65–75.

Higgins, J.P.T. and Green, S. (eds) (2006) Assessment of Study Quality. *Cochrane Handbook for Systematic Reviews of Interventions 4.2.6*. The Cochrane Library, Issue 4, 2006. John Wiley & Sons, Ltd., Chichester.

Hill, S.P., Flynn, J. and Crawford, E.J.P. (2000) Early discharge following total knee replacement – a trial of patient satisfaction and outcomes using an orthopaedic outreach team. *Journal of Orthopaedic Nursing*, **4**(3), 121–126.

Hodgins, M.J., Ouellet, L.L., Pond, S., Knorr, S. and Geldart, G. (2008) Effect of telephone follow-up on surgical orthopedic recovery. *Applied Nursing Research*, **21**(4), 218–226.

Jadad, A.R., Moore, R.A., Carroll, D. *et al.* (1996) Assessing the quality of reports of randomized clinical trials: Is blinding necessary? *Control Clinical Trials*, **17**(1), 1–12.

Jester, R., Santy, J. and Rogers, J. (2011) *Oxford Handbook of Orthopaedic and Trauma Nursing*. Oxford University Press, Oxford.

Judd, J. (2005) Strategies used by nurses for decision-making in the paediatric orthopaedic setting. *Journal of Orthopaedic Nursing*, **9**(3), 166–171.

Khan, F., Ng, L., Gonzalez, S. and Turner-Stokes, L. (2009) *Multidisciplinary Rehabilitation Programmes Following Joint Replacement at the Hip and Knee in Chronic Arthropathy (Review) 48*. The Cochrane Collaboration: John Wiley and Sons, Ltd., Chichester.

Lowe, J. and Prior, M. (2008) *A Systematic Review of the Literature on Rxtended Scope of Practice Physiotherapy: Physiotherapy Extended Scope of Practice Project*. ACT Government Health Directorate: ACT Government; 2008. Available at: http://www.health.act.gov.au/c/health?a=sendfile&ft=p&fid=1378078168&sid= (accessed 22 April 2014).

Lucas, B. (2002a) Orthopaedic patient journeys: a UK perspective. *Journal of Orthopaedic Nursing*, **6**(2), 86–89.

Lucas, B. (2002b) Developing the role of the nurse in the orthopaedic outpatient and pre-admission assessment settings: a change management project. *Journal of Orthopaedic Nursing*, **6**(3), 153–160.

Lucas, B. (2006) Judgement and decision making in orthopaedic nursing practice related to chronic knee pain. *Journal of Orthopaedic Nursing*, **10**(4), 206–216.

Lucas, B., Cox, C., Perry, L. and Bridges, J. (2013) Pre-operative preparation of patients for total knee replacement: an action research study. *International Journal of Orthopaedic and Trauma Nursing*, **17**(2), 79–90.

Lusardi, M.M., Jorge, M. and Nielsen, C.C. (2012) *Orthotics and Prosthetics in Rehabilitation*, 3rd edn. Elsevier Saunders, St Louis.

Mooney, M. and Ireson, C. (2009) *Occupational Therapy in Orthopaedics and Trauma*. John Wiley & Sons, Ltd., Chichester.

Murray, M.M. (2011) Reflections on the development of nurse-led back pain triage clinics in the UK. *International Journal of Orthopaedic and Trauma Nursing*, **15**(3), 113–120.

Newey, M., Clarke, M., Green, T., Kershaw, C. and Pathak, P. (2006) Nurse-led management of carpal tunnel syndrome: an audit of outcomes and impact on waiting times. *Annals of the Royal College of Surgeons of England*, **88**(4), 399–401.

Paulson, D.S. (2004) Taking care of patients and caring are not the same. *Association of periOperative Registered Nurses Journal*, **79**(2), 359–360.

Price, R. (2012) Forming a strategy for hospital pharmacy success. *European Journal of Hospital Pharmacy*, **19**(1), 5–6.

Randall, A., Grigg, L., Obideyi, A. and Srikantharajah, I. (2008) Fascia Iliaca compartment block: A nurse-led initiative for preoperative pain management in patients with a fractured neck of femur. *Journal of Orthopaedic Nursing*, **12**(2), 69–74.

Shepperd, S., Doll, H., Broad, J., Gladman, J. *et al.* (2009) Hospital at home early discharge. *Cochrane Database of Systematic Reviews* 1 (Art. No.: CD000356). DOI: 10.1002/14651858.CD000356.pub3.

Solheim, K., McElmurray, B. and Kim, M. (2007) Multidisciplinary teamwork in US primary health care. *Social Science and Medicine*, **65**(3), 622–634.

Tzenalis, A. and Sotiriadou, C. (2010) Health promotion as multi-professional and multi-disciplinary work. *International Journal of Caring Sciences*, **3**(2), 49–55.

Wainwright, T. and Middleton, R. (2010) An orthopaedic enhanced recovery pathway. *Current Anaesthesia and Critical Care*, **21**(3), 114–120.

Wardman, C. (2002) Nurse-led fracture review clinic: an innovation in practice. *Journal of Orthopaedic Nursing*, **6**(2), 90– 94.

Webster, J., Connolly, A., Paton, F. and Corry, J. (2011) The effectiveness of protocol drive, nurse-initiated discharge in a 23-h post-surgical ward: A randomized controlled trial. *International Journal of Nursing Studies*, **48**(10), 1173–1179.

Webster-Gandy, J., Madden, A. and Holdsworth, M. (2011) *Oxford Handbook of Nutrition and Dietetics*, Oxford Medical Handbooks, 2nd edn. Oxford University Press, Oxford.

Wiecha, J. and Pollard, T. (2004) The interdisciplinary eHealth Team: chronic care for the future. *Journal of Medical Internet Research*, **6**(3), 22.

CHAPTER 6

Rehabilitation and the orthopaedic and musculoskeletal trauma patient

Rebecca Jester

London South Bank University, London, UK; Dudley Group NHS Foundation Trust, Dudley, West Midlands, UK

Introduction

The aim of this chapter is to provide an evidence-based discussion of rehabilitation of the orthopaedic and trauma patient. There are many who require and will benefit from rehabilitation and some specific examples will be provided within this chapter and within other condition-specific chapters. Where robust evidence exists there will be a critical application of research to approaches to rehabilitation. However, to date there is limited high level evidence to support many aspects of patient rehabilitation within trauma and orthopaedics. There are two relevant Cochrane systematic reviews relating to rehabilitation; Cameron *et al.'s* (2009) review included nine studies comparing coordinated multidisciplinary approaches to rehabilitation of older patients with proximal femoral fractures to usual orthopaedic care (this review is discussed in more detail within the team approaches to rehabilitation section) and Mason *et al.'s* (2012) review which included two trials related to rehabilitation following hamstring injuries. In addition, a search revealed seven studies comparing rehabilitation settings (which are critically discussed within the rehabilitation settings section). The information within this chapter is, therefore, in the main based upon evidence from the following sources: formal education, symposia, conference presentations, non-research publications, expert opinion and reflections on clinical experience (of the author and other clinical experts).

History and context of rehabilitation

Rehabilitation is a process which aims to optimise a patient's full recovery potential following an episode of illness, trauma or surgery. Mauk (2012) offers the following definition:

> (Rehabilitation is a process of adaptation or recovery through which an individual suffering from a disabling or functionally limiting condition, whether temporary or irreversible, participates to regain maximal function, independence and restoration.) (p2).

There are two key misconceptions about rehabilitation to be cognisant of. Firstly, rehabilitation is not a place; it is a process. Hence, to state "the patient is waiting to go to rehabilitation" is a misnomer and furthermore is detrimental to the patient as the rehabilitation process should begin as soon as the patient is medically stable. Secondly, there is frequently a misconception that rehabilitation is about restoring the individual to their pre-injury/surgery status. This is not always possible and a significant aspect of rehabilitation is to support the patient and their family to adapt to a change in their functional ability. Rehabilitation has a number of key goals including:

- restoration of optimum function (physical, social and psychological)
- promote and sustain maximum independence and provide assistance where care deficits exist
- facilitation of adaptation when return to former health status or function is not possible

Orthopaedic and Trauma Nursing: An Evidence-based Approach to Musculoskeletal Care, First Edition. Edited by Sonya Clarke and Julie Santy-Tomlinson.

- psychological support for the patient and their family who have experienced trauma, change or loss (in the context of loss of the former self)
- prevention and early detection of complications
- supporting the patient to meet their short-, medium- and long-term goals
- creating enabling environments to facilitate independence and social integration
- education of the patient and informal carers to understand their condition and ongoing treatment and management strategies
- promote self-management and patient empowerment
- optimising health and quality of life (including pain management).

The concept of rehabilitation in healthcare is not a new phenomenon. The importance of restoring function following trauma in particular has been evident over many centuries, particularly during war and conflict. Florence Nightingale pioneered rehabilitation as a nursing concept during the Crimean War. Many developments in prosthetics, assistive devices, mobility aids, new treatments and therapies have been as a direct result of the need to support those wounded in conflict either as service men and women or civilian causalities and to facilitate, when possible, military personnel's return to active duty. Sadly, in contemporary society, the world continues to be plagued by conflict, war and terrorism and the need for evidence-based rehabilitation has never been greater.

Models of care

Many of those requiring rehabilitation will have either a permanent or temporary disability. In recent years there has been a realisation and acknowledgement that disabled people are not the problem, the problem is the way that society is organised to discriminate against those individuals with a disability (Jester 2007). In the UK (and reflected in the law in other parts of the world), the Disability Discrimination Act of 1995 has supported the view that it is a societal responsibility to prohibit less favourable treatment of people with a disability. The Act gave new rights in relation to access to goods, services and facilities, employment and buying or renting land or property and has supported the social model of disability where the onus is on society to make adjustments and support those with a disability. Crosby and Jackson (2000) summarised what disabled people have identified as their fundamental needs in order to be able to live independently:

- information about choices
- peer support and counselling
- appropriate housing, which you can get into, move about in, live in and is in the right place
- equipment to support you to do the things you want to do
- personal assistance to facilitate independence
- accessible transport
- access to the built environment.

Healthcare practitioners have a key responsibility to provide information about enabling environments, patient's rights under the Disability Discrimination Act and to signpost patients and their families to further information and services to optimise their independence. Apart from the social model of disability, practitioners need to have an applied working knowledge of frameworks and models that embrace maximising patient independence, promote a focus on health and wellbeing and support patients and families to cope with change and make adaptations. Neuman's Systems Model (Neuman 1982) focuses on the impact of illness and disability on both the patient and the informal caregiver and is based upon their identification of inherent stressors and personal strengths which can be recruited to aid coping and adaptation. Roy's Adaptation Model (Roy 1984) focuses on modes of adaptation, which include physiological role function, self-concept and interdependence modes. Both of these models lend themselves well to orthopaedic and trauma care generally, but are particularly pertinent in the rehabilitation phase.

There has been a realisation that it is both undesirable and unfeasible to promote paternalistic models of healthcare support for individuals with chronic disease and/or disability. A self-management (SM) model is preferable where individuals with chronic disease and/or disability embrace an internal locus of control for their own health and wellbeing. Self-management requires education and preparation of the individual and Redman (2004) suggests SM programmes must use problem-based learning approaches and include skill development in problem solving, development of clinical judgement, self-efficacy building and belief modification and symptom reinterpretation.

The rehabilitation process

Rehabilitation should begin as soon as the patient is medically stable enough to engage with it. It is important to emphasise that the patient and their family (if appropriate) are viewed as equal partners with practitioners within the rehabilitation process and not as passive recipients. Rehabilitation is best viewed as a cyclical process beginning with comprehensive assessment, agreeing short-, medium- and long-term goals, development of a collaborative plan to work toward the goals and evaluation of progress. As the patient achieves goals either partially or fully then the cycle begins again with re-assessment.

Assessment

Comprehensive assessment is the first stage of the rehabilitation process. It is essential to gather data to form a baseline to measure progress against and ascertain the patient's support systems and home situation. The patient may be entering the rehabilitative phase within the same unit as their acute episode of treatment. In that case the team will already have assessed the patient and have relevant information about the health status and social situation. If the patient is, however, transferred from acute services to rehabilitation in another setting, a more comprehensive rehabilitation-focused assessment will be needed. A comprehensive discussion of assessment in trauma and orthopaedics is provided in Chapter 7, but an assessment within the context of rehabilitation needs to have a stronger psycho/social focus than the typical medical model. Hoeman (2008) suggests that assessment within the rehabilitation phase should have a specific focus on functional skills, psychosocial status, environment and financial status. There are a number of models that lend themselves to rehabilitation including Roy's adaptation model (Roy 1984) and Orem's (Orem 2001) self-care deficit model.

Goal setting

Goal setting is not generally used in the acute care setting where the nursing process tends to focus on the identification of actual or potential patient problems. Goals have the following characteristics:

- Goals are positive statements of intent with associated time frames.
- Goals should be realistic and achievable, but at the same time provide appropriate challenge to the patient to give them something to strive and work toward.
- Goals should be discussed and agreed with the patient and family/significant others if appropriate and progress toward goals regularly reviewed and documented.

It is good practice for the goals to be a combination of short-, medium- and long-term as achievement of short-term goals can help to motivate the patient to push toward the medium- and long-term goals. For example, the patient with a traumatic amputation of a lower limb may have a short-term goal of being able to stand for a short period with their new/temporary prosthesis, a medium-term goal of walking up and down stairs with their prosthetic limb and a long-term goal of returning to a sport such as horse riding using their prosthesis.

Developing an implementation plan and evaluation

Once goals have been mutually agreed between the patient and multidisciplinary team (MDT) a plan to support the achievement of the goals needs to be developed and reviewed on a daily basis. The plan should make explicit the roles and required actions of the patient/family and each member of the MDT to achieve the goals. It must be agreed which member/s of the team has the best skills and expertise to support the patient with each particular goal (Jester 2007). Often nurses will have an important continuing function with all of the goals due to their 24-hour presence with the patient. Realistic time scales should also be agreed between the MDT and the patient and then documented. It is important that the plan minimises the use of jargon and is understandable to the lay person. Treatment and therapies planned should be evidence-based and advantages, potential disadvantages and associated risk should be discussed with the patient in order for their consent to participate to be considered informed.

Progress toward achievement of the agreed goals needs to be reviewed on a regular basis. The process of evaluation should be shared between the MDT, patient and family where appropriate. Evaluation involves both the gathering of objective and subjective measurements to make an informed decision regarding change in the patient's function and status. Subjective data include seeking the patient's own perceptions, typically through self-reported generic Health Related Quality of Life (HRQoL) and disease-specific measures (which are discussed later within this chapter and are defined in Chapter 7) along with pain assessment. Objective data include clinician-measured function, movement and physiological parameters; examples of these are provided later within this chapter. Once evaluation has been completed new goals can be set or adjustments made to existing goals.

Team approaches to rehabilitation

Effective team working is one of the most important factors in successful rehabilitation, but it is important to understand what is meant by team working and the different approaches such as multidisciplinary, interdisciplinary and transdisciplinary and their cognate advantages and disadvantages (see Box 6.1). A description and comparison of these approaches is provided in Table 6.1. There is a move away from multidisciplinary working. As more care and rehabilitation is provided in the community setting there is a growing realisation that team members need to share skills and knowledge to have a wider repertoire of skills than the traditional professional-specific model. Multi-skilling between nurses and therapists is becoming common, particularly in 'Hospital at Home' schemes as it is not cost-effective or desirable for the patient for discreet professions to make multiple visits. The team involved in rehabilitation of the trauma/orthopaedic patient typically involves nurses, healthcare and therapy assistants, physiotherapists, occupational therapists, social workers, medical practitioners and orthotists. Other professionals such as the dietician and psychologist may be included if the patient's goals require their input. It is essential that practitioners fully embrace the patient and if appropriate family or informal carers as legitimate members of the team.

Box 6.1 Evidence digest: Multidisciplinary approaches for inpatient rehabilitation

Co-ordinated multidisciplinary approaches for inpatient rehabilitation of older patients with proximal femoral fractures (Review) (Cameron *et al.*, 2009).

A Cochrane systematic review conducted by Cameron *et al.* (2009), which included nine trials, examined the effects of co-ordinated multidisciplinary inpatient rehabilitation, compared with usual (orthopaedic) care, for older patients with hip fracture and concluded there tended to be better combined outcomes (mortality and reduced function necessitating institutional care) for patients receiving co-ordinated inpatient rehabilitation, but the results were not statistically significant and the results were heterogeneous.

Table 6.1 Description and summary of key differences between MDT, IDT and TDT approaches to team working

MDT (Multidisciplinary team)	IDT (Interdisciplinary team)	TDT (Transdisciplinary team)
Independent profession-specific assessments of the patient	Shared assessment documentation and sharing of assessment data to avoid repetition.	The primary clinician will lead the assessment but draw on expertise of other team members as appropriate
Clearly demarcated role boundaries	Blurring of professional boundaries and more multi-skilling between professional groups	Members of team cross-train and develop a portfolio of skills that transcend traditional professional role descriptors
Communication is more vertical than lateral and team conferences do not usually take place.	Regular communication in the form of goal review and case conferences	The primary clinician acts as the communication coordinator, but communication is open and non-hierarchal
Each member of the team usually works independently to achieve discipline specific goals	Goals are patient-centred and shared with all members to work toward	Goals are patient-centred and team members are often cross-trained to work toward the goals
Each member of the team retains their own records for individual patients	Use of integrated care pathways and shared documentation	Records tend to be patient held and updated in partnership with patient and family
Team leader tends to nearly always be a medical doctor	Team leader not profession-specific, but based on the leader having the most appropriate experience, skills and leadership and co-ordination abilities	One team member designated as the primary clinician for the patient, but is guided by other professionals as required

The role of the nurse

Nurses make a unique contribution to the rehabilitation process and yet continue to struggle to articulate what their contribution and role are. Conversely the contribution of therapists, social workers, physicians and psychologists is well defined within the literature (Jester 1997). Waters (1996) considered the role of nurses to be secondary to other members of the MDT and comprising three main components:

- general maintenance – including overall ward management and maintenance of patients' physical wellbeing in terms of nutrition, hygiene and skin care
- Expertise in areas such as tissue viability, continence and pain management
- Carry-on role – nurses maintain the progress made by therapists over the 24 hour period e.g. mobility and dressing practice.

The description of the nurse's role offered by Waters (1996) underestimates the essential nature of these fundamental aspects of the rehabilitation process. Specifically, the patient who has unmanaged pain or develops sepsis from pressure ulcers is not going to be able to fully commit to working toward their rehabilitation goals. Nurses also have a fundamental role in assessing and managing the risk of complications such as infection, pressure ulcers and venous thromboembolism which pose a serious threat to the patient's wellbeing and ability to progress with their rehabilitation.

Nurses are still predominantly the only professional group to have a 24-hour presence and work over the 7-day week. This allows them to develop a strong therapeutic relationship with the patient and be sensitive and observant to small, but potentially significant changes in the patient's condition. Nurses are likely to be the only profession available to speak to and update families during visiting times about progress in the rehabilitation process. This unique 24-hour presence also enables the nurse to see how the patient functions over the 24-hour period. This can provide a valuable insight into the patient's readiness for discharge. For example, the patient who is safe and independent during the day may become disorientated and have a propensity to fall during the night.

Traditionally nurses working with patients in the acute phase of their care will provide assistance with the activities of daily living that the patient is too unwell to do for themselves. Within the restorative phase, however, the nurse needs to optimise independence and to encourage the patient to do as much for themselves as possible. The transition from direct caring to a more supportive 'hands-off' approach can be difficult for both patients and nurses to come to terms with. A study by Ellul *et al.* (1993) reported that when nurses incorporated the skills patients were learning in therapy sessions into everyday aspects of the patient's care, it resulted in a 55% increase in the time that patients spent engaged in meaningful therapeutic activity contributing toward achievement of their goals.

To date the nursing role in rehabilitation remains underdeveloped, partly through a relatively low emphasis on rehabilitation within the pre-qualifying nursing curriculum and few opportunities at postgraduate/post registration level. This may also be due to nursing being unable to clearly articulate the value of its role in rehabilitation compared to other professionals such as therapists. However, rehabilitation as a specialism is gaining momentum. The potential role of nurses in rehabilitation, if they were afforded better support and education to develop the requisite skills, was summarised in the work of Nolan *et al.* (1997) who suggested the following role contributions:

- assessment of physical condition, delivery of evidence-based care and prevention of complications
- education/counselling
- psychosocial interventions
- support and education of family carers
- coordinating, liaison and facilitating transition.

The RCN (2007) guidance on the role of the rehabilitation nurse outlined eight categories where the nurse can positively influence rehabilitation:

- essential nursing skills
- therapeutic practice
- coordination
- education
- empowerment and advocacy
- clinical governance
- political awareness
- advice and counselling.

Psychological support in rehabilitation

Both the work of Nolan (1997) and the RCN guidelines (2007) have emphasised the importance of the nurse in providing psychological support to patients engaged in rehabilitation. Many trauma and orthopaedic patients who

Box 6.2 Body concepts (Price 1990a). Reproduced with permission from Prentice Hall

Body concepts

1 Body reality – the body as it really is
2 Body ideal – beliefs about how the body should be
3 Body presentation – how the body is presented to the outside world (how we dress, use of cosmetics, wigs etc)

require rehabilitation will have some degree of altered body image. Body image is defined by Schilder (1935) as:

> (the picture of our body which we form in our mind, that is to say the way in which our body appears to ourselves.) (p17)

Price (1990) identifies dimensions of body image; perception, cognition, social and aesthetic and proposes a 5-dimensional model of body image comprising three body concepts (Box 6.2) and two mitigating personal responses to change or threat to the body concepts which are personal coping strategies and our social support network.

Price (1990) recommends that for the individual to have an acceptable self-body image, an equilibrium needs to be maintained between the three concepts and two personal responses. The trauma and orthopaedic patient may have severe threats to their body concepts due to temporary or permanent changes to their body such as scoliosis, limb shortening due to hip pathology, amputation, scarring from surgery or trauma, need for an external fixator, casts and use of walking/mobility aids. The impact of alterations of body image should be explored with the patient and appropriate support put in place. This may be to empower the patient to optimise self-help and informal support through support groups and family/social support or referral to counselling and psychotherapy.

Trauma and orthopaedic conditions that may benefit from rehabilitation

The need for rehabilitation will exponentially rise as the demographic profile of the population continues to age. Those requiring trauma and orthopaedic care will range from the very young child to the very elderly and will often have a number of co-morbid conditions. For example, the infant born with congenital orthopaedic conditions such as osteogenesis imperfecta (brittle bone disease) will need lifelong support to optimise function and minimise disability. Broadly, the type of conditions that require rehabilitation to optimise function can be categorised as:

- acute onset – for example fractures, bone tumours, osteomyelitis and soft tissue injury such as ligament ruptures
- gradual onset with relapsing course – for example rheumatoid arthritis and low back pain
- acute onset with constant course – such as spinal cord injury, traumatic amputation and ankylosing spondylitis
- gradual onset and progressive course – such as osteoarthritis, bone and joint tuberculosis and degenerative spondylolisthesis.

Nurses working within trauma and orthopaedics with very young infants through to the very elderly require knowledge, skills and competence in rehabilitation no matter where the care setting might be.

Rehabilitation settings

Traditionally, rehabilitation for trauma and orthopaedic patients was delivered within the in-patient setting either within the same unit as the acute phase of care or following transfer to a specialist rehabilitation facility. The second of these options frequently led to the rehabilitation phase not being instigated until the patient was transferred and had a deleterious impact on patient outcomes and length of stay. There is, however, an increasing shift of rehabilitation into the community setting. This shift has, in part, been due to a systematic reduction in the number of hospital beds available and the realisation that prolonged hospitalisation is not therapeutically beneficial for many – specifically children and older adults. Another influencing factor is that community rehabilitation is less costly and is also more realistic in the patient's own home (Jester 2007). There is a gradual move away from rehabilitation services being medically led with community-based services often being led by specialist nurses and therapists. There is a growing evidence base to support the superiority of home-based rehabilitation compared to in-patient models within trauma and orthopaedics.

There also appears to be a growing body of evidence to support home-based rehabilitation compared to hospital-based alternatives. A summary of the evidence is

Box 6.3 Evidence digest: The setting for rehabilitation

A study by Jester and Hicks (2003a) of Hospital at Home (HaH) services and in-patient units in the rehabilitation phase following hip and knee replacement surgery (THR and TKR) reported that HaH was found to be significantly more effective in terms of patient satisfaction and reduced joint stiffness and at least as effective as in patient care in relation to levels of joint pain, joint function and incidence of post operative complications. The study also included the views of family carers and reported that of the 21 family carers interviewed all would choose HaH in preference to in-patient care. Jester and Hicks (2003 b) also reported HaH was more cost-effective than in-patient models because of a reduction of hospital bed days offset against community service costs. A RCT by Siggeirsdottir *et al.* (2005) also reported home-based rehabilitation was safer and more effective in improving function and quality of life after THR than in-patient rehabilitation.

Mahomed *et al.* (2008) concluded from a comparison of home and hospital based rehabilitation following primary THR and TKR in Canada that there was no difference in pain, functional outcomes, or patient satisfaction between patients receiving home-based rehabilitation and those that had inpatient rehabilitation, but found the home-based intervention to be more cost-effective.

Grant *et al.* (2005) compared a home and hospital based rehabilitation programme for patients undergoing anterior cruciate ligament reconstruction and reported improved outcomes at 3 months postoperatively for the home-based rehabilitation group.

provided in Box 6.3. However, it is important to remember that home-based interventions often require the patient to have sufficient family/informal carer support to be eligible for 'Hospital at Home' (HaH) type schemes. Smith (1999) recommended that decisions about location of rehabilitation services should consider:

- Appropriateness — or relevance of the service for the patient. For example home-based rehabilitation may be more realistic for some individuals, but for others their levels of social support may present risk for home-based interventions.
- Equity — there should be equal access to rehabilitation, not dependent on locality.
- Accessibility — this relates to issues of physical accessibility as discussed earlier within this chapter and issues such as waiting times for specialist rehabilitation services.
- Acceptability — the degree to which the rehabilitation service meets the expectations of the patient.

Within contemporary healthcare, commissioners often make decisions about setting up or discontinuation of services based on cost-effectiveness and patient choice and preference may not be always be considered. Jester (2003) urged that decisions regarding rehabilitation setting following joint arthroplasty of the knee and hip should take into consideration patient preference, their locus of control and support systems and that the orthopaedic nurse has a key role in advocating for patient choice regarding location of their rehabilitation.

Summary

This chapter has aimed to demonstrate that most trauma and orthopaedic patients will require some form of rehabilitation and therefore the nurse needs to optimise their role and contribution to the rehabilitation process. Rehabilitation has been defined as a goal-orientated process that should be begin as soon as the patient is medically stable following trauma or elective interventions. A relatively strong evidence base has been presented regarding the choice of rehabilitation settings, with home-based models proving a more cost-effective alternative to inpatient approaches, although the importance of patient choice and consideration of suitability were emphasised. Nurses will need to work across the interface of hospital and community settings to support patients through the rehabilitation journey and should ensure they have the requisite skills and knowledge to facilitate this. Also the benefits of transdisciplinary team working have been explored where nurses and therapists share and expand their collective repertoire of skills and underpinning knowledge.

Recommended further reading

Hoeman, S. (2008) *Rehabilitation Nursing: Prevention, Intervention and Outcomes*, 4th edn. Mosby Elsevier, St Louis.

Jester, R. (2007) *Advancing Practice in Rehabilitation Nursing*. Wiley Blackwell, Oxford.

Mauk, K. (2012) *Rehabilitation Nursing: A Contemporary Approach to Practice*. Jones and Bartlett. Sudbury, MA.

References

Cameron, I., Handoll, H., Finnegan, T., Madhok, R. and Langhorne, P. (2009) *Co-ordinated multidisciplinary approaches for inpatient rehabilitation of older patients with proximal femoral fractures (Review)*. John Wiley and Sons Ltd. *Cochrane Database of Systematic Reviews*, Issue 4.

Crosby, N. and Jackson, R. (2000) *The Seven Needs and the Social Model of Disability*. Coalition for Inclusive Living, Derbyshire.

Ellul, J., Watkins, C., Ferguson, N. and Barer, D. (1993) Increasing patient engagement in rehabilitation activities. *Clinical Rehabilitation*, **7**, 297–302.

Grant, J.A., Mohtadi, N.G., Maitland, M.E. and Zernicke, R.F. (2005) Comparison of home versus physical therapy-supervised rehabilitation programs after anterior cruciate ligament reconstruction: a randomized clinical trial. *The American Journal of Sports Medicine*, **33**(9), 1288–1297.

Hoeman, S. (2008) *Rehabilitation Nursing: Prevention, Intervention and Outcomes*, 4th edn. Mosby Elsevier, St. Louis.

Jester, R. (2003) Early discharge to Hospital at Home: Should it be a matter of choice? *Journal of Orthopaedic Nursing*, *b* (**2**), 64–69.

Jester, R. (2007) *Advancing Practice in Rehabilitation Nursing*. Wiley Blackwell, Oxford.

Jester, R. and Hicks, C. (2003) Using cost-effectiveness analysis to compare hospital at home and in-patient interventions. Part 1. *Journal of Clinical Nursing*, **12**, 13–19.

Jester, R. and Hicks, C. (2003) Using cost-effectiveness and analysis to compare hospital at home and in-patient interventions. Part 2. *Journal of Clinical Nursing*, **12**, 20–27.

Mahomed, N.N., Davis, A.M., Hawker, G. *et al.* (2008) Inpatient compared with home-based rehabilitation following primary unilateral total hip or knee replacement: a randomized controlled trial. *The Journal of Bone and Joint Surgery (American)*, **90**(8), 1673–1680.

Mason, D., Dickens, V. and Vail, A. (2012) Rehabilitation for hamstring injuries. *Cochrane Database of Systematic Reviews* **12** (Art. No.: CD004575). DOI: 10.1002/14651858.CD004575.pub3.

Mauk, K. (2012) *Rehabilitation Nursing: A Contemporary Approach to Practice*. Jones and Bartlett, Sudbury, MA.

Neuman, B. (1982) *The Neuman Systems Model: Application to Nursing Education and Practice*. Appleton Century Crofts, Norwalk, CT.

Nolan, M., Booth, A. and Nolan, J. (1997) *New Directions in Rehabilitation: Exploring the Nursing Contribution*. Research Report Series No 6. English National Board for Nursing, Midwifery and Health Visiting, London.

Orem, D.E. (2001) *Nursing: Concepts of Practice*, 6th edn. Mosby, London.

Price, B. (1990) *Body image. Nursing Concepts and Care*. Prentice Hall, London.

Redman, B.K. (2004) *Patient Self Management for People with Chronic Diseases*. Jones and Bartlett, Massachusetts.

Roy, C. (1984) *Introduction to Nursing: An Adaptation Model*, 2nd edn. Prentice Hall, Englewood Cliffs, NJ.

Royal College of Nursing (2007) *The Role of the Rehabilitation Nurse: RCN Guidance*. RCN Publishing, London.

Schilder, P. (1935) *Image and Appearance of the Human Body*. Kegan Paul, London.

Siggeirsdottir, K., Olafsson, O., Jonsson, H. *et al.* (2005) Short hospital stay augmented with education and home-based rehabilitation improves function and quality of life after hip replacement: randomized study of 50 patients with 6 months of follow-up. *Acta Orthopaedica*, **76**(4), 555–562.

Smith, M. (1999) *Rehabilitation in Adult Nursing Practice*. Churchill Livingstone, Edinburgh.

Waters, K. (1996) Rehabilitation: core themes in gerontological nursing, in *A Textbook of Gerontological Nursing: Perspectives on Practice* (eds L. Wade and K. Waters), Baillere-Tindall, London.

PART II
Specialist and advanced practice

CHAPTER 7

Clinical assessment of the orthopaedic and trauma patient

Rebecca Jester

London South Bank University, London, UK; Dudley Group NHS Foundation Trust, Dudley, West Midlands, UK

Introduction

The aim of this chapter is to provide an evidence-based discussion of assessment of the orthopaedic and trauma patient. The chapter adopts a person centred approach to the subject of assessment as it is important to remember that, although a person's chief complaint will be a musculoskeletal problem, most are likely to have co-morbidities and psycho/social issues that relate to their problem. Practitioners will be using their assessment skills throughout the patient's journey from initial presentation in primary care, emergency room or outpatients department to on-going evaluation following intervention or change in medical status. Throughout the chapter, where robust evidence exists, there will be critical application of research to approaches to assessment and examination. However, to date there is very little high level evidence to support many aspects of patient assessment/clinical diagnostics within trauma and orthopaedics affirmed by a dearth of systematic reviews. Therefore the information within this chapter is in the main based upon evidence from the following sources: formal education, symposia, conference presentations, non-research publications, expert opinion and reflections on clinical experience (the author's and other clinical experts').

Principles of clinical assessment

Clinical assessment can be defined as gathering both objective and subjective data for the purposes of generating differential diagnoses, evaluating progress following a specific procedure or course of treatment and evaluating the impact of a specific disease process. Examples of objective and subjective data can be found in Table 7.1.

There are some important key principles related to assessment including:

- introducing yourself
- confirming the patient's identity
- explaining what the assessment is going to involve
- gaining the patient's consent for the assessment
- establishing if the patient wants a family member or carer to be present during the assessment
- good hand hygiene prior to and on completion of assessment/examination.

It is important to establish, either prior to or early in the assessment, if the patient has any degree of cognitive dysfunction. Communicating with patients with impaired cognition requires management of the immediate environment to reduce accessory noise and constant re-orientation to what you are doing and why. It is also important to establish that the patient has the mental capacity to consent to the assessment before proceeding. People with learning disabilities often are not supported well in acute hospitals (MENCAP 2007). Thoughtful communication involves minimising healthcare jargon, use of pictorial aids if appropriate and including a family carer. These can all help to alleviate anxiety during the assessment process. Non-verbal and para-verbal communication play a key role in putting patients with cognitive impairment or learning difficulties at ease during the assessment and enhancing the accuracy and quality of information elicited during the assessment.

Orthopaedic and Trauma Nursing: An Evidence-based Approach to Musculoskeletal Care, First Edition. Edited by Sonya Clarke and Julie Santy-Tomlinson.

Table 7.1 Types of subjective and objective data

Subjective data	Objective
History – dependent on accuracy of patient and/ or family as historians Patient reported outcome measures (PROMS), patients' subjective perceptions of their symptoms and the impact on their quality of life and functional ability, mental health status Pain assessment	Radiographic and other clinical investigations such as blood tests, MRI, CT Measurement of range of movement (ROM) using goniometry Base line observations such as blood pressure, weight, height, body mass index (BMI), temperature, heart rate Measurements of limb length and muscle strength Physical assessment including muscle, strength, palpation, auscultation and inspection. Clinician measures such as timed get up and go test.

It is important to:

- Ensure the patient is comfortable and their privacy and dignity are maintained at all times during the assessment. Patients of either sex should be asked if they would like a chaperone present during any physical examination and unless the patient refuses (this should be documented) a chaperone should always be present during intimate examinations of patients of the opposite sex. The name and signature of any chaperone should be clearly documented.
- Check the patient is not in pain, thirsty, hungry or needing the toilet prior to embarking on the assessment process. Also be mindful not to overtire older or frail patients with prolonged questioning, examination and clinical investigations. Patients may require a break and the assessment process may need to be phased to accommodate their needs.
- When documenting the assessment ensure you record negative as well as positive findings. For example *'patient reports no locking or giving way of the knee joint'*.

Models and frameworks of patient assessment

It is important to adopt a systematic approach to patient assessment to avoid missing valuable information and to minimise repetition. Patient assessment should be interprofessional and a shared assessment document adopted. This approach enables the multidisciplinary team (MDT) to share information and avoid wasting the patient's time by several health care professionals attempting to collect the same information. Approaches to patient assessment will vary depending upon patient needs; for example, whether the patient is presenting as an emergency with multiple trauma or a non-emergency with a painful joint/s or musculoskeletal dysfunction.

Emergency presentation

The patient presenting in the Emergency Department (ED) with severe or multiple injuries must have an urgent and systematic assessment to identify life threatening issues using Advanced Trauma Life Support (ATLS). In most healthcare organisations these observations will be recorded on a Modified Early Warning Score (MEWS) chart. See Chapter 16 for further detail regarding assessment of the patient following trauma.

Non-emergency, elective or planned presentation

Within orthopaedic care the medical model of assessment has predominated, with the main aim of the assessment being to understand the patient's chief complaint/problem and arrive at a differential diagnosis. Traditionally, this has been solely within the remit of the medical profession, but in recent years a growing number of specialist and advanced nurse and physiotherapy practitioners have taken on this role. The medical model comprises:

- taking a history to elicit the chief complaint or presenting problem
- observation and inspection
- physical examination using palpation, percussion and auscultation

- assessing movement and strength
- clinical investigations.

The medical model lends itself to the patient who is presenting with a clearly defined orthopaedic problem with minimal co-morbidities or without complex social or psychological issues. However, many patients within the orthopaedic setting have more problems than just a single chief complaint and require a more person-centred rather than disease-centred approach to their assessment. The medical model of assessment tends to focus on the disease process rather than the impact of the disease on an individual and the ideology of holistic health assessment is to review the individual as a whole, with a focus on their overall health needs rather than the disease.

There are several assessment frameworks or models that lend themselves to the person with multiple physical, social and psychological issues and which nurses may find useful to structure their assessment. Assessment is the first part of the nursing process (comprising assessment, planning, implementation and evaluation of care). Nursing models and theories seem to have lost favour in contemporary clinical practice which has become mainly target-orientated, but it remains important that nurses promote a holistic approach to assessment and care. An overview of the assessment component of these nursing or psychological models is presented below.

Roy's Adaptation Model

This model, developed by Roy (1984), is based upon four modes; *physiologic, self-concept (including body image and self-concept), role function and interdependence mode*. This model lends itself particularly well to patients who are in the restorative phase following musculoskeletal trauma or spinal cord injury or those suffering with chronic conditions such as back pain and arthritis (see Chapter 6 for further reading on rehabilitation). The model focuses on assessing the patient's behaviour and stimuli toward adaptation in each of the four modes. The physiologic mode includes:

- oxygenation
- nutrition
- elimination
- activity and rest
- skin integrity
- the senses
- fluid and electrolytes
- neurological function and
- endocrine function.

The role function model includes:

- primary role (age, sex, development level)
- secondary role (relatively permanent positions requiring performance such as spouse, parent, sibling) and
- tertiary role (freely chosen and relatively temporary such as employee, student).

The self-concept mode includes:

- the physical self
- body image
- body sensations
- the personal self – comprising self-ideal and self-expectancy and the
- moral–ethical–spiritual self.

The interdependence mode is about:

- support systems, both intrinsic and extrinsic to the individual, and their receptive/contributive behaviours.

Wellness framework

The wellness framework (Pinnell and de Meneses 1986) can be used to provide a systematic approach to data collection during the assessment process. It focuses on health and wellness rather than disease or ill health and uses the following categories:

- Degree of fitness: exercise patterns, muscle strength, muscle and joint flexibility, body proportions (fat and muscle).
- Level of nutrition: analysis of nutritional intake, patient's knowledge of healthy nutrition, sociocultural beliefs about diet.
- Risk appraisal/level of life stress: identification of patient's risk factors to health, identification of sources of stress to the patient, the patient's perception of stress and their coping patterns.
- Life-style and personal health habits: habits regarding health behaviours, regular health screening, dental checks, alcohol/drug/smoking consumption, sleep and weight management.

The role of the nurse in orthopaedic care must incorporate promotion of healthy life styles and supporting patients to minimise risk such as the link between obesity and joint problems and the wellness framework lends itself well to this aspect of orthopaedic assessment.

Maslow's hierarchy of needs

Maslow (1954) first developed his theory of motivation and personality. From this seminal work, a hierarchy of needs can be used to structure the assessment process. The needs are arranged in a pyramid based on the premise that until the lowest or most fundamental needs of the individual are addressed they are unable to move to higher levels of functioning. These levels of need are presented below in order (lowest to highest):

- Physiological (survival needs) – Assessment of oxygenation, nutrition status, fluid balance, body temperature, elimination, shelter (home conditions and support) and sex (assessing individual's concerns about resuming sexual activity following procedures such as spinal fusion or hip arthroplasty).
- Safety and security (need to be safe and comfortable) – Physical safety: assess risk of falls; pressure sores, infection, VTE, pain assessment. Psychological security should be assessed in terms of the patient's need for information and inclusion in decisions about their care and treatment.
- Love and belonging – Elicit information about the patient's social and family support.
- Esteem and self- esteem – assess issues around body image and adaptation and coping and eliciting what the patient's goals are.
- Self-actualisation – assess the extent to which the patient's full potential is being reached, their levels of autonomy and motivation.

The medical model

History taking

Taking a history has three principal functions:

- Provision of data to inform decision making around differential diagnosis and treatment planning.
- Initiates a medium by which a therapeutic bond is formed between patient and practitioner.
- Creates a forum for education.

The importance of thorough and accurate history taking has been recognised for many years. It is very tempting for busy practitioners to try and steer the patient's presenting signs and symptoms to fit a particular disease pattern by asking leading questions, but this can lead to an inaccurate diagnosis. Silverman and Hurst (1991) suggest that history alone can provide the correct diagnosis in approximately 80% of patients.

History taking comprises ten stages which should be followed in order:

1 **Chief complaint** – elicit the chief complaint, using an open-ended question such as 'What brings you here today'?

2 **History** of the chief complaint –

P Provocative or palliative – what makes it worse or better?

Q Quantity or quality – how often do you experience the problem?

R Region or radiation – is the problem localised or more diffuse?

S Severity or scale – how would you rate your problem?

T Timing – is there a particular time of the day or night associated with your problem? When was the onset of your problem and has it been constant or intermittent?

3 **Recapitulation** – re-affirm with the patient at this stage that you have understood what their main problem is and the history of that problem as this allows any misconceptions to be resolved before proceeding further with the history.

4 **Family history** – some musculoskeletal conditions have a genetic disposition such as rheumatoid arthritis. A genogram is the most systematic and succinct way to record a family history.

5 **Past medical history** (PMH) – including all major illnesses, surgery and treatments. Patients may often forget significant aspects of their PMH and you may need to triangulate information with accessory information from the patient's notes, further questioning based on their medication, and findings from inspection such as scarring indicating previous trauma or surgery.

6 **Psychosocial and occupational history** – frequently musculoskeletal problems can be associated with patients' previous or current occupation, for example often severe osteoarthritis of the knee is related to occupations such as HGV driving, climbing up and down ladders or carpet fitters. Repetitive strain injury of the wrists and hands is often found in people who use computers for long periods of time on a daily basis. A social history will elicit what the patient's home situation is in terms of living accommodation and support from family and friends. This is very important for discharge planning and ascertaining if any adaptations to the home or work environment are needed to alleviate the patient's symptoms and increase independence.

7 **Review of symptoms** – although the patient will be presenting with a chief complaint of a musculoskeletal problem/s in certain situations such as preoperative assessment, it is necessary to review all the body systems to rule out any co-morbidities that may present as a risk during surgery/anaesthesia (see Chapter 5 for further detail on pre-operative assessment). The review of systems should also include a review of the individual in terms of rest and sleep patterns, smoking and alcohol habits. Table 7.2 provides guidance on reviewing the body systems. To review the systems in a systematic way it is best to take a head-to-toe approach.

8 **Allergies** – ascertaining if the patient has any known allergies to medications, dressings/adhesive or latex. Historically patients were tested for sensitivity to nickel, cobalt or chromium, but the clinical significance of metal sensitivities following prosthetic replacements is questionable and therefore routine metal allergy testing is no longer recommended. However, it is still important to question patients about metal skin sensitivity, specifically nickel as the patient may have a skin reaction from clips or staples following surgery. The evidence base for the value of routine metal allergy testing is equivocal as a study by Frigerio *et al.* (2011) concluded that objective determination of metal sensitivity at preoperative assessment should be considered when planning joint arthroplasty, as it would help the surgeon determine the most appropriate prosthesis.

9 **Medications** – including prescribed, over the counter (OTC) and homoeopathic medicines. Patients can often be unsure of the names, doses and function of their medications so it is important to cross-verify with accessory information such as prescription printouts.

10 **Education** – this stage of the history taking process facilitates the opportunity for the patient and/or their family if present to ask questions and also to provide health promotion advice. For example if the patient reports smoking then smoking cessation advice can be provided. Also, if the patient is obese or morbidly obese, information and support for weight reduction can be offered. It is also important to offer the patient and/or family member the opportunity to ask any questions or raise any issues they feel have not been covered during the history taking/assessment.

Table 7.2 Review of Systems

Body system	Example questions
Integmentary	Do you have any skin lesions, sores, unhealed wounds, pressure sores, rashes, fungal infections of nails?
Mental health/psychological well-being	Do you currently suffer with anxiety or depression?
Neurological	Do you suffer with fits, faints, blackouts, headaches, muscle weakness/ wasting or altered or loss of sensation?
Respiratory	Do you suffer with shortness of breath either at rest or on exertion or suffer with wheezing, bronchitis, asthma, chest infections or dry or productive cough?
Cardiovascular	Do you have any problems with chest pain, circulatory problems, leg ulcers, blood clots or varicose veins?
Musculoskeletal (The chief complaint will have been explored earlier in the history, but additional musculoskeletal problems may be present.)	Do you have any joint pain, swelling, locking or giving way, limitations to movement, fractures or muscle/tendon/ligament injury?
Gastrointestinal	Do you have any gastric bleeding, ulcers, abdominal pain, oesophageal reflux, loss of appetite, unintentional weight loss or gain. Ascertain bowel habits and if there has been any recent change.
Genitourinary	Do you have any problems passing urine such as urgency, frequency, incontinence, hesitancy, nocturia or urine infection?

Principles of physical examination

Based on information gained during the history, the practitioner can then focus the physical examination. Which body systems to include in the assessment will depend on both information from the history and the nature of the assessment. For example if the patient is presenting postoperatively with deteriorating vital signs a thorough examination of several systems including cardiovascular, respiratory, neurological and abdominal may be needed. If the patient is presenting in the orthopaedic or primary care clinic with a specific localised musculoskeletal problem then the examination can focus on the joint of concern, bearing in mind that musculoskeletal pain can often be referred and therefore it is important to include examination of joints above the specific site of the problem and to always compare both limbs. The important principle is to have a sound rationale for which systems and specific elements of systems you decide to include and exclude and this should be documented within your assessment.

It is important to use all senses during assessment including sight, smell, hearing and touch. There are several techniques used within physical examination which are observation, inspection, palpation, percussion, auscultation and measurement.

Observation

The first step of assessing a patient is through observation of them. Observation involves the senses of sight, smell and hearing. A good tip is to start observing the patient as you approach them (or them you) to observe:

- How they rise from a chair, transfer from bed to chair etc
- Facial expressions indicating pain/discomfort, anxiety or low mood
- Use of a walking aid and if they are using it correctly
- Gait analysis e.g. Trendelenburg gait indicating a potential hip problem, stiff knee gait or a drop foot
- Crepitus from movement of the joints or wheezing/rattles from the chest
- Does the patient look flushed, hot, pale, sweaty or jaundiced?
- Does the patient look well cared for or unkempt?
- Smell of acetone from the breath indicating ketosis
- Smell of urine or faeces.

Your initial observations should be recorded within the assessment and explored with the patient during the history.

Inspection

Inspection is much more detailed than general observation and focuses on detecting specific issues in musculoskeletal examination such as the presence or absence of swelling, bruising, scarring, skin discoloration, oedema, muscle wasting, alteration of shape, posture or deformity.

Inspection for swelling/s should note if it is localised or diffuse and confined to the joint or extending beyond the joint. Swelling confined to the joint itself can indicate either effusion due to excessive synovial fluid or non-pyogenic conditions such as rheumatoid or osteoarthritis. Swelling beyond the joint may indicate infection of the limb such as cellulitis, tumours, vascular or lymphatic problems. It is important to be precise in recording the location and extent of any swelling observed and to affirm by further questioning the onset, duration and pattern of swelling e.g. intermittent, fluctuating in severity, relieving or exacerbating factors. There are specific tests to confirm swelling which are discussed under palpation and special tests.

Inspection should also include the identification of any bruising or abrasions suggesting recent trauma and scarring from previous surgery or trauma. Changes to skin colour should also be noted, specifically erythema (redness), which may indicate a localised response to trauma or infection, or pallor possibly indicating compromised vascular function. Any muscle wasting should be noted, usually indicating limited use due to pain or injury or impaired nerve supply (denervation). For example, muscle wasting of the quadriceps can be very common in patients with knee trauma or pathology and wasting of the thenar eminence (of the thumb) in conditions of the hand/wrist such as carpal tunnel syndrome (median nerve compression). Inspection should also be used to detect deformity, altered posture or shortening; these can result from either a congenital abnormality, trauma or destructive joint disease.

Palpation

Palpation should be used to detect changes in temperature of the limbs/joints/spine and detect any tenderness. The back of the hand rather than the practitioner's palms should be used to detect localised or diffuse changes in temperature. Increased heat over a joint is indicative of inflammatory processes, whereas diffuse heat away from the joint may indicate a tumour or infection such as cellulitis. Coolness of a limb is generally indicative of arterial pathology such as atherosclerosis.

Identifying the exact location of tenderness is important in identifying precisely which underlying structures may be involved. Observing the patient for signs of distress or discomfort during palpation is important; as is documenting precisely the exact location and extent of tenderness and or alteration in skin temperature.

Assessing movement

Many orthopaedic conditions result in loss or restriction of movement. Assessing the range of joint movement requires knowledge of the normal range possible (Chapter 4). Restriction in movement can be due to contraction of joint capsules, tendons and muscles or lodging of loose bodies between the articulations of the joint. A resultant fixed flexion deformity of the joint can occur; most commonly an inability to fully flex the joint. Movement of the joint controlled by the patient is known as *active range of movement* and *passive movement* is when the practitioner controls the movement of the joint; the latter being appropriate when the muscles responsible for movement of the joint are paralysed. It is important to observe and listen to the patient when conducting measurement of range of movement, observing for signs of pain and distress. There is an unequivocal evidence base regarding the best method of measuring range of joint movement.

Assessing muscle strength

Assessing strength of muscle contraction is indicative of the strength of each joint movement and therefore should be included within the examination process. A scale developed by the Medical Research Council (MRC 1975) is used to record muscle strength and is shown in Box 7.1

Box 7.1 MRC Scale for Recording Muscle Power (MRC 1975)

0 = No muscle power
1 = Flicker of activity
2 = Movement with effect of gravity eliminated i.e. in a place at right angles to gravity but not against resistance
3 = Movement against gravity but not against applied resistance
4 = Movement against applied resistance but less than full power
5 = Normal power

Assessing for shortening of the lower limbs

As part of examination of the hip and lower limb it is important to determine the presence or absence of shortening (McRae 2010). True shortening, where the limb is physically shorter, may be caused by a number of pathologies including loss of articular cartilages caused by arthritis, displaced hip fracture, dislocation of the hip, epiphyseal trauma and old fractures of the tibia or femur. In apparent shortening the limb length is not altered but appears shorter because of contracture of the adductor muscles resulting in tilting of the pelvis. To measure for true shortening the first stage is to ask the patient to lie flat on a couch with the pelvis positioned squarely and both legs stretched out as straight as possible with heels flat to the couch. In the normal patient the heels and the anterior iliac spines are level. If a discrepancy is noted by this visual check it is necessary to measure the limbs with a tape measure which should be of material that does not stretch. Measure from the inferior edge of the anterior superior iliac spine to the middle of the medial malleolus and then extend the measurement down to the bottom of the heel with the ankle in the neutral position. Compare both sides and repeat the measurements until accuracy is assured. To measure for apparent shortening, measure between the umbilicus or xiphisternum down to the middle of both medial malleoli.

Gait assessment

There are many causes of abnormal gait patterns, including neurological and musculoskeletal disorders. There are a number of orthopaedic conditions that may produce gait abnormalities including Trendelenburg gait (waddling gait) due to hip pathology, stiff knee gait due to knee pathology and drop foot gait due to damage to the nerves responsible for dorsi-flexion of the foot. Gait analysis is most commonly undertaken by the physiotherapist or orthopaedic surgeon, but nurses working within specialist or advanced roles may carry out gait analysis as part of their assessments.

Special tests

There are a number of specific tests that may be included as part of examination of the patient. Clinical reasoning based upon the patient history and prior aspects of the examination including observation, inspection, palpation and measurement of motion will determine if special tests are required to assist in making a differential diagnosis. The most common of these include testing for valgus instability of the knee joint using the anterior draw test, testing for varus instability using the Lachman test and the Trendelenburg test for weakness of the abductor muscles of the hip. The Trendelenburg test involves the patient standing on one leg and then the tilt of the pelvis on the opposite side is observed – if the pelvis drops below the horizontal plane then the test is said to be positive.

Assessing deep tendon reflexes

Deep tendon reflexes are tested by gently tapping over a tendon using a patellar hammer and observing for movement of the associated muscles. When examining the spine for suspected prolapsed intervertebral disc, both the knee and ankle reflexes should be tested. When testing the knee reflex, the knee should be supported by the clinician's arm and the infra patellar tendon gently tapped observing for contraction of the quadriceps. A diminished or absent contraction indicates a possible prolapse at the level of L3/L4. The ankle reflex is assessed by positioning the ankle in the mid position, knee bent and hip slightly externally rotated then lightly tapping the Achilles tendon and observing for plantar flexion of the foot. An absent or diminished ankle reflex is indicative of pathology at vertebrae S1/S2. It is important when assessing deep tendon reflexes that there is no muscle contraction in the area being assessed so the patient must be relaxed. Reflexes are recorded as follows:

0 = absent
+ = reduced
++ = normal
+++ = increased
++++ = increased with clonus

Clinical investigations

Once the history and examination have been completed the practitioner needs to decide what clinical investigations are needed to arrive at a differential diagnosis and/or treatment plan. Clinical investigations including X-Rays, MRI and CT scans or blood investigations have associated costs and risks to the patient e.g. cumulative doses of radiation, and so should be requested only with a clear justification of their need. Nurses working in trauma and orthopaedics should have an understanding of the common investigations to offer support and explanation to the patient. Nurses working in specialist and advanced roles often undertake the requesting and interpretation of clinical tests within their scope of practice. The most common investigations include:

- Radiographic imaging (X-ray) – the most commonly used diagnostic imaging in trauma and orthopaedics. AP and lateral views are the most frequently requested view, but other views include: comparison images, oblique views, localised views and stress films. All clinicians requesting X-Rays must undertake specific radiology safety training and be judicious in requesting X-Rays in relation to the cumulative dose of radiation the patient is receiving.
- Computed tomography (CT scan) – still uses beams of radiation, but provides a more detailed view of tissue slices from different angles and more detailed differentiation of different tissue types.
- Magnetic resonance imaging (MRI) – avoids any exposure to radiation, using high strength magnetic fields and electrical impulses to create detailed images of bone and soft tissue. These are increasingly used in the investigation of spinal problems such as suspected prolapsed intervertebral discs and damaged structures such as meniscal and ligament tears in the knee and shoulder.
- Ultrasound imaging – is regarded as being risk-free and comparatively inexpensive. Its main value is to detect fluid in and around joints and therefore is useful in identifying heamarthrosis or the presence of infected or inflamed tissue.
- Dual energy X-ray absorptiometry (DEXA) – A non-invasive scan to test the density of bones for diagnosis of osteoporosis.
- Common haematological investigations – including full blood count (FBC) (which includes red and white cells and platelets), tests for inflammatory processes include C-reactive protein (CRP), erythrocyte sedimentation rate (ESR) and plasma viscosity (PV). It should be noted that these markers of inflammation can also be present due to infection. Serum uric acid and serum calcium, phosphate and alkaline phosphate may also be requested.

Boxes 7.2 and 7.3 provide examples of the underpinning evidence for two modes of physical assessment.

Box 7.2 Evidence digest: Goniometry

Goniometry has for many years been considered the gold standard in measuring range of joint movement; indeed if performed correctly it provides a very accurate measure of joint motion. Watkins *et al.* (1991) reported that use of a long-armed goniometer (LAG) in measuring flexion and extension of the knee joint had greater accuracy and inter-rater reliability than visual estimations. The measurements are obtained by placing the parts of the measuring instrument along the proximal and distal bones adjacent to the joint concerned and the movement should be free of any muscle contraction. It is important to align the goniometer carefully with appropriate anatomical landmarks such as the greater trochanter of the femur and lateral malleous for measuring motion of the knee joint and to ensure the goniometer stays in position as the patient moves their joint. The measurement should be taken three times and the average ROM recorded to five degree increments. However, new technologies are being introduced to further improve accuracy in measuring joint movement. A study by Hambly *et al.* (2012) compared the accuracy of the traditional LAG and a new novel smart phone application (iGoniometer) in measuring active knee flexion in a healthy adult population, and reported the iGoniometer demonstrated high relative and absolute reliability, although they recommended that further evaluation was required on a population with knee pathology.

Box 7.3 Evidence digest: Assessment findings

A 3-year prospective longitudinal study of 68 patients with OA of the knee joint reported a significant correlation between diminished joint space width and patient-reported symptoms of pain, but found no correlation between increased osteophyte formation visible on X-ray and patient reported symptoms (Fukui *et al.*, 2010). An earlier study by Neogi *et al.* (2009) also reported a strong correlation between radiographic evidence of diminished joint space in patients with OA knee and pain symptoms, but did not find a significant relationship between osteophyte changes on X-ray and patient reported symptom. This research emphasises the necessity of use of self-report outcome measures to gain the subjective perspective of the patient regarding the impact of the pathology on their quality of life and functional ability and also their view on their health status following a particular treatment or procedure.

Assessing the impact of disease on the individual

It is important, as part of the assessment process, to evaluate the impact of a particular disease on the individual to inform the treatment or management plan. There may be little correlation between what clinical investigations and examination reveal and the perception of the individual. Patients with severe osteoarthritic changes on X-Ray may report minimal disruption to their activities of daily living. Conversely patients with minimal radiographic changes may report their symptoms to be intolerable with a dramatic impact on their quality of life and functional ability (Swagerty and Hellinger 2001). This is explored in more detail in Box 7.4.

Self-report outcome measures can be broadly categorised into general health-related quality of life tools (HRQoL) and disease-specific tools. HRQoL measures aim to measure the multifaceted nature of health including physical, social and psychological health and can be used across many different types of diseases and health issues (Jester *et al.*, 2011). Their main limitation is that they lack the sensitivity to detect relatively small changes in health status for a particular disease process (Bowling, 2001) and therefore should be used in conjunction with disease-specific measures. Examples of HRQoL measures include: Sickness Impact Profile, The Nottingham Health Profile and Short Form 36 Health Survey Questionnaire (SF 36). There are many disease-specific self-report measures developed for patients with musculoskeletal conditions including; the Arthritis Impact Measurement Scale, the Oxford Hip and Knee Scores, the WOMAC index and the Harris Hip Score. The practitioner should ensure that any HRQoL or disease-specific measure used as part of the assessment

Box 7.4 The Abbreviated Mental Test Score (AMTS) (Qureshi and Hodkinson 1974). Reproduced with permission from OUP

- How old are you?
- What is the time to the nearest hour?
- Name the place
- Recognition of two persons e.g. a nurse and a doctor
- Date and month of birth
- Date of first world war (start or end)
- Queen's name
- Count 20-1 backwards
- 5-minute recall of a full street address

process has undergone rigorous testing to ensure it is valid, reliable, sensitive, specific and patient-friendly.

Assessing cognitive function

A significant number of patients presenting with musculoskeletal problems may have a degree of cognitive dysfunction this may already be noted in the patient's records. As part of a comprehensive assessment process the nurse should ensure that cognitive dysfunction is detected and its cause investigated and managed. It should never be assumed that because a patient is elderly their confusion is due to dementia. It is vital to ascertain the onset of the patient's confusion, specifically if it is an established diagnosed problem due to dementia, head injury or stroke or whether there has been a recent onset. Acute confusional states must be thoroughly investigated by taking a history of the onset from the patient if possible, family members or informal carers and then carrying out appropriate clinical investigations and observations to elicit the cause. Acute confusion (delirium) can be caused by many factors including urea and electrolyte (U and E) imbalance, sepsis, hyper- or hypoglycaemia, adverse reaction to prescribed medications, raised intracranial pressure (ICP) and drug/alcohol related. The practitioner should inform the medical team of the onset of acute confusion and commence observations using the MEWS chart and Glasgow Coma Scale (Chapter 16) to determine if any vital signs fall outside of normal parameters. Then the practitioner, in collaboration with the medical team, should begin to collect information to contribute towards determining the cause of confusion including:

- blood tests for U and E, capillary blood sugar (CBS), liver function tests, blood cultures, CRP and ESR
- urinalysis for protein, ketones and glucose and send a MSU if a urine infection is suspected
- oxygen saturation rates
- accurate monitoring of fluid input and output
- review medication with medical and pharmacy team for possible interactions or adverse reactions.

Once delirium has been ruled out based on these investigations then the patient's cognitive status should be assessed using a valid and reliable tool such as the Abbreviated Mental Test Score (AMTS, Qureshi and Hodkinson 1974) or the Mini Mental State Examination (MMSE, Folstein *et al.*, 1975). The AMTS comprises ten items as detailed in Box 7.4; the best possible score is 10/10 with each correct item scoring 1. The diagnostic cut-off point varies between authors, but generally <6 indicates cognitive dysfunction (Jester *et al.*, 2011). Although widely used in clinical practice and well tested for their psychometric properties, both the MMSE and AMTS have their limitations as they are developed for a specific age and ethnic group. Explain to the patient why you are asking the questions comprising the MMSE and AMTS and ensure privacy and an environment that has minimal background noise and disruption to get the best results.

Assessing risk

An integral part of the assessment process is to assess patient's risk of harm or injury including risk of: falls, pressure sores, malnutrition and VTE. Specific risk assessment tools are presented and discussed within the related chapters of this text. However, the predictive accuracy of all risk assessment tools must be evaluated to ensure that the practice associated with them is evidence-based. Predictive accuracy is the ability of a tool to be both sensitive and specific; to minimise the number of false positives (over prediction) and false negative (under prediction). A pilot study by Jester *et al.* (2005) found the predictive accuracy of two falls assessment tools (FRASE and STRATIFY) with older hip fracture patients to be poor, reporting Receiver Operator Characteristic scores to be 0.560 and 0.629 respectively, indicating significant over-prediction when using the tools.

Summary

This chapter has discussed best practice in assessment of orthopaedic and trauma patients. The content has included the traditional medical approach to assessment including physical examination, but has also offered a number of alternative models rooted in nursing and psychology theory. Where available there has been critical application of research and the deficit of high level evidence to underpin clinical assessment has been highlighted. Good assessment skills are fundamental to nursing practice as they generate data from which our care and treatment is planned and implemented.

Recommended further reading

McRae, R. (2010) *Clinical Orthopaedic Examination*, 6th edn. Churchill Livingstone Elsevier, Edinburgh.

References

Bowling, A. (2001) *Measuring Disease*, 2nd edn. Open University Press, Maidenhead.

Folstein, M., Folstein, S. and McHugh, P. (1975) 'Mini-Mental State' a practical method for grading the cognitive state of patients for the clinician. *Journal of Psychiatric Research*, **12**, 189–198.

Frigerio, E., Pigatto, P., Guzzi, G. and Altonare, G. (2011) Metal sensitivity in patients with orthopaedic implants: a prospective study. *Contact Dermatitis*, **64**(5), 273–279.

Fukui, N., Yamane, S., Ishida, S. *et al.* (2010) Relationship between radiographic changes and symptoms or physical examination findings in subjects with symptomatic medial knee osteoarthritis: a three-year prospective study. *BMC Musculoskeletal Disorders*, **11**, 269–279.

Hambly, K., Sibley, R. and Ockendon, M. (2012) Agreement between a novel smartphone application and a long arm goniometer for assessment of knee flexion. *International Journal of Physiotherapy and Rehabilitation*, **54**(October), 4–6.

Jester, R., Wade, S., and Henderson, K. (2005) A pilot investigation of the efficacy of falls risk assessment tools and prevention strategies in an elderly hip fracture population. *Journal of Orthopaedic Nursing*, **9**(1), 27–34.

Jester, R., Santy, J. and Rogers, J. (2011) *Oxford Handbook of Orthopaedic and Trauma Nursing*. Oxford University Press, Oxford.

Maslow, A. (1954) *Motivation and Personality*. Harper, New York.

McRae, R. (2010) *Clinical Orthopaedic Examination*, 6th edn. Churchill Livingstone Elsevier, Edinburgh.

Medical Research Council (MRC) (1975) *Aids to the Investigation of Peripheral Nerve Injuries*. HMSO, London.

MENCAP (2007) *Death by Indifference*. MENCAP, London. Available at: http://www.nmc-uk.org/Documents/Safeguarding/England/1/Death%20by%20Indifference.pdf (accessed 21 May 2013).

Neogi, T., Felson, D., Niu, J. *et al.* (2009) Association between radiographic features of knee osteoarthritis and pain, results from two cohort studies. *British Medical Journal*, **339**, b2844.

Pinnell, N. and de Meneses, M. (1986) *The Nursing Process: Theory, Application and Related Processes*. Appleton-Lange, Norwalk, CT.

Qureshi, K. and Hodkinson, H. (1974) Evaluation of a 10 question mental test in the institutionalized elderly. *Age and Ageing*, **3**, 152–157.

Roy, C. (1984) *Introduction to Nursing: An Adaptation Model*, 2nd edn. Prentice-Hall, New Jersey.

Swagerty, D. and Hellinger, D. (2001) Radiographic assessment of osteoarthritis. *American Family Physician*, **64**(2), 279–287.

Watkins, M., Riddle, D., Lamb, R. and Personius, W. (1991) Reliability of goniometric measurements and visual estimates of knee range of motion obtained in a clinical setting. *Physical Therapy*, **71**, 90–96.

CHAPTER 8

Key musculoskeletal interventions

Lynne Newton-Triggs[1], Hannah Pugh[2], Jean Rogers[3] and Anna Timms[4]

[1] *Bedford Hospital, Bedford, UK*

[2] *University College Hospital, London, UK*

[3] *Stepping Hill Hospital, Stockport, UK*

[4] *Royal National Orthopaedic Hospital, Stanmore, Middlesex, UK*

Introduction

There are a number of key interventions used in the orthopaedic and trauma setting, mainly to support and immobilise limbs while bone and soft tissue healing take place. The three interventions most frequently met by the orthopaedic practitioner are casts, traction and external fixation. Caring for patients with any one of these interventions requires highly specialised, in-depth knowledge of the theory, application, care and complications so that safe, effective care can be provided. The following three sections consider casts, external fixation and traction with a focus on providing an overview of how each works and outlining the care and support required for safe, effective patient care whilst taking into account limitations in the evidence base.

The principles of casting

The aim of this section is to provide an overview of the principles of casting and the care of the patient with a cast. The application of a cast is a specialised technical skill that requires education, training, practice and constant review of competence to ensure patients receive safe, high quality care. Most casts should be applied by practitioners with a specialist casting qualification and experience. It is important, however, that all practitioners working with patients with casts have an in-depth understanding of care needs once the cast has been applied.

A cast is a rigid device used to provide support and protection following injury and surgery and for other musculoskeletal conditions that require immobilisation (Table 8.1). Casts are constructed from flexible bandages impregnated with material which hardens when 'cured' following contact with water. The bandage is usually dipped in water, wrapped around the limb or body part and then held in position until the material hardens. This provides a firm support that follows the contours of the area it encases.

A number of materials are used for casting (Table 8.2). Plaster of Paris casts are most often used immediately following injury or surgery as they are relatively cheap and easy to apply. A lighter, more robust, synthetic cast can then be applied for a longer period of time once swelling has subsided. The choice of cast depends on applier preference and the instructions of the consulting surgeon.

Health and safety is an important consideration for both patients and staff whether a cast is applied in a casting room or other area. Employers and staff have a duty to ensure safety through systems that provide:

- training and education in safe cast application
- staff with the correct skills and experience
- appropriate, well-maintained equipment.

Ideally casting should take place in a casting room where specialist facilities are available. Casting materials and equipment should always be used in accordance with the manufacturer's instructions and there should be a regular and recorded equipment maintenance programme. The application of casts involves the use of substances which might be hazardous to health.

Orthopaedic and Trauma Nursing: An Evidence-based Approach to Musculoskeletal Care, First Edition. Edited by Sonya Clarke and Julie Santy-Tomlinson.

Table 8.1 The functions of casts

Support	Supporting and restricting movement following fracture until healed
Rest	Resting soft tissues following fracture, strain or sprain to reduce swelling and muscle spasm
Immobilisation	To rest a joint in disease or hold a joint in place following dislocation, particularly if ligaments are damaged. Also used following muscle or tendon surgery to aid healing
Positioning	To correct, stabilise and maintain alignment of a limb with a bone disorder or deformity
Prevention	To prevent bone deformity
Healing	To assist healing of wounds i.e. leg ulcers
Comfort	For the comfort of patients to aid pain relief

Table 8.2 Types of casting materials

Type of material	Properties	Advantages	Disadvantages
Plaster of Paris	Gauze bandages impregnated with powdered calcium carbonate	Relatively inexpensive Easily moulded Very strong Permeable, allowing the skin to breathe Supple at the edges	Poor strength to weight ratio Disintegrates when wet Requires 24 hours to fully set Affects the visibility of radiographs
Synthetic	Flexible fibreglass and polyester substrate impregnated with polyurethane resin	Lighter weight More durable Breathable and porous Radiolucent Water resistant Reaches full rigidity quickly	More expensive Abrasive and rough May cause skin reactions for patients and staff

Appropriate risk assessment must, therefore, take place. Manufacturers of casting materials have a legal responsibility to provide information and guidance which must be adhered to. Important precautions include:

- Plaster of Paris application and removal results in dust which can be inhaled by patients and staff. Oscillating saws must be fitted with a vacuum and staff and patients should wear a face mask.
- Gloves need to be worn, particularly when applying synthetic materials as the resin can cause irritation.
- The noise produced by the oscillating cast saw is below the required daily exposure limit for personnel. However, it becomes louder on contact with casting materials and ear defenders should be worn if the saw is to be used for prolonged periods of time.

There must be enough staff available to apply casts safely. Ideally, there should be one person to hold and position the patient's limb and reassure the patient whilst the other applies the cast.

Casting technique

The basic principles of cast application are the same whether applying plaster of Paris or synthetic casts. Casting is a highly skilled and technical activity that requires great manual dexterity. It should only be undertaken by staff with the knowledge and skills required and who practice the skills regularly. Even so, all staff working in orthopaedic and trauma settings should have a working understanding of the principles of cast application.

A good cast should always:

- Be applied in the recommended position – providing the best possible support of the limb.
- Be functional – not restricting joint movement unnecessarily and not restricting movement of joints that are not within the cast.
- Fit well – to provide adequate splintage but not be too tight. Casts that are too tight restrict blood and nerve supply and must be smooth inside without ridges that cause pressure.

- Be 'just enough' – sufficient casting material should be applied to achieve the support necessary whilst keeping the cast as light as possible
- Be complete – the cast should not be a succession of layers but should be moulded so that the materials involved are fully bonded together.

Before applying a cast it is essential to:

- check the patient's details and the written instructions for the cast
- prepare the area to be used and ensure all equipment is ready for use
- provide verbal and written information and gain consent
- provide reassurance and pain relief prior to any casting
- position and support the patient and limb correctly and comfortably
- maintain privacy and dignity
- assess the condition of the patient's skin
- ensure that jewellery has been removed from the limb to be casted.

Cast application follows general principles:

- Stockinette and appropriate padding is applied that is not excessive, but adequately protects bony prominences and vulnerable skin.
- Casting materials should be applied in accordance with the manufacturer's instructions for timings and water temperature.
- The casting material should be applied by starting at one end of the area to be covered and each turn of the casting bandage should be approximately one third of the previous turn.
- All the bandages should be applied carefully, but rapidly; smoothing continuously so that the cast layers laminate together.
- The cast should be applied without tension so that it is not too tight or too loose.
- The cast is then moulded to the shape of the area. This should be done with the palm of the hand and not the fingers, which can cause indentations leading to pressure under the cast.
- Once the cast has set, the edges should be trimmed and the stockinette should be folded back and secured with casting material.

Application of a synthetic cast is very similar but with the following exceptions:

- Padding is used but stockinette is not required.
- Extra strips of adhesive padding are applied at ends where the cast will start and terminate so that it can be turned back over the edges of the cast.
- The bandages are rolled out covering half of the previous turn with controlled tension.
- During the final moulding the cast needs to be held in place until set, otherwise the shape will not be held.

Following completion of the cast:

- The patient's skin should be cleansed and dried.
- Cast edges should be checked and trimmed as necessary to ensure that joints maintain their full range of movement and that edges do not rub the skin. The edges should then be padded and the stockinette secured in place.
- Cast setting depends on the type of cast applied and the patient should be advised how long this will take and instructed to rest the area and not bear weight on the cast during this time. All limbs in casts should be elevated and rested on pillows.
- The cast should be left uncovered for 48 hours to allow it to dry and should be handled as little as possible to prevent denting and cracking.
- Neurovascular assessment should be undertaken for all limb casts (see Chapter 9) and clearly documented.
- Documentation of any assessment, intervention and follow-up must be clear and precise.
- All advice given verbally should also be given in written format to the patient and carer. It should include care of the cast preventing complications and exercise sheets.
- If equipment such as crutches is required, advice and demonstration/practice should be given in writing and verbally on how to use them both. A physiotherapy referral may be advised.

Cast complications

If a cast is poorly or inappropriately applied the patient is at risk of injury and professional and legal action can be taken. A good quality cast is the best way to make sure that complications do not occur. The complications of casts along with mode of recognition and management are listed in Table 8.3. These complications can also be prevented by making sure the patient knows how to seek help immediately if they have any problems at all.

Table 8.3 Complications of casts

Complication	Recognition	Management
Cracking, softening, breakdown	The cast has not been applied or treated correctly. Patients and carers must be given clear verbal and written instructions	• Observe the cast hourly until dry • Reapply or reinforce only following medical review
Bleeding through the cast	If the cast is over an open or surgical wound or if the cast is causing a sore	• Seepage through a cast to be marked and observed • Excessive or odorous seepage requires medical review • Removal or bi-valving may be necessary
Pressure or cast sores	Due to a poorly fitted cast or because the patient has tried to relieve itching under the plaster by using foreign objects. There may be burning under the cast and/or localized heat and with possible swelling and discharge from the cast. Sleep is often disturbed	• Easing back of the edge of the cast for observation may be possible • Splitting or bi-valving may be necessary • Remove the cast on medical advice if there is a severe sore or a foreign body is retained inside the cast
Circulatory and/or nerve impairment	Causes: • the cast is too tight • swelling within the cast These can lead to increased pressure within the limb	• Patient and carers must know what to look for and when and who to report any change to • Hourly colour, movement and sensation (CSM) and capillary refill monitoring • Immediate medical advice must be sought • Removal or bi-valving of the cast may be necessary. Elevation of the limb unless compartment syndrome is suspected • Gentle exercise of the joints above and below the cast to improve circulation
Cast syndrome (fluid volume deficit)	A patient with a body cast may exhibit nausea, vomiting and abdominal pain. Caused by hyperextension of the spine causing the duodenum to be compressed between the superior mesenteric artery and the aorta which can lead to intestinal obstruction. This can occur weeks or months after the cast has been applied.	• Information to patients and carers about how to recognise the condition. • Immediate medical attention • Window or bivalve the cast to allow for abdominal distention • The patient should be positioned onto their abdomen • If the patient is vomiting a nasogastric tube may be required
Joint stiffness	Patient complains of pain and stiffness on movement at a joint	• Clear verbal/written instructions for exercising affected and unaffected joints
Skin reactions	Patient complains of itching or has non-localising burning pains or rashes. The skin can also blister. This is unusual and is generally a reaction to the padding	• Medical advice must be sought and the cast may need to be removed and different padding and material applied

Living with a cast

It is important that practitioners have an understanding of how a patient will cope with life in a cast (Box 8.1). A comprehensive assessment by the multidisciplinary (MDT) team may be required to ensure the patient will be able to manage safely after discharge. This will depend on previous levels of independence, the ability to accept a different level of self-care than before, availability of assistance from others and the practical advice they are given.

Assistance may be required with some activities of daily living including:

Toileting – a stool to place the leg on if in a long leg cast and a commode and/or hoist if mobility is poor.

Eating and drinking – food and fluids within easy reach; making sure the patient has their food cut up if their arms are in casts; equipment such as non-slip mats and adapted cutlery.

Dressing – advice on the best clothing to wear or adaptations to be made such as Velcro fastenings.

Mobility – assessment of mobility and aids required with instructions for use.

Sleeping – can be difficult. Extra pillows and bed cradles may help along with short term medication to help re-establish a sleep pattern.

Box 8.1 Evidence digest

Living in a plaster cast

The number of casts applied in any orthopaedic department each year is enormous, but there is only a very limited evidence base regarding supporting and caring for patients living with a cast. A qualitative research study by Williams (2010) describes the patient's experiences of living in a below-knee cast. Data were collected from patients who had been in a lower limb cast for at least four weeks using unstructured interviews and transcriptions were analysed using interpretive phenomenological analysis. Seven main themes were identified: 'hard work' illustrated how difficult everyday tasks became; 'it gets you down' described how the participants began to feel frustrated and sorry for themselves; 'different circumstances' showed how participants put their situation in context in order to cope. Other themes were: 'making it better', 'back to normal', 'pain' and 'getting through it'. It is important that practitioners have an understanding of this experience from the patient's perspective and such qualitative research is an ideal medium for this.

Socialising – living with a cast can result in significant isolation and additional support is needed in leaving the home such as temporary use of a wheelchair and contact with voluntary organisations to provide transportation.

Cast removal, splitting and bi-valving

Casts may be removed or bi-valved at the end of treatment, when a new cast is needed or if there is a problem with the cast or limb causing neurovascular compromise. Every orthopaedic practitioner should be able to safely remove or bi-valve a cast. Bi-valving involves cutting the cast in half along both sides so that one half of the cast can be removed whilst the limb is still supported with the other half. The same process should be used when removing a cast, allowing the bottom half of the cast to be used as a splint while the limb is inspected. The limb can then be carefully lifted out of the cast to remove it.

Casts are bi-valved or removed using either plaster shears or an oscillating plaster saw. Practitioners must receive training and be competent in the use of either piece of equipment. Prior to cutting, the cast should be marked on the medial and lateral sides so that the cutting lines do not pass over any bony prominences or fragile skin.

Before removing a cast it is important to:

- Check the patient's details and the written instructions for removal.
- Prepare the area and equipment to be used.
- Give verbal information prior to removal to gain the patient's cooperation and consent.
- Demonstrate the equipment to be used on the patient prior to use to allay anxiety.
- Adequate pain relief must be provided.
- The patient must be positioned comfortably and the part of the body to have the cast removed must be supported in the correct position.
- Privacy and dignity must be maintained at all times.
- The patient's cast should be carefully assessed prior to removal to ensure the correct equipment is used for cast removal.
- Mark the cutting area medially and laterally avoiding bony prominences.
- Written information must be given to the patient following cast removal.

All types of casts can be removed with plaster shears or an oscillating saw. Synthetic casts require special saw blades made of tungsten.

Plaster shears are blunt, and crush plaster of Paris between two hinged 'jaws'. The blade of the shears should be passed between the cast and the padding with the hand nearest the cast being kept parallel to the limb and kept still. If the shears are tilted they can dig in or catch the patient's skin. The other hand is then used to push the shears together to cut through the cast. Once the cast is cut through on both sides it can be opened with the plaster spreaders and the padding cut all the way through with bandage scissors. Shears are often used to remove children's casts as the oscillating plaster saw may frighten them. Shears are often not effective with synthetic casts.

Plaster saws have an oscillating circular blade which vibrates back and forth at high speed rubbing through the casting material. It must have a vacuum attached to ensure the dust is collected in keeping with health and safety regulations. The blade is held at right angles to the cast and light pressure is applied to make it cut without dragging the saw along the cast. The blade is then removed and reapplied above or below the original cut in an in-and-out motion. The saw must not be used by someone with wet hands and care must be taken as the blade can become hot and burn the skin if:

- a dragging motion is used instead of the in and out motion
- the saw is used continually for a long period of time
- even in normal use the patient may feel the heat through the padding
- if there is a large cast and it is taking a long time to remove it.

The patient's skin can also be damaged if:

- the cast is bloodstained and the padding and gauze has hardened
- the patient's skin is taught through swelling
- the blade of the saw is blunt or damaged
- the cast is unpadded as extra care then needs to be taken to avoid damaging the patient's skin.

The patient's limb should be placed back in the remaining half of the cast until it has been assessed and permission is given to remove it.

It is important that the patient is warned that their skin will have flaky yellow scales where the upper layers have been unable to shed. The limb will also appear thin and withered as muscles lose their tone from lack of use. The skin should be carefully inspected and assessed and any signs of pressure or soreness should be reported and documented. The patient should be encouraged to wash and dry the area gently and if the skin is very dry, oils or emollient cream can be applied. The skin will be more sensitive to sunlight.

Orthotics, braces, prosthetics and appliances

Orthotics is a specialty that deals with the design, manufacture and supply of orthoses – a general term for splints, appliances and braces. These are externally applied devices that are used to modify the structural or functional characteristics of the neuromuscular and skeletal systems (BAPA 2000). They can be used for acute injuries, chronic conditions and prevention of injury. Prosthetics are devices used to replace either a whole or part of an absent or deficient limb. An orthosis may be used to:

- control, guide or immobilise a limb, joint or body segment
- restrict movement in a given direction
- assist movement and/or posture
- reduce weight-bearing forces for a particular purpose
- assist with rehabilitation following fractures after the removal of a cast
- provide easier movement capability or reduce pain by correcting the shape and/or function of the body
- act as part of fixed or balanced traction
- prevent or correct deformity
- prophylactically for athletes in contact sports.

The orthotist is a healthcare professional with a key role in an orthopaedic and trauma multidisciplinary team (Chapter 5). They design and fit a variety of orthoses under prescription from a licensed healthcare provider. Orthotists also provide ongoing support and information to the patient and the carers.

Caring for a patient with an orthosis is very much like caring for a patient in a cast. Patients and carers can be taught to undertake their own skin care and advised how to seek help if there are problems. Advice also needs to be given regarding preventing and recognising neurovascular problems, exercising and mobilising safely using the orthosis or prosthesis to prevent joint stiffness and swelling. Verbal and written information and advice on how to care for the orthosis and how to recognise complications must be given to both patients and carers. Adjustments to any orthosis should only be undertaken by staff who have the knowledge and skills required. The complications that can occur for patients with an orthosis are related to poorly fitted devices and are similar to those experienced with casts.

External fixation and pin site care

External fixation is a powerful surgical technique, which involves the use of pins and tensioned wires attached to an external scaffolding framework to hold bones in place. The types of frames used in limb reconstruction correct deformity in children and adults, stabilise high-energy fractures in near-fatal trauma and grow bone lost due to trauma or bone tumours where the only other alternative is amputation.

Stabilisation of fractures using external fixation has been in use for thousands of years and mummified remains of humans with long bone fractures with external splintage have been found. It evolved in the 1950s to include deformity correction following the work of Gavril Abramovich Ilizarov (1921–1992) who first used circular frames with threaded rods and wires to help postwar amputees to overcome flexion contractures. One such patient had an undiagnosed fracture. Rather than distracting the contracture itself, distraction occurred at the fracture site. Subsequent X-rays showed bone formation in the gap. This was termed *distraction osteogenesis*, a previously unknown phenomenon. Bone actively forms in the endosteum, periosteum and bone marrow when compression and distraction is applied in the presence of stable external fixation. Connective tissue only forms bone by distraction osteogenesis; this is the process by which fibroblasts lay down type 1 collagen, orientated along the line of tension. The tension is supplied through the external fixator gradually distracting the bone ends, normally at a rate of 1mm per day, Osteoblasts then invade the periphery and start laying down bone in columns.

Types of fixator

Many types of external fixator now exist, but they generally fall into two categories: *monolateral* and *circular*. Figures 8.1 and 8.2 illustrate just two of many different types of frames. 'Hybrid' fixators are a combination of both circular and monolateral fixators. Monolateral fixators are biomechanically less stable than circular fixators.

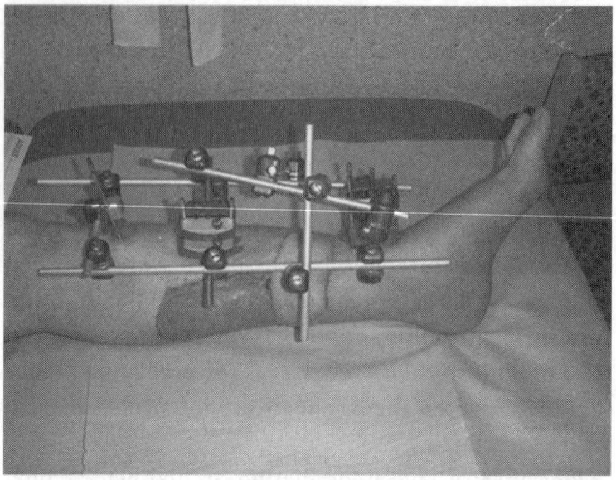

Figure 8.1 Hoffman (monolateral) external fixator frame

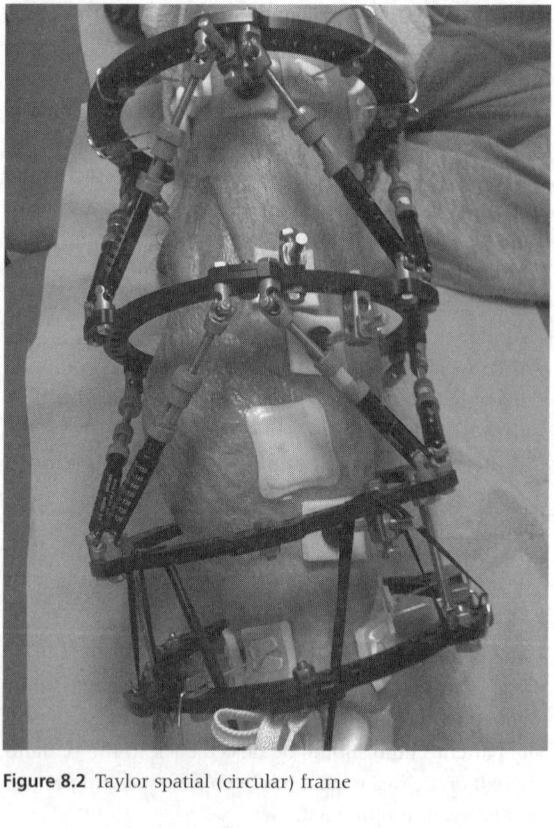

Figure 8.2 Taylor spatial (circular) frame

Monolateral fixators (e.g. Figure 8.1) are usually modular devices used to stabilise a fracture. They enable the surgeon to build their own frame and position half-pins away from any soft tissue injury. Some monolateral fixators can also be used for deformity correction; these usually involve a rail system. Often used for femoral lengthening, they are arguably more comfortable for the patient than a circular fixator, but may not allow early weight bearing.

Circular external fixators (see for example Figure 8.2) are used for both fracture stabilisation and deformity correction. They can be used to correct:

- angulation
- rotation
- translation
- limb length discrepancy.

The circular frame is easily adjustable. Adding load, through early weight bearing to the already tensioned wires, stiffens the frame. Weight bearing increases blood flow to the limb and promotes healing. There are two main types of circular fixator: the *Ilizarov* and the *hexapod*. The Ilizarov has straight rods and hinges. The patient or their carer adjusts the fixator (usually with a set of spanners) in four increments per day of 0.25 mm. Hexapods are based on the Gough Stuart platform which is also used in industry, for example in parallel robotics and aircraft simulators. Six telescopic struts are adjusted once daily according to a computer calculated prescription. Depending on the manufacturer of the fixator, it may be single or multi-use. The practitioner should establish if the equipment can be re-used and should the patient be transferred to another hospital, or in the case of death, it is important to ensure its return, as lost or mislaid equipment can lead to considerable financial loss (Timms *et al.*, 2010).

Biomechanics

The biomechanical properties of the frame in addition to its fixation to the bone are important to the success of the treatment. A frame which is either unstable or too stiff can lead to non-union. The skill of the surgeon is of prime importance as poor application of the fixator will lead to failure of the treatment. The fixator can also become unstable due to failure of the hardware. Components of the fixator, wires and half pins may occasionally loosen or break. Pin loosening and pin site infections are known to be related (Saithna 2010). An unstable fixator needs urgent review. If the wire or pin breaks at the interface between the wire and the fixator, it may be possible to 're-fix' the wire. If the wire breaks at the interface with the bone, it will need to be removed and, depending on the stage of treatment, the patient may need further surgery to replace the broken wire or pin. The patient may describe:

- hearing the metal break
- the pin site may have become increasingly painful
- the wire may move freely depending upon where it has broken
- the fixator may feel unstable.

It is important to inform the surgeon of this as one broken wire affects the overall fixator stability which may lead to further wire or pin breakage and a failure of the fixator.

Complications

Pain

Pain is an anticipated result of limb reconstruction and patients should be prepared to deal with some degree of discomfort, particularly in the early stages. Modern analgesic drugs allow much more control of pain and offer several alternatives if a particular drug is found to be unsuitable.

Pin site infection

This is arguably the second most likely complication after pain (Patterson 2006) and should take up a large part of pre-operative counselling. Teaching patients to recognise the signs and symptoms of infection is essential as following discharge from hospital it is unlikely that the patient will see a health professional daily. It is important to explain that should infection occur it is not a failing on the patient's or clinician's part; rather a common outcome of having metal work penetrating the protective barrier of the skin for prolonged periods of time (see pin site care below).

Joint stiffness

Prolonged periods of immobility will lead to joint stiffness. Patients should be encouraged, with physiotherapist support, to mobilise and exercise joints not constrained by the frame. In some cases the frame will span a joint – most commonly the knee or ankle – because of the fracture site and it is important to inform the patient that following frame removal a great deal of work will be necessary to regain joint function. Managing expectations is very important as the joint in question may never be as flexible as it was pre-injury.

Swelling

The majority of patients will experience some swelling during the treatment. This is partly a natural biophysical reaction to the presence of metalwork within the body. With lower limb frames, most commonly the swelling is due to the loss of the 'pumping action' supplied by the calf muscles when mobilising. Weight bearing through the affected limb can help reduce this. In some circumstances the limb may swell to a degree that the rings are in contact with the skin and steps must be taken to protect the area from pressure damage.

Nerve and blood vessel injury

A complication of any orthopaedic surgery and where the insertion of a particular wire or pin proves to be a problem, it may be necessary to remove and possibly re-site this.

Compartment syndrome

Because frame surgery is often minimally invasive, compartment syndrome is rare. However the same neurovascular assessments should be undertaken throughout treatment and the immediate post-operative period with frame surgery as any other orthopaedic procedure (Chapter 9). Some of the temporary, monolateral fixators are applied following high impact trauma where risk is greatly increased.

Venousthromoboembolism

Any procedure which limits mobility and function puts the patient at risk of VTE (Chapter 9). Pre-operative preparation gives the clinician the opportunity to advise the patient on the signs and symptoms to look out for.

Re-fracture

Although X-rays may look adequate and the patient is reporting positively, a frame is sometimes removed too early. This can result in re-fracture. This will present in a gradual 'bend' at the fracture/regenerate site and increased pain. This is why may surgeons are now opting to remove the interlocking struts for a couple of weeks prior to complete removal, if bending occurs the struts can be reinserted and the limb can be left to heal for longer. Others will choose to protect the limb in a cast or orthotic for a few weeks preceding removal. It is considered preferable to remove the frame late rather than too early.

Nursing care

Nursing care for patients with frames can be time-intensive and both physically and emotionally draining for both the patient and carers. Pre-operative counselling improves patient understanding and acceptance, but in cases of new trauma this is not an option. Those with chronic injuries may be facing the decision of having a frame fitted or amputation, raising a discussion about when to abandon limb salvage treatment and offer amputation. This involves intense psychological support, especially given that the patient may have many months or years of treatment in a frame for it to then fail, with the end result being amputation. Therefore, it is worth bearing in mind the work of the Lower Extremity Assessment Project (LEAP) (MacKenzie and Bosse 2006), demonstrating the importance of managing patients' expectations. Patients should be made aware that following severe trauma, function of the affected limb may never return to its pre-injury state.

Patients, with support from family and friends, will cope with limb reconstruction better than those without a support network (Patterson 2006), especially concerning factors such as reduced mobility, fixator adjustments and getting to multiple hospital appointments. Patient support groups are not widespread, so many will turn to websites and social networking for information. Whilst this should be encouraged, patients should be made aware that much of this information is opinion and not evidence-based.

Box 8.2 Evidence summary

Factors influencing outcome of following limb salvage surgery and amputation

MacKenzie and Bosse (2006) *Factors Influencing Outcome Following Limb-Threatening Lower Limb Trauma: Lessons Learned From the Lower Extremity Assessment Project (LEAP).*

At 2- and 7-year follow-ups, the LEAP study found no difference in functional outcome between patients who underwent either limb salvage surgery or amputation. However, outcomes on average were poor for both groups. This study and others provide evidence of wide-ranging variations in outcome following major limb trauma, with a substantial proportion of patients experiencing long-term disability. Outcomes are often more affected by the patient's economic, social, and personal resources than by the initial treatment of the injury – specifically, amputation or reconstruction and level of amputation.

Another consideration is the frequent X-rays required to monitor bone regeneration. Poor regeneration may result in the need to reduce the rate of adjustment or distraction or it may be appropriate to speed up the adjustment process. Where regeneration is slow or in patients having treatment for non-union, it is especially important to advise on the effects of smoking and non-steroidal anti-inflammatory use. Cigarette smoke contains toxic chemicals which affect both respiratory parenchyma and the fracture healing process as nicotine in the blood supply causes the vessels to constrict by approximately 25% of normal diameter and decreased levels of nutrients are supplied to the bones. This is potentially catastrophic for a patient undergoing further surgery for a non-union. See Box 8.3 for further discussion.

Non-steroidal anti-inflammatory drugs (NSAIDs) are commonly used in orthopaedic trauma and surgery. A lesser known side effect is that of decreased fracture healing. Although much of the available literature is based on animal studies, it demonstrates that NSAID administration in the early stages of fracture healing delays the process (Beck *et al.*, 2003), causing decreased osteoblastic activity, although there is also some dispute of this (Huo *et al.*, 1991). NSAIDs also reduce the synthesis of type I collagen (Ou *et al.*, 2012) and osteocalcin mRNA and diminish angiogenesis (Jones *et al.*, 1999), so many surgeons are now recommending that patients avoid these drugs for a period of time after injury. This may be difficult for patients and it is important that patients are informed of the rationale. A sound knowledge of other analgesics which could be offered as an alternative is important and specialist pain practitioners should be sought. Newer anti-inflammatory drugs, COX inhibitors, act in a different manner to NSAID's and so may be considered as an alternative.

Box 8.3 Evidence summary

Smoking and bony union after ulna-shortening osteotomy

A study examined the relationship between cigarette use and occurrence of delayed union and non-union after ulna-shortening osteotomy for ulnar impaction syndrome. Chen *et al.* (2001) examined healing data from 39 patients who had undergone wrist surgery in 40 wrists. The mean union rates were 7.1 months in smokers and 4.1 months in non-smokers. Six smokers (30%) and no non-smokers experienced delayed union or non-union. Given the adverse effects of smoking on bony union, they recommend that smoking history be considered when selecting patients for such procedures.

Mobilising

With the majority of circular frames the patient will be able to fully weight bear and this should be encouraged as controlled stress at the fracture site stimulates fracture healing. Mobilisation also contributes to the patient's psychological wellbeing at a time when patients may be suffering with feelings of loss of control. It will take time for a patient to be able to fully weight bear through an affected limb, ranging from days to months. Often a good place to build up confidence is in a swimming pool, although this needs to be timed with pin site care.

Work

Returning to work will have a positive psychological impact but may not be practical and a thorough social history will assist in being able to provide advice. Someone who is desk-based is more likely to be able to return to work than a builder, but care will still have to be taken that the environment is suitable; for example, the patient must be able to elevate the limb throughout the day and perhaps alter their method of transport to work.

Sleeping

Sleep can be severely affected following application of a frame. Support of the limb, comfort measures and good pain management may help. Care should also be taken to protect the rest of the body from the frame using padding.

Sexuality

Patients sometimes have a frame for a substantial period of time and may have undergone years of failed treatments, placing considerable strain on relationships. The patient should be given the opportunity to discuss this openly. They may enquire about sexual activity during treatment. It is important the nurse is prepared for this and can offer appropriate guidance when required.

Pin site wounds

The pin site is the point at which the pin or wire penetrates the soft tissues. The nature of the pin site is affected by many biopsychosocial factors and can be influenced by all members of the multidisciplinary team and the patient. These factors include:

- The patient or their carers need to commit to caring for their limb and the fixator, either through self-care, allowing others into their home and/or attending their GP surgery and hospital appointments on a regular basis.
- Pins and wires should be inserted using a slow pulsed technique to prevent the wire becoming overheated and causing thermal necrosis to the soft tissues and bone, providing an ideal environment for bacteria to flourish. Untensioned wires, frames and loose pins are also known to be related to pin site infection (Saithna 2011).
- The nurse is the majority stakeholder in the patient's care so needs to ensure the patient and their carers feel confident with basic frame care through assessment and education.
- The physiotherapist ensures mobility is maintained wherever possible and educates the patient on the prevention of contractures. Exercise may irritate the pin sites and strategies such as applying more padding with compression to the sites may help alleviate this.
- The occupational therapist assesses the patient and provides aids such as a shower seat to help maintain the patient's hygiene needs. This is important because there is evidence that a patient's skin is a major source of bacterial infection contributing to postoperative wound infection (Florman and Nichols, 2007).

Pin site infection

The prevention, identification and treatment of any infection is of prime importance. With pins and wires passing through the skin, muscle and bone, pin site infection is a constant risk. The presence of a foreign body in the wound interrupts the normal healing process, Parallels between the general infection guidelines and the 2010 RCN pin site guidance can be seen (Box 8.3). Pin site care is an area lacking in sufficient high quality research. Cochrane Systematic Reviews (Lethaby *et al.*, 2011) have concluded that there is little or no evidence on which to base practice. In the absence of such research practitioners should implement strategies to minimise infection. Despite there being limited literature regarding pin site infection, there is currently no validated assessment tool. This is important because it affects the validity and comparison of research trials. There is some consensus amongst practitioners (Clint *et al.*, 2010, Santy-Tomlinson *et al.*, 2011) that pin sites appear to fall into three categories:

- A healthy, 'calm' or 'good' pin site, one which is not inflamed, is dry and resembles a piercing.
- An infected or 'ugly' pin site, a site which is painful, inflamed and is heavily discharging, possibly with frank pus.
- The third category being the hardest to quantify but lies at an unknown point between the other two; Santy-Tomlinson *et al.*, (2011) describe these sites as being 'irritated.'

Wound swabs do not help in the distinction between 'irritated' and 'infected' sites as they do not distinguish between colonisation and infection. See Box 8.4 for a summary of recommendations for the care of pin sites.

Box 8.4 Evidence digest

Pin site care

Guidance on pin site care. Report and recommendations from the 2010 consensus project on pin site care (Timms *et al.*, 2011). This consensus study is based on expert opinion. Although the lowest form of evidence, the lack of high quality studies makes this an appropriate way to guide practice. The recommendations from the consensus reflect current infection control guidance for percutaneous insertion sites as well as findings from studies cited in the Cochrane review.

The recommendations of the consensus are:

- In the absence of allergy or skin sensitivity, pin sites should be cleaned once weekly using an alcoholic Chlorhexidine solution and non-shedding gauze.
- The frequency of dressing changes should be increased if infection is confirmed or suspected or if strikethrough occurs on the pin site dressing.
- Pin sites should be kept covered with a dressing that is non-shedding and which also keeps excess exudate away from the wound.
- Dressings should be held in situ with a clip attached to the wire or half pin to apply light compression.
- Patients with pin sites should not soak in a bath of water, but may shower immediately prior to dressing changes.
- Infection should be diagnosed using patient-reported signs and symptoms and patient perceptions of the presence of infection should be taken seriously.
- Increasing pain at the pin site, decreased mobility, spreading erythema, increased swelling and discharge are indicators of the presence of infection.

Contemporary traction

Traction is now used much less commonly due to improved implants and surgical techniques for the treatment of fractures. The result of this is that the skills needed to care for patients with traction are often not maintained. However, management by traction remains essential for those patients whose age or condition means that surgical treatment is not appropriate. It is vital that orthopaedic nurses have a basic understanding of the principles of traction, the ability to apply the most common types of traction and the knowledge to care for patients with traction. The evidence base for both the benefits of traction and the care required is very limited because it is now such a small, but important, part of orthopaedic care. This presents the practitioner with little evidence-based guidance and much advice is based on experience and trial and error.

Principles of traction

Traction is the application of a pulling force to a part or parts of the body for the treatment of bone and muscle disorders or injuries. Traction in the opposite direction, *counter-traction*, is also necessary in accordance with Newton's third law of motion – that for every action there is an equal and opposite reaction. Control of the injured part by traction facilitates bone and soft tissue healing based on simple mechanical principles but this can lead to complications. Traction can be used to:

- relieve pain due to muscle spasm
- restore and maintain alignment of bone following fracture or dislocation
- rest injured or inflamed joints whilst maintaining a functional position
- allow movement of joints during fracture healing
- prevent or gradually correct deformities due to contraction of soft tissue caused by disease or injury.

Methods of application

In order to apply traction a satisfactory grip must be obtained on a part of the patient's body via the skin or bone for a specified period of time. This can be achieved manually or via skin or skeletal traction:

- **Manual** – the pulling force is applied manually usually by the hands; for example when the fracture is being reduced or held in alignment while a cast or a more permanent form of traction is applied. Manual traction is also required during any adjustments to the traction arrangement which necessitates the temporary release of the traction weight.
- **Skin** – the application of a traction force over a large area of skin which is then transmitted via the soft tissues to the bone. The maximum pull should not exceed that recommended by the manufacturer of the traction appliance. The grip on the body is less secure than with skeletal traction. Skin traction can be adhesive or non-adhesive. Non-adhesive traction is preferable if the traction is only to be on for a short period of time. Adhesive traction should not be used with fragile or damaged skin as removal may cause further skin injury.
- **Skeletal** – the application of a traction force directly to the bone through metal pins or wires allowing large forces to be transmitted directly to the bone. It is used if traction is to be maintained for a significant amount of time and when greater weight is required. Sites for the insertion of metal pins for skeletal traction include the proximal end of the tibia, the calcaneum, the distal femur, the skull and the olecranon.

There are two mechanisms that can be used for skin and skeletal traction:

- **Fixed** – the pull is between two fixed points such as Thomas splint traction (Figure 8.3).
- **Balanced or sliding** – the pull is between the weights and the body weight of the patient (Figure 8.4).

These two forms of traction can be applied in several ways – fixed or sliding skin traction; fixed or sliding skeletal traction; combined fixed and balanced traction and modified skeletal traction. The method that is chosen depends on the condition or injury being treated.

Principles of applying traction

Essential principles must be observed if traction is to be effective:

- the grip or hold on the body must be secure
- there must be counter-traction
- the weights used should be prescribed and documented
- there must be minimal friction from cords and pulleys
- frequent checks of the patient and traction equipment should be made and documented to ensure that:
  - the traction setup is functioning as planned and is safe
  - the patient is not suffering any injury or deterioration due to the traction treatment

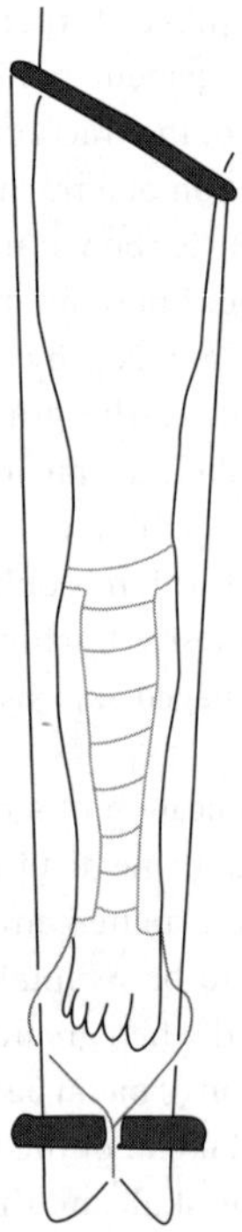

Figure 8.3 Fixed skin traction with a Thomas splint

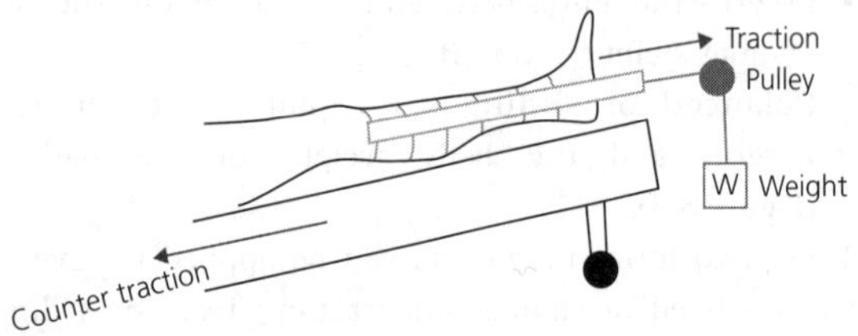

Figure 8.4 Skin traction

  ○ the traction system once set up is maintained at all times.

Traction that is poorly or incorrectly applied and maintained can cause discomfort and further injury.

Mechanics of traction

Traction systems have a number of mechanical components which it is important to understand when providing care:

- **Counter-traction** – it is essential in any traction system that there is a pull in the opposite direction in order to overcome muscle spasm and to prevent the patient from being dragged towards the traction pull. Counter-traction can be achieved in two ways; balanced sliding traction or fixed traction:
  ○ *Balanced (sliding) traction* – a system of weights and pulleys are used to apply and direct the traction pull. Counter-traction is exerted by the weight of the patient aided by gravity when the bed is tilted away from the traction pull by elevating the foot or head end of the bed (Figure 8.4).
  ○ *Fixed traction* – traction and counter-traction is exerted between two fixed points. An appliance such as the Thomas splint is used to gain purchase on the body proximally to the muscles in spasm/injury. Skin extensions on the leg are then tied firmly to the end of the Thomas splint and counter-traction forces are transmitted up the sides of the Thomas splint to the ring encircling the limb. This is a self-contained system that does not require weights or bed elevation to achieve traction and counter-traction (see Figure 8.3). It can be used when transferring patients. A balanced system is sometimes added to elevate the limb and for ease of movement of the patient.
- **Position of pulleys** – the position of pulleys within the traction system determines the direction of the traction pull and the angle. The number of pulleys used and their position affects the amount of pull that is exerted. For example, in a single pulley system the amount of traction pull is virtually equal to the amount of traction weight used, whereas two pulleys in the line of the same traction weight almost doubles the pull exerted because of the 'block and tackle' effect. This can be seen in Hamilton Russell traction where the amount of horizontal pull exerted on the leg is double that of the weight applied (Figure 8.5).
- **Vector forces** – traction forces in two different, but not opposite, directions to the same body part create a resultant force. The direction of the resultant force is determined by the position of the pulleys which direct the traction cords to the weight. In Hamilton Russell traction, for example, one force – the weight – is broken up into multiple forces to achieve a specific resultant force on the fracture site. The vector forces created can only act in the direction of the traction cords and include an upward force applied directly to the knee by means of the sling and two forces distal to the foot which reaches the femur through the leg (Figure 8.5). Changes and adjustments can

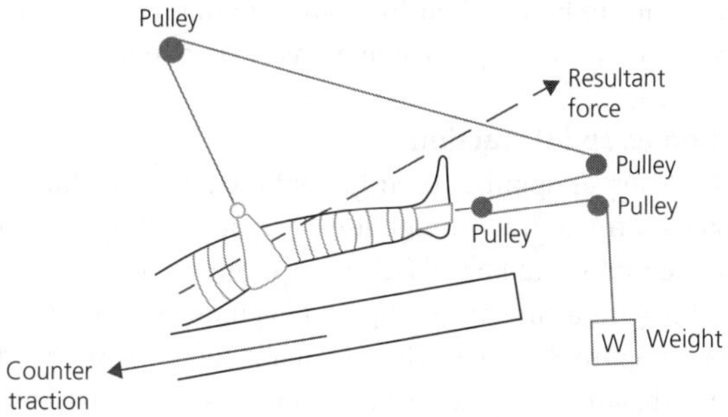

Figure 8.5 Hamilton Russell traction

be made by altering the weights or the position of the pulleys.

- ***Friction*** – the force that acts between any two surfaces and is present within the traction system. It gives resistance to the traction pull and reduces the efficiency of the traction force. Friction cannot be eliminated but can be minimised by ensuring that:
  - the pulley wheel runs freely
  - the traction cord runs centrally over the groove of the pulley
  - the weights are not resting against the bed or on the floor
  - the bedclothes are not resting against the traction cords.

Care of traction

In addition to the fundamental holistic care of the patient with traction there are a number of checks that should be made on the traction system. These checks should be carried out by a practitioner who has appropriate competence, skill and knowledge:

- Traction equipment should be checked daily to ensure that beams and clamps have not become loose.
- Traction should be checked at least once every shift and following interventions such as movement of the patient, physiotherapy and X-ray as the traction system may have been inadvertently altered.
- Traction cords must be attached securely using standard non-slip knots such as the 'clove-hitch' or 'two-half-hitches'. Only traction cord should be used as it is designed not to stretch and the ends of the cords should be short and bound back on themselves to prevent fraying. The knot should not be covered. Short cords should not be joined together by knots – this prevents the smooth running over pulleys.
- The alignment of the cords should be checked to ensure the maintenance of the appropriate pulling forces and the cord should be running freely over the groove.
- The pulleys must be checked at least once each shift to ensure they are running freely to minimise friction and that the cords are sitting in the groove. There should only be one traction cord per pulley wheel.
- Weights should be hanging freely and not resting on the floor or any other surface as this compromises the efficiency of the traction system. They should also be securely attached.
- Weights should not be hung directly over the patient.
- Bed cradles should be in use to prevent bed clothes from interfering with the free running of traction cords.
- Counter-traction should be maintained at all times.
- If skin traction is in use the skin should be checked at least four-hourly for rubbing or sore areas and the bandages should be monitored to ensure they are not too tight and don't become loose or slip.
- If skeletal traction is being used the sharp ends of the pins should be covered to prevent injury and the pins should be checked to ensure they have not become loose or moved. In addition the pin sites should be checked for signs of infection as discussed above.
- If a Thomas splint is in use it should fit correctly. Skin under the ring should be kept clean and dry and should be checked and gently moved to prevent skin injury. The traction system may need to be adjusted to avoid increasing pressure under the ring.

Common types of traction

Hamilton Russell traction

A balanced traction system using vectors to effect a pull along the long axis of the femur (Figure 8.5). It is used to:

- maintain the joint space at the hip
- Manage fractures of the acetabulum
- Support fractures of the shaft of femur

Traction can be applied using below-knee skin traction or a skeletal pin.

Gallows/Bryant traction

This is used in the management of fractures of the shaft of femur in very young children and in the preliminary management of congenital dislocation of the hip. It is only safe to use for children who are under two years of age and weigh less than 14 kg due to the risk of vascular complications. Traction is exerted by full length skin extensions to both legs and the child is positioned with the hips flexed to 90° and both legs are suspended vertically. Enough weight is applied so that the child's pelvis is lifted just clear of the mattress ensuring that counter-traction is provided by the weight of the child's body (Figure 8.6). Due to the risk of vascular complications a set of baseline neurovascular observations should be documented prior to the application of the traction and these should be repeated hourly for the first 24 hours, then 2-hourly for a further 24 hours and then 2–4 hourly thereafter. The feet should be checked for colour, temperature, capillary return, pulses and active/passive movement.

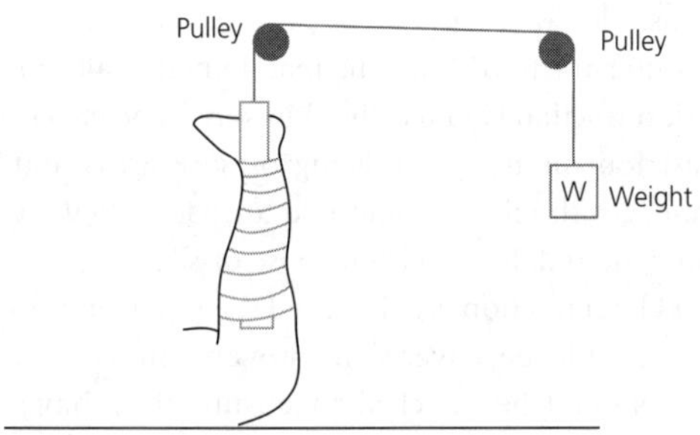

Figure 8.6 Bryants/Gallows traction

Thomas splint traction

The Thomas splint is used in conjunction with skin or skeletal traction to immobilise and position fractures of the femur. It can be used in all age groups. It is a long leg splint with a ring at the hip and extends to beyond the foot (Figure 8.3). The Thomas splint can be suspended in a balanced system using skin or skeletal traction either as a sliding system of traction or as fixed traction. This type of traction allows the injured limb to be maintained and moved in a gravity-free environment (Figure 8.7). The Thomas splint can also be used with fixed traction to transport patients between wards/departments and hospitals.

Dunlop traction

Dunlop traction is now rarely used for the gradual reduction of supracondylar and transcondylar fractures of the humerus in children and adolescents. The shoulder is abducted 45° and the elbow is flexed to 45°. Lateral pull is exerted on the forearm via the skin extensions and a second force is directed downwards on the distal humerus by the use of a weighted sling. These two forces act in different but not opposite directions and counter-traction is achieved by the weight of the patient's body when the side of the bed or mattress is elevated (Figure 8.8).

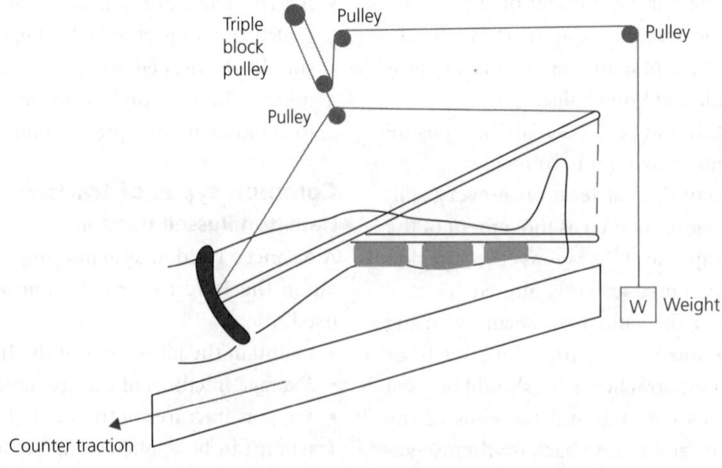

Figure 8.7 Balanced Thomas splint traction with Pearson attachment

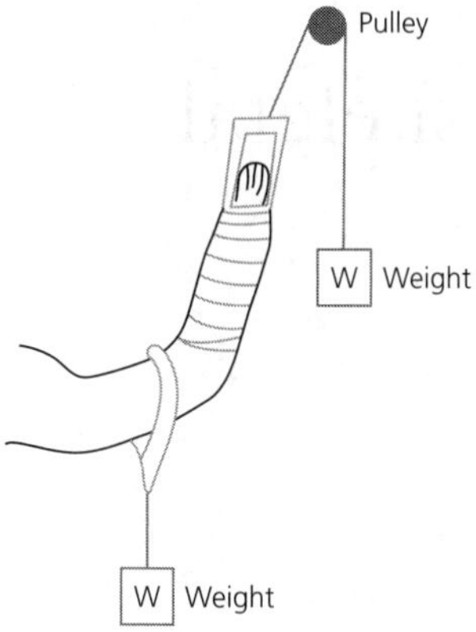

Figure 8.8 Dunlop traction

Recommended further reading

Jester, R., Santy, J., and Rogers, J. (2011) *Oxford Handbook of Orthopaedic and Trauma Nursing*. Oxford University Press, Oxford.

Royal College of Nursing (RCN) (2002) *Traction Manual*. RCN Publishing, London.

References

Beck, A., Krischak, G. and Sorg, T. (2003) Influence of diclofenac (group of nonsteroidal anti-inflammatory drugs) on fracture healing. *Archives of Orthopaedic and Trauma Surgery*, **123**, 327–332.

British Association of Prosthetists and Orthotists (BAPA) (2000) *Guidelines for Best Practice*. BAPA, Paisley.

Chen, F., Osterman, A.L. and Mahony, K. (2001) Smoking and bony union after ulna-shortening osteotomy. *American Journal of Orthopaedics*, **30**(6), 486–489.

Clint, S.A., Eastwood, D.M., Chasseaud, M., Calder, P.R. and Marsh, D.R. (2010) The "good, bad and ugly" pin site grading system: a reliable and memorable method for documenting and monitoring ring fixator pin sites. *Injury*, **14**(2), 147–150.

Florman, S. and Nichols, R.L. (2007) Current approaches for the prevention of surgical site infections. *American Journal of Infectious Diseases*, **3**(1), 51–61.

Huo, M.H., Troiano, N.W., Pelker, R.R., Gundberg, C.M. and Friedlaender, G.E. (1991) The influence of ibuprofen on fracture repair: biomechanical, biochemical, histologic, and histomorphometric parameters in rats. *Journal of Orthopaedic Research*, **9**, 383–390.

Jones, M.K., Wang, H., Peskar, B.M. *et al.* (1999) Inhibition of angiogenesis by nonsteroidal anti-inflammatory drugs: insight into mechanisms and implications for cancer growth and ulcer healing. *Nature Medicine*, **5**(12), 1418–1423.

Lethaby, A., Temple, J. and Santy, J. (2011) Pin Site Care for Preventing Infections Associated With External Bone Fixators and Pins. *Cochrane Database of Systematic Reviews* **12** (Art. No.: CD004551). DOI: 10.1002/14651858.CD004551.pub3.

MacKenzie, E. and Bosse, M.J. (2006) Factors influencing outcome following limb-threatening lower limb trauma: lessons learned from the Lower Extremity Assessment Project (LEAP) *Journal of the American Academy of Orthopaedic Surgeons*, **14**(10), S205–S210.

Ou, Y.S., Tan, C. An, H. *et al.* (2012) The effects of NSAIDs on types I, II, and III collagen metabolism in a rat osteoarthritis model. *Rheumatology International*, **32**(8), 2401–2405.

Patterson, M. (2006) Impact of external fixation on adolescents: an integrative research review. *Orthopaedic Nursing*, **25**(5), 300–308.

Saithna, A. (2010) The influence of hydroxyapatite coating of external fixator pins on pin loosening and pin track infection: a systematic review. *Injury*, **41**(2), 128–132.

Santy-Tomlinson, J., Vincent, M., Glossop, N., Jomeen, J. and Pearcey, P. (2011) Calm, irritated or infected? The experience of the inflammatory states and symptoms of pin site infection and irritation during external fixation. A grounded theory study. *Journal of Clinical Nursing*, **20**(21/22), 3163–3173.

Timms, A., Sorkin, T., Pugh, H., Barry, M. and Goodier, W.D. (2010) "No-one has ever asked for it back!" A survey assessing the fate of reusable external fixation equipment in mortuaries. *Injury*, **41**(2), 141–143.

Timms, A., Vincent, M., Santy-Tomlinson, J. and Hertz, K. (2011) RCN Guidance on pin site care. Report and recommendations from the 2010 Consensus Project on Pin Site Care. Royal College of Nursing. 004 137. Available at: http://www.rcn.org.uk/__data/assets/pdf_file/0009/413982/004137.pdf (accessed 30 March 2014).

Williams, M. (2010) The patient's experience in a plaster cast. *International Journal of Orthopaedic and Trauma Nursing*, **14**(3), 132–141.

CHAPTER 9
The complications of musculoskeletal conditions and trauma

Julie Santy-Tomlinson[1], Sonya Clarke[2] and Peter Davis MBE[3]

[1] *University of Hull, Hull, UK*
[2] *Queen's University Belfast, Belfast, UK*
[3] *Newark, Nottinghamshire, UK*

Introduction

The aim of this chapter is to provide evidence-based guidance for the identification of risk, detection, prevention and management of those complications which most frequently affect the patient with musculoskeletal injuries and conditions, and following orthopaedic and trauma surgery. The development of preventable complications is a major cause of both morbidity and mortality and is an area of considerable significance in providing evidence-based care. The death of a patient following musculoskeletal care and procedures is almost always the result of one or more complications which can also lead to significant delays in recovery, patient distress and discomfort. Much care provided in both the acute, rehabilitation and community setting is aimed at minimising the potentially harmful effects of four factors which lead to complications:

- *tissue injury* – to bone and/or soft tissue due to trauma or surgery
- *surgery* – the effects of anaesthesia and surgical procedures
- *reduced mobility* as a result of musculoskeletal conditions, injury or surgery and associated care
- *stasis* – of major body systems as a result of reduced mobility.

These issues are also mitigated by increasing age, with the older patient more likely to suffer from all complications. While there are a large number of potential complications for the orthopaedic and trauma patient, this chapter will focus on those which are either the most common or most dangerous.

Infection

The human body is constantly exposed to microorganisms both from the environment and those resident organisms which live naturally on or within the body, mostly without causing infection. Infections can occur whenever damaged or vulnerable tissue is exposed to harmful pathogens; leading to a complex tissue response brought about by the multiplication and attack by such microorganisms depending on the susceptibility of the patient and the virulence of the organism. Potentially harmful organisms such as bacteria, viruses and fungi may *contaminate* an area. Multiplication of the organisms may then lead to *colonisation*. Infection is not, however, considered to be present until attack from a pathogenic organism results in an acute or chronic tissue reaction. Bacteria may contaminate or colonise tissue without causing infection. When the patient's immune system is compromised due to factors such as ill health or depleted nutrition, colonisation is more likely to progress to *infection*.

Both tissue injury and infection result in an inflammatory reaction which is part of the human immune response. This is a distinct reaction brought about by both chemical and physical phenomena and results in the appearance of what are often called the 'cardinal' signs of inflammation/infection: redness, pain, swelling and heat. If the organism causing infection is 'pyogenic' (pus producing) collections of pus may also form as abscesses. There may also be increased exudate.

Orthopaedic and Trauma Nursing: An Evidence-based Approach to Musculoskeletal Care, First Edition. Edited by Sonya Clarke and Julie Santy-Tomlinson.

Infection is most often diagnosed through a detectable tissue response to microbial invasion. The symptoms of infection are a manifestation of the inflammatory response and vary according to the type of infection and the tissue or system affected, resulting in significant distress and discomfort for the patient. They can include:

- pain, swelling, redness and heat at the site of infection and/or in the surrounding area
- loss of function of the area affected, particularly if pain and/or swelling affect joints and other musculoskeletal structures
- tissue exudate which may or may not contain pus
- pyrexia and/or
- generally feeling unwell, with malaise or lethargy.

A diagnosis of infection should be made based on the manifested symptoms. This can be augmented, but not replaced by, culture and analysis of wound samples in the microbiology laboratory.

The orthopaedic and trauma patient is particularly vulnerable to the following types of infection:

- soft tissue infection, most often wound infection (Chapter 12) with surgical site and traumatic wound infection being a significant risk
- bone infection (osteomyelitis) and joint infection (infective arthritis) (Chapter 13)
- urinary tract infection and
- respiratory tract infection.

Healthcare-associated infection is the main cause of infection in orthopaedic and trauma patients, acquired by transfer from one person or surface to another. The way by which an infection can spread involves five links in the 'chain of infection (HPA 2013).' Understanding how the links are made is important in understanding the ways in which the chain can be broken and infection prevented:

1. *A causative organism* – a pathogenic organism is present which is capable of causing infection.
2. *A reservoir of infection* – a place (human or environmental) which provides ideal conditions for the causative organism to multiply including a supply of nutrients.
3. *A portal of exit* – allows the organism to leave the reservoir, e.g. in body fluids, on the skin (particularly the hands), in various body fluids such as respiratory droplets.
4. *A mode of transmission* – a method through which the organism is spread to another person and acquired by them. The most common methods of transfer are through body fluids, on the hands of patients and healthcare workers and ingestion along with airborne transmission of organisms during surgery.
5. *A susceptible patient* – who is vulnerable to infection because their immune response is compromised. This risk is greater in hopitalised patients, those who are injured and/or undergo surgery, those of greater or of very young age or with concurrent medical conditions that cause a reduction in the immune response and those who are malnourished.

The prevention of orthopaedic infections is particularly important because of the potentially devastating consequences of transfer of infection to bone and resultant osteomyelitis which is difficult to eradicate and results in long term pain and distress. The avoidance of osteomyelitis is a central aim of infection control in the orthopaedic and trauma setting. A major concern is the ability of remote infections such as urinary tract infections and surgical site infections to transfer to sites of orthopaedic implants as a result of 'seeding' of bacteria to implant sites.

The prevention and control of infection

Prevention and control of infection measures have been standardised as a result of a large body of amassed evidence which demonstrates the most effective approaches (See Box 9.1. for an example of evidence-based guidelines). These include the following (Pratt *et al.*, 2007):

- *Environmental hygiene* through rigorous cleaning processes
- *Hand hygiene*: many healthcare-associated infections are transferred from one person to the other on the hands of healthcare staff
- The use of *personal protective equipment* to provide a barrier between the healthcare provider and a source of infection
- The *safe use and disposal of sharps*: high risk of blood borne infection from accidental inoculation with contaminated sharps
- Preventing infections associated with the use of *short-term indwelling urethral catheters*, which provide a major portal for infection
- Preventing infections associated with *central venous catheters* – with a significant danger of blood-borne infection.

Evidence has shown that effective hand hygiene is the most effective method of preventing the transfer of infection. Compliance, however, is much lower than the

Box 9.1 Evidence digest

Evidence-based guidelines for preventing health-care associated infections

Many counties have developed national guidelines for the prevention of healthcare-associated infection. The 'epic 2' guidelines (Pratt *et al.*, 2007) provide an example from England. These were commissioned by the Department of Health (England) and revised, reviewed and updated in 2007. They were created by a nurse-led multi-professional team who undertook extensive consultation, using multiple systematic reviews of the evidence and other guidelines as well as expert opinion – demonstrating use of all levels of evidence available at that time.

The guidelines describe in detail the interventions and precautions practitioners should take to prevent HCAI, which include recommendations for:

- hospital environmental hygiene
- hand hygiene
- the use of personal protective equipment
- the safe use and disposal of sharps
- preventing infections associated with the use of short-term indwelling urethral catheters and
- preventing infections associated with central venous catheters.

These precautions are designed to break the 'chain of infection'. The authors point out that effective infection prevention and control are an essential feature of ensuring patient protection. The orthopaedic and trauma team should incorporate such national, regional and local guidelines into everyday practice in order to reduce the risk of infection during episodes of musculoskeletal care and intervention.

target of 100% (see Table 9.1 and Box 9.2) and measures must be taken to ensure that compliance is as high as possible (Tromp *et al.*, 2012). All staff should undergo regular education to support compliance and to ensure that skills are up to date and embedded in their practice.

Prophylactic prevention of infection, using antibiotics in the orthopaedic and trauma setting is standard practice and has been shown to reduce rates of infection where risk is high, such as in traumatic wounds and surgery which involves implantation (Gillespie and Walenkamp 2010). However, resistance is an increasing problem across all healthcare settings and the careful and prudent use of antibiotic therapy is increasingly important. This reinforces the need for measures which minimise all infections (Dohmen 2008).

Table 9.1 The 'five moments for hand hygiene' (WHO 2006). Reproduced with permission from the World Health Organisation

1 Before patient contact	When? Clean your hands before touching a patient when approaching him or her Why? To protect the patient against harmful germs carried on your hands
2 Before an aseptic task	When? Clean your hands immediately before any aseptic task Why? To protect the patient against harmful germs, including the patient's own germs, entering his or her body
3 After body fluid exposure risk	When? Clean your hands immediately after an exposure risk to body fluids (and after removing gloves) Why? To protect yourself and the healthcare environment from harmful patient germs
4 After patient contact	When? Clean your hands after touching a patient and his or her immediate surroundings when leaving Why? To protect yourself and the surroundings from harmful patient germs
5 After contact with patient suroundings	When? Clean your hands after touching any object or furniture in the patient's immediate surroundings, when leaving – even without touching the patient. Why? To protect yourself and the surroundings from harmful patient germs

Shock

Shock is a complex life-threatening state resulting in a significant reduction in systemic tissue perfusion and subsequent reduced oxygen (O_2) delivery to the tissues. Early recognition and management are vital in increasing the patient's chance of survival. This physiological syndrome creates cellular dysfunction with an imbalance between O_2 delivery and O_2 consumption. Oxygen deprivation leads to cellular hypoxia and derangement of critical cellular processes which can progress to organ failure and death (Kleinpell 2007). The circulatory system no longer sustains essential functions such as the provision of nutrients and O_2 to cells and removal of waste. Without intervention, the result is sequential cell death, end-organ damage, multi-system organ failure and death.

Garretson and Malberti (2007) describe four distinct stages of shock which are initially reversible but then rapidly become irreversible:

Box 9.2 Evidence digest

Study of hand hygiene compliance (Lee *et al.*, 2011). Reproduced with permission from Elsevier.

This large study (Lee *et al.*, 2011) was conducted in 33 surgical (including orthopaedic) departments across ten hospitals in nine countries. Hand hygiene practices using the 'five moments' for hand hygiene (WHO 2006) were examined in surgical wards using direct observation of practice by a standard method of observation developed by the World Health Organization. A minimum of 100 hand hygiene opportunities were observed in each department, resulting in a total of 4649 opportunities being observed by the study team. The statistical analysis showed that compliance with hand hygiene guidance ranged from 8% to 72% amongst medical staff and 15% to 84% amongst nurses. When staff had been exposed to risk (e.g. after touching a patient or being in contact with body fluids) the compliance rates were higher than before exposure such as touching a patient or undertaking a procedure. The authors argue that this shows that behavioural factors such as perceived risk to oneself have an impact on compliance.

Practices varied across hospitals in terms of whether handwashing was practised or hand rubbing (e.g. with alcohol gel). Higher workload was measured by nurse to patient ratios and was shown, as in many previous studies, to be a significant factor in hand hygiene compliance. There was no evidence, in this study, that recent educational campaigns had an effect on compliance.

The authors acknowledge that observational data may not be the most reliable and that other measures for compliance such as monitoring of dispenser use may be more accurate.

This study shows the relevance of healthcare staff's compliance with recommended hand-hygiene practice and demonstrates that there are a number of complex factors that result in lack of compliance, resulting in increased risk of infection for the patient.

Stage 1 Initial stage of shock This is reversible, but easily overlooked due to an absence of clinical signs to indicate impending shock. There is a reduction in cardiac output with a change from aerobic to anaerobic metabolism, which can lead to lactic acidosis (due to the inadequate clearance of lactic acid from the blood).

Stage 2 Compensatory stage of shock There is an attempt to regain homeostasis and improve the perfusion of tissues. The sympathetic nervous system produces catecholamine which dilates the bronchi and constricts peripheral blood vessels. Water conservation is initiated by the release of aldosterone by the adrenal/renal system.

Stage 3 Progressive stage of shock The body has lost the compensatory mechanism that sustains the perfusion of tissues, resulting in metabolic and repository acidosis along with electrolyte imbalance. There is a visible deterioration.

Stage 4 - Refractory stage of shock This presents with irreversible cellular and organ damage. The condition becomes unresponsive to treatment and death is imminent (Hand 2001).

Hypovolaemic shock (HS)

Hand (2001) defines hypovolaemic shock as:

> (a life threatening condition due to failure of the body to provide the tissues with sufficient oxygen and nutrients to meet cellular needs.) (p 45)

There is excessive fluid loss, (e.g. the blood loss from bleeding). Prevention requires ensuring adequate cardiac output and circulation volume. With a blood loss of 750 ml the body may enter the compensated stage and changes to vital signs will occur (Bench 2004). A 40% fluid loss threatens life.

The patient will present with:

- anxiety, restlessness and altered mental state due to decreased cerebral perfusion and subsequent hypoxia
- hypotension due to decreased circulatory volume
- rapid, weak, thready pulse and tachycardia due to decreased blood flow
- cool, clammy skin due to vasoconstriction
- mottled skin, especially in the fingers and toes due to insufficient perfusion
- rapid, deep respirations due to sympathetic nervous system stimulation and acidosis
- hypothermia resulting from decreased perfusion and evaporation of sweat
- thirst and dry mouth, due to reduced fluid and urinary output
- fatigue due to inadequate oxygenation
- systolic blood pressure <90 mm Hg or 40 mm Hg below baseline.

Management includes accurate patient assessment and fluid balance with fluid/blood replacement. Bleeding must be controlled to restore blood volume with infusions of hypertonic crystalloid solutions and/or blood products (Docherty 2002). Blood replacement with packed red cells is administered if there is blood loss to prevent hypoxia. Accurate fluid assessment and documentation are essential with accurate measurement and documentation of intake and output. Treatment can include vasopressors to stimulate contraction of the muscular tissues of the heart, capillaries and arteries. Physical assessment should not depend totally on the 'monitoring equipment' but 'looking' at the patient holistically – observing for the signs of shock. Supplementary oxygen may be prescribed to counteract the respiratory effects of shock.

Cardiogenic shock

Cardiogenic shock is associated with a decline in cardiac output and tissue hypoxia, despite adequate fluid volume. A damaged left ventricle is unable to pump effectively and cardiac output is reduced to less than 2.2 L/min (normal being 4–8 L/min) (Bench 2004). McLuckie (2003) reports the older female patient to be at a higher risk of developing this type of shock, as well as those with a history of MI and diabetes. It can be a complication of either acute myocardial infarction (MI) and other cardiac conditions, often resulting in death.

The clinical presentation is similar to hypovolaemic shock but the patient can deteriorate more quickly. There may be:

- Raised central venous pressure (CVP), chest pain, anxiety and feelings of doom and demise (Hand 2001). Pain relief and reducing anxiety will help reduce the patient's cardiac workload.
- Absent pulse with tachyarrhythmia.
- There may be evidence of distended jugular veins due to increased jugular venous pressure.

The main goal is to re-establish circulation to the myocardium, minimise heart muscle damage and improve the heart's effectiveness as a pump (Garretson and Malberti 2007). Evaluation of arterial blood gases (ABG) and cardiac monitoring are essential. Intervention includes oxygen therapy to reduce the workload of the heart by reducing tissue demands for blood flow. The myocardium can be reperfused by thrombolysis (e.g. injection of streptokinase). Early intervention is pivotal as the effect is reduced within hours of onset and development of shock. Mechanical vascularisation such as percutaneous coronary intervention (PCI) and coronary artery bypass grafting (CABG) (Man and Nolan 2006) is advocated for those patients less than 75 years (Sleeper *et al.*, 2005). The administration of cardiac drugs to increase the heart's pumping action is also used as a treatment option e.g. inotropics (e.g. Dopamine) and vasopressors (nitroglycerin).

Septic shock

Septic shock is a serious condition that occurs when an overwhelming infection leads to low blood pressure and low blood flow. The brain, heart, kidneys and liver may not work properly or fail. Sources of infection include septicaemia, osteomyelitis in bone, endocarditis and pericarditis of the heart, cellulitis and wound infections and urinary tract infections. The mortality rate is estimated to be around 40–50% (Oppert *et al.*, 2005). Early recognition may be difficult and the practitioner's role central in recognising condition changes and seeking medical attention.

A classic sign of septic shock is absolute and relative hypovolaemia (Garretson and Malberti 2007):

- absolute – result of vomiting, sweating or oedema
- relative – result of vasodilatation and peripheral blood pooling.

Presentation includes hypotension, altered coagulation, inflammation, impaired circulation at a cellular level, anaerobic metabolism, changes in mental status and multiorgan failure. There may also be alteration in coagulation due to the inflammatory response.

Fluid resuscitation is central in management, but fluid type remains under debate (Vincent and Gerlach 2004). Other treatment options include vasopressor therapy and continuous and accurate blood pressure (BP) monitoring using an arterial catheter. Blood transfusion may be necessary when central venous oxygen saturation is less than 70% and haematocrit less than 30%. Alternatively, if greater than 30% the inotrope Dobutamine may be used alongside supplemental O_2 therapy. It is necessary to identify and control/remove the source of infection and to administer antibiotics when a diagnosis has been confirmed, with drug type dependent on pathogen. However, controversy remains over the actual time frame. A broad spectrum antibiotic should be administered within three hours of entering an accident and emergency department (Garretson and Malberti 2007). Corticosteroid therapy may be used for the anti-inflammatory effect but high doses have not been shown to more effective (Oppert *et al.*, 2005).

A Surviving Sepsis Campaign (SCC) now common practice within UK hospitals was a 2002 initiative of the European Society of Intensive Care Medicine, the International Sepsis Forum, and the Society of Critical

Care Medicine. The 'bundles' approach is intended to simplify the complex processes of the care of patients with severe sepsis. This set of care interventions are derived from a collection of evidence-based practice guidelines. When implemented in their entirety they are likely to have an enhanced effect when compared to implementing each individual guideline The SSC aims to reduce mortality from sepsis via a multi-point strategy, primarily by:

- building awareness of sepsis
- improving diagnosis
- increasing the use of appropriate treatment
- educating healthcare professionals
- improving post-ICU care
- developing guidelines of care
- facilitating data collection for the purposes of audit and feedback.

For further information visit the http://www.surviving-sepsis.org website.

Venous thromboembolism

Venous thromboembolism (VTE) is a condition in which a blood clot (thrombus) forms in a vein. Blood flow through the affected vein can be limited by the clot, and may cause swelling and pain. Venous thrombosis occurs most commonly in the deep veins of the leg or pelvis; this is known as a deep vein thrombosis (DVT). An embolism occurs if all or a part of the clot breaks off from the site where it forms and travels through the venous system. If the clot lodges in the lung, a potentially serious and sometimes fatal condition, pulmonary embolism (PE) occurs. Venous thrombosis can occur in any part of the venous system. However, DVT and PE are the commonest manifestations of venous thrombosis. The term VTE embraces both the acute conditions of DVT and PE and also the chronic conditions which may arise after acute VTE, such as post-thrombotic syndrome and pulmonary hypertension; both problems being associated with significant ill-health and disability.

Orthopaedic patients are often predisposed to be at significant risk of developing a VTE due to the nature of their disease and condition. The most significant risk factors are outlined in the UK by the National Institute for Health and Clinical Excellence (NICE 2010):

- active cancer or cancer treatment
- age over 60 years
- critical care admission
- dehydration
- known thrombophilias
- obesity (body mass index [BMI] over 30 kg/m^2)
- one or more significant medical comorbidities (for example: heart disease; metabolic, endocrine or respiratory pathologies; acute infectious diseases; inflammatory conditions)
- personal history or first-degree relative with a history of VTE
- use of hormone replacement therapy
- use of oestrogen-containing contraceptive therapy
- varicose veins with phlebitis.

These risk factors are reflected globally and lead to 25 000 patient deaths per year in UK hospitals alone; the largest proportion of these deaths being in the orthopaedic patient (NICE 2010). There are three factors responsible for the development of VTE:

- venous stasis
- vein injury
- blood chemistry changes.

These factors were first described by Rudolph Virchow and are commonly referred to as 'Virchow's Triad'. It is now generally accepted that it is usually a combination of these factors that causes a thrombus to form, rather than one factor in isolation. The inherent impaired physical mobility and activity intolerance that affects orthopaedic patients gives rise to circulatory stasis. If they also have existing conditions of, or have experienced trauma, to the circulatory system and in addition have alterations in blood coagulation then they are in real danger of developing a VTE (Davis 2004a).

Although there have been numerous trials, there remains uncertainty about how to prevent VTE (NICE 2010, Davis 2004a). The true incidence of DVT and PE is very hard to calculate. More patients have less invasive surgery and emphasis is placed on early mobilisation and early discharge from hospital. Prophylaxis (both mechanical and pharmacological) is widely used, but practice varies and implementation is patchy. There is a strong sense that DVT and PE are less of a problem than they used to be in surgical patients but this may be hidden from the clinicians by early discharge rather than being truly reduced; 80% of DVT are subclinical and the average DVT occurs on the 7th postoperative day, often after the patient has left hospital (NICE 2010).

Risk assessment

The majority of hospitalised orthopaedic patients would be considered at risk of developing a VTE and should receive appropriate prophylactic interventions. Those in the community or following discharge are also at risk. Assessment is based on some, but not all, of the predisposing factors referred to previously. See NICE (2010) guidance on VTE in the hospitalised patient for a current example of a risk assessment tool for the UK. All surgical patients are recommended to be assessed.

Methods of prevention

Due to the characteristic uncertainty of the evidence currently available, prevention is contentious, but recommendations do exist that identify those preventative methods most likely to be successful. Guidance often relates to specific fields such as orthopaedics and even specific forms of surgery such as hip fracture and hip and knee replacement.

Pharmacological

These include (Autar 2009a):

- fondaparinux
- heparins
- vitamin K antagonists
- aspirin
- dabigatran
- rivaroxaban.

Mechanical

- anti-embolism or graduated compression stockings (Autar 2009b)
- intermittent pneumatic compression devices (Davis and O'Neill 2002)
- foot impulse devices (Davis and O'Neill 2002).

Care

- early mobilisation and leg exercises
- hydration (but through the oral route not intravenous).

Current guidelines recommend the use of these interventions in combination. They also increasingly highlight the patient's view such as the difficulty and discomfort associated with graduated compression stockings (NICE 2010). All prophylactic interventions carry risk as well as benefit and these must be balanced in any care decisions for individual patients. The risk of bleeding is an example with pharmacological interventions for VTE.

The linking of evidence through an EBP approach to orthopaedic nursing practice is well illustrated by the issue of VTE. Research, such as in areas of early mobilisation and hydration is often lacking or the research is so poor quality that it cannot be relied upon to direct practice decisions. Even when evidence is strong it has to be applied consistently and with knowledge and understanding. Davis (2004b) discusses ways in which the problems of translation and utilisation can be overcome with respect to VTE.

Fat embolism syndrome (FES)

The term 'fat embolism' (FE) denotes the presence of fat globules in the peripheral circulation and lung parenchyma most commonly following fracture of long bones, pelvis or other major trauma. 'Fat embolism syndrome' is a severe manifestation of FE where the patient presents with a triad of dyspnoea, petechiae (rash) and mental confusion. It is usually asymptomatic, but a few patients will develop signs and symptoms of multiorgan dysfunction, particularly involving the triad of lungs, brain and skin. A variety of theories to explain FES are reported within the literature. Jain *et al.* (2008) report three:

- *Mechanical theory* suggests a mechanical obstruction in the pulmonary capillaries resulting from fat emboli within the marrow or adipose tissue. Some fat particles then pass into the systemic circulation via cardiac or pulmonary routes to embolise in the renal, cerebral, skin or retinal capillaries.
- *Toxic theory* proposes that free fatty acids (FFA), released at the time of trauma or during breakdown of fat in the lung, directly affect the pneumocytes, resulting in an inflammatory response and acute respiratory distress syndrome. The FFA may originate from lipid stores mobilised by circulating catecholamines.
- *Obstructive theory* proposes that a chemical event at the trauma site releases mediators that affect the solubility of circulating lipids, resulting in coalescence and subsequent embolisation. Normally chylomicrons may coalesce into fat globules large enough to occlude pulmonary capillaries.

Risk factors include young age, closed and multiple fractures, conservative intervention for long bone fractures along with intramedullary nailing and nailing or reaming of medullary cavities. The clinical features of FES often develop 24–72 hours after trauma when fat droplets acting as emboli become impacted in the pulmonary microvasculature and other microvascular beds such as in the brain (Shaikh 2009). Long bone fractures should be reduced as soon as possible after injury and any reaming of the bone conducted with great care in an effort to prevent further emboli.

Reports of mortality and morbidity vary:

- A mortality rate of 5–15% is reported by Shaikh (2009) and Jain *et al.* (2008). It is also reported that, even with severe respiratory failure associated with FE, it seldom leads to death (Shaikh, 2009).
- Coma, ARDS, pneumonia and congestive heart failure are poor prognostic signs.
- Shaikh (2009) reports that patients with increased age and multiple co-morbidities and/or decreased physiologic reserves have worse outcomes.

Fat embolism occurs rarely in paediatric trauma patients. A 'lethal case report' discusses a case of FES in a nine-year-old boy after a direct blunt trauma and a pelvic fracture. On the second day post-trauma, the child showed signs of bowel perforation and septic shock which led to an acute aggravation of the pulmonary symptoms of FES, cardiac arrest and death – illustrating the potentially disastrous sequelae. The response to the case was to advocate prevention by early fracture stabilisation (Teeuwen *et al.*, 2009).

Diagnosis

Shaikh (2009) proposes that a high level of suspicion is needed to diagnose FES. A combination of clinical criteria and MRI of the brain will enable early and accurate diagnosis. The condition is commonly diagnosed on the basis of the clinical features and by excluding other causes. Gurd and Wilson's diagnostic criteria are shown in Box 9.3 where identification of FES requires the presence of at least one major criterion and at least four minor criteria.

Alternative diagnostic tools include:

- Schonfeld *et al.* (1983) proposed a quantitative measure to diagnose FES; a score of more than five points is required to diagnose FES. The measures include a scoring system where Petechiae is awarded 5 points, X-ray chest diffuse infiltrates 4, hypoxemia 3, with fever, tachycardia, tachypnoea and confusion all awarded a score of 1.
- According to Lindeque *et al.* (1987) FES can be diagnosed on the basis of respiratory system involvement alone, as noted in Box 9.4.

Laboratory findings will show: thrombocytopenia, anaemia, high ESR and fat macroglobulinaemia. A series of chest X-rays within 24–48 hours will show a 'snow storm' appearance and dilation of the right side of the heart (Shaikh 2009). CT findings may be normal or reveal haemorrhages consistent with microvascular injury.

Box 9.3 Signs of Fat Embolism Syndrome (Gurd and Wilson 1974. Reproduced with permission from The British Editorial Society of Bone & Joint Surgery.)

- *Major* signs:
  - petechial rash
  - respiratory insufficiency
  - cerebral involvement.
- *Minor* signs:
  - tachycardia >120BPM
  - fever >39.4°C
  - retinal signs – fat or petechiae
  - jaundice
  - renal signs – anuria/oliguria.

Box 9.4 Lindeque et al.'s criteria (1987). Reproduced with permission from The British Editorial Society of Bone & Joint Surgery

Sustained pO_2 < 8 kpa
Sustained pO_2 > 7.3 kpa
Sustained respiratory rate >35/min, in spite of sedation
Increased work of breathing, dyspnoea, tachycardia, anxiety

Interventions

Non-drug: High flow rate oxygen is given to maintain arterial tension within the normal range. Mechanical ventilation may be required, necessitating transfer to the intensive care unit. Restriction of fluids/use of diuretics can minimise fluid accumulation in the lungs as long as circulation is sustained. Maintenance of intravascular volume with 'IV' fluids or blood is vital as shock can exacerbate lung injury caused by FES.

Drugs: Heparin, steroids, alcohols and dextran have been reported to be ineffective by Enneking (1995). More recently Al-Khuwaitir *et al.* (2002) report a high dose of corticosteroids are effective in preventing FES. The use of steroids is a controversial issue (see Box 9.5 for exploration of the evidence).

Acute compartment syndrome

Compartment syndrome (ACS) is a clinical condition that occurs when there is an increase in pressure and/or a decrease in the size of a muscle compartment resulting in reduced capillary blood flow and leading to cell death. If the pressure is not relieved within hours, irreversible damage to the tissues and nerves may result in contractures, paralysis, loss of sensation

Box 9.5 Evidence digest. Reproduced with permission from Canadian Medical Association

Cochrane review library: Independent high quality evidence for health care decision making (Bederman *et al.*, 2009)

***Question**: Do corticosteroids reduce the risk of fat embolism syndrome in patients with long-bone fractures? A meta-analysis*

This systematic review of seven trials found that corticosteroids may be beneficial in preventing fat embolism syndrome and hypoxia in patients with long-bone fractures. The authors' conclusions are based on the evidence, but small sample sizes, randomisation failures and lack of generalisability to a modern multiple trauma setting engender some uncertainty in the reliability of the conclusions. Randomised and quasi-randomised trials of patients with at least one long-bone fracture that compared prophylactic corticosteroid intervention with no pharmacological treatment were included. Clinically important associated head, chest or abdominal injuries studies were excluded. Included patients were predominantly male, with mean age ranging from 22 to 42 years. Assessment of study quality considered the randomisation method and blinding of outcome assessors in addition to the use of a 21-point quality assessment scale converted to a score out of 100.

Six trials (389 patients) reported the primary outcome, with a further trial reporting mortality. Sample size ranged from 20 to 87 patients. There was considerable variation in both quality (two trials were quasi-randomised) and the dose and duration of corticosteroid treatment. Corticosteroids reduced the risk of fat embolism syndrome by 78%. Corticosteroids also reduced the risk of hypoxia by 61%, but did not have a statistically significant effect on petechiae, mortality or infection. No trials measured avascular necrosis. There were neither significant differences between subgroups based on dose, quality score, degree of blinding or randomization nor heterogeneity between trials.

The review suggested that corticosteroids may be beneficial in preventing fat embolism syndrome and hypoxia, but not mortality, in patients with long-bone fractures without increased risk of infection. A large RCT is required to corroborate the results of this meta-analysis. The authors concluded that no change in current practice is recommended.

and amputation (Judge 2007). The most common site is the anterior compartment of the lower leg. Any compartment can be affected, although the majority of cases present with a tibial fracture. The condition can be difficult to diagnose in all patients but especially in children, with delays in diagnosis leading to disastrous outcomes (Bae *et al.*, 2001).

The patient can present with ACS as a result of:

- *trauma* – fracture, haematoma, vascular damage, electrical injuries
- *oedema-related* – frostbite, burns
- *coagulopathies* – genetic, iatrogenic, acquired
- *other* – external compression.

In acute compartment syndrome, limb compression leads to local pressure with local tamponade (blockage). This results in capillary necrosis and oedema with increased compartment pressure and muscle ischaemia. This then leads to compartment tamponade, nerve injury and muscle infarction.

Symptoms can vary, but the patient will most often present with parasthesia, tingling and numbness as pressure increases within the compartment of the limb which will feel tense and warm on palpation. The skin will feel tight and appear shiny. Pain will usually appear '*out of proportion to the injury*' even at rest and can be elicited or worsened by passive stretching of the involved compartment. The pain may be throbbing, increases with elevation of the extremity and is unrelieved by opioids.

Late signs may include a pale limb, greyish or whitish in tone with a prolonged capillary refill time. In the latter stages the skin will feel cool on palpation with paralysis another late sign. The patient may also not respond to direct neural stimulation due to damage to the myoneural junction and a weak pulse or pulselessness to the effected limb. These late signs demonstrate that neurovascular and muscle damage have already occurred and the priority for the practitioner is to recognise the condition from the early signs so that permanent damage can be prevented.

Bandages and dressing should be removed if ACS is suspected and the limb should not be elevated even though this is a common principle of care for the orthopaedic/trauma patient with swelling and pain.

Measurement of the compartment (C) pressure is helpful but not standard practice in all clinical units. The normal resting pressure within a closed compartment varies with Edwards (2004) reporting 0–8 mm Hg and Nye (1996) 0–10 mm Hg. The pressure of a compartment can be established percutaneously using a wick/slit catheter or wick catheter attached to a pressure transducer. The Stryker intra-compartmental monitor system is commonly used in conjunction with an 18 gauge needle to determine C pressure. McQueen (1996) suggested that there is inadequate tissue perfusion when tissue pressure rises within compartment to within 30 mm Hg of the patient's diastolic B/P >30 mm Hg.

Neurovascular assessment

All patients who have a musculoskeletal injury, undergone orthopaedic surgery or cast immobilisation of a limb are at risk of developing neurovascular compromise which can lead to compartment syndrome. Peripheral neurovascular assessment involves the systematic assessment of the neurological and vascular integrity of a limb, with the aim of recognising any neurovascular deficit promptly (Judge 2007). Tissue damage deteriorates with time, therefore prompt identification and intervention is necessary. There does not however appear to be a consensus on best practice and frequency in completing and documenting neurovascular assessment with a view to reducing patient risk and promoting early identification of neurovascular compromise.

In keeping with the most common symptoms of ACS, Dykes (1993) recommends a 5-P approach to neurovascular assessment with a focus on:

- pain
- pulses
- pallor
- parasthesia
- paralysis.

Judge (2007) more recently recommends that neurovascular observations should include the assessment of pain, paralysis (movement), paraesthesia (sensation), presence of pulses and/or capillary refill and swelling. Pain is central to all neurovascular assessment as the most common, earliest and important presenting symptom of compartment syndrome. Empirical, review and discussion literature all suggests pain as the only true warning symptom of acute compartment syndrome. Grottkau *et al.*'s (2005) retrospective study of 133 cases of compartment syndrome reported that 90% of patients complained of pain. A multidimensional approach should be applied encompassing the use of a valid (ability to measure) and reliable (consistency) pain assessment tool (Clarke 2003). Shields and Clarke (2011) also recommend the use of a dedicated chart to record pain intensity and type, alongside warmth, sensation, colour, capillary refill time and the movement of the affected and unaffected limb as an important method of collecting and comparing data from baseline onwards.

A central aspect of care of the patient with suspected ACS is to treat any suspicion as a medical emergency requiring immediate medical attention. It is essential that the practitioner informs a senior member of medical staff immediately so that intervention can be instigated.

Surgical intervention

Fasciotomy is the management option of choice for ACS; the fascia is divided along the length of the compartment to release pressure. The pressure at which fasciotomy is performed is based on the clinical picture/rising pressure. Following the procedure the wound is usually left open for approximately five days until the soft tissues have recovered and swelling has begun to subside. Muscle and skin grafting may be required.

Urinary tract infection (UTI)

The urinary tract is the most common source of healthcare-associated infection. Because of stasis in the urinary system during anaesthesia, surgery and post-operative recovery the risk is high in all surgical patients and in those with restricted mobility. In the orthopaedic and trauma patient, such stasis may be prolonged.

The urinary tract is usually sterile above the distal 1 cm of the urethra although the perineum is colonised with resident bacteria from the skin and bowel which can gain entry through the urethral meatus. Emptying the bladder usually removes any potential pathogens (Weston 2008), but if the urethra is opened by a urethral catheter, a method of transmission for invading organisms to enter the bladder is provided. This risk of infection is, therefore, significantly increased by bladder catheterisation, so this should be avoided in orthopaedic patients because of the link between bacteriuria and implant site infection (Heaney 2011). It has been shown that the longer the catheter is in situ, the greater the likelihood of UTI (Stephan *et al.*, 2008). If there are unavoidable reasons for catheterisation (e.g. urinary retention) it is essential that a closed drainage system is maintained with meticulous regard for hygiene and asepsis during insertion of the catheter and subsequent care and that the catheter is removed as soon as possible. Other risk factors for UTI include dehydration and this is one of many reasons for ensuring that adequate oral or intravenous fluids are administered.

The prevention of UTI involves early mobilisation and ensuring that the patient has good fluid balance in order to reduce urinary stasis and ensure that urine does not become concentrated. Older people sometimes voluntarily restrict fluid intake as do those with any degree of urinary incontinence or difficulty in getting to the toilet and it is important to discuss the implications of this with the patient. There is some limited evidence that drinking cranberry juice prevents UTI, but the amount that is required and the timing is uncertain (Jepson and Craig 2009). It is possible that the right amount of any oral fluid is useful and the presence of a moderate amount of vitamin C in cranberry and other fruit juice is also beneficial in supporting the immune system as a whole. Ensuring a good standard of perineal/penile hygiene, especially in the immobile patient, is also important as is early mobilisation and a return to normal toileting habits as soon as possible. Research also suggests that the existence of a UTI pre-operatively can predispose the patient to surgical site infection (SSI) following orthopaedic surgery even if there are no symptoms (Ollivere *et al.*, 2008). This confirms the possibility of UTI as a remote source for SSI and possible implant infection and highlights the need for preoperative screening for UTI by urinalysis (identifying protein and blood).

Identifying and treating UTI as early as possible is essential in order to prevent any likely transmission to remote sites and to the ureters and kidneys. The main symptoms which might alert the practitioner to the presence of UTI are:

- a need to urinate frequently – often passing small amounts
- pain on passing urine
- lower abdominal/pubic pain.

The first two are less likely to be evident in the patient with an indwelling urinary catheter and other symptoms might include pyrexia, general feeling of being unwell and mild to severe confusional state/delirium. The presence of blood or protein on urinalysis is also indicative of infection. If UTI is suspected a mid-stream sample of urine should be taken for culture and sensitivity.

Treatment of UTI involves treatment with an appropriate course of antibiotics along with adequate pain relief and good oral or 'IV' hydration.

Urinary retention

A significant reason for urinary catheterisation in the orthopaedic patient is urinary retention which is frequently reported following orthopaedic surgery. It is defined as an inability to pass urine even though the patient has a full bladder. This can result in a great deal of pain and distress for the patient and can lead to bladder distention and urinary tract infection. Retention can also lead to UTI, adverse autonomic responses such as vomiting, hypotension and cardiac dysrhythmia and permanent damage to the bladder with resultant future urinary problems (Baldini *et al.*, 2009). Early recognition of the problem is, therefore, essential and should be included as an aim for all postoperative care. There is no evidence that routine catheterisation intraoperatively as a method of prevention is beneficial and the risk of haematogenous spread of infection to the surgical site is too great for this to be advised.

The main symptom of urinary retention is pain and discomfort in the lower part of the abdomen in a patient who is unable to pass urine in spite of good fluid balance. This can, however, be masked postoperatively by the effects of general and regional anaesthesia, nerve blockade and analgesia. Bladder catheterisation can also be used as a method of assessing bladder volume and diagnosing retention through measurement of residual volume of urine. This, however, carries with it the risk of infection associated with perurethral catheterisation. The literature suggests that the use of nurse-led ultrasound to assess bladder volume is a relatively simple and appropriate way for the practitioner to monitor bladder volume and identify retention whilst avoiding unnecessary catheterisation (Edmond 2009).

Once retention has been identified, the treatment usually involves bladder catheterisation. It is recommended that this is done as an in-out catheterisation rather than with an indwelling catheter and that antibiotic prophylaxis is essential (Baldini *et al.*, 2009). It may be necessary for the bladder volume to be monitored for up to 48 hours postoperatively, but most problems tend to resolve once the patient begins to mobilise and is able to visit the toilet to void.

Respiratory tract infection

Pneumonia (lower respiratory tract infection) is a potentially fatal hospital-acquired infection in orthopaedic and trauma patients. It is the most common cause of hospital deaths for patients following hip fracture. Mucosal surfaces in the respiratory tract contain large numbers of resident flora which combat pathogenic attack. The upper respiratory tract is lined with ciliated epithelium which, along with the cough reflex, helps to expel bacteria (Weston 2008) and other particles. It is when these mechanisms are suppressed that the patient is prone to respiratory tract infection. Inhaled pathogens are able to combat these mechanisms and reach the lungs. Patients who have undergone surgery or suffered trauma are at risk. The risk is also increased by advanced age, concurrent medical conditions, general anaesthesia, depleted nutrition and immobility.

Measures for prevention of respiratory tract infection in the orthopaedic patient include:

- avoidance of elective surgery in patients with pre-existing respiratory infections (usually viral) through preoperative screening
- post-operative pain relief to facilitate coughing and deep breathing
- early post-operative mobilisation
- since chest infection is often hospital-acquired, universal infection control precautions are an essential aspect of prevention.

Observation of the at-risk patient for symptoms of pneumonia is essential in enabling early management. Symptoms may be insidious or develop quite suddenly and include:

- shortness of breath/rapid and/or shallow breathing
- a cough which may or may not be productive initially
- sputum which may be yellow, green, brown or blood stained – a specimen should be obtained for culture
- chest pain
- pyrexia
- tachycardia
- acute confusion
- general malaise and fatigue
- loss of appetite.

A diagnosis of pneumonia is made based on the above symptoms along with chest auscultation (abnormal lung sounds can be hard) and chest X-ray (demonstrating lung consolidation). There will also be a raised white cell count. A positive sputum culture will help to identify the causative organism and direct treatment.

Management of pneumonia should be commenced immediately due to the potentially life-threatening nature of the infection. This should include the following considerations:

- Antibiotic therapy according to the nature and sensitivity of the pathogen causing the pneumonia. The timeliness and appropriateness of this is central to the recovery of the patient along with other supporting measures but may be complex if a resistant strain of bacteria is the causative organism.
- Constant monitoring of vital signs of the patient with a view to detecting and acting upon any further deterioration.
- Maintenance of hydration using intravenous infusion of fluids if necessary.
- Optimum nutrition – using nutritional supplementation, nasogastric or enteral feeding as necessary.
- The patient should be cared for sitting up or in the semi-recumbent position, providing their orthopaedic condition allows.
- Deep breathing exercises and chest physiotherapy.

Constipation

Constipation is a very common and significant complication which can either be acute or chronic. In the orthopaedic and trauma patient it is often caused by a decrease in bowel action due to a combination of factors that lead to hard, dry stools that are difficult and/or painful to pass. The problem is defined by the patient and may include what they feel to be 'unsatisfactory' or incomplete defecation. Constipation is known to be more common in women, possibly due to hormonal factors. Although it is thought there is a link between the incidence of constipation and increasing age, this is most likely because of the greater incidence of other precipitating factors in older people. Some other common causes of constipation in the orthopaedic and trauma patient include:

- *Dehydration* – leading to desiccated stools.
- *Reduced mobility* – resulting in weakness in the accessory muscles which help bowel evacuation.
- *Reduced or changed dietary intake* – resulting in a diet which is depleted or lacking in fibre.
- *Pharmacological agents* – one of the main side effects of many drugs is constipation: in the orthopaedic and trauma patient both opioid and non-opioid analgesic agents are implicated, but other drugs such as antidepressants can also contribute to because of the slowing effect on peristaltic action (Richmond and Wright 2004).

Hospitalised patients and those reliant on others for toileting needs often resist the urge to pass bowel movements because of embarrassment or pain associated with the required activity – particularly if they require a bed pan (Cohen 2009). Because of embarrassment patients may not be willing to inform a health professional of the problem. These are issues which it is essential the practitioner is sensitive to.

Impaction, where faeces become trapped in the lower part of the large bowel, is very distressing for the patient. The most serious consequence of untreated constipation and impaction is bowel obstruction by a volvulus which becomes a surgical emergency and can be fatal. It is essential that this is avoided through careful assessment and prevention.

The most important aspect of the prevention and management of constipation is the early and continuous assessment of bowel activity. Because nearly all orthopaedic and trauma patients have at least one risk factor for constipation and because of the reluctance of patients to discuss difficulties with the nurse it is essential that a proactive daily assessment of bowel activity is made. Box 9.6 discusses evidence related to the development of a constipation risk assessment scale. 'Normal' bowel habits vary from one person to another and the practitioner must take this into account when assessing bowel function – considering the patients' normal frequency of opening their bowels. If constipation lasts more than a few weeks and/or is associated with other symptoms such as abdominal mass/pain or blood in the stools, then a medical referral is made to rule out other more serious causes of constipation.

Proactive prevention of constipation is an important aspect of the care of the orthopaedic and trauma patient. It is important that this is incorporated into the standard care of all patients at risk of constipation and is not left until constipation has begun to occur. Prevention involves management of the causes and risk factors for constipation. This generally includes helping to provide conditions for toileting routines which are as near to normal for the patient as possible with due consideration of privacy and position:

- *Monitor* – daily assessment and recording of bowel activity.
- *Diet* – ensuring the diet contains or is supplemented with foodstuffs high in dietary fibre.
- *Hydration* – ensuring that the patient takes plenty of oral fluids.
- *Exercise* – within the limits and abilities of the patient; when unable to walk there may be benefit from abdominal exercise such as pelvic tilt (JBI 2008).

It is important that any tendency to constipation is managed as soon as possible after symptoms occur. The management of constipation generally involves the use of pharmacological laxatives. There are several different types of laxative which work in different ways:

- *Bulking agents* – contain fibrous material which absorb water in the bowel and make stools softer.
- *Peristaltic stimulants* – useful where peristaltic action is reduced.
- *Osmotic laxatives* – encourage the absorption of fluid into the stools.
- *Stool softeners* – lubricate and moisten stools.

Box 9.6 Evidence digest. Reproduced with permission from John Wiley & Sons

Developing and validating a constipation risk assessment scale (Richmond and Wright 2004, 2006 and 2008)

Richmond and Wright (2004, 2006 and 2008) undertook the development and validation of a constipation risk assessment scale and published their findings in a series of three papers:

The first paper (Richmond and Wright 2004) outlines a literature review which aimed to identify the risk factors for constipation so that these could inform the development of an assessment tool using standard literature search and review processes – an important first step in tool development.

The second paper (Richmond and Wright 2006) reports on the development of a constipation risk assessment scale based on the previous literature review. The independent variables for constipation were allocated a score that reflected their relative contribution to the development of constipation. The risk factors were then organised to produce a user-friendly and comprehensive tool. The tool was subjected to content and face validity assessment and the instrument modified accordingly.

The third paper in the series (Richmond and Wright 2008) aimed to test the reliability of the instrument developed in the 2006 study. Tests for stability, equivalence and internal consistency showed that the tool was stable over the passage of time and provided equivalent results when different raters used the tool. Construct validity was assessed by contrasting constipated and non-constipated subjects.

Although this work was based on work with patients with cancer, it is relevant to the orthopaedic and trauma patient in that it demonstrates how a reliable and valid instrument can be developed that can help practitioners to identify those patients most at risk of constipation so that preventive action can be taken.

When constipation is opiate-induced it is advisable to begin treatment with a combination of an osmotic laxative and a peristaltic stimulant. If this treatment fails to resolve constipation or faecal impact is suspected, treatment with suppositories or enemas along with peristaltic stimulants may be required.

Recommended further reading

Dellinger, R.P., Levy, M.M., Rhodes, A. *et al.* (2013) Surviving Sepsis Campaign: International guidelines for management of severe sepsis and septic shock: 2012. *Critical Care Medicine*, **41**(2), 580–637.

Hilton, A.K., Pellegrino, V.A. and Scheinkestel, C.D. (2008) Avoiding common problems associated with intravenous fluid therapy. *The Medical Journal of Australia*, **189**, 509–513.

National Institute for Health and Clinical Excellence (NICE) (2010) *Venous thromboembolism: Reducing the Risk*. CG92 Available at: http://guidance.nice.org.uk/CG92/NICEGuidance/pdf/English (accessed 30 March 2014).

Royal College of Nursing (RCN) (2013) *Right Blood, Right Patient, Right Time: RCN Guidance for Improving Transfusion Practice*. London: RCN. Available at: http://www.rcn.org.uk/__data/assets/pdf_file/0009/78615/002306.pdf (accessed 30 March 2014).

References

Al-Khuwaitir, T.S., Al-Moghairi, I.M., Sherbeeni, M.N. and Subh, H.M. (2002) Traumatic fat embolism. *Saudi Medical Journal*, **22**(12), 1532–1536.

Autar, R. (2009a) New oral anticoagulants to revolutionise VTE management. *Journal of Orthopaedic Nursing*, **13**, 165–171.

Autar R (2009b) A review of the evidence for the efficacy of anti-embolism stockings in VTE prevention. *Journal of Orthopaedic Nursing*, **13**, 41–49.

Bae, D., Kadiyala, K. and Waters, P. (2001) Acute compartment syndrome in children: contemporary diagnosis, treatment, and outcome. *Journal of Pediatric Orthopaedics*, **21**(5), 680–688.

Baldini, G., Hema, B., Aprikian, A. and Carli, F. (2009) Postoperative urinary retention: anaesthetic and perioperative considerations. *Anesthesiology*, **110**(5), 1139–1157.

Bederman, S.S, Bhandari M., McKee M.D. and Schemitsch, E.H. (2009) Do corticosteroids reduce the risk of fat embolism syndrome in patients with long bone fractures. A meta-analysis. *Canadian Journal of Surgery*, **52**(5), 386–393.

Bench, S. (2004) Assessing and treating shock: an evidenced based review. *British Journal of Nursing*, **13**(12), 715–721.

Clarke, S.E. (2003) Orthopaedic paediatric practice: an impression pain assessment. *Journal of Orthopaedic Nursing* **7**(3), 132–136.

Cohen, S. (2009) Orthopaedic patient's perceptions of using a bed pan. *Journal of Orthopaedic Nursing*, **13**(2), 78–84.

Davis, P. (2004a) Venous thromboembolism prevention – an update. *Journal of Orthopaedic Nursing*, **8**: 50–56.

Davis, P. (2004b) A critical exploration of practice improvement with reference to VTE prevention. *Journal of Orthopaedic Nursing*, **8**: 208–214.

Davis, P. and O'Neill, C. (2002) The potential benefit of pneumatic compression in the prevention of DVT. *Journal of Orthopaedic Nursing*, **6**, 95–100.

Docherty, B. (2002) Cardiorespiratory physical assessment for the acutely ill: Part 1. *British Journal of Nursing*, **11**(11), 750–758.

Dohmen, P.M. (2008) Antibiotic resistance in common pathogens reinforces the need to minimize surgical site infections. *Journal of Hospital Infection*, **70**(52), 15–20.

Dykes, P.C. (1993) Minding the five P's of neurovascular assessment. *American Journal of Nursing*, **93**(6), 38–39.

Edmond, L. (2006) A brief literature search and clinical audit of postoperative urinary retention following total joint replacement. *Journal of Orthopaedic Nursing*, **10**(22), 77–72.

Edwards, S. (2004) Acute compartment syndrome. *Emergency Nurse*, **12**(3), 32–38.

Enneking, F.K. (1995) Cardiac arrest during total knee replacement. *Journal of Clinical Anaesthesia* **7**(3), 253–263.

Garretson, S. and Malberti, S. (2007) Understanding hypovolaemic, cardiogenic and septic shock. *Nursing Standard*, **50**(21), 46–55.

Gillespie, W.J. and Walenkamp, G.H.I.M. (2010) Antibiotic prophylaxis for surgery for proximal femoral and other closed long bone fractures. *Cochrane Database of Systematic Reviews* **3** (Art. No.: CD000244). DOI: 10.1002/14651858.CD000244.pub2.

Grottkau, B.E., Epps, H.R. and DiScala, C. (2005) Compartment syndrome in children and adolescents. *Journal of Pediatric Surgery*, **40**(4), 678–682.

Gurd, A.R. and Wilson, R.E. (1974) The FES. *Journal of Bone and Joint Surgery (British)*, **56**, 408–416.

Hand, H. (2001) Shock. *Nursing Standard*, **15**(48), 45–52.

Health Protection Agency (HPA) (2013) *General Information on Healthcare Associated Infections (HCAI)*. Available at: http://www.hpa.org.uk/Topics/InfectiousDiseases/InfectionsAZ/HCAI/GeneralInformationOnHCAI/ (accessed 10 May 2014).

Heaney, F. (2011) Nurse decision to insert a urinary catheter in a female patient in orthopaedic specialty: the development of a protocol to guide care. *International Journal of Orthopaedic and Trauma Nursing*, **15**(4), 212–219.

Jain, S., Nagpure P.S., Singh R. and Garg, D. (2008) Minor trauma triggering cervicofacial necrotizing fasciitis from odontogenic abscess. *Journal of Emergency Trauma Shock*, **1**, 114–118.

Jepson, R.G., Williams, G. and Craig, J.C. (2012) Cranberries for preventing urinary tract infections. *Cochrane Database of Systematic Reviews* **10**(Art. No.: CD001321). DOI: 10.1002/14651858.CD001321.pub5.

Joanna Briggs Institute (JBI) (2008) *Management of Constipation in Older Adults*. Best Practice **12**(7). Available at: http://connect.jbiconnectplus.org/ViewSourceFile.aspx?0=45 (accessed 30th March 2014).

Judge, N.L. (2007) Neurovascular assessment. *Nursing Standard*, **21**(45), 39–44.

Kleinpell, R.M. (2007) Recognising and treating five stages of shock states cited in Garretson, S. and Malberti, S. (2007) Understanding hypovolaemic, cardiogenic and septic shock. *Nursing Standard*, **50**(21), 46–55.

Lee, A., Chalfine, A., Daikos, G.L. *et al.* (2011) Hand hygiene practice and adherence determinants in surgical wards across Europe and Israel: A multicenter observational study. *American Journal of Infection Control*, **39**(6), 517–520.

Lindeque, B.G., Schoeman,H.S., Dommissen, G.F., Boeyens, M.C. and Vlok, A.L. (1987) Fat embolism syndrome: a double blind therapeutic study. *Journal of Bone and Joint Surgery (British)*, **69B**(1), 128–131.

Man, H.J. and Nolan, P.E. (2006) Update on the management of cardiogenic shock. *Current Opinion in Critical Care*, **12**(5), 431–436.

McLuckie, A. (2003) Shock: an overview, in *Oh's Intensive Care Manual*, 5th edn (eds Oh, T.E., Bernsren, A.D. and Soni, N.) Butterwort Heinemann, London, pp. 71–77.

McQueen, M.M., Christie. J. and Court-Brown, C.M. (1996) Acute compartment syndrome in tibial diaphyseal fractures. *Journal of Bone and Joint Surgery (British)*, **78**(1), 95–98.

National Institute for Health and Clinical Excellence (NICE) (2010) Venous thromboembolism; Reducing the risk. CG92. Available at: http://guidance.nice.org.uk/CG92/NICEGuidance/pdf/English (accessed 30 March 2014).

Nye, P.J. (1996) Complications in *NAON Core Curriculum for Orthopaedic Nursing*, 3rd edn. National Association of Orthopaedic Nurses, Pitman, NJ.

Ollivere, B.J., Ellahee, N., Logan, K., Miller-Jones, J.C.A. and Allen, P.W. (2008) Asymptomatic urinary tract colonisation predisposes to superficial wound infection in elective orthopaedic surgery. *International Orthopaedics*, **33**(3), 848–850.

Oppert, M., Schilnder, R. and Husung, C. (2005) Low dose hydrocortisone improves shock reversal and reduces cytokine levels in early hyperdrynamic septic shock. *Critical Care Medicine*, **33**(11), 2457–2464.

Pratt, R.J. Pellowe, C.M. and Wilson, J.A., (2007) Epic 2: National evidence-based guidelines for preventing healthcare-associated infections in NHS hospitals in England. *Journal of Hospital Infection*, **65**(Suppl 1), S1–S64.

Richmond, J.P. and Wright, M.E., (2004) Review of the literature on constipation to enable development of constipation risk assessment scale. *Journal of Orthopaedic Nursing*, **8**(4), 192–207.

Richmond, J.P. and Wright. M.E. (2006) Development of a constipation risk assessment scale. *Journal of Orthopaedic Nursing*, **10**(4), 186–197.

Richmond, J.P. and Wright, M.E. (2008) Establishing reliability and validity of a constipation risk assessment scale. *Journal of Orthopaedic Nursing*, **12**(3–4), 129–150.

Schonfeld, S.A., Ploysongsang, Y., DiLisio, R. *et al.* (1983) Fat embolism prophylaxis with corticosteroid: a prospective study in high-risk patients. *Annals of Internal Medicine*, **99**(4), 438–443.

Shaikh, N. (2009) Emergency management of fat embolism syndrome. *Journal of Emergency Trauma Shock*, **2**(1), 29–33.

Shields, C. and Clarke, S. (2011) Neurovascular observation and documentation for children within accident and emergency: a critical review. *International Journal of Orthopaedic and Trauma Nursing*, **15**(1), 3–10.

Sleeper, L.A., Ramanathan, K. and Picard, M.H. (2005) Functional status and quality of life after emergency revascularization for cardiogenic shock complicating acute myocardial infarction. *Journal of American College of Cardiology*, **46**(2), 266–273.

Stephan, F., Sax, H., Wachsmuth, M. *et al.* (2006) Reduction of urinary tract infection and antibiotic use after surgery: a controlled, prospective before-after intervention study. *Clinical Infectious Diseases*, **41**(1 June), 1544–1551.

Teeuwen, P.H., Sloots, P.C., de Blauw, I., Wijnen, R. and Biert, J. (2009) A lethal case of fat embolism syndrome in a nine-year-old child: options for prevention. *European Journal of Trauma and Emergency Surgery*, **35**(3), 311–313.

Tromp, M., Huis, A., de Guchteneire, I. *et al.* (2012) The short-term and long-term effectiveness of a multidisciplinary hand hygiene improvement program. *American Journal of Infection Control*, **40**(8), 732–736.

Vincent, J.L. and Gerlach, H. (2004) Fluid restriction in severe sepsis and septic shock: an evidenced based review. *Critical Care Medicine*, **32**(11), 451–454.

Weston, D. (2008) *Infection Prevention and Control. Theory and Clinical Practice for Healthcare Professionals*. John Wiley and Sons, Chichester.

World Health Organization (WHO) (2006) *Your Five Moments for Hand-hygiene*. Version 1. WHO, Geneva. Available at: http://www.who.int/gpsc/tools/5momentsHandHygiene_A3.pdf (accessed 30th March 2014).

CHAPTER 10

Nutrition and hydration

Rosemary Masterson

Cappagh National Orthopaedic Hospital, Finglas, Dublin, Ireland

Introduction

Nutrition and hydration are influenced by many factors. These include cultural, personal and psychological (beliefs, attitudes and emotions), biological and physiological (age, gender, pregnancy, activity), socio-economic (availability and cost), cultural and religious, educational (nutritional knowledge), extrinsic (media, time, foods in season) and food (taste and appearance) (Geissler and Powers 2005). Good nutrition plays an important role in recovery from orthopaedic injury or surgery. Musculoskeletal health can be impacted upon by poor nutrition; failure to get enough nutrients can lead to poor skeletal tissue development or rickets while the impact of a poor quality diet can contribute to obesity or osteoporosis. Poor nutrition can increase the healing time in wounds and fractures, increase the risk of infection, decrease muscle strength plus leading to constipation and delayed recovery. This can prolong the treatment and may prevent the patient returning to work or to independent living while increasing the cost to the patient and the health service.

Maintaining good hydration is also critical to maintaining good health and especially with advancing age. Poor hydration can lead to multiple problems, tendons and ligaments become less resilient, repeated urinary tract infections, constipation and fatigue can occur. Dehydration can delay recovery and discharge.

This chapter will examine the role of diet in musculoskeletal health, discuss the metabolic response of the body to trauma and surgery, analyse the importance of a nutritional assessment, the subsequent interventions and the role of hydration and dehydration.

Diet and musculoskeletal health

Healthy eating requires planning and knowledge. A balanced diet is essential for health and provides the appropriate amount of nutrients needed to meet the requirements of the body. This can be achieved by eating a variety of foods with no single food having the correct proportions of all essential nutrients. If a deficiency or an excess of a nutrient is consumed, it can have an impact on health; potentially leading to obesity, anaemia, rickets or osteoporosis. A well balanced diet containing the major components is important in maintaining musculoskeletal health, preventing disease and promoting recovery and healing.

Energy is central to recovery and healing and consideration should be given to the amount of energy required to meet individual needs. Several factors can influence daily energy requirements; for example age, gender, activity levels and basal metabolic rate.

Basal metabolic rate refers to activity within the body that maintains function (e.g. respiratory function, cardiac function, body temperature) and is affected by:

- ***metabolism*** – the processing of nutrients within our bodies.
- ***catabolism*** – the reactions that release energy and
- ***anabolism*** – the building of new tissue.

Energy requirements increase depending on demand, for example while a fracture is healing or an infection is present. Recommended daily amounts of all nutrients, including energy, are based on the average healthy adult and need to be adjusted for the individual.

Six major dietary components are considered essential: carbohydrates, fats, proteins, vitamins, minerals and

Orthopaedic and Trauma Nursing: An Evidence-based Approach to Musculoskeletal Care, First Edition. Edited by Sonya Clarke and Julie Santy-Tomlinson.

water. Carbohydrates, proteins and fat are called macronutrients and are required in larger amounts than the micronutrients (vitamins and minerals). Although micronutrients are required in smaller amounts, they remain essential for metabolism, normal growth and well-being.

Carbohydrates are mainly made up of sugars and starches. They are essential in providing energy and heat, sparing the use of protein to provide energy and as an energy store (as glycogen and fat) when eaten in excess of needs.

Fats provide energy and are made up of different types of fatty acids, some of which are essential for health in small amounts. Fatty acids are classified as saturated, monounsaturated or polyunsaturated depending on their structure. Fats are a carrier for fat-soluble vitamins and are necessary for their absorption. A high intake of saturated or trans fatty acids can have adverse effects on health.

Proteins are essential for growth and repair of tissues and cells and play a role in the production of enzymes, plasma proteins, immunoglobulins and some hormones. They also are involved in the provision of energy (when there is not enough carbohydrate in the diet).

Vitamins are chemical compounds required in small quantities and are divided into two groups; the fat soluble vitamins (D, A, E & K) and the water soluble vitamins (B & C). Vitamins relevant to musculoskeletal health include:

- **Vitamin D** regulates calcium and phosphate metabolism by increasing their absorption from the gut and stimulating their retention by the kidneys, promoting the calcification of bones. A deficiency in children can cause rickets and osteomalacia in adults. Vitamin D is manufactured in the skin through exposure to sunlight and/or obtained in the diet from sources such as eggs, butter, cheese and fish liver oils. Cereals and margarine are fortified with vitamin D. Some groups of people such as those of Asian descent, black people, older, institutionalised and housebound people and those who habitually cover the skin (for religious reasons) are vulnerable to vitamin D deficiency as a result of limited exposure to sunlight.
- **Vitamin A** (retinol/carotenoids) is found in whole milk, egg yolks, liver, fish oil, cheese, butter, carrots, dark leafy green vegetables and orange-coloured fruits (e.g. mangos and apricots). It is responsible for cell growth and differentiation, promotion of immunity, as a defence against infection and promotion of growth in bones. Large amounts of retinol can cause bone damage. Some food products are now fortified with vitamin A such as margarine and reduced fat spreads.
- **Vitamin B complex** is divided into B_1, B_2, B_3, B_6, B_{12}, folate, pantothenic acid and biotin. Thiamin (vitamin B_1) is found in nuts, yeast, egg yolk, liver, legumes and meat. Deficiency can result in severe muscle wasting, delayed growth in children and increased susceptibility to infections. Other B vitamins do not impact directly on musculoskeletal health but have an effect on health generally.
- **Vitamin C** is found in fresh fruit and green vegetables. It is associated with protein metabolism e.g. laying down of collagen fibres in connective tissue. A deficiency can delay wound healing and inhibit bone repair.

Minerals are inorganic substances required by the body in small amounts for a variety of different functions. They are involved in the formation of bones and teeth, are essential constituents of body fluids and tissues and are components of enzyme systems. They are also involved in normal nerve function. Minerals relevant to musculoskeletal health include:

- **Calcium** is the most abundant mineral in the human body and is found in dairy products, eggs, green vegetables and some fish (e.g. sardines). An adequate supply is obtained from a well-balanced diet but certain groups can require more such as teenagers and pregnant or nursing mothers. It is absorbed from the intestines and is an essential structural component of bone where we find approximately 99% of our calcium (with the other 1% found in blood). Calcium is required for vascular contraction and vasodilation, muscle function, nerve transmission, intracellular activity and hormonal secretion. It also provides rigidity in bones in the form of calcium phosphate. Calcium regulation is controlled by the action of parathyroid hormone, vitamin D and calcitonin (Geissler and Powers 2005) with less than 1% of vitamin D and calcitonin needed to support metabolic function. As it is tightly regulated, the levels in the body do not fluctuate with dietary changes; instead the body uses bone tissue as a source of calcium to maintain concentrations. A negative calcium balance occurs when net calcium absorption fails to compensate for urinary calcium losses. Signs of calcium deficiency include stunted growth, poor quality bones,

Table 10.1 Daily recommended intake of calcium in healthy subjects (Office of Dietary Supplements (US), 2012). Reproduced with permission from US Federal Government

Age	Calcium intake (mg)	
	Male	Female
0–6 months	200	200
7–12 months	260	260
1–3 years	700	700
4–8 years	1000	1000
9–13 years	1300	1300
14–18 years	800	800
19–50 years	1000	1000
51–70 years	1000	1200
71 plus	1200	1200

Pregnant and lactating women in the age group of 14–18 years and 19–50 years should take the recommended intake for that group.

Table 10.2 Daily recommended intake of calcium (Expert group on Vitamins and Minerals 2003). Reproduced with permission from Food Standards Agency

Age	Calcium intake (mgs)
1– 3 years	350
4–6 years	450
7–10 years	550
11–18 years (girls)	800
11–18 years (boys)	1000
19–50 years	700
50 + years	700
Pregnant women	700
Breastfeeding women	As per the above recommendations for their age group plus an additional 550 mg

teeth and bone malformation. Bone undergoes continuous remodelling with constant resorption and deposition into new bone. The balance between these two actions can change with age. For example, in a period of growth (in children and adolescents), formation exceeds absorption. In adulthood both actions are relatively equal but in the aging population, particularly post-menopausal women, bone resorption exceeds formation resulting in bone loss and an increased risk of osteoporosis. During these periods, this results in a change in the recommended daily intake. Recommended daily calcium intakes vary from country to country. The recommended daily intake for the USA and United Kingdom are shown in Tables 10.1 and 10.2.

- **Phosphorus** is essential for skeletal development and is found in cheese, oatmeal, liver and kidney. It is also added to foods and drinks such as cola as polyphosphates or phosphoric acid. Where there is a normal level of calcium a deficiency of phosphorus is unlikely as bone mineral consists of calcium phosphate. Along with calcium and vitamin D, it is involved in the hardening of bones.
- **Iron** is an essential trace element. Sources include liver, beef, lamb, soya beans, tofu, lentils, kidney beans and green leafy vegetables. The recommended daily intake varies according to sex and age e.g. for females aged 19–50 years, 18 mg daily is advised while for males of the same age 8 mg daily is advised (Office of Dietary Supplements 2007) with only a small proportion absorbed (less than 15%). Iron is essential for the formation of haemoglobin (oxygen-carrying component) in red blood cells. Iron deficiency is a condition that causes anaemia if iron stores are depleted and is the most common nutritional deficiency. Mild anaemia in many individuals is of little health consequence due to compensatory mechanisms in the body (such as increased cardiac output, diversion of blood flow and increased release of oxygen from haemoglobin), but the body cannot compensate in severe anaemia which results in poorer oxygen delivery to the tissues and impacts on body function. Work performance is limited and this will influence the participation of patients in rehabilitation post injury and after surgery. It is essential that the patient's haemoglobin is within an acceptable range to facilitate recovery and rehabilitation.
- **Zinc** can be obtained from shellfish, meat and whole grains with the recommended intake being 10–12 mg daily. Reduced growth is the only clearly demonstrated consequence of mild zinc deficiency although it is thought that zinc plays a central role in turnover and metabolism of connective tissue so a deficiency may have a negative influence on bone formation (Geissler and Powers 2005).
- **Sodium** is found in most foods and can also be added to food. It helps regulate water content in the body. A diet high in sodium increases urinary calcium excretion. Sodium occurs as an extracellular action and is involved in muscle contraction, transmission of nerve impulses

along the axons and water and electrolyte balance. The British Nutrition Foundation (2012) recommends a salt intake (sodium chloride) of no more than 6g daily. Currently intakes of sodium are high and although some is essential, a substantial reduction in intake is required.

- **Potassium** is found in fruit and vegetables and other foods. As with sodium, it is also involved in muscle contraction, transmission of nerve impulses and water and electrolyte balance and occurs as an intracellular action.
- **Fluoride** is involved in the mineralisation of bones. Fluoride is present in the majority of foods. Adding fluoride to drinking water is controversial; low fluoride levels may be beneficial but higher levels are toxic, resulting in fluorosis leading to joint pain and spinal defects (Geissler and Powers 2005). Fluorosis is rare in the Western world but is common in parts of Africa, China and India.
- **Magnesium** is important in calcium homeostasis and in the metabolism and/or action of vitamin D so is essential for the synthesis and secretion of the parathyroid hormone. A deficiency results in impaired parathyroid hormone secretion, disturbed calcium homeostasis and hypocalcaemia is a common symptom of a moderate to severe deficiency (Expert Group on Vitamins and Minerals 2003).
- **Aluminum** toxicity occurs in chronic renal failure or in patients receiving parenteral nutrition, or when drinking or ingesting substances that are high in aluminium, or living or working in an environment that contains high levels of aluminium or is very dusty. Osteoblast function is impaired in this toxic environment and there is reduced bone remodelling and osteomalacia.
- **Manganese** is required for bone health. It is found in vegetables, cereals and nuts and tea provides a rich resource. A deficiency is rare.

Fibre is found in cereals, beans, pulses, fruit and vegetables and although not a nutrient, it facilitates movement in the gut and helps prevent constipation. Other dietary components can also influence bone health. Excessive alcohol consumption can affect bone quality and increase the risk of fracture. A suggested link between an increased intake of caffeine and fracture is noted in publications on bone health; however, Heaney (2002) reported in a large prospective study of caffeine intake and fracture risk that, while there was a three times greater risk of hip fracture for women consuming more than 817mg caffeine a day (five cups of coffee), the number of hip fractures in the study were small. It is possible that this intake is not a cause of fractures but may be associated with a change in calcium intake when less milk is ingested. A high intake of carbonated beverages is also associated with a lower bone mineral density due to lifestyle and dietary factors. SIGN (2004) although supportive, report the evidence as inconclusive and do not make any recommendations in this area.

Metabolic response to tissue injury and trauma

The metabolic effect of trauma and surgery is catabolism of stored body fuels. The size and time span of this response is proportional to the injury and any complications (Desborough 2000), so energy requirements will increase depending on the demand created by the processes of recovery and healing. It is essential, therefore, that the nutritional needs of the patient are considered in the post-trauma, preoperative, perioperative and post-operative periods. The increased demands placed upon the body during recovery from surgery, injury and associated complications can lead to malnutrition and delayed recovery and warrants careful consideration by the multidisciplinary team.

The dietary needs of children and adolescents must take into account their age, growth and development which can make them susceptible to nutritional imbalance and deficiencies. Consideration needs to be given to additional demands related to exercise, sport and training programmes. As individuals age, the risk of chronic disease increases and nutrition plays a role in the development of, susceptibility to and outcome of disease. Other groups at risk of under nutrition and malnutrition include those with learning disabilities, dementia and other mental health conditions. Lee and Kolasa (2011) identify the difficulties of providing adequate nutrition to people with advanced dementia who need assistance with feeding.

Nutrition assessment and intervention

Malnutrition refers to both under-nutrition and over-nutrition. Nutrition deprivation does not imply a lack of food, but the provision of a diet that does not meet the physiological needs of the patient (Kneale 2005). Patients are at risk of malnutrition if the intake of nutrients is affected by comorbidities, surgery or underlying problems that affect appetite or absorption of food. Malnutrition can have a wide range of consequences including impaired immune response, muscle fatigue, impaired wound healing and growth (BAPEN 2011). Patients at risk of malnutrition remain in hospital for longer than those who are well nourished and are more likely to be discharged to alternative settings rather than home. The risk of malnutrition is increased in the older person, leading to impaired coordination with an increased risk of falls. Nutritional support is essential for those who are malnourished; i.e. with a *Body Mass Index* (BMI) of less than 18 kg/m^2, unintentional weight loss of >10% in the previous 3–6 months or a BMI of <20 kg/m^2 and an unintentional weight loss greater than 5% within 3–6 months (NICE 2006).

Obesity is a common nutritional problem in many developed countries. It exists where there is an excess accumulation of body fat when the BMI exceeds 29.9 (Box 10.1) and associated with high morbidity and mortality rates. Obese patients may prove challenging during all phases of care due to an associated risk of complications. The role of the nurse during preparation for surgery is critical in providing support and advice with respect to achieving weight loss.

Measuring nutritional status can be predictive of health outcomes and the assessment of nutritional intake is required if there may be a need to provide advice to the person or interventions such as enteral or parenteral support. Nutritional assessment approaches include dietary assessment, the use of anthropometry (physical measurement of aspects of human body size) and the use of biochemical, functional and clinical measures or indices. Biochemical status measures are defined for each nutrient and assess the concentration of the nutrient or its derivative in body fluid. Functional indices are assessments of the metabolic processes that are nutritionally dependent. Clinical indices are the signs and symptoms of a nutritional deficiency.

Dietary assessment involves attaining a dietary history from the individual or carer for the previous 24 hours or by administering a questionnaire to determine the frequency of different food groups eaten over the previous week. Anthropometry includes the measurement of body weight and height from which the BMI is calculated (Box 10.1). The percentage of body fat can be estimated by measuring the sum of the thickness of skinfolds over the biceps, triceps, subscapular and supra-iliac sites. The fat content varies with age and gender. It is now recognised that intra-abdominal fat measurement has a greater influence on the development of heart disease and diabetes than fat measurement in subcutaneous sites and is useful in orthopaedic assessment in preparation for surgery.

Box 10.1 Body Mass Index (BMI)

WHO Classification

Calculation of BMI

$$BMI = \frac{Weight(Kg)}{Height(m^2)}$$

Interpretation of BMI

<16	Severely underweight
16–18.4	Underweight
18.5–24.9	Normal range
25–29.9	Overweight
30–39.9	Obese
>40	Severely obese

The 'Malnutrition Universal Screening Tool' (MUST) (BAPEN 2011) involves five steps. The first three gather nutritional measurements, noting the percentage of unplanned weight loss and consider the effect of acute disease providing a score for each. An overall risk score or category of malnutrition is determined by adding the score obtained from steps 1 to 3 (step 4). The patient is then considered to be either at low, medium or high risk. Step 5 involves using guidelines and local policy to form an appropriate action plan for the patient. Actions can involve repeat screening (low risk), observation and nutritional support (medium risk) and referral to a dietician, regular monitoring and nutritional support (high risk). Those in all categories must have any underlying condition treated and be provided with help and advice on food choices and with eating and drinking. Training for staff on the use of such a tool is an important part of its implementation.

Nutritional support includes methods to improve or maintain nutritional intake and may involve simple assistance at meal times or the provision of a diet deemed appropriate to the patient's needs after a nutritional assessment. Support can include oral nutrition supplements, enteral tube feeding, PEG (percutaneous endoscopic gastrostomy) or parenteral nutrition. NICE (2006) provide a protocol for nutritional, anthropometric and clinical monitoring of nutritional support. This includes provision of nutrients, monitoring weight and BMI, observing gastrointestinal function, monitoring feeding tubes or catheter entry sites, observing the patient's clinical condition, setting goals and laboratory monitoring.

If the nutrition of a patient is shown to be compromised, a plan of care needs to be put in place. This can involve all or some of the multidisciplinary team depending on individual need. This can include the nursing team, dietician, speech therapist, occupational therapist, pharmacist and catering team. The nursing team has the most contact with the patient through observing and monitoring patients at meal times and providing assistance where appropriate, plus contribute to the provision of a balanced diet. Making sure patients are eating, recognising poor appetite, documenting and reporting dietary intake are all essential. Providing an environment conducive to better nutrition is also part of the nurse's role. This may include restricting visiting at mealtimes but ensuring carers and relatives can participate in helping patients to eat, ensuring that non-essential nursing and medical procedures are not carried out at mealtimes and avoiding the organisation of investigations or tests at mealtimes. Patients also need advice on a diet that is balanced to promote their individual recovery which can be facilitated by nurses in conjunction with the dietician. Good practice includes identifying and supporting 'at risk' patients, monitoring dietary intake, providing appetising and attractive food and having food, snacks and high calorific drinks available around the clock.

Additional support can be sought from a dietician who can apply their knowledge in order to promote health, prevent disease and aid in the treatment of illnesses. They can also assess the nutritional status of the patient, advise on appropriate therapeutic diets or feeding regimens while monitoring and instigating appropriate changes in the nutritional care plan. A speech therapist may be involved if the patient has swallowing or chewing difficulties or is considered at risk of aspiration. Occupational therapists assess the patient's range of movement and mobility in relation to managing independence at home, provide appropriate aids which can be used in hospital and then in the community. Pharmacists can provide advice around dietary supplements, enteral and parenteral feeds. The catering team's role is to provide a variety of foods with appropriate nutritional value, taking into account the needs of the patient recovering from injury or surgery or those with dietary restrictions. The presentation, texture and consistency of food produced by the team also contribute to a better service and patient outcome. A balanced diet can be achieved by such multidisciplinary team working. A member of the catering team meeting with patients on a regular basis can provide good feedback on which to continue a good service or provide information that can lead to improvements.

The move towards creating a healthier environment in hospitals with respect to nutrition is essential. The Council of Europe (2003) identified 10 key characteristics of good nutritional care in hospitals and these were endorsed by many organisations. Issues such as screening on admission and adoption of a multidisciplinary approach to nutritional care are highlighted. In the drive to improve standards, national governments must be involved. One such example is the Essence of Care initiative (DoH 2010) which identified twelve benchmarks to address the fundamentals of nutritional care (Table 10.3).

Oral health problems such as dental caries, oral disease, gum disease and infection can affect food choices and ultimately nutritional status with ill-fitting dentures a potential sign of recent weight loss. Practitioners can help their patients by asking about oral health problems and recommending dental consultation where appropriate (Palmer *et al.*, 2010). Other interventions can include inspection of the oral cavity, noting any ulceration or abnormality alongside a plan that considers frequent oral hygiene, cleaning of dentures and use of a mouthwash.

Hydration and dehydration

Good hydration involves ensuring an adequate amount of water is available to body tissues. Dehydration is a depletion of water content in the tissues resulting from either loss of fluid or inadequate intake. Maintaining hydration is critical to maintaining good health especially in advancing age. Poor hydration can lead to multiple problems such as tendons and ligaments becoming less resilient, constipation, dry and itchy skin, acne, nose bleeds, repeated urinary tract infections, dry coughs, sneezing, sinus pressure, headaches and daytime fatigue. These are often as a result of build-up of toxins as excretory mechanisms fail to function properly. Dehydration can also

Table 10.3 Essence of Care Benchmarks for Nutrition (Department of Health 2010). Reproduced with permission from Crown copyright

Benchmarks for the management of food and drink in the health care setting and the community	
Factor	**Benchmark of best practice**
1. Promoting health	People are encouraged to eat and drink in a way that promotes health
2. Information	People and carers have sufficient information to enable them to obtain their food and drink
3. Availability	People can access food and drink at any time according to their needs and preferences
4. Provision	People are provided with food and drink that meets their individual needs and preferences
5. Presentation	People's food and drink is presented in a way that is appealing to them
6. Environment	People feel the environment is conducive to eating and drinking
7. Screening and assessment	People who are screened on initial contact and identified at risk receive full nutritional assessment
8. Planning, implementation, evaluation and revision of care	People's care is planned, implemented, continuously evaluated and revised to meet individual needs and preference to food and drink
9. Assistance	People receive care and assistance when required with eating and drinking
10. Monitoring	People's food and drink intake is monitored and recorded.

weaken the body's immune system and leads to chemical, nutritional and pH imbalances. Insufficient hydration fatigues muscles, reduces coordination and causes muscle cramps, restricting the patient's ability to maintain physical function and mobility.

Water is essential for life. It makes up about 55–60% of body weight with adequate fluid intake essential for healthy organ function. Water is lost during respiration (about 300–400 ml per day) and urination (1–2 L per day with a general rule of thumb of 1 ml/kg/hr with boundaries of 0.5 ml–2 ml/kg/hr). Water is also lost through the skin by evaporation (600 ml per day) and faeces (100–200 ml per day). This loss depends on age, body size, physical activity, health and environmental conditions and is normally balanced by the intake of food and water. Water has many functions, the moistening of food for swallowing, regulation of body temperature, transport of substances around the body, a medium for excretion of waste products, dilution of water products in the body; provision of a moist environment required by cells and the facilitation of metabolic reactions.

The recommended fluid intake is 1.2 litres per day for adults (British Nutrition Foundation 2012). For children, the recommended fluid intake varies with age (NICE 2010) (Table 10.4).

Fluid and electrolyte balance can be affected by the physiological response to the stress of surgery or injury, with glucocortoid secretion increasing reabsorption of sodium and water in the kidneys with a corresponding loss of potassium and hydrogen ions. Increased levels of antidiuretic hormone also increase water reabsorption while high aldosterone levels further increase sodium reabsorption in order to maintain circulating volumes and renal perfusion. As a result of trauma to the tissue from injury or surgery, intracellular potassium is released, resulting in an exchange for retained sodium. Levels of potassium need careful monitoring and should be replaced as appropriate (Alexander *et al.*, 2006).

Table 10.4 Recommended daily fluid intake for Children (NICE 2010)

Age	**Sex**	**Total daily intake (mls)**
4–8 years	F	1000–1400
	M	1000–1400
9–13 years	F	1200–2100
	M	1400–2300
14–18 years	F	1400–2500
	M	2100–3200

Nausea and vomiting

Post operative nausea and vomiting (PONV) is a common unpleasant experience, with patients at risk of aspiration, electrolyte imbalance, pain, increased length of stay and significant discomfort. Risk factors identified for PONV include obesity, older age, female gender, children, prior history, anxiety, inadequate pain relief, prolonged fasting and post-operative hypotension. Simple measures such as hydration, supplemental oxygen and sitting the patient upright can be effective along with the appropriate use of anti-emetics.

Starvation/fasting

Periods of fasting or starvation related to trauma and surgery can be as a result of ill health, fasting prior to and after surgery and loss of appetite associated with trauma, surgery or ill health. Although metabolic adaptation can sustain the normal energy requirements of the body for approximately 10 hours during starvation, minimising the length of fasting periods is essential in promoting good nutrition and recovery. In the past, surgical patients were fasted routinely from food and drink for long periods of up to 12 hours before anaesthesia to reduce the risk of aspiration and pneumonitis. Despite evidence (Brady *et al.*, 2003, Brady *et al.*, 2009) that shorter preoperative fasting does not increase the risk of this complication, practice continues to vary. Long fasting times for surgery can impact on hydration and nutrition, therefore surgery should be planned to ensure fasting/starvation times can be kept to a minimum and intravenous hydration implemented.

Preoperative fasting is often in excess of the recommended 2 hours for fluids and 6 hours for milk or food. The '2–6' rule applies to adults; water can be drunk up to two hours before induction of anaesthesia along with a minimum preoperative fasting time of six hours for food (solids, milk and milk-containing drinks). The volume of administered fluid does not appear to have an impact on patients' residual gastric volume and gastric pH when compared to a standard fasting regime. It is suggested that the anaesthetic team should consider further interventions for patients at the highest risk of regurgitation and aspiration. For children, the 2-4-6 rule applies. The intake of water or other clear fluid should cease two hours before induction of anaesthesia with breast feeding ceasing four hours and formula milk, cow's milk or other solids ceasing six hours before anaesthesia (RCN 2005). See Box 10.2 for further discussion of the evidence.

Box 10.2 Evidence digest. Reproduced with permission from The Cochrane Collaboration

Preoperative fasting

Preoperative Fasting for Adults to Prevent Peri-operative Complications. A Cochrane Review (Brady *et al.*, 2003)

This review was undertaken to systematically review the effect of different on preoperative fasting regimes on peri-operative complications and patient wellbeing in different adult populations. Randomised controlled trials which compared the effect on post-operative complications of different fasting regimes on adults were selected.

Results

Thirty eight randomised controlled comparisons were identified from 22 trials. Most were based on healthy adult participants who were not considered at increased risk of complications. There was no evidence that a shortened fluid fast time increased the risk of complications compared with the standard nil-by-mouth regime from midnight. In fact, participants given a drink of water preoperatively were found to have a significantly lower volume of gastric contents than the groups who followed a standard fasting regime.

Preoperative Fasting for Children to Prevent Peri-operative Complications. A Cochrane Review (Brady *et al.*, 2009)

This review was undertaken to systematically review the effect of different preoperative fasting regimes on perioperative complications and patient wellbeing in children. Randomised and quasi-randomised controlled trials of preoperative fasting regimens for children were identified.

Results

Forty seven randomised controlled comparisons were identified from 25 trials involving 2543 children. One incident of aspiration and regurgitation was reported. Children permitted fluids up to 120 minutes preoperatively were not found to experience higher gastric volumes or lower gastric pH values than those who fasted. The children permitted fluids were less thirsty and hungry, better behaved and more comfortable than those who fasted. There is no evidence that children who are denied oral fluids for more than six hours preoperatively benefit in terms of intraoperative gastric volume and pH compared with children permitted unlimited fluids up to two hours preoperatively.

Minimising the length of fasting times combined with appropriate fluid management during surgery is a key factor in improving patient and surgical outcomes after major surgery. Oesophageal Doppler guided fluid management is a minimally invasive procedure that can enable the anaesthetist to accurately administer IV fluids during surgery and reduce post-operative complications (Callow 2010). Post-operatively, patients should be encouraged to drink as soon as they are ready providing there are no contra-indications (RCN 2005). Intravenous fluid replacement should be administered as prescribed and discontinued when the patient is drinking adequate fluids.

Many serious fluid balance problems can be averted by keeping careful assessment of the intake and output of the patient and maintaining good records (Methany 2000) so that appropriate and timely action can be taken. Accurate fluid balance recording allows the practitioner to monitor intake and output and calculate the balance or discrepancy. Accuracy in both measurement and documentation is fundamental to patient care and outcomes, but this is often neglected, is inaccurate and does not give a clear account of the patient's input and output.

Summary

Good nutrition and hydration play a key role in the patient's recovery. By ensuring that consideration is given to nutrition and hydration in conjunction with other aspects of care, good patient outcomes can be achieved while reducing delays in the patient returning to their previous level of independence.

Recommended further reading

Council of Europe (2003) Food and Nutritional Care in Hospitals. Available at: https://wcd.coe.int/ViewDoc.jsp?id=85747 (accessed 29 October 2013).

Desborough, J.P. (2000) The stress response to surgery and trauma. *British Journal of Anaesthesiology*, **85**(1), 109–117.

Hilton, A.K., Pellegrino, V.A. and Scheinkestel, C.D. (2008) Avoiding common problems associated with intravenous fluid therapy. *The Medical Journal of Australia*, **189**, 509–513.

References

Alexander, M., Fawcett, J. and Runciman, P.J. (2006) *Nursing Practice: Hospital and Home*, 3rd edn. Churchill Livingstone Elsevier, Edinburgh.

BAPEN (2011) The MUST Explanatory Booklet (Online). Available at: http://www.bapen.org.uk (accessed 12 October 2012).

Brady, M.C., Kinn, S., Stuart, P. and Ness, V. (2003) Preoperative Fasting for Adults to Prevent Perioperative Complications. *Cochrane Database of Systematic Reviews* **4** (Art. No.: CD004423). DOI: 10.1002/14651858.CD004423.

Brady, M.C., Kinn, S., Ness, V. *et al.* (2009) Preoperative fasting for preventing perioperative complications in children. *Cochrane Database of Systematic Reviews* **4** (Art. No.: CD005285). DOI: 10.1002/14651858.CD005285.pub2.

British Nutrition Foundation (2012) (Online). Available at: http://www.nutrtion.org.uk (accessed 6 November 2012).

Callow C. (2010) Doppler monitoring reduces hospital stay, The Clinical Services Journal, (March), 41–43.

Council of Europe (2003) Food and Nutritional Care in Hospitals. Available at: https://wcd.coe.int/ViewDoc.jsp?id=85747 (accessed 29 October 2013).

Department of Health (DoH) (2010) *Essence of Care: Benchmarks for Food and Drink*. The Stationery Office, Norwich.

Desborough, J.P. (2000) The stress response to surgery and trauma. *British Journal of Anaesthesiology*, **85**(1), 109–117.

Expert Group on Vitamins and Minerals (2003) *Safe Upper Limits for Vitamins and Minerals*. Food Standards Agency, London.

Geissler, C. and Powers, H. (2005) *Human Nutrition*, 11th edn. Elsevier Churchill Livingstone, Edinburgh.

Heaney, R.P. (2002) Effects of caffeine on bone and the calcium economy. *Food and Chemical Technology*, **40**(9), 1263–1270.

Kneale, J. (2005) The importance of nutrition, in *Orthopaedic and Trauma Nursing*, 2nd edn (eds J. Kneale and P. Davis). Elsevier Churchhill Livingstone, Edinburgh, pp.164–179.

Lee, T.J. and Kolassa, K. (2011) Feeding the person with late stage Alzheimers Disease. *Nutrition Today*, **46**(2), 75–79.

Methany, N. (2000) *Fluid and Electrolyte Balance: Nursing Considerations*, 4th edn. Lippincott, Philadelphia.

National Institute for Health and Clinical Excellence (NICE) (2006) *Nutrition Support in Adults CG32*. NICE, London.

National Institute for Health and Clinical Excellence (NICE) (2010) *Nocturnal Enuresis and Bedwetting in Children and Young People CG111*. NICE, London.

Office of Dietary Supplements (2007) Iron Factsheet. Available at: http://ods.od.nih.gov/factsheets/IronHealthProfessional/ (accessed 31 October 2013).

Office of Dietary Supplements (2012) Calcium Factsheet. Available at: http://ods.od.nih.gov/factsheets/CalciumHealthProfessional/ (accessed 4 November 2012).

Palmer, C.A., Burnett, D.J. and Dean, B. (2010) Its more than just candy: important relationship between nutrition and oral health. *Nutrition Today*, **45**(4), 154–156.

Royal College of Nursing (RCN) (2005) *Perioperative Fasting in Adults and Children*. RCN, London.

SIGN (2004) Managing Osteoporosis, Guidelines 71. Available at: www.sign.ac.uk (accessed 4 November 2012).

CHAPTER 11

Pain assessment and management in orthopaedic and trauma care

Carolyn Mackintosh-Franklin
University of Hull, Hull, UK

Introduction

Pain is the most frequently reported initial symptom in up to 91% of all trauma patients and is the commonest reason for self-referral to accident and emergency or community health services (Berben *et al.*, 2008), but the high variability in pain experiences between individuals means that the extent of and reaction to pain is unpredictable. The individual and unique nature of this experience makes it essential for all patients to be rigorously assessed prior to initiating appropriate pain management treatments/techniques. To ensure optimal standards of patient care, this requires practitioners working with patients in pain to be fully informed of the evidence base for best practice in this area.

The nature of pain

Pain is frequently reported as having an elusive quality which is difficult to quantify and is highly variable between individuals. This has led to great difficulty in establishing explanations for pain as an emotion or a physical sensation.

The Gate Control theory of pain

In 1946, based on experiences in the Second World War, Dr H Beecher published a seminal paper which ignited debate on the nature of pain as a purely physical phenomenon and argued that the meaning of pain to the individual experiencing it was a key component (Beecher 1959). The first scientific evidence to support this was published by Melzack and Wall (1965) in their outline of what continues to be known as the Gate Control Theory of pain (Figure 11.1). This has undergone a number of subsequent modifications, but the overall premise of the theory is generally accepted and provides a workable explanation for this complex phenomenon that marries both mechanistic physiological explanations with myriad individual variables. It can be broken down into four key segments: peripheral sensitisation, spinal modulation, central modulation and conscious recognition. Together these are called nociception (Parsons and Preece 2010).

Peripheral sensitisation

- At the point of trauma/injury the body's initial response is to initiate a chemical reaction which is known as an "inflammatory response."
- Once this reaches a critical threshold it activates a chain of nerve impulse reactions that propel the message towards the central body systems.
- Two key types of nerve fibres are specifically responsible for the transmission of pain messages – A-delta fibres and C fibres.
- A-delta fibres transmit 'fast' messages commonly associated with acute, sharp stabbing pain and reflex responses and are present in large quantities in the somatic areas of the body.
- C fibres transmit 'slow' messages and are present in both the somatic areas of the body, but also in the viscera and are commonly associated with slower throbbing pain sensation and chronic pain conditions.
- A third peripheral nerve fibre A-beta is not involved in transmission of pain but does play a role in moderating the pain experience.
- A-delta and C fibres are commonly referred to as nociceptors that transmit noxious messages.

Orthopaedic and Trauma Nursing: An Evidence-based Approach to Musculoskeletal Care, First Edition. Edited by Sonya Clarke and Julie Santy-Tomlinson.

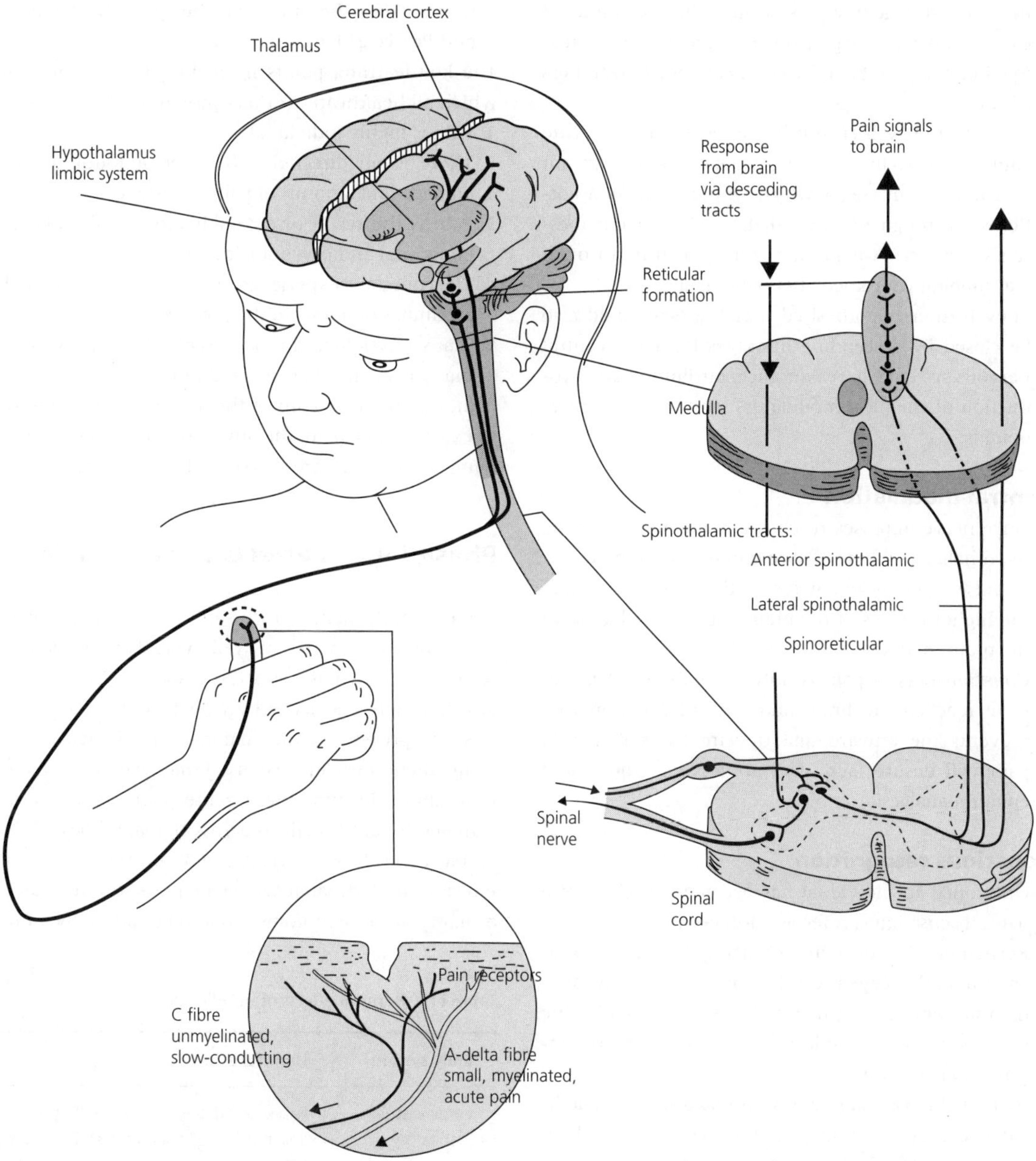

Figure 11.1 Gate control theory of pain

Spinal modulation

- Once messages from the peripheral nerves reach the spinal column they enter an area of the dorsal horn, known as the substantia gelatinosa.
- Impulses cross over in the spinal tract and are sent upwards to the hypothalamus in the brain.
- Impulses may be modified upon entry into the substantia gelatinosa and this can impact on the amount of pain experienced.
- Modification at this stage was initially hypothesised as a 'gate' similar to a garden gate which, when open, allows unimpeded entry for nerve impulses to

transmit message upwards through the spinal tract. If closed, however, the gate prevents the onwards transmission and results in a lack of conscious awareness of pain.

- Melzack and Wall (1965) hypothesised that the gate could be closed by activating A-beta fibres to transmit non-noxious messages which would result in a bottleneck through the gate that would prevent messages from the A-delta and C fibres getting through e.g. rubbing your knee after banging it.
- They further hypothesised that the gate could also be closed by descending messages from the central nervous system e.g. reassurance, attribution and production of chemical modulators such as endogenous opioids.

Central modulation

- Once nerve impulses reach the brain they enter the hypothalamus where C fibre impulses terminate.
- Impulses from A-delta fibres continue to be relayed to the higher centres of the brain and enter all areas of the brain matrix.
- Consciousness of pain is only gained once impulses have reached the brain and any intervention that prevents the onward and upward transmission of pain will ensure lack of awareness e.g. spinal and epidural analgesia.

Conscious recognition

- Only once an individual has become conscious of a painful sensation can recognition occur.
- Recognition is crucial in modulating the pain experience, as at this stage the individual will not only identify that they have pain, but place some form of value on it which will significantly affect their interpretation and behaviour.
- Acute pain (associated with trauma and orthopaedic surgery) may mean the pain is associated with a high anxiety or a highly emotional situation such as fear of death, making an individual highly vigilant about their pain, interpreting any pain sensations as severe and highly significant.
- Alternatively, pain could equally be interpreted as non-threatening and this may allow an individual to minimise the experience and treat symptoms lightly.
- It is hypothesised that this interpretation can lead to direct physiological modulation of pain impulses through changes to the inflammatory chemicals present in both the brain and the spinal tract (Parsons and Preece 2010).

The key learning points from the gate control theory which all healthcare workers should be aware of are:

1 Pain is highly individual.
2 There is no direct link between amount of tissue damage and amount of pain experienced.
3 Pain is the result of a combination of physiological, emotional and psychological factors.
4 The conscious experience of pain can be modulated at a number of points in the process.
5 Many physiological processes are still unproven with many exact mechanisms unknown.

Although the gate control theory works relatively well to explain acute pain, the physiological processes underlying chronic pain are still subject to much debate.

Physiological effects of acute pain

Aside from the actual process of nociception, acute pain also provokes a series of well-evidenced physiological responses known as the 'stress response.' This is generally considered a means by which the body can minimise or prevent further damage and is activated by sympathetic nervous activity. Prolonged stress such as that caused by unrelieved acute pain can result in a number of harmful effects across all major body systems (Table 11.1). It is especially important to recognise the effects of undertreated acute pain in the trauma patient, as many of the symptoms can also be caused by a range

Table 11.1 Harmful effects of unrelieved pain

Body system	Harmful effect
Cardiovascular	Raised blood pressure and heart rate
Respiratory	Splinting – small tidal volumes, high inspiration and expiration pressures and decreased vital capacity – hypoxemia, pneumonia and confusion
Endocrine	Release of hormones, carbohydrate, protein and fat catabolism, hyperglycaemia and increased inflammatory response
Gastro intestinal	Decrease in gastric emptying and motility – paralytic ileus
Reduced physical activity	Delayed mobilisation and increased inpatient stays

of other factors which may also be affecting the patient e.g. hypovolaemia. Although action may be taken to correct one element, undertreated pain can reduce the effectiveness any interventions.

Types of pain

Acute pain is commonly associated with traumatic injury and orthopaedic surgery. It can be defined as pain of sudden specific onset of limited duration and is identified as having a number of key features. It is:

- incident-specific
- serves a function
- objective clinical signs
- commonly associated with trauma
- of known duration
- responsive to a range of analgesics
- affects only the individual
- limited financial implications.

Acute pain is also commonly regarded as serving as an alarm warning about impending or actual bodily damage, motivation to escape from the cause of pain and to protect an injured area (Parsons and Preece 2010).

In contrast, chronic pain is associated with chronic musculoskeletal conditions and can be defined as pain of long or indeterminate duration which may persist beyond the time of normal healing or without specific causation (Mackintosh and Elson 2008). It can be identified as being:

- not incident-specific
- uncertain causal factors
- unknown duration
- of limited functionality
- unresponsive to a range of treatments
- affects a wider social group
- can have severe financial implications
- closely associated with depressive illness.

The clear difference between the two experiences can have a major impact on the individual pain sufferer and their family as well as affecting the central modulation of the pain experience (Mackintosh and Elson 2008). It is also important to note that acute and chronic pain do not necessarily occur in isolation from each other. Patients with chronic pain conditions can also suffer from acute pain episodes (e.g. hip fracture in a patient with osteoarthritis) and poorly treated acute pain is now a well recognised precursor of chronic pain with 50–60% of trauma patients reporting moderate to severe injury-related pain 6–12months after their trauma (Clay *et al.*, 2010).

Pain is also commonly classified into two major types (Parsons and Preece 2010):

1 Nociceptive pain – pain as a direct result of injury to somatic substances e.g. skin, bone, muscle and connective tissues and as a direct result of injury to the viscera e .g. gastrointestinal obstruction, pancreatitis.
2 Neuropathic pain – pain as a direct result of damage to the sensory or peripheral nervous system; this can be centrally generated i.e. sympathetically maintained pains (SMP's) or peripherally generated e.g. nerve root compression.

These two types of pain do not occur in isolation and it is common for patients to experience both types of pain from the same trauma e.g. both somatic and nerve damage from a compound fracture.

This means the orthopaedic/trauma practitioner will encounter patients experiencing a wide range of pain symptoms and reacting to these in highly variable and unpredictable ways. This places great importance on the individual assessment of pain to ensure treatment is both appropriate and effective.

Pain assessment

The individual and highly variable nature of pain makes pain assessment an essential element of good quality care. Without it the treatment and management of pain is likely to be ineffective. A large body of evidence continues to suggest that pain assessment is poorly and infrequently carried out. Reasons for the failure to adequately assess patients' pain are many and varied and include: lack of knowledge of why or how to assess pain, pain assessment as a low priority, failure to believe patients' self-reports of pain and failure of patients to report pain (Gillaspie 2010).

Knowledge of how to assess pain is fundamental. Accurate assessment can provide many indicators that aid diagnosis of both the condition and the pain and facilitate appropriate and effective treatment. Guidelines for the management of hip fractures (NICE 2011) state that the first point of assessment is to 'assess the patients pain' followed immediately by offering analgesia to all patients regardless of cognitive state.

Nine Key areas should be considered when taking a pain history (ANZCA 2005):

1 site of pain – where it hurts
2 how the pain started

3 what the pain feels like – its character
4 how much it hurts – its intensity
5 symptoms associated with it – nausea
6 effect of pain on activities and sleep
7 any current treatment for the pain
8 any past medical history
9 other factors influencing symptoms – beliefs, expectations, coping mechanisms.

These can be used simply as direct questions when in conversation with a patient, but answers provide important clues to treatment and management. This is especially important if trying to differentiate between nociceptive pain and neuropathic pain. The patient's own descriptive words are essential. Nociceptive pain from somatic damage is commonly described as: sharp, hot, vice-like, and is easily localised. Nociceptive pain (from viscera) is more likely to be described as; dull, cramping or colicky and it is more difficult for the patient to identify the exact spot which hurts. Instead it is characterised by a more generalised overall tenderness. Neuropathic pain may be described as burning, shooting and stabbing. It can happen spontaneously and can be associated with hypersensitivity of surrounding tissue (hyperalgesia).

Formal pain assessment

Although speaking directly to a patient to identify the nature of their pain is both common sense and best practice, because of the long history of failings in this area formalised pain assessment tools are now commonly used and there is clear evidence that they lead to improvements in patients' pain experiences (Parsons and Preece 2010). These take a variety of forms, measure a range of pain dimensions and have been developed for use across a wide range of different patients from pre-verbal infants to those with advanced dementia. Some of these tools focus on the patient's own self-report, whilst others use behavioural indicators to arrive at algorithmically derived measures of an individual's pain. It is generally accepted that using the patient's self-report of pain is best practice.

The commonest used pain assessment tools in the acute setting are self-reported uni-dimensional tools, which measure one element of the pain experience – its intensity. These take three forms: Descriptive scales, numerical scales and visual analogue scales (VAS) (Box 11.1).

Box 11.1 Example of descriptive scales, visual analogue scale and numerical scales

Verbal rating scale

No pain	Mild pain	Moderate pain	Severe pain	Very severe pain

Pain intensity scale

0 no pain
1 mild pain
2 discomforting
3 distressing
4 horrible
5 excruciating

Visual analogue scale

No pain ______________________ Worst pain imaginable
(Note: this line should be exactly 10cm long when used in practice)

Verbal analogue scale

No pain	Mild pain	Moderate pain	Severe pain	Very severe pain

Numerical rating scale

1	2	3	4	5	6	7	8	9	10

Descriptive scales consist of a range of words which can be used to describe the intensity of pain along a continuum e.g. from no pain to unbearable pain:

- Numerical scales require a patient to give their pain a rating based on a number with 1 normally being the least and 10 the highest pain intensity.
- Visual Analogue Scales consist of a 10 cm long line with no pain at one end and the worst pain imaginable at the other and the patient is asked to mark or indicate on the line where their pain currently sits.

Another commonly used uni-dimensional tool is the "Wong Baker Faces" rating scale which consists of pictures of stylised faces ranging from smiling to crying, which can be used in children who are able to point to the appropriate picture.

The key advantage for these tools is:

- The speed with which they can be used (particularly for the patient following acute traumatic injury).

- They provide a baseline against which the effect of treatments can be measured.
- Their repeatability over a period of time/treatment.

They also suffer from a number of disadvantages (Parsons and Preece 2010):

- Their uni-dimensional nature severely limits their scope.
- Some patients have difficulty in conceptualising their pain as a number or a line on a rating scale.
- Some patients prefer to use their own choice of descriptive words and find others restricting.
- They commonly assume the patient has only one source of pain.
- They are entirely reliant on the patients self-report.
- They cannot be used with a patient who is unable to communicate.
- They are not liked by some practitioners.

A useful adjunct to the uni-dimensional pain tool is the addition of body pictures, normally showing the front and back of the body. These allow either the patient or the nurse to draw exactly where the pain is, if it moves to indicate where this occurs and, where a patient has multiple sources of pain, to document each individually (Mackintosh and Elson 2008).

In order to overcome some of these disadvantages more complex multi-dimensional self-report pain assessment tools have been developed. A commonly used example of a more structured self-report scale is the McGill Pain Questionnaire (Mackintosh 2007) which assesses a range of aspects about the pain experience besides simple intensity. Its effectiveness in the acute situation is limited as it is lengthy to administer and is more commonly associated with chronic pain assessment.

In the United Kingdom chronic pain is now frequently assessed using the SF36 scale (available in the public domain from www.RAND.org) which seeks to link quality of life with pain intensity and physical functionality and has tended to replace the Brief Pain Inventory as the assessment tool of choice. Although these tools may be useful for assessing pain in the longer-term orthopaedic patient who has a complex trajectory of interventions and treatments, they are of little value in acute pain situations. They are also limited to use with patients who are able or willing to self-report. Where patients cannot self-report, a range of other tools have been developed focusing on two key groups: preverbal infants and young children and patients who are cognitively impaired or suffer from dementia. These tools focus on observational data gained from analysis of the patient's behaviour and can include characteristics such as: facial grimacing or frowning, agitation, aggression, verbal expressions such as moaning and physiological indicators of increased heart rate and raised blood pressure. The Abbey Dementia Scale is a commonly used example and is freely available from www.dementiacareaustralia.com. The effectiveness of these tools is hard to establish as they are used on a group of patients who are unlikely to provide feedback. Where these have been used to initiate improved pain management regimes for patients with dementia in care homes, there is evidence of decreased agitation and aggression, which is assumed to be evidence of reduced pain (Cunningham 2006).

When considering pain assessment tools, important points can be summarised as:

- Regular pain assessment using a tool improves acute pain management.
- Self-reporting of pain is best practice and should be used whenever possible.
- The pain assessment tool used should be appropriate to the individual patient.

Successful pain assessment

For pain assessment to be effective in minimising pain, it must focus beyond the use of a pain assessment tool and must be carried out frequently. It must be documented and unacceptable levels of pain must result in action to alleviate the pain. Pain should be assessed immediately upon presentation to the hospital and within 30 minutes of administering initial analgesia, followed by hourly pain assessment until settled and then assessed routinely (NICE 2011). The International Association for the Study of Pain (IASP) (Schugg 2011) has led a campaign since 2000 to have pain assessment included as the 'fifth vital sign' in conjunction with routine temperature, blood pressure, heart rate and respiration rate (TPR), highlighting the importance of regular, routine pain assessment for all patients.

Parsons and Preece (2010) identify four key times when pain assessment should be carried out:

1 initially to gain a base line observation
2 at intervals following an intervention e.g. 15–30 minutes
3 at regular intervals after a treatment begins
4 following any reported change in the description, location and intensity of the pain.

Box 11.2 Evidence digest. Reproduced with permission from LWW

A systematic investigation to improve post-operative pain management for orthopaedic patients (Gillaspie 2010)

Gillaspie (2010) identified that patients undergoing total joint replacement surgery had a high incidence of unsatisfactory pain which made this a 'high risk for pain' procedure. In order to increase satisfaction with post-operative pain a 'GEMBA' approach was used which looked specifically at one physical setting, the orthopaedic 'floor' (ward/unit). Data were gathered from patients, nurses, physical therapy staff and anaesthetists. This exposed gaps in current practice with a specific focus on patient education. Pre-operative information failed to prepare patients for actual post-operative experiences. As a direct result of this a new bedside patient information tool was developed. This was evaluated in three cycles of; Plan, Do, Study, Act (PDSA), with additional refinements added at each stage of the cycle. Evaluation of the new tool demonstrated improved patient-staff communication, more accurate pain assessment and increased patient satisfaction with post-operative pain.

Parsons and Preece (2010, p. 75) also highlight six golden rules for pain assessment:

1 always assess pain
2 always ask the patient
3 all people should always use the same pain assessment tool on the same patient
4 always assess pain on movement or deep breathing or coughing and not just at rest
5 always document the patient's pain assessment
6 always evaluate the intervention using the same pain assessment tool.

All pain assessment which is reliant on the patient's self-report assumes that the patient's self-reports will be believed. As McCaffery (1979) is frequently quoted as saying 'pain is what the person says it is and exists when they say it does.' Unfortunately, a growing body of evidence suggests that, in many situations, practitioners are reluctant to believe patients and frequently use their own subjective judgements of a person's pain in preference to the patient's. Progress in pain assessment and management can only be made if practitioners are prepared to accept the patient's self-report and this is fundamental to all forms of pain assessment. Evidence focused on pain assessment is explored in Boxes 11.2 and 11.3.

Box 11.3 Evidence digest. Reproduced with permission from Elsevier

Incidence of trauma pain in emergency departments (Berben *et al.*, 2008)

Under-treatment of pain in emergency departments has been frequently reported. This observational study (Berben *et al.*, 2008) over three months in two emergency departments in the Netherlands describes the prevalence, intensity, location and course of pain in trauma patients. 450 patients were included in the study, with no differences between the two departments. 91% of patients reported pain on admission and 86% reported pain on discharge, with an average pain intensity of 5.9 (out of 10 maximum) on admission and 5 on discharge. Nearly half of all patients reported no change in pain on discharge. Only 49% of patients reported receiving information on pain management and 19% received pharmacological pain treatments. Pharmacological pain treatments consisted of local anaesthetics (40%) and systemic pain medications (60%).

Overall management of pain was considered a low priority with a key focus on 'anatomical' injury treatment. Even simple pain alleviation methods such as ice packing and elevation of body parts were infrequently observed. The researchers concluded that pain in the emergency department continues to be under-treated and requires to be addressed systematically including assessment using recognised tools and treatment with basic pharmacological and non-pharmacological methods initiated at the earliest stage.

Pain management

Once pain has been assessed it can be managed in a number of ways, and it is now commonly accepted that in most instances a multi-modal or balanced approach towards pain management is likely to be the most effective (Malchow and Black 2008). A multi-modal approach involves treating the pain using a variety of approaches and methods designed to work on different components of the pain experience. A variety of models of treatment are used in practice normally focusing on: systemic analgesics, local and regional anaesthetics, adjuvant drugs and non-pharmacological management of pain. All of these approaches have some benefit to the management and treatment of acute traumatic and orthopaedic pain (Clark *et al.*, 2009). An example of such benefits is explored in Box 11.4.

Box 11.4 Evidence digest. Reproduced with permission from LWW

An intervention to improve the post-operative pain experience for orthopaedic patients (Napier and Bass 2007)

This study used a retrospective chart review to compare reports of post-operative pain, ambulation and length of stay in 41 patients who received intrathecal injections prior to total knee replacement and 44 patients who had general anaesthetic (GA) only. Epidemiological differences between the two groups did not account for any of the observed differences in the three variables under review. Findings indicated that post-operative pain scores were consistently higher for the duration of the inpatient stay for patients who had GA only. Pain on initial ambulation was also higher for the GA group and length of ambulation shorter. By the third ambulation session mean distances were similar for both groups. In total the GA group ambulated for an overall shorter distance. The authors support the use of intrathecal injections to reduce post-operative discomfort, increase ambulation and ultimately reduce length of inpatient stay.

Pain management interventions at the site of trauma

Treatments to minimise pain can be focused at the site of trauma itself and can combine systemic, local and non-pharmacological techniques. Knowledge of pain physiology highlights the importance of the inflammatory response at the point of trauma and any intervention which reduces this response can produce pain relief.

The most common interventions which focus on the site of trauma are non-steroidal anti-inflammatory medications (NSAIDs) as these are particularly useful where there is extensive tissue damage or musculoskeletal pain. They can be taken orally, per rectum, in slow relief preparations or topically. However NSAIDs are not inherently analgesics and provide pain relief simply through reducing the inflammatory response. This means that except in cases of mild pain, they should normally be used in combination with other forms of pain treatment, for their opioid sparing properties. NSAIDs work by reducing prostaglandin production through the inhibition of the cyclo-oxygenase (COX) system, and newer NSAIDs have been developed which work more selectively, targeting COX-2 which is associated with trauma-related inflammation, although due to gastro intestinal side effects NSAIDs should be used with caution and they should not be used in patients with a history of gastric ulceration. There is also some concern about the effect of NSAIDs on bone healing and this should be taken into account.

Local anaesthetics can also be extremely useful for reducing pain at the site of trauma as their basic mode of action is to inhibit sodium influx preventing the nerve membrane from depolarising, hence preventing nerve impulses from achieving action potential and halting the onward transmission of pain messages to the dorsal horn of the spine. Infiltration is also a commonly used local anaesthetic method normally used during surgical procedures. A local anaesthetic agent is injected into a wound (surgical or traumatic) during suturing or wound closure and also has a longer term effect of reducing the total amount of opioid analgesia required (Girdhari and Smith 2006). Local anaesthetics can also be used to target specific nerve pathways through direct injection to create specific nerve blocks. A variety of these are available depending on the point of trauma e.g. femoral nerve block for a hip fracture. They are normally limited to pain from trauma to a limb as blocks in the abdomen, pelvis and trunk are much more difficult to achieve.

Non-pharmacological methods for relieving pain at the site of trauma should also be attempted. These include a range of simple measures which could be utilised by all practitioners (Smith and Colvin 2005):

- positioning
- splinting/supporting
- application of heat or cold
- general comfort measures.

Pain management interventions to block onwards transmission

As well as targeting the site of trauma, pain management interventions can also be used to prevent the onward and upward transmission of pain from the dorsal horn of the spine to the hypothalamus.

Although the use of transcutaneous electrical nerve stimulator (TENS) machines are not considered suitable for the relief of acute pain, they can have some efficacy once the initial acute phase has subsided and may be useful for patients with longer term orthopaedic conditions. TENS machines are hypothesised to work by producing mild non-noxious (non-painful) stimuli in the form of electrical impulses. Electrodes are placed above the level of injury. A mild electrical impulse then stimulates A-beta fibres to activity and these messages enter the dorsal horn of the spinal column either at the same level or above that of the A-delta and C fibres in an attempt to 'crowd' the 'gate' and prevent onwards transmission of pain messages through the spinal tract. The efficacy of TENS machines is debatable with limited evidence. As they have no known side effects and are considered effective by some patients they are always worth consideration (Mackintosh and Elson 2008).

More commonly used epidural or spinal analgesias are used to block onwards transmission of pain messages. Epidural analgesia produces pain relief by continuous administration of pharmacological agents into the epidural space via an indwelling catheter. For orthopaedic trauma and surgery the catheter is commonly inserted into the lumbar epidural space, although it can also be inserted into the thoracic space following bowel and abdominal surgery and in patients with multiple rib fractures. Spinal or intrathecal analgesia differs from epidural as it is only used for short-term pain relief and normally as part of a surgical procedure.

Commonly used pharmacological agents include local anaesthetics, normally in combination with an opioid analgesic. A range of combinations have been advocated and although it is now recognised that a combination of the two types of drugs achieves the highest efficacy for pain relief, the exact combination is subject to ongoing debate (Smith and Colvin 2005).

Epidural and spinal analgesia can produce effective pain relief, but are subject to a number of constraints:

- They are both highly invasive techniques that require a skilled physician.
- They require carefully monitoring as serious side effects can occur.
- The nerve block achieved is non-discriminatory and although it will halt onward transmission of pain it also prevents all messages from reaching the higher senses – this means patients will be unable to mobilise or have reduced mobility, bladder and bowel emptying and need enhanced pressure area care.
- They cannot be used for prolonged periods of time.

Pain management interventions to affect conscious recognition

Once pain messages have reached the higher centres of the brain, conscious recognition of the experience takes place. However, this awareness can be modulated through use of systemic analgesics, adjunctive analgesia and non-pharmacological methods.

Systemic analgesia

Systemic analgesia is commonly used for the treatment of all pain types. This involves the use of paracetamol and opioids and inhalational analgesia such as nitrous oxide.

Paracetamol has limited anti-inflammatory action and should not be confused with aspirin which is part of the NSAID family. It is useful in mild to moderate pain, it can be safely used in combination with NSAIDs and opioids and is considered to have 'opioid sparing' properties i.e. when used in combination a lower opioid dose is required to achieve the same effect.

Opioids are the collective name for a group of drugs with opium-like properties which are similar to the endogenous substances the body is known to produce in response to pain. They have no peripheral action but bind to receptor sites in the central nervous system such as mu, kappa and delta receptors in the mid-brain and spinal cord where they suppress or inhibit pain transmission. Morphine is the commonest and most frequently used opioid analgesia and is the first-line systemic analgesic drug of choice for severe acute pain. It can be administered intravenously (IV), intra muscularly (IM), translingually, transdermally, orally and rectally (PR) as well as administered continuously in the form of an infusion or slow-release preparation or intermittently.

In acute pain, IV administration is the most effective way to produce fast-acting effective pain relief and should be the method of choice. IM administration should be avoided where possible as rate of take-up and action is slower and less certain than IV administration in acute situations. Once acute pain has been stabilised, transdermal or oral administration of morphine is preferred as its efficacy may be more closely monitored.

Individual opioid requirements vary up to a factor of 30 and for safe and effective use the dose should be titrated to the desired effect while minimising side effects. Side effects of systemic analgesia are frequently reported. Doses of paracetamol should be carefully monitored to ensure overdosing does not occur, as irreversible liver damage can occur. The use of opioids also engenders a range of side effects from the most commonly reported: constipation and gastric irritation, to sedation, confusion and respiratory depression. The more severe side effects are frequently over-represented and fears and misconceptions about these can lead to under-treatment of pain with opioids. Fear of addiction is also a factor which limits the appropriate and effective use of opioids. This has arisen due to misconceptions and misinformation. Addiction is extremely unlikely to occur following use of opioids for pain management in opioid-naïve patients. It should only be considered as problematic when a patient has had previous opioid use either prescribed or through illegal drug use. In either instance, where a patient has acute pain, it should not be withheld (Smith and Colvin 2005).

Nitrous oxide is more commonly known as Entonox in the UK and consists of a 50:50 mixture of oxygen and nitrous oxide which produces quick-acting, short-lasting pain relief. It is commonly used as a self-administered inhalation and is extremely useful for systemic pain relief when no other options are available i.e. at an accident site or for relief of short-lasting incident-specific pain following a procedure e.g. dressing change. It has minimal short term side effects, but cannot be used as a long term inhalation as nitrous oxide can lead to the breakdown of red blood cells.

Adjuvant analgesics may also have a place in the management of traumatic and orthopaedic pain, although their use is more commonly limited to patients with longer-term or chronic pain conditions thought to derive from underlying neuropathic damage. The exact mode of action of these drugs is not fully known and continues to be subject to extensive research; however they are well recognised as having an important effect in reducing the levels of pain reported by patients with neuropathic damage (Parsons and Preece 2010). The two commonest drug groups used are: antiepileptic drugs and tricyclic antidepressants.

Carbamazapine is the commonest of the antiepileptic drugs used and has been used for the treatment of phantom limb pain. Amitriptyline has a long history of use in chronic pain, although it has now been superseded by a new generation of trycyclics, most notably gabapentin and pregabalin. Clinical guidelines for the use of these drugs are available from NICE (2010).

Both these groups of adjuvant drugs can take up to two weeks to have any noticeable effect on reducing pain, which means they are not suitable for the treatment of acute pain, but where neuropathic pain is suspected treatment should be initiated as soon as possible to allow for this delayed onset.

Table 11.2 Relative efficacy of commonly used analgesics (adapted from Smith and Colvin 2005 p. 4 with permission). Reproduced with permission from Elsevier

Drug	Number needed to treat (NNT)
Paracetamol 1 g	4.6
Paracetamol 1 g+codeine 60 mg	2.2
Dihydrocedine 30 mg	10.0
Tramadol 100 mg	4.8
Diclofenac 50 mg	2.3
Ibuprofen 400 mg	2.4
Morphine 10 mg (IM)	2.9

When considering the use of pharmacological preparations for pain management the relative efficacy of different drugs should also be considered (Table 11.2). This is especially important when amending prescriptions for patients who may have an existing analgesia regime (e.g. undergoing arthroplasty for osteoarthritis) or who require adjustment to gain optimum pain relief.

When considering pain management the main points can be summarised as:

1 A multi-modal or balanced approach will always produce the most effective pain relief.
2 This can be achieved by using management approaches that focus on managing pain, peripherally at the site of trauma, interfering with the transmission of pain, and altering conscious perception of pain.
3 Where pain management is suboptimal this is nearly always due to poor pain management practices and produces unnecessary suffering.

Summary

Pain assessment and management in orthopaedic and trauma patients adheres to the same principles regardless of the underlying condition. The varied nature of pain experienced by these patients ensures that all nurses involved in their care must be familiar with best practice across the full range of pain that an individual can experience. The management of pain is a humanistic imperative and poorly managed pain exposes patients to unnecessary suffering and is a symptom of poor practice, rather than a necessary consequence of physical trauma. Nurses should ensure that their practice reflects the current principles of best practice and that pain assessment and management for all patients is at optimum levels.

Recommended further reading

National Institute for Clinical Excellence (NICE) (2010) Neuropathic Pain. *The Pharmacological Management of Neuropathic Pain in Adults in Non-specialist Settings*. NCG 96. NICE, London.

National Institute for Clinical Excellence (NICE) (2011) *Hip Fracture: The Management of Hip Fracture in Adults*. NCG 124. NICE, London.

Parsons, G. and Preece, W. (2010) *Principles and Practice of Managing Pain. A Guide for Nurses and Allied Health Professionals*. McGraw Hill, Maidenhead.

References

Australian and New Zealand College of Anaesthetists (ANZCA) and Faculty of Pain Medicine (2005) *Acute Pain Management: Scientific Evidence*. National Health and Research Council, Canberra Australia.

Beecher, H.K. (1959) *Management of Subjective Responses*. Oxford University Press, New York.

Berben, S.A.A., Tineke, H.J.M., Meijs, R.T.M. *et al*. (2008) Pain prevalence and pain relief in trauma patients in the Accident and Emergency Department. *Injury*, **39**, 578–585.

Clark, M.E., Scholten, J.D., Walker, R.L. and Gironda, R.J. (2009) Assessment and treatment of pain associated with combat related polytrauma. *Pain Medicine*, **10**(3), 456–469.

Clay, F.J., Newstead, S.V., Watson, W.L. *et al*. (2010) Biopsychosocial determinants of persistent pain 6 months after non-life threatening acute Orthopaedic trauma. *The Journal of Pain*, **11**(5), 420–430.

Cunningham, C. (2006) Managing pain in patients with dementia in hospital. *Nursing Standard*, **20**(46), 54–58.

Gillaspie, M. (2010) Better pain management after total joint replacement surgery. A quality improvement approach. *Orthopaedic Nursing*, **29**(1), 20–24.

Girdhari, S. and Smith, S.K. (2006) Assisting older adults with orthopaedic outpatient acute pain management. *Orthopaedic Nursing*, **25**(3), 188–195.

Mackintosh, C. (2007) Assessment and management of patients with post-operative pain. *Nursing Standard*, **22**(5), 49–55.

Mackintosh, C. and Elson, S. (2008) Chronic pain: clinical features, assessment and treatment. *Nursing Standard*, **23**(5), 48–56.

Malchow, R.J. and Black, I.H. (2008) The evolution of pain management in the critically ill trauma patient: emerging concepts from the global war on terrorism. *Critical Care Medicine*, **36**(7 suppl): S346–S357.

McCaffery, M. (1979) *Nursing Management of the Patient with Pain*, 2nd edn. Lippincott, Philadelphia, PA.

Melzack, R. and Wall, P.D. (1965) Pain mechanisms, a new theory. *Science*, **150**, 971–979.

Napier, D.E. and Bass, S.S. (2007) Postoperative benefits of intrathecal injection for patients undergoing total knee arthroscopy. *Orthopaedic Nursing*, **26**(6), 374–378.

National Institute for Clinical Excellence (NICE) (2010) *Neuropathic Pain. The Pharmacological Management of Neuropathic Pain in Adults in Non-specialist Settings NCG 96*. NICE, London.

National Institute for Clinical Excellence (NICE) (2011) *Hip Fracture: The Management of Hip Fracture in Adults*. NCG 124. NICE, London.

Parsons, G. and Preece, W. (2010) *Principles and Practice of Managing Pain. A Guide for Nurses and Allied Health Professionals*. McGraw Hill, Maidenhead.

Schugg, S.A. (2011) 2011 – the global year against acute pain (Editorial) *Anaesthesia and Intensive Care*, **39**(1), 11–14.

Smith, C.M. and Colvin, J.R. (2005) Control of acute pain in postoperative and post traumatic situations. *Anaesthesia and Intensive Care*, **6**(1), 2–6.

On-line resources:

International Association for the Study of Pain: http://www.iasp-pain.org/am/template.cfm?Section=Home

British Pain Society: http://www.britishpainsociety.org/

CHAPTER 12

Wound management, tissue viability and infection

Jeannie Donnelly[1], Alison Collins[2] and Julie Santy-Tomlinson[3]

[1] *Queens University Belfast/Belfast Health and Social Care Trust, Belfast, UK*
[2] *Belfast City Hospital, Belfast, UK*
[3] *University of Hull, Hull, UK*

Introduction

This chapter provides an outline of the knowledge and skills required by practitioners caring for patients with the main types of acute and chronic wounds in the field of trauma and orthopaedics. Recommendations for practice will often be pragmatic as empirical research is, in many instances, lacking. The chapter is divided into two sections. Section 1 focuses on the nursing management of wounds. This will include consideration of both surgical and traumatic wounds, an overview of the wound healing process and will discuss current thinking with regards to dressing techniques. Section 2 will consider issues relating to the prevention and management of pressure ulceration.

Whilst all wound types move through the three main stages of wound healing (inflammation, proliferation and contraction), speed and efficiency of healing is affected by a range of local and systemic factors. Key factors (according to wound type) will be highlighted. These must not, however, be viewed as mutually exclusive as all factors e.g. smoking and infection, will affect all wound types.

Wound management

Surgical wounds

A simple surgical wound is a healthy and uncomplicated break in the continuity of the skin resulting from surgery. It is expected to follow a rapid and predictable pathway towards healing with minimal tissue loss, scarring and loss of function. Surgeons take great care to protect as much tissue as possible from injury, carefully considering the placement of the incision, managing blood loss (to prevent haemorrhage and haematoma) and considering the best way to bring each layer of tissue (muscle, fascia, subcutaneous tissue and skin) into approximation through wound closure (Coulthard *et al.*, 2010). Approximation speeds time to healing, reduces scaring and helps prevent infection. The wound is said to heal by primary intention.

Traumatic wounds

Traumatic wound care is an integral part of the care of the patient following musculoskeletal trauma as soft tissue wounds are often consistent with the rest of the pattern of injury. Such wounds present a number of additional challenges. A compound fracture wound with full thickness tissue loss, for example, requires careful assessment (as there may be damage to nerves, tendons or muscles) and debridement of devitalised tissue. Often the wound cannot be closed immediately due to the risk of or presence of infection or excessive oedema. Closing very oedematous tissue will result in a taut wound leading to stress which can cause tissue ischaemia (reduced blood flow), particularly at the wound edge, potentially leading to tissue death or wound dehiscence (gaping or bursting open). To prevent this from happening body cavities and deeper structures are sutured closed and the layers of the skin left open to allow for free drainage of foreign material or pus or

Orthopaedic and Trauma Nursing: An Evidence-based Approach to Musculoskeletal Care, First Edition. Edited by Sonya Clarke and Julie Santy-Tomlinson.

whilst waiting for swelling to decrease. The patient will normally return to surgery after 3–4 days for a further wound assessment, followed by irrigation and debridement and wound closure if it is safe to do so. This is known as delayed primary closure. The wound is said to heal by tertiary intention (Lorenz and Longaker 2008).

Some wounds cannot be closed using surgical techniques due to one or more of the following reasons: (a) the patient is not well enough to undergo surgery, (b) the wound is small or superficial (c) the wound is heavily contaminated, infected or chronic or (d) the wound is deep with a 'dead space' and lack of subcutaneous tissue. If the skin is left open it is important to prevent the dead space filling with blood as haematoma is the perfect medium for bacteria to multiply and as it does not have a blood supply to initiate the immune system. Healing is by secondary intention.

The wound healing process

Wound healing is the process by which damaged tissue is replaced and function restored. The wound healing process is dynamic and can be divided into three overlapping phases: haemostasis/inflammation, proliferation and maturation (remodelling).

During haemostasis damaged blood vessels constrict and blood leaking from them begins to coagulate. Platelets in the vicinity are 'activated' by collagen fibres in the damaged vessels and clump together forming a relatively unstable plug. The activated platelets release vasoconstrictors and other chemicals which stimulate the clotting cascade and attract other platelets to the area. The end result is a clot (platelets intertwined with fibrin).

The goal of the inflammatory phase of wound healing is to limit the amount of tissue damage and prepare the wound for healing by removing unhealthy tissue and foreign matter such as bacteria. White blood cells (basophils, neutrophils and monocytes) play a major role. Basophils release heparin and histamine. Neutrophils and monocytes (converted to macrophages) migrate from the blood vessels and congregate at the site of injury, engulfing and destroying microorganisms. The inflammatory process is a necessary part of healing. Visible signs of the process are redness, heat, swelling, pain, loss of function and increased exudate.

The goal of the proliferation phase is to close the defect as quickly as possible. The wound fills with granulation tissue (unless it is very superficial in which case it will simply re-epithelialise), contracts down in size and epithelialises. Viable epidermal cells divide and migrate from the wound edges. Migration ceases when the epidermal cells come into contact with each other.

Granulation tissue is a network of collagen fibres, new blood vessels and white blood cells and peaks between five and nine days post-operatively, presenting as a 'healing ridge' along the margins of the wound (Doughty and Defriese 2007). New blood vessels form by the process of 'angiogenesis'. New capillaries (containing oxygen-rich blood and micronutrients) give the tissue a bright red granular appearance. Oxygen is important for cellular activity and any condition that impedes oxygenation of the tissues (e.g. smoking, peripheral vascular disease) slows healing and can lead to wound breakdown (Knuutinen *et al.*, 2002). Dark coloured granulation tissue, which bleeds easily, can be indicative of infection, poor perfusion or ischaemia.

Good nutrition (see Chapter 10) is central to successful wound healing. Malnutrition may involve a deficiency or excess (or imbalance) of energy, protein and other nutrients which can be a significant factor in wounds failing to heal or succumbing to infection.

Maturation occurs once the wound has re-epithelialised and strengthens the scar tissue. Weak Type III collagen fibres (produced by fibroblasts during granulation) are changed into or replaced by strong Type I collagen. As the wound has essentially healed there is a downturn in cellular activity and the need for extra oxygen and nutrients decreases.

In a simple surgical wound, the inflammatory phase is usually complete within 36–48 hours and the proliferative phase is complete in 28 days. Maturation can take around 100 days. A surgical wound is usually 'sealed' within 48 hours and will be dry (no bleeding or exudate) and can be exposed. The time frame is variable and may be extended depending on the complexity of the surgery, local wound conditions and the health of the patient. A patient whose wound continues to produce a high amount of exudate five days post-operatively, or who is complaining of increasing pain may have a surgical site infection (SSI). Wounds which are open or continue to 'weep' (exude) will need to be carefully monitored and dressed.

The phases of wound healing are dynamic; wounds may move forwards or backwards through each phase depending on the health of the patient. For example, a wound which was healing well (showing signs of granulation) but becomes infected, will move back into the inflammatory stage. A chronic wound is often described as a wound which is 'stuck' in the inflammatory or proliferative phase of wound healing.

Factors affecting wound healing

Factors affecting wound healing are often referred to as intrinsic (internal – specific to the individual) or extrinsic (external – applied to the individual). Any systemic condition which results in poor perfusion, a lack of essential micronutrients, the ability to fight infection or tissue wasting/destruction can delay wound healing (Table 12.1).

To aid wound healing, the general health and well-being of the patient must be optimised. This is achieved by creating a care plan which takes into account relevant health and psychosocial issues. Nurses, as 'gatekeepers' of care, have a responsibility to use their knowledge of the patient's needs and refer to other practitioners when help is needed.

Extrinsic factors that affect healing can be mechanical (pressure, shear, friction), chemical (wound exudate, cleansing solutions etc.) or thermal (heat, cold, radiation). Some of these factors (such as a moist wound environment) can aid healing, whilst others can delay healing.

Table 12.1 Factors and conditions affecting wound healing

Factor	Relevant conditions
Poor perfusion	• Respiratory and cardiovascular disorders • Arthrosclerosis, cardiovascular disorders such as cerebral vascular disease, angina and peripheral vascular disease • Diabetes – elevated blood glucose stiffens arteries and causes narrowing of the blood vessels leading to decreased blood flow • Smoking (nicotine) – causes blood vessels to constrict • Sepsis – leads to microvascular and macrovascular thrombosis • Medications – have a variety of effects on circulation • Poor social circumstances – especially homelessness, heat poverty • Stress – excess levels of noradrenaline are released leading to vasoconstriction
Micronutrient deficiency	• Malabsorption disorders, e.g. ulcerative colitis • Inability to eat or drink effectively, e.g. swallowing difficulties • Poor diet due to poverty or poor dietary choices • Alcoholism • Malignancy/cancer, the body is in a state of catabolism, the patient may be malnourished (nausea and vomiting)
Immunodeficiency/ suppression	• Neonate • Advanced age • Rheumatoid arthritis • HIV, AIDS • Stress • Cushings syndrome • Malignancy (myeloma, leukaemia, sarcoma etc.) • Diabetes – a high glucose level causes the immune cells to function ineffectively • Medications, e.g. cytotoxic drugs, corticosteroids
Tissue wasting/destruction	• Malignancy • Diabetes – neuropathy leads to inflammation and degeneration of peripheral nerves, which may interfere with circulation • Multiple sclerosis, spinal injury • Some conditions such as a stroke or spinal injury may result in the patient being unable to reposition themselves leading to pressure damage • Genetic disorders • Physical abuse, neglect or self harm • Certain medicaments, e.g. Nicorandil

Moist wound healing

Surgical wound dressings are applied to stem bleeding, absorb exudate and provide protection but there is constant debate about which dressing product best achieves such functions. Dry dressings may adhere to the wound (as fibres integrate into the clot matrix) causing pain and trauma on removal. Woven dressings are commonly used with the objective of absorbing wound moisture. It is claimed, however, that moist wounds heal more quickly than those left to dry out under textile-based dressings because epithelialisation is retarded by the formation of a dry scab (Winter 1962). A dressing which facilitates an optimal level of wound moisture, on the other hand, promotes wound healing (Harle *et al.*, 2005). Orthopaedic wound dressings should therefore have the attributes of the ideal dressing (Box 12.1) in addition to being absorbent and protective. The ability of a wound dressing to stretch with movement to avoid restricting limb movement and accommodate postoperative oedema is also important especially after hip and knee arthroplasty which requires a degree of force on behalf of the surgeon to position the prosthesis firmly, thereby resulting in postoperative bruising and swelling around the joint (Jester *et al.*, 2000).

Permeability and transparency

The permeability of a dressing refers to its ability to permit gaseous exchange (including water vapour) between the wound and external environment. Transparent films allow wound exudate and peri-wound skin to be inspected without dressing removal, minimising the risk of accidental wound contamination and trauma. Exudate, however, can pool under film dressings and cause maceration of the wound and surrounding skin (Cutting and White 2002) and peri-wound blister formation (Harle *et al.*, 2005). Absorbent central pad dressings with an adhesive border are quicker and easier to apply than traditional dressing pads, but offer no additional advantages in terms of permeability. Vapour-permeable film dressings transmit moisture away from the wound bed to varying degrees, but should not be applied as the primary dressing at sites of profuse drainage since absobency is limited. 'Film plus fabric' dressings combine transpiration and absorbency, helping to prevent accumulation of fluid (Aindow and Butcher 2005). The moist and relatively hypoxic environment produced by semi-occlusive and occlusive dressings accelerates angiogenesis and promotes tissue repair (Holm *et al.*, 1998). See Box 12.2 for further discussion of wound moisture balance.

Box 12.1 The properties of an ideal dressing (Cosker *et al.*, 2005). Reproduced with permission from MA Healthcare Limited

- Permeability – to control the rate of air exposure and the gaseous exchange between the wound and the outside environment
- The ability to remain in situ during bathing
- Transparency – to allow the monitoring of any fluid accumulation and other complications
- Low adherence – to facilitate removal from susceptible thin skin
- The ability to act as a complete barrier to bacteria and water, but not to moisture vapour

Box 12.2 Evidence digest: Wound moisture balance

Several studies examine the concept of moisture balance, facilitating an arthroplasty wound free of complications (Battacharyya *et al.*, 2005; Cosker *et al.*, 2005; Harle *et al.*, 2005; Abuzakuk *et al.*, 2006; Ravenscroft *et al.*, 2006). According to Cosker *et al.* (2005) 'fabric plus film' island dressings perform better (in terms of less blistering) compared to adhesive central pad dressings, film dressings and traditional wound pads and tape alone. Bhattacharyya *et al.* (2005) noted a lower incidence of both postoperative blistering ($p=0.24$) and superficial inflammation of surrounding skin ($p<0.001$) when a 'fabric plus film' island dressing was used versus an adhesive central pad dressing post arthroscopy of the knee. This reduction in blister formation (whilst not statistically significant) is arguably clinically significant, given the association of peri-wound skin trauma with superficial wound infection (Harle *et al.*, 2005; Polatsch *et al.*, 2004) and the fact that minor wound sepsis potentially increases the risk of deep wound sepsis (Blaylock *et al.*, 1995; Gaine *et al.*, 2000). The use of a vapour-permeable film to retain a hydrofibre dressing also appears to offer clinical advantages (less skin injuries such as blistering and epidermal stripping) when compared with a conventional wound pad and tape (Harle *et al.*, 2005) or adhesive central pad dressing (Abuzakuk *et al.*, 2006; Ravenscroft *et al.*, 2006).

Ability to act as a bacterial barrier

Traditional absorbent dressings provide limited protection against microbial ingress and may shed fibres into the wound, causing a focal point for infection (Jones 2006). Microbes pass through the dressing rapidly when it is damp and are dispersed into the environment on dressing removal, increasing the risk of cross-infection (Cooper and Lawrence 1996). Vapour-permeable films, incorporated into a fabric-island dressing or used as a retention dressing, have the advantage of being impermeable to bacteria (Pudner 2001). Hydrocolloids protect the wound from exogenous bacteria and have the advantage of lowering the pH of wounds to slightly acidic, inhbiting the growth of microbes (Bryan 2004). Hydrofibre dressings protect the wound from bacterial invasion by absorbing and retaining large amounts of exudate (including microbes) (Clarke *et al.*, 2009), reducing the need to change the dressing (Ravenscroft *et al.*, 2006) and lessening dispersal of microbes on dressing removal (White 2001).

Bathing and showering

There is a strong correlation between patient satisfaction with the postoperative dressing and ability to perform their usual personal hygiene routine (Bhattacharyya *et al.*, 2005). There is arguably no need to apply any dressing to a surgical wound after the early postoperative period since a natural bacteria-proof barrier (fibrin seal) is quickly re-established. Patient hygiene is facilitated and worry about the wound reduced by use of a vapour-permeable film until the wound is sealed with fibrin and drainage has ceased. Environmental moisture has a minimal effect on waterproof dressings providing it does not migrate under the surface. For this reason showering is preferable to bathing.

Ease of removal

Patients may experience pain where traditional gauze dressings adhere to the wound bed. Paraffin tulle gras also has a tendency to dry out and may result in postoperative wound trauma (Voegeli 2008). According to Gupta *et al.* (2002), spirit-soaked gauze lifts off the wound as it dries. However, spirit-soaked gauze is likely to cause pain on contact with broken skin due to the astringent properties of alcohol-based preparations. Alcohol solutions delay wound healing and usage should be restricted to prophylactic skin disinfection (Morgan 2004). Ravenscroft *et al.* (2006) found removal of hydrofibre and film combined to be less painful than an adhesive fabric dressing.

Wounds can exhibit a wide combination of different characteristics, e.g. deep tissues may be exposed or the wound may be malodourous with a high or low exudate. There is no one product which is 'smart' enough to manage all of these. Characteristics change as they move through the healing continum and practitioners must use their assessment to set realistic treatment objectives and make evidence based dressing choices.

Wound assessment

The first part of a wound assessment is to take a history of all factors leading to the cause of the wound. This information will provide clues to the underlying aetiology, the amount and type of tissue damage as well as potential complications such as infection. The five questions listed in Table 12.2 will help in this process. The second part of the assessment is to carefully observe the wound and the surrounding tissues to guide care and the choice of dressing. Results of the assessment should be recorded on a wound observation chart.

Wound measurement

The length, width and depth of the wound should be recorded as accurately as possible using a sterile disposable tape measure (which must not touch the wound). The length and width of the wound should be measured using the body axes as a reference point (as opposed to the longest and shortest part of the wound). Dimensions can change rapidly and over time measurements can become confused. In a wound where depth is easily visualised, a sterile probe can used to measure the distance from the bottom of the wound to the surface of the skin. Some wounds consist of extensive cavities or extremely narrow sinuses and the skin can be undermined, leading to exposure of fragile structures (blood vessels, nerves, organs). Wounds should not be probed unnecessarily as these fragile structures can be easily damaged. A surgeon or a tissue viability nurse may be able to map out the wound to assess the direction/depth of cavities. The dimensions of a wound which contains necrosis or slough will increase as 'dead' tissue is autolysed.

Wound bed

The wound bed tends to be described by the colour of tissue observed (black/brown, yellow, red and pink) (Table 12.3), indicating underlying problems such as ischaemia or tendon exposure. For example, if hard black necrosis is noted on the heel (Figure 12.1) it would be wise to assess the blood supply to the lower limb before wound debridement. If there is no blood supply, tissue cannot regenerate or mount an effective host response to infection. Tendons on the other hand, need to be kept moist to prevent dessication and loss of function. If there is no blood supply the practitioner should keep the wound dry and seek specialist help. As wounds can contain a mixture of tissues it can be difficult to accurately quantify what can be seen. Clinical judgement can be

Table 12.2 Wound history questions for wound assessment

Question	Rationale
Why is it there?	• i.e. trauma due to a fall, surgery etc. ○ Following trauma, determine the type and amount of tissue damage by asking questions about the characteristics of the mechanism involved • When the aetiology is unclear further investigations should determine the cause, e.g. a tissue biopsy
Where is the wound?	• The position may suggest aetiology e.g. a wound over a bony prominence may be linked to pressure damage • Wounds next to the anus may be at risk of faecal contamination • Wounds on the feet will raise issues around mobility • Wounds in awkward areas may be more difficult to dress, e.g. perineal area, joints, head • Accurate record keeping is esential, particularly if the patient has a number of wounds
When did it appear?	• The greater the time between wounding and good wound care, the greater the risk of infection especially for traumatic wounds • To determine if the wound has become chronic or not progressing to healing
Who is looking after the patient/client and their wound?	• It is important to communicate with practitioners, e.g. surgeons, district nurses, carers, who have been involved in the patients care, particularly if the patient is a poor historian • They will provide important additional information about the patient's health and socal status • Assess whether the patient's treatment regime is effective and identify allergies
What would the patient/client like to achieve?	• It is very important in establishing a realistic treatment objective, e.g. the patient may state that they want the wound healed in time for a special event. This may not be achievable and requires clarification so that the patient has time to accept the reality of their situation • This can help clarify the wound characteristic which is causing the patient the most distress, e.g. malodour, pain, or exudate

Table 12.3 Wound bed assessment – tissue colour

Colour	Definition	Differential rationale
Black	Tissue is necrotic (dead). There is no blood supply. Hard black necrosis is called eschar.	Dressings and ointments which contain silver (Ag) can stain the tissues a black colour but staining is superficial and temporary
Yellow	This tissue is sloughy. Slough is made up of dead cells and wound debris.	Tendons, fascia, bone and fat can also appear yellow.
Red	This tissue is healthy. Granulating tissue is comprised of collagen fibres (Type III) and new blood vessels. The new capillaries give the tissue its bright red colour and slightly uneven 'bumpy' texture. Dark red granulation tissue is a sign of poor perfusion or infection (Figure 12.2).	Muscles, organs (such as bowel) and dermis will also be red. Sometimes tissue can over-granulate; often referred to as 'proud flesh' as it sits above the level of the skin. It is often seen around trache and peg tube sites.
Pink	This tissue is healthy and is re-epithelialising.	The skin surrounding a wound can become very wet and macerated due to excess exudate. This skin can appear pinkish/white in colour.

used to make a subjective calculation of each tissue type. This is then expressed as a precentage, e.g. 20% black, 50% yellow, 30% red. During dressing changes the percentages are recalculated and compared to the previous assessment. Changes help to determine improvement or deterioration. Photographs can also be useful in charting the progress of extensive wounds.

The practitioner must have an understanding of the evidence-based rationale behind dressing selection to enable setting realistic wound management objectives.

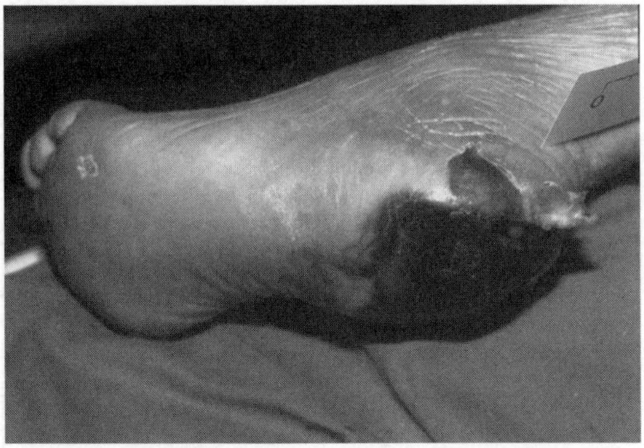

Figure 12.1 Heel pressure ulcer with necrosis and hard, black eschar

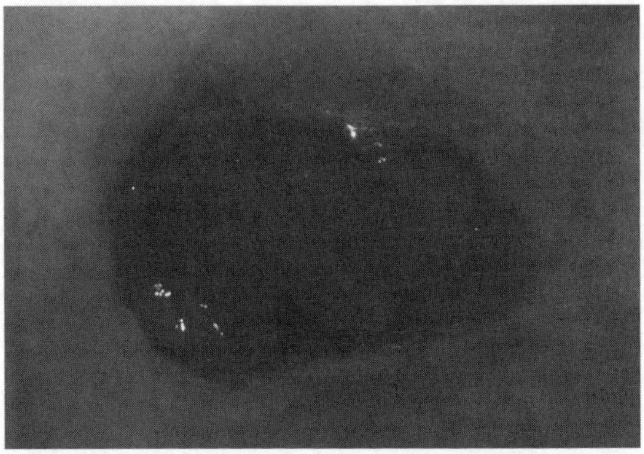

Figure 12.2 Wound containing over-granulation tissue

Dressing products range from those that actively donate moisture to a wound (hydrogels) to those that absorb or contain moisture. Some are impregnated with antimicrobial agents which should not be used unless there are clinical signs of infection or the patient is immunocompromised and there is a very high risk of infection. It is also important that general advice and support is given to the patient with respect to promoting healing and preventing infection.

Surgical site infection

Healthcare-associated infections (HAIs) collectively affect approximately one in ten hospital patients every year (DoH 2006). Such infections are costly complications of heath care that cause pain and discomfort, complicated and delayed recovery and sometimes death (Srinivasaiah 2007). Surgical site infection alone has been reported by NICE (2008) to be responsible for over one-third of perioperative deaths, increased healthcare costs and a significant impact on patient quality of life. Surveillance and prevention of infection are a major focus of health care and are seen as a care quality indicator.

Any infection is the outcome of complex interactions between a host, a pathogen and the environment (EWMA 2005) and is defined as:

> (The deposition of organisms in tissues and their subsequent growth and multiplication along with an associated tissue reaction.)
>
> (Ayliffe *et al.*, 2001)

Bacteria cannot penetrate intact skin, but can enter easily if the skin is damaged or an incision is made such as in the case of a surgical or traumatic wound. Infection is a painful and distressing complication that impairs the process of wound healing and is instrumental in delayed recovery. If it is allowed to progress it can lead to death through the spread of infection, septicaemia and organ failure.

The colonisation of any wound with microorganisms is unavoidable. The human body is host to a large number of bacteria and fungi that are part of the normal homeostatic mechanisms and are essential to many physiological processes. Harmful pathogenic organisms, however, are ever-present on the human body, in the atmosphere and in the environment. Ordinarily, the human immune system prevents these potential pathogens from entering the human body and causing harm. Organisms that are normally relatively harmless can become problematic when conventional preventive mechanisms fail.

In the orthopaedic patient the major risk from the spread of infection is osteomyelitis (infection of bone tissue) which is extremely difficult to eradicate. Osteomyelitis is also associated with biofilms attached to implanted devices or haematogenous seeding (spread of bacteria from the blood stream to implant sites) (Trampuz and Zimmerli 2006) and is a much feared complication of bone injury and surgery as the condition often becomes chronic and prevents bone from healing, leading to long-term pain and disability. The prevention of infections, including surgical site infection which may lead to osteomyelitis, is particularly central to the care of all orthopaedic patients.

Surgical site infection (SSI) is defined as:

> (Infection occurring up to 30 days after surgery (or up to one year after surgery in patients receiving implants and affecting the incision or deep tissue at the operation site.)
>
> (Owens *et al.*, 2008)

An estimated average of 2–5% of surgical patients develop SSI during their recovery and up to a year following orthopaedic implant surgery (NICE 2008). Most SSIs are caused by skin-derived bacteria, primarily *staphylococcus aureus* (Dohmen, 2008). Studies of SSI in orthopaedic patients report the incidence of serious deep infections associated with SSIs and highlight consequential increases in the length of hospital stay (Coello *et al.*, 2005). For example, deep wound infection occurs in up to 3% of patients following hip fracture repair. Surveillance data focus on high volume orthopaedic procedures such as arthroplasty and internal fixation of fractures (Morgan *et al.*, 2005). Although rates are dropping each year, SSIs in this group remain a significant problem. In many countries surveillance of SSI rates following orthopaedic surgery for total hip replacement, total knee replacement, hemiarthroplasty and open reduction of long bone fracture is mandatory. Many patients are now discharged from hospital before the surgical wound has healed, so it is likely that the symptoms of SSI may not appear until after discharge from hospital. Following orthopaedic implant surgery, deep surgical site infections may take up to one year to manifest (Health Protection Agency 2008).

Box 12.3 Evidence digest: Wound dressings to prevent wound surgical site infection

Several studies examine whether the choice of wound dressing impacts on the incidence of SSI after hip and knee surgery. Cosker *et al.* (2005) concluded that the incidence of SSI associated with adhesive fabric dressings or film plus fabric dressings was broadly similar. Ravenscroft *et al.* (2006), however, recorded a higher incidence of dressing failure (defined in part by the development of wound infection) with adhesive fabric dressings compared to hydrofibre and film. A similar trend in SSI reduction was noted when a Jubilee dressing was compared to an adhesive fabric dressing after arthroplasty of the hip and knee (Dillon *et al.*, 2007; Emmerson *et al.*, 2007). The component primary dressings for both the Jubilee and standard adhesive fabric dressings were the same (a liquid film-forming skin protectant and hydrofibre). Thus, any reduction in SSI should be attributed to the secondary hydrocolloid dressing, since this was the only known factor that differed between the two patient groups. Clarke *et al.* (2009) also reported low wound infection incidence rates when Jubilee dressings were applied with and without a liquid film-forming skin protectant.

Preventing surgical site infection

The use of the most recent evidence-based guidelines for preventing HAIs is central to the prevention of surgical site infection. This should focus on local and national guidance (Chapter 9). Specific measures for the prevention of surgical site infection include:

- Evidence-based preoperative preparation and perioperative care including skin preparation and antibiotic prophylaxis.
- Strict aseptic technique when dressing or handing wounds and wound drains.
- Wound drains should be removed as soon as possible, preferably within 24 hours of surgery.
- Keeping wounds covered in the hospital environment and until the proliferation phase of healing is complete (Box 12.3) and tampering with the wound/dressing as little as possible.
- Ensuring the patient's general health status and tissue perfusion is optimised through good nutrition and hydration.
- Close postoperative assessment and surveillance of the wound for signs of infection until recovery is complete and immediate medical referral if infection is suspected.

A frequent change of dressings is a potential risk factor for SSI (Leaper 2000) as exogenous bacteria may contaminate the wound during the dressing procedure. The rate of miotic cell division and leucocyte activity (necessary for wound healing and bacterial defence) is increased under wound dressings which facilitate near to core body temperatures (Xia *et al.*, 2000). Frequent cooling associated with changing the dressing should therefore be avoided as a means of reducing the risk of SSI.

Recognising surgical site infection

There are two common approaches to diagnosing infection:

1. Assessment of the clinical symptoms of infection based on observation of the wound and the localised and systemic inflammatory response and generalised systemic patient symptoms.
2. The laboratory analysis of samples taken from the wound used to identify the type and amount of growth of organisms (microbial load) in the wound.

Clinical assessment findings are widely considered to be a reliable approach to identifying infection in most wounds (Serena *et al.*, 2006) (Table 12.4). Damage to tissue causes an inflammatory reaction that is manifested as symptoms which provide potentially useful indicators

Table 12.4 Signs of surgical site infection which should be considered as part of the clinical assessment. Reproduced with permission from The Cochrane Collaboration

Sign	Rationale
Wound site/pain	Pain may reappear after the pain following injury or surgery has subsided. It may also last beyond that which would normally be expected for that injury or surgery.
Exudate	Excessive wound exudate which does not settle may be clear serous exudate or a purulent discharge. Discharge may also be dark brown if it arises from infection of a haematoma deep within the surgical site.
Foul odour	Indicates the presence of pathogenic microorganisms.
Wound breakdown	This may become apparent at the time of removal of sutures or clips and can be the result of an infected haematoma which acts as a barrier to wound healing.
Systemic symptoms	The patient may feel generally unwell with flu-like symptoms such as aches, lethargy, pyrexia and hot or cold shivers, disturbed sleep and loss of appetite.

of infection. There are four 'cardinal' signs of acute inflammation; redness, heat, swelling and pain. An important factor to consider is that, in deep surgical site infections, redness and heat at the base of the wound cannot be seen and may only manifest as pain. Hence any patient report of increasing or unresolved pain must be taken seriously. The presence or drainage of pus is an additional sign of infection in some wounds where the causative organism is 'pyogenic' (pus-forming).

The use of 'film plus fabric' dressings and films (as retention dressings), does not permit clear visual assessment of the wound area for early signs of wound infection such as spreading erythema to be identified (Mansha *et al.*, 2005). Additional signs of infection such as unexpected wound pain or tenderness, malodour, dehiscence, purulent discharge, localised swelling or heat in conjunction with microbiological analysis (Santy 2009) aid differentiation between the normal postoperative inflammatory response and that of inflammation due to infection.

A wound that exhibits clinical signs of infection may instigate sampling of the wound. Laboratory analysis of wound samples can provide the clinician with information about the microbial load within the wound. It cannot, however, differentiate between a colonised wound and an infected wound, so cannot diagnose infection. It can only confirm the presence of organisms in or around the wound and does not provide any information about whether this is having a detrimental effect on the host tissue (Sibbald 2003). Hence, diagnosis of infection should be based on clinical signs. Wound sampling should only be considered in wounds not responding to chosen antibiotics.

Pressure ulcers

Pressure ulcers (PUs, decubitus ulcers, bedsores, pressure sores/injuries) are localised areas of tissue damage that result from pressure or a combination of pressure and shear forces (EPUAP and NPUAP 2009). They usually occur over bony prominences, most commonly the sacrum and the heel bone, but can occur at any site that is subjected to pressure. Global incidence and prevalence surveys show that pressure ulcers remain a common problem. Prevalence rates are influenced by numerous factors such as mortality, length of stay and the influx of admissions, which vary considerably, but can help measure the burden of the problem and help in decision making regarding resource allocation. Incidence studies, which are based on the accumulation of new pressure ulcers, reflect the nosocomial (acquired in hospital/during care) problem and are particularly useful in determining patients at risk and allow inferences regarding the effect of preventive care measures (International Guidelines 2009). Some patient groups are at a higher risk than the general hospital population including those who are critically ill, older adults (>65 years) and people who have reduced mobility such as many orthopaedic patients.

It is difficult to determine the true cost of pressure-related tissue damage but a high prevalence or incidence of pressure ulcers leads to human suffering, lost opportunity costs, extra resources used and potential litigation. It is important that nurses act to reduce the number and severity of ulcers through the delivery of evidence-based care. The physical, social and psychological suffering experienced by patients with pressure ulcers is immense. Hopkins *et al.* (2006) used a phenomenological approach to explore the 'endless pain' and 'restricted life', which patients suffer. This distress is caused by: (1) local factors such as pain, wound exudate and malodour, often leading to social isolation; (2) delayed rehabilitation, which may result in economic hardship and (3) serious complications such as cellulitis, osteomyelitis, septicaemia, limb amputation and even death.

Classification of pressure ulcers

In order to improve written and verbal communication amongst practitioners the EPUAP/NPUAP (2009) scale is widely used to classify pressure ulcers. Ulcers are classified into four (six in the USA version) categories depending on the depth of tissue damage:

- The wound is assessed as category/stage I when there is observable erythema that is non-blanchable or persistent along with pain and raised tissue temperature.
- Category/stage II is denoted by partial thickness skin loss with a shallow, open, red/pink ulcer without slough or bruising. This stage might also present as a fluid-filled blister.
- Category/stage III presents as full thickness skin or tissue loss in which subcutaneous fat may be visible. The ulcer may, however, be either shallow or deep and there may also be slough, but not to any great depth (Figure 12.3).
- Category IV refers to deep ulcers in which there is full thickness tissue loss in which there may be exposed bone, tendon or muscle. There may also be slough or eschar present within the wound along with undermining or tunnelling.

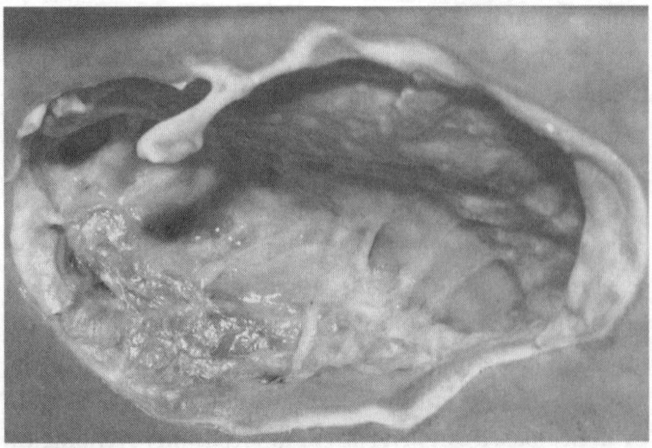

Figure 12.3 Pressure ulcer containing slough

In the USA two further categories are often used. Unstageable/unclassified ulcers are those in which there is full thickness skin or tissue loss but the depth is unknown as the wound may be obscured by slough and/or eschar. Suspected deep tissue injury is a further category referring to other wounds in which the depth is unknown. A localised area of purple or maroon but intact skin is recognised as denoting damage to the underlying tissue but the full depth of tissue damage cannot be ascertained.

A quick reference guide to this scale can be viewed and downloaded at:

http://www.npuap.org/wp-content/uploads/2012/02/Final_Quick_Prevention_for_web_2010.pdf which offers the practitioner further advice and evidence-based rationale for use of the system.

Pressure ulcer formation

When an external load is applied to the skin, autoregulatory processes allow the internal capillary pressure to rise so that blood flow is reduced. It is believed that pressure damage occurs when the blood supply to the skin is occluded by an external perpendicular force which supersedes internal capillary closing pressure. Intense pressures of short duration are as injurious to tissues as lower pressures applied for a longer period. This demonstrates that, in order to prevent pressure damage, it is essential to reduce the intensity and duration of pressure by, for example, repositioning immobile patients and the use of pressure-redistributing support surfaces.

Other forces such as friction and shear can significantly decrease the tolerance of tissue to directly applied pressure. Extrinsic factors, such as moisture, friction and shear impinge upon the surface of the skin and intrinsic factors reduce the sensation or perception response mechanism or alter the structural constituents and perfusion of tissues. More than 200 contributing factors have been identified in the development of pressure ulcers.

Superficial ulceration

It has been suggested that superficial pressure ulcers occur in one of two ways: (1) the epidermis is simply stripped away from the dermis; this typically occurs as a result of skin being abraded through, for example, repetitive rubbing or poor 'moving and handling' techniques (frictional forces); or (2) shear forces distort and damage the microvasculature, which feeds the epidermal basal layer. The basal layer becomes ischaemic and sloughs off.

Deep ulceration

There are two main ways in which deep tissue can suffer significant damage. A typical stage 4 pressure ulcer occurs when the fascia between fat and muscle is unable to block the pressure from damaging underlying muscle and bone (Black *et al.*, 2007). This force directly occludes blood vessels, causing ischaemia. It may also affect arteries that penetrate into bone marrow, sometimes resulting in aseptic necrosis of underlying bone. Meanwhile the dermal capillaries remain largely unaffected, possibly because of other factors such as shear. Shear forces disrupt arterioles in the muscle but, since muscle is a well vascularised tissue, the resulting haematoma is likely to be large and well beyond the capacity of the body to absorb. The lesion will track towards the skin surface. Tissue insult does not end when the pressures and forces are withdrawn, as rapid reperfusion may also contribute to injury.

Preventative care

The detection of early or superficial tissue damage along with the instigation of appropriate and timely care can prevent or reverse the majority of impending pressure ulcers. Guidance for preventative care is enshrined in local, national and international guidelines that highlight that pressure ulcer prevention begins on admission with a baseline skin assessment to determine the presence or absence of pressure damage. This is followed by a holistic assessment to identify factors that may heighten susceptibility.

Risk assessment scales numerically rate a range of risk factors which are added together to indicate the likelihood of pressure damage. Many risk assessment scales, however, have not been tested for predictive ability and factors such as the client group and preventive care can affect sensitivity and specificity. It is important to use scales as a framework for assessment as opposed to the sole indicator of risk. The level of risk can change along with the patient's condition and it is vital that risk is reassessed at regular intervals. Most healthcare providers have a standard risk assessment format that is used by all staff and local guidelines often govern the frequency and triggers for this.

Following each assessment a care plan must be tailored to address risk factors such as pressure, shear, friction, incontinence, pain and malnutrition with the goal of:

1 Maintaining and improving tissue tolerance to pressure through evidence-based skin care and addressing malnutrition.
2 Protecting against the adverse effects of external mechanical forces.

Moisture (urine, faeces, perspiration and wound drainage) adversely affect skin in one of five ways:

1 It may make skin more susceptible to tissue damage by enhancing the frictional component of a shearing force (Sprigle 2000)
2 It can irritate and macerate skin, making it more prone to infections and rashes, resulting in superficial skin loss (Kotter and Halfens 2010).
3 Elevated humidity at the skin surface may cause discomfort and agitation, leading to abrasions (Clark 1996).
4 Many skin cleansers contain products that remove sebum and surface lipids, drying skin, rendering it vulnerable to water-soluble irritants and increasing friction (Gray *et al.*, 2002).
5 Moisture may interact with chemical residues left on bed linen following the laundering process (Alberman 1992) resulting in chemical burn that leads to skin damage.

In order to combat these problems, clinical guidelines highlight the importance of:

- Daily systematic skin assessments, paying attention to bony prominences.
- The promotion of continence and immediate cleansing at time of soiling.
- Mild cleansing agents (pH 5.5) and judicious use of moisturisers that keep skin well hydrated.
- Minimising friction and shear forces through careful positioning, transferring and turning techniques.

Malnutrition, particularly protein–calorie malnutrition, increases an individual's risk of developing pressure ulcers. This point has been supported by Langer *et al.* (2003) who carried out a systematic review in order to (a) summarise the best available research and (b) enable evidence-based guidance on the role of nutritional interventions in pressure ulcer prevention and treatment (Box 12.4 and Chapter 10).

The adverse effects of external mechanical forces can be minimised in two ways:

1 Completely remove pressure (offload) from the pressure areas using manual repositioning techniques, devices such as pillows and splints and/or alternating mattresses.

Box 12.4 Evidence digest: The role of nutritional interventions in pressure ulcer prevention and treatment (Langer *et al.*, 2003)

Only four studies met Langer *et al.*'s (2003) review inclusion criteria and for various reasons entitled 'Methodological weaknesses of studies designed to detect the impact of nutritional interventions on pressure ulcer incidence'; none of these were deemed to be sufficiently scientifically robust to detect the true impact of nutritional interventions on pressure ulcer incidence. Patient groups, interventions, outcome measurements and follow-up periods (ranging from 14–180 days), were too heterogeneous to allow for meta analysis.

Despite these problems, it was noted that all of the studies, which looked at the effect of mixed nutritional supplements in people recovering from hip fractures, reported a lower incidence of pressure ulcers in the groups receiving dietary supplements. It was also noted that in the acute phase of a critical illness elderly people appeared to develop fewer pressure ulcers when given two daily supplement drinks. Other independent risk factors for pressure ulceration were also noted and included low serum albumin, a lower limb fracture, a Norton score <10 or a low Kuntzman score.

Given these findings and the fact that (a) collagen degradation occurs following injury, (b) essential nutrients are required for collagen synthesis and stability during healing (Nixon 2001), it is reasonable to hypothesise that the skin of critically ill malnourished patients may be particularly vulnerable to the effects of pressure, shear and friction but requires further investigation.

Box 12.5 Evidence digest: Preventive schemes to assess the effects of turning (Defloor *et al.*, 2005)

A study by Defloor *et al.* (2005) used a four-arm experimental design (over a 4-week period) to compare four preventative schemes to assess the effects of turning with different intervals on the development of pressure ulcers. Subjects were recruited from 11 nursing homes caring for older people (n = 838). Of these:

- 65 patients were allocated to 2-hourly turns on a standard institutional mattress
- 65 patients were allocated to 3-hourly turns on a standard institutional mattress
- 67 patients were allocated to 4-hourly turns on a viscoelastic polyurethane foam mattress
- 65 patients were allocated to 6-hourly turns on a viscoelastic polyurethane foam mattress
- 576 patients were allocated to the standard care group.

Using logistic regression, the investigators found that the incidence of non-blanchable erythema was not significantly different between groups. However, the incidence of grade II and higher pressure ulcers was significantly less in the 4-hour interval group (3.0% compared with incidence figures in the other groups varying between 14.3% and 24.1%). The authors concluded that 4-hourly turns are a feasible preventive method in terms of effect, effort and cost. Interestingly, further data from this study presented by Vanderwee *et al.* (2005) indicated that 29.1% of the pressure ulcers were located at the heels. The authors concluded that elevating the heels from the mattress could have prevented these ulcers.

2 Use a conforming support surface to distribute the body weight over a larger surface area (pressure reduction) and reduce the magnitude and/or duration of pressure between a patient and their support surface (the "interface pressure") (McInnes *et al.*, 2011).

Turning

The traditional 2-hourly turn originates from attempts to prevent pressure damage in a spinal injury unit (Clark 1998). While there appears to be very little scientific evidence to support its efficacy, research by Moore *et al.* (2011) indicates that 3-hourly repositioning using the '30-degree tilt' reduced the incidence of pressure damage when compared to a 6-hourly turn. It is not always possible, however, to reposition patients if their underlying physiological condition is critical and unstable. One study that has examined this issue is considered in Box 12.5. Furthermore, 2-hourly repositioning can lead to sleep disruption, which can lengthen recovery, suppress immune function and pre-dispose patients to infection (Carskadon 2005). Gillespie *et al.* (2012) note that whilst regular movement is important, unnecessary repositioning may cause increased discomfort for people with wounds, stiff joints, bony pain or contractures.

30-degree tilting regime

It has been argued that the 30° tilt is more effective in off-loading bony prominences than a 90° body turn (Figure 12.4). Each time the patient needs to be repositioned, they are gently rolled 20–30° medially or laterally from the starting point onto 'soft sites' (e.g. the side of the buttock) as opposed to bony prominences. Pillows are used to support the body and to act as space fillers. One corner of the pillow is placed under the ankle (to elevate the heel) and the rest of the pillow is

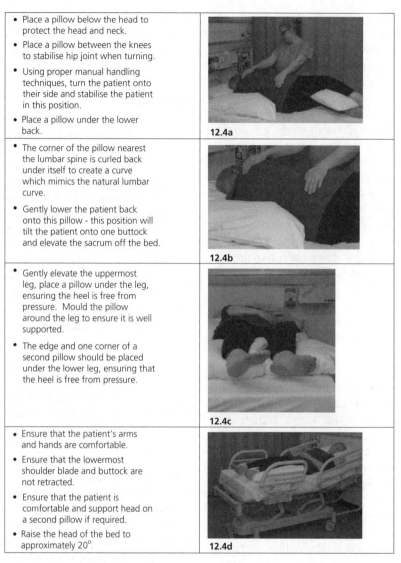

• Place a pillow below the head to protect the head and neck. • Place a pillow between the knees to stabilise hip joint when turning. • Using proper manual handling techniques, turn the patient onto their side and stabilise the patient in this position. • Place a pillow under the lower back.	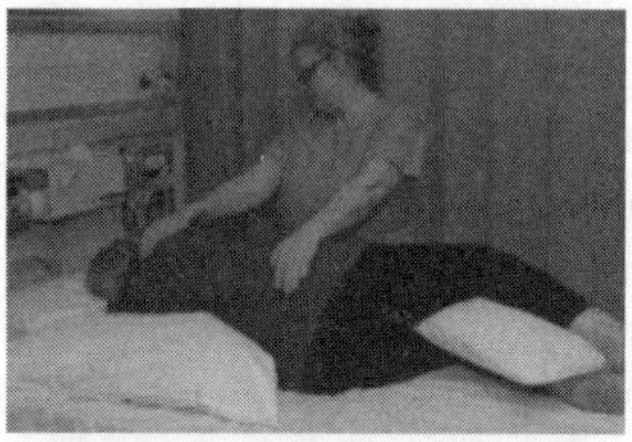 **12.4a**
• The corner of the pillow nearest the lumbar spine is curled back under itself to create a curve which mimics the natural lumbar curve. • Gently lower the patient back onto this pillow - this position will tilt the patient onto one buttock and elevate the sacrum off the bed.	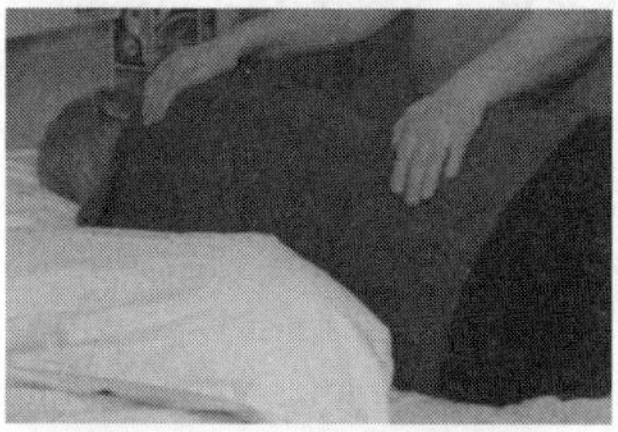 **12.4b**
• Gently elevate the uppermost leg, place a pillow under the leg, ensuring the heel is free from pressure. Mould the pillow around the leg to ensure it is well supported. • The edge and one corner of a second pillow should be placed under the lower leg, ensuring that the heel is free from pressure.	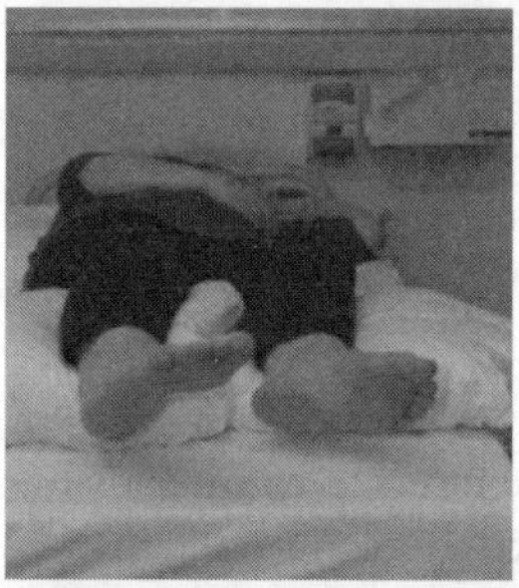 **12.4c**
• Ensure that the patient's arms and hands are comfortable. • Ensure that the lowermost shoulder blade and buttock are not retracted. • Ensure that the patient is comfortable and support head on a second pillow if required. • Raise the head of the bed to approximately 20°.	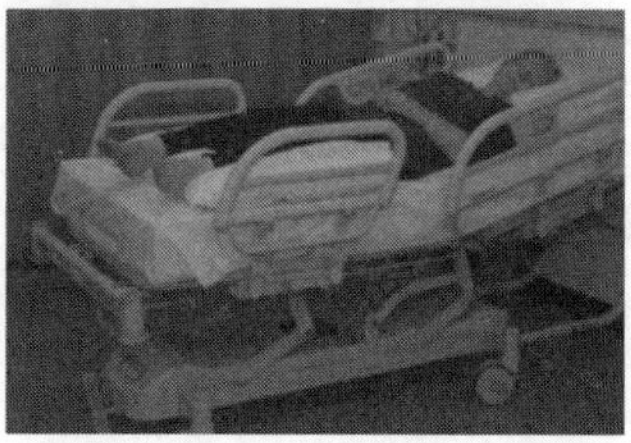 **12.4d**

Figure 12.4 (a, b, c, and d) Performing the 30 degree tilt

moulded into any gaps made by the contour of the limb to create more uniform pressure loads. This should, in theory, reduce the pressure over any one area. Defloor (2000) used $TCPO_2$ measurements to show the benefits of offloading bony prominences using the 30° tilt technique and Moore *et al.* (2011) showed that it reduced the incidence of pressure damage in elderly at-risk patients in comparison to standard care. The technique is not, however, suitable for all patients; it is contraindicated, for example, in patients with an acute spinal injury and may be contraindicated in patients following a hip arthroplasty due to the risk of iatrogenic injury and contractures.

Pillows

The benefits and risks associated with the use of pillows as a pressure relieving device is under-researched. Heels which project beyond pillows are subject to zero pressure (Smith 1984), suggesting that carefully placed pillows (Figure 12.4c) can be a cost-effective way of offloading the heel. Smith, however, believed that pillows were unacceptable due to the increased risk of deep venous thrombosis and there are also concerns about the pressure which may be exerted over the Achilles tendon. Sigel *et al.* (1973), however, noted that a body tilt to a 10-degree foot-up position increased venous flow by 30%, suggesting that with a pillow in situ simply tilting the bed could offset any risk of deep venous thrombosis. In acutely ill bed-bound patients any potential risk of a venous thromboembolism would be minimised through the current standard treatment (Chapter 9). Concern that inappropriately placed pillows can lead to knee contractures can be overcome by placing pillows lengthways, i.e. from just below the crease of the knee to the ankle or using the pillow as a 'space-filler'. Both of these techniques should maximise the surface contact area and reduce pressure on all parts of the lower leg. In addition, bending the knee section of a profiling bed helps to reduce the risk that the knee will become hyperextended. Pillows are easily 'kicked' out of the safe position; heels may lie on the pillow rather than over the edge of the pillow and the heel area will be subject to pressure and tissue could become damaged (Donnelly 2005).

Collars

Cervical collar related pressure ulcers remain relatively common. They commonly occur on the occiput, the chin and the shoulders. Risk factors include ICU admission ($P=0.007$), mechanical ventilation ($P=0.005$), the necessity for cervical MRI ($P \leq 0.001$) and time to cervical spine clearance ($P \leq 0.001$) (Ackland *et al.*, 2007). Interestingly, the time to cervical spine clearance was the major indicator, with a 66% increase in risk of tissue damage for every one day increase in cervical collar time (Chapter 19). There are a number of actions which nurses can take to reduce the risk of pressure damage:

- change the patient from a rigid to a semi-rigid collar as soon as possible
- ensure the collar is fitted correctly and is the right size
- remove the collar every 4 hours for skin assessment and hygiene
- hair should be parted and hidden pressure points such as the occiput inspected for signs of redness or discolouration
- check the chin, mandible, ears, shoulders, sternum and laryngeal prominence for pressure damage
- wash and dry the skin carefully
- men should be shaved for comfort and to prevent skin irritation.
- check the collar padding – this must be changed if it is wet or soiled
- if necessary adjust the pad so that no plastic touches the skin.

Heel splints

Devices which completely offload the heel, appear to be more effective than support surfaces in reducing the incidence of heel pressure ulcers. In a recent study (Donnelly *et al.*, 2011), older patients with a fracture of the hip were randomly allocated to receive heel elevation plus use of a pressure-redistributing support surface or standard care (pressure-redistributing support surface alone). Findings indicated that subjects in the control group (heels down) were more likely than those in the intervention group (heel elevation) to suffer pressure damage. The challenge with current devices is that many patients find them uncomfortably warm and too heavy. Further consideration is given to safe care of casts and traction in Chapter 8.

Alternating support surfaces

Alternating pressure redistributing devices (mattresses replacements, overlays and cushions) contain a number of air-filled 'cells', which alternately inflate and deflate beneath the patient, mimicking normal body movement. As these cells inflate they generate high interface pressures, but because these are only sustained for a short period of time, the body is (arguably) able to withstand the pressure. As soon as the cells deflate, the hypoxic tissue is reperfused by the normal hyperaemic response. Allen *et al.* (1993) noted, however, that no studies have shown that bony prominences such as the heel are completely offloaded and remain vulnerable to damage. As most immobilised patients experience reduced blood flow, alternating pressure may also have an effect on tissue perfusion, resulting in improved blood flow and facilitating the prevention of pressure ulcers.

Pressure-reducing support surfaces (constant low pressure devices)

Pressure-reducing support surfaces are designed to mould around the shape of the patient. They increase the amount of contact that the body has with the support surface, thus reducing the magnitude of interface pressures at any given anatomical location. Although many different types of pressure-reducing devices are available, a systematic review of the literature has been unable to determine which is most effective with regards to pressure ulcer prevention (McInnes *et al.*, 2011). The review determined that higher specification foam mattresses offer more protection than standard hospital foam mattresses and that air-fluidised beds may improve pressure ulcer healing rates. Pressure-redistributing equipment presently used to prevent pressure ulcers has not been fully and reliably evaluated.

Management of pressure ulcers

Inevitably, most orthopaedic practitioners will continue to care for patients with pressure ulcers. Good fundamental care which includes nutritional support and hydration remains central to this. Without the pressure ulcer prevention measures discussed above no pressure ulcer will heal. Hence it is only when all possible prevention measures are in place that a focus on good wound management practice can be made with a view to healing the ulcer. Practitioners must make intelligent use of wound management guidelines discussed in the first section of this chapter.

Recommended further reading

Bryant, R.A. and Nix, D.P. (eds) (2011) *Acute and Chronic Wounds: Current Management Concepts*, 4th edn. Mosby, St. Louis.

Dealey, C. (2012) *The Care of Wounds. A Guide for Nurses*, 4th edn. Wiley Blackwell, Oxford.

European Pressure Ulcer Advisory Panel and National Pressure Ulcer Advisory Panel (EPUAP/NPUAP) (2009) Treatment of Pressure Ulcers: Quick Reference Guide. Washington DC: National Pressure Ulcer Advisory Panel (online). Available at: http://www.npuap.org/wp-content/uploads/2012/02/Final_Quick_Prevention_for_web_2010.pdf (accessed 2 January 2014).

Flanagan, M. (2013) *Wound Healing and Skin Integrity. Principles and Practice*. Wiley Blackwell, Oxford.

References

Ackland, H.M., Cooper, J., Malham, G.M. and Kossmann, T. (2007) Cervical Spine Factors Predicting Cervical Collar-Related Decubitus Ulceration in Major Trauma Patients. *Spine*, **32**(4), 423–428.

Aindow, D. and Butcher, M. (2005) Films or fabrics: is it time to reappraise postoperative dressings? *British Journal of Nursing*, **14**(19), S15–S20.

Alberman, K. (1992) Is there any connection between laundering and the development of pressure sores? *Journal of Tissue Viability*, **2**(2), 55–56.

Allen, V., Ryan, D.W. and Murray, A. (1993) Potential for bed sores due to high pressures: influence of body sites, body position, and mattress design. *British Journal of Clinical Practice*, **47**(4),195–197.

Ayliffe, G.A., Babb, J.R. and Taylor, L.J., (2001) *Hospital Acquired Infection. Principles and Prevention*, 3rd edn. Arnold, London.

Bhattacharyya, M., Bradley, H., Holder, S. and Gerber, B. (2005) A prospective clinical audit of patient dressing choice for post-op arthroscopy wounds. *Wounds UK*, **1**(1), 30–34.

Black, J., Baharestani, M., Cuddigan, J. *et al.* (2007) National Pressure Ulcer Advisory Panel's Updated Pressure Ulcer Staging System. *Urologic Nursing*, **27**(2), 144–150.

Bryan, J. (2004) Moist wound healing: a concept that changed our practice. *Journal of Wound Care*, **13**(6), 227–228.

Carskadon, M.A. and Dement, W.C. (2005) Normal Human Sleep: An Overview, in *Principles and Practice of Sleep Medicine*, 4th edn. (eds M.H. Kryger, T. Roth and W.C. Dement), Elsevier Sanders, Philadelphia.

Clark, M. (1996) The aetiology of superficial sacral pressure sores, in *Proceedings of the 6th European Conference on Advances in Wound Management* (edsD.L. Leaper, Cherry, G.W. and C. Dealey), MacMillan Press, Amsterdam, pp. 167–170.

Clark, M. (1998) Repositioning to prevent pressure sores – what is the evidence. *Nursing Standard*, **13**(93), 58–64.

Clarke, J. V., Deakin, A.H., Dillon, J.M., Emmerson, S. and Kinninmonth, A.W.G. (2009) A prospective clinical audit of a new dressing design for lower limb arthroplasty wounds. *Journal of Wound Care*, **18**(1), 5–11.

Coello, R., Charlett, A., Wilson, J. *et al.* (2005) Adverse impact of surgical site infections in English hospitals. *Journal of Hospital Infection*, **60**(2), 93–103.

Cooper, R. and Lawrence, J. C. (1996) The prevalence of bacteria and implications for infection control. *Journal of Wound Care*, **5**(6), 291–295.

Coulthard, P., Esposito, M., Worthington, H.V., van der Elst, M., van Waes, O.J.F. and Darcey, J. *Tissue adhesives for closure of surgical incisions. Cochrane Database of Systematic Reviews* **5**(Art. No.: CD004287). DOI: 10.1002/14651858.CD004287.pub3.

Cosker, T., Elsayed, S., Gupta, S., Mendonca, A. and Tayton, K. (2005) Choice of dressing has a major impact on blistering and healing outcomes in orthopaedic patients. *Journal of Wound Care*, **14**(1), 27–29.

Cutting, K.F. and White, R.J. (2002) Maceration of the skin and wound bed 1: its nature and causes. *Journal of Wound Care*, **11**(7), 275–278.

Defloor, T. (2000) The effect of position and mattress on interface pressure. *Applied Nursing Research*, **13**(1), 2–11.

Defloor, T. and Clark, M. (2005) Pressure ulcer classification tool (PULCLAS), EPUAP, Oxford (online). Available at: http://www.epuap.org (accessed 21 April 2013).

Department of Health (DOH) (2006) *The Health Act 2006: Code of Practice for the Prevention and Control of Healthcare Associated Infection*. DoH, London.

Dillon, J.M., Clarke, J.V., Emmerson, S. and Kinninmonth, A.W.G. (2007) The Jubilee method: A novel, effective wound dressing following total hip and knee arthroplasty, Poster presentation, in *Proceedings of the American Academy of Orthopaedic Surgeons Annual Meeting, San Diego*, California.

Dohmen, P.M. (2008) Antibiotic resistance in common pathogens reinforces the need to minimise surgical site infections. *Journal of Hospital Infection*, **70**(S2), 15–20.

Donnelly, J. (2005) The Importance of a Pilot Study in Informing a Main Study Design, Poster Presentation, in *National Pressure Ulcer Advisory Panel 9th National Conference: Merging Missions*. Salt Lake City, USA. *February 25–26*.

Donnelly, J., Winder, J., Kernohan, W.G. and Stevenson, M. (2011) An RCT to determine the effect of a heel elevation device in pressure ulcer prevention post-hip fracture. *Journal of Wound Care*, **20**(7), 309–312, 314–318.

Doughty, D.B. and Defriese, B. (2007) Wound-healing physiology, in *Acute and Chronic Wounds: current Management Concepts*, 3rd edn (eds R.A. Bryant and D.P. Nix), Mosby, St. Louis.

European Pressure Ulcer Advisory Panel and National Pressure Ulcer Advisory Panel (EPUAP/NPUAP) (2009) *Treatment of Pressure Ulcers: Quick Reference Guide*. National Pressure Ulcer Advisory Panel, Washington DC. Available at: www.npuap.org (accessed 21 April 2013).

Gaine, W.J., Ramamohan, N.A., Hussein, M.G., Hullin, M.G. and McCreath, S.W. (2000) Wound infection in hip and knee arthroplasty. *The Journal of Bone and Joint Surgery (British)* **82-B**(4), 561–565.

Gillespie, B.M., Chaboyer, W.P., McInnes, E., Kent, B. and Whitty, J.A. (2012) Repositioning for pressure ulcer prevention in adults (Protocol). *Cochrane Database of Systematic Reviews* **4**(Art. No.: CD009958). DOI: 10.1002/14651858.CD009958.pub2.

Gray, M., Ratliff, C. and Donovan, A. (2002) Perineal skin care for the incontinent patient. *Advances in Skin and Wound Care*, **15**(4), 170–175.

Gupta, S., Lee, S. and Moseley, L. (2002) Postoperative wound blistering: is there a link with dressing usage? *Journal of Wound Care*, **11**(7), 271–273.

Harle, S., Korhonen, A., Kettunen, J. and Seitsalo, S. (2005) A randomised clinical trial of two different wound dressing materials for hip replacement patients. *Journal of Orthopaedic Nursing*, **9**(4), 205–210.

Health Protection Agency (2008) *Protocol for Surveillance of Surgical Site Infection*. Version 3.4 Surgical Site Infection Surveillance Service. Available at: http://www.hpa.org.uk/webc/hpawebfile/hpaweb_c/1194947388966 (accessed 17 April 2014)

Holm, C., Petersen, J. S., Gronboek, F. and Gottrup, F. 1998 Effects of occlusive and conventional gauze dressings on incisional healing after abdominal operation. *European Journal of Surgery*, **164**:179–183.

Hopkins, A., Dealey, C., Bale, S., Defloor, T. and Worboys, F. (2006) Patient stories of living with a pressure ulcer. *Journal of Advanced Nursing*, **56**(4), 345–353.

International Guidelines (2009) *Pressure Ulcer Prevention: Prevalence and Incidence in Context. A Consensus Document*. MEP Ltd, London. Available at: http://www.woundsinternational.com/pdf/content_24.pdf (accessed 17 April 2014)

Jester, R., Russell, L., Fell, S., Williams, S. and Prest, C. (2000) A one hospital study of the effect of wound dressings and other related factors on skin blistering following total hip and knee arthroplasty. *Journal of Orthopaedic Nursing*, **4**(2), 71–77.

Jones, V.J. (2006) The use of gauze: will it ever change? *International Wound Journal*, **3**(2), 79–86.

Kotter, J. and Halfens, R. (2010) Moisture lesions: Inter-rater agreement and reliability. *Journal of Clinical Nursing*, **19**,716–720.

Knuutinen, A., Kokkonen, N., Risteli, J. *et al.* (2002) Smoking affects collagen synthesis and extracellular matrix turnover in human skin. *British Journal of Dermatology*, **146**,588–594.

Langer, G., Knerr, A., Kuss, O., Behrens, J. and Schlömer, G.J. (2003) Nutritional interventions for preventing and treating pressure ulcers. *Cochrane Database of Systematic Reviews* **4**(Art. No.: CD003216). DOI: 10.1002/14651858.CD003216.

Leaper, J. (2000) Wound Infection, in *Bailey and Love's Short Practice of Surgery*, 23rd edn. Arnold, London, pp. 87–98.

Lorenz, P. and Longaker, M.T. (2008) Wounds: biology, pathology and management, in *Surgery: Basic Science and Clinical Evidence* (eds J.A. Norton, P.S. Barrie, R.R., Bollinger *et al.*), Springer, New York, pp. 191–205 .

Mansha, M., Sharif, K., Sharif, Z., Kashif, F.A. and Diggory, P. 2005 The impact of different methods of wound closure and dressing on the rate of wound infection in patients with fracture neck of femur. *Journal of Orthopaedic Nursing*, **9**(4), 195–198.

McInnes, E., Jammali-Blasi, A., Bell-Syer, S.E.M., Dumville, J.C. and Cullum, N. (2011) Support surfaces for pressure ulcer prevention. *Cochrane Database of Systematic Reviews* **4**(Art. No.: CD001735). DOI: 10.1002/14651858.CD001735.pub4.

Moffat, C.J (2005) *Identifying Criteria for Wound Infection*. European Wound Management Association (EWMA) Position Document. MEP Ltd., London.

Moore, Z., Cowman, S. and Conroy, R.M. (2011) A randomised controlled clinical trial of repositioning, using the 30° tilt, for the prevention of pressure ulcers. *Journal of Clinical Nursing*, **20**, 2633–2644.

Morgan, D.A. (2004) *Formulary of Wound Management Products. A Guide for Healthcare Staff*, 9th edn. Euromed Communications Limited, Surrey.

Morgan, M., Black, J., Bone, F. *et al.* (2005) Clinician-led surgical site infection surveillance of orthopaedic procedures: a UK multi-centre pilot study. *Journal of Hospital Infection*, **60**(3), 201–212.

National Institute for Clinical Excellence (NICE) (2008) *Surgical Site Infection: Prevention and Treatment of Surgical Site Infection.* NICE, London.

Nixon, J, (2001) The Pathophysiology and Aetiology of Pressure Ulcers, in *The Prevention and Treatment of Pressure Ulcers*, 2nd edn (ed. M.J. Morison), Mosby, Edinburgh, pp. 17–36.

Owens, C.D. and Stoessel, K. (2008) Surgical site infection: epidemiology, microbiology and prevention. *Journal of Hospital Infection*, **70**(S2), 3–10.

Pudner, R. (2001) Postoperative dressings in wound management. *Journal of Community Nursing*, **15**(9), 33–37.

Ravenscroft, M., Harker, K. and Buch, K. (2006) A prospective, randomised, controlled trial comparing wound dressings used in hip and knee surgery: Aquacel® and Tegaderm™ versus Cutiplast™. *Annals of the Royal College of Surgeons of England*, **88**(1), 18–22.

Santy, J. (2009) Recognising infection in wounds. *Nursing Standard*, **23**(7), 53–4, 56, 58.

Serena, T., Robson, M.C., Cooper, D.M. and Ignatius, J. (2006) Lack of reliability of clinical/visual assessment of chronic wound infection: the incidence of biopsy-proven infection in venous leg ulcers. *Wounds*, **18**, 197–202.

Sibbald, R.G., Orsted, H., Schultz, G.S., Coutts, P. and Keast, D. (2003) Preparing the wound bed 2003: focus on infection and inflammation. *Ostomy Wound Management*, **49**(11), 24–51.

Sigel, B., Edlestein, A.L., Felix, R. and Memhardt, C.R. (1973) Compression of the deep venous system of the lower leg during inactive recumbence. *Archives of Surgery*, **106**, 38–43.

Smith, I. (1984) Heel aids. *Nursing Times*, **80**(36), 35–39.

Sprigle, S. (2000) Effects of forces and the selection of support surfaces. *Topics in Geriatric Rehabilitation*, **16**(2), 47–62.

Srinivasaiah, N. Dugdall, H., Barrett, S. and Drew, P. (2007) A point prevalence survey of wounds in the north-east of England. *Journal of Wound Care*, **16**(10), 413–419.

Trampuz, A. and Zimmerli, W., (2006) Diagnosis and treatment of infections associated with fracture fixation devices. *Injury*, **37**(2 Suppl), S56–S59.

Vanderwee, K., Grypdonck, M.H.F. and Defloor, T. (2005) Effectiveness of an alternating pressure air mattress for the prevention of pressure ulcers. *Age and Ageing*, **34**(3), 261–267.

Voegeli, D. (2008) The effect of washing and drying practices on skin barrier function. *Journal of Wound, Ostomy and Continence Nurses*, **35**(1), 84–90.

Winter, G.D. (1962) Formation of the scab and the rate of epithelialisation of superficial wounds in the skin of the young domestic pig. *Nature*, **193**, 293–294.

White, R. (2001) New developments in the use of dressings on surgical wounds. *British Journal of Nursing*, **10**(6), S70.

Xia, Z., Sato, A., Hughes, M.A. and Cherry, G.W. (2000) Stimulation of fibroblast growth in-vitro by intermittent radiant warming. *Wound Repair Regeneration*, **8**(2), 138–144.

PART III

Common orthopaedic conditions and their care and management

CHAPTER 13

Key conditions and principles of orthopaedic management

Elaine Wylie[1] and Sonya Clarke[2]

[1] *Craigavon Area Hospital, Craigavon, Northern, Ireland*

[2] *Queen's University Belfast, Belfast, UK*

Introduction

This chapter provides an overview of the knowledge required to promote optimal care for patients presenting with common orthopaedic conditions in the young adult (and child when appropriate), adult and older person. Osteoarthritis, arthropathies, rheumatoid arthritis, the metabolic condition osteoporosis, osteomyelitis, low back pain, scoliosis, spinal stenosis and intervertebral disc disease are considered. Each condition is discussed in relation to its definition, epidemiology, diagnosis, clinical presentation and management. It will have a central nursing focus but also within the wider context of the 'specialist nurse' and multidisciplinary team (MDT). Management and care options will be explored with reference to best available evidence and national guidance.

Arthritis is an umbrella term that covers all forms of joint and muscle pain. Musculoskeletal diseases are widespread in the community with around 20 million people in the UK suffering from one of the many forms of arthritis. An Arthritis Research Campaign report (2002) found that nearly nine million people (19% of the population) consulted their GP for arthritis in the previous year. These conditions result in higher levels of disability and patient self-reported limitations of quality of life than heart disease or cancer. They are the commonest cause of work-limiting health problems, long standing illness and sickness absence in the UK.

Osteoarthritis

The name 'osteoarthritis' (OA) (also known as osteoarthrosis/degenerative joint disease) comes from three Greek words meaning bone, joint and inflammation. It is a non-inflammatory disorder of synovial joints that results in loss of hyaline cartilage and remodelling of surrounding bone. It is a chronic, progressive disorder, commonly affecting hands, hips, knees, shoulders and spine. Approximately eight million people in the UK have OA but only around one million of them will seek treatment. It is estimated that more than six million people in the UK have painful OA of the knee and more than 650 000 have painful OA of the hips (Arthritis Research UK 2011). The condition is more common in women except in hip OA, which affects men equally (Doherty *et al.*, 2006). The prevalence of radiographic and symptomatic OA increases with age (Fransen *et al.*, 2010) although many people with radiological evidence of OA remain asymptomatic and it is, therefore, not an inevitable consequence of ageing.

Pathogenesis

OA is a dynamic process that involves tissue production and remodelling of the joints, with a loss of hyaline cartilage, typically at the point of maximum load-bearing rather than widespread destruction. Osteophyte formation (abnormal outgrowth of cartilage that becomes ossified) occurs at the joint margin and cysts may develop in the bone – small areas of osteonecrosis caused by increased

Orthopaedic and Trauma Nursing: An Evidence-based Approach to Musculoskeletal Care, First Edition. Edited by Sonya Clarke and Julie Santy-Tomlinson.

pressure on the bone when the cartilage is no longer adequate in its load distributing function (Doherty *et al.*, 2006). Other primary and secondary pathological changes include subacromial sclerosis, thickening of the joint capsule and evidence of osteochondral bodies in the synovium.

Primary OA has no known cause, although inheritance is a considerable factor, especially in the hands (Doherty *et al.*, 2006). Other factors include:

- being female
- congenital joint abnormalities
- genetic polymorphisms
- ethnicity with susceptibility in particular joints varying between ethnic groups
- ageing.

Secondary OA occurs as a result of:

- obesity
- high level/high impact sport or occupational activities
- repetitive and long-term occupational factors, such as repeated kneeling, twisting and handling heavy weights while standing.

Signs and symptoms

The main symptoms of OA are pain and stiffness. In the early stages, pain may be transient or even absent and progression is often slow. Pain is variable with patients having good days and bad days with pain best at the start of the day or after rest and worst with joint use and at the end of the day. Severe OA can cause pain at rest and mobility, self-care and leisure. Morning stiffness or stiffness after a period of inactivity generally lasts less than 15 to 30 minutes. Pain is typically described as dull, aching or throbbing and localised to a specific region. Crepitus may be noticeable on movement due to roughened articular surfaces and the joint may be painful on palpation. Restricted movement can be caused by pain, joint capsule thickening or the presence of osteophytes.

Squaring of the first carpal metacarpal (CMC) joint may be evident in hand OA due to osteophyte formation. Changes often occur in the distal interphalangeal joints (Heberden's nodes) and at the proximal interphalangeal joints (Bouchard's nodes). Once nodes have fully formed, pain and tenderness at the distal interphalangeal joints and proximal interphalangeal joints often improve but pain at the CMC joint will not improve. Hand OA can reduce grip strength, having significant implications for numerous functional activities and cause considerable frustration for patients who are no longer able to perform tasks with the same precision and strength (Hill *et al.*, 2010).

Pain from OA of the hip is typically felt in the groin, although it can radiate down to the knee. This is often associated with reduced lower limb muscle strength due to lack of use. Patients commonly have an abnormal pattern of walking caused by weakness of the abductor muscles. OA of the foot commonly affects the first metatarsal phalangeal joint and may result in a hallux rigidus or hallux valgus deformity. This, and associated deformities, can cause pain on walking or difficulty with finding appropriate footwear. Lack of comfortable footwear or diminished strength and fitness discourages many people from pursuing usual activities, such as shopping or going out walking.

Diagnosis is usually based on history and examination. The two most important diagnostic clues are the pattern of joint involvement and the presence or absence of fever, rash or other symptoms outside the joint. As part of the physical examination, the joint should be evaluated for swelling, limitations of range of movement, pain on movement and crepitus. There is no laboratory test that is specific for osteoarthritis. Treatment is usually based on the results of diagnostic imaging. In patients with OA, X-rays may indicate narrowed joint spaces, abnormal density of the bone and presence of subacromial cysts or bony spurs. The patient's symptoms, however, do not always correlate with X-ray findings. It is important to exclude other medical conditions that may be present. Differential diagnoses may include pseudogout, bursitis, rheumatoid arthritis and reactive arthritis.

A management plan should be considered in relation to the person's quality of life, functional limitations and pain experience. It should aim to reduce pain and maintain or improve the individual's mobility and encourage self-management as this provides a greater sense of self-empowerment and reduces reliance on health services and pharmacological therapies. A range of options are available that can be used in multiple combinations to achieve maximum outcome for the individual. Core treatments recommended in the Clinical Guidelines for the Management of Osteoarthritis (NICE 2008a) include exercise, appropriate weight loss and access to information.

Exercise is important in managing OA irrespective of age, comorbidity, pain severity and disability because it may reduce pain and help to improve function. It can be designed to strategically improve general mobility, function and self-efficacy. An exercise programme needs to be carefully tailored to individual needs and preferences and should not hinder the persons' ability and enthusiasm and, consequently, delay positive behavioural change. Many individuals experience an exacerbation of pain and stiffness after exercise, although most will not have any adverse reaction to controlled exercise (Hurley *et al.*, 2007). A reduction in weight transferred through joints, such as knees, hips and feet, may reduce the severity of the symptoms a person experiences. This may be achieved through the transfer of weight by using a walking stick or through sensible weight loss if the patient's body mass index is excessive. Patients should be encouraged to lose weight by eating healthily and adopting a sensible programme of exercise. However, this approach is difficult for many older people struggling with basic mobility or shopping and preparing meals. It is important to consider a holistic approach to OA and its effects on lifestyle and functional abilities before advocating strict regimes of diet and exercise. The use of insoles or knee braces can improve pain, stiffness and function in the knee, while hand splints can improve function in the hand and should be considered with those experiencing symptoms (NICE 2008a). Referral to orthotics and occupational therapy services can provide assessment of biomechanical problems and appropriate orthoses to support painful joints and reduce joint pain.

Pharmacological management

Medications helpful in the management of pain include simple analgesics, *non-steroidal anti-inflammatory drugs (NSAIDs)* and opioids. Paracetamol is usually the first line of pharmacological pain management as it has few side effects; although anti-inflammatories provide better pain relief, paracetamol has fewer side effects. Paracetamol and codeine combinations have no demonstrable benefit over paracetamol alone (NICE 2008a). NICE (2008a) recommends using non-steroidal anti-inflammatory drugs (NSAIDs) to manage pain, but around 10–20% of people who use oral NSAIDs experience dyspepsia and risk gastric complications, which are reduced when NSAIDs are used topically and these are now the first line of treatment (Zhang *et al.*, 2010). The development of the Cox-2 selective anti-inflammatory drug has reduced the incidence of gastric effects, but add to the risk of thrombus formation. They are also associated with a slight increase in risk of renal failure (Adam 2011).

Opioids can be very effective but their benefits can be outweighed by side effects: nausea, vomiting, dizziness and constipation. Even though the use of extended release opioids in OA improves sleep, patients can be fearful about addiction. Intra articular steroid injections of knees can be an adjunct to other pain relieving treatments (NICE, 2008a). Hyaluronan acid can also be injected into the knee joint, however, there is a lack of placebo controlled trials and some trials suggest efficacy is limited and these are not recommended by NICE (Avouac *et al.*, 2007). Capsaicin, a topical cream based on chilli peppers, causes localised burning pain, but is then followed by pain relief and has been shown to alleviate mild to moderate pain caused by OA knee (Kosuwon *et al.*, 2010).

Steroid or hyaluronic acid injections into the knees can bring partial pain relief for up to three months (NICE 2008a). However, there is a lack of placebo controlled trials and some trials suggest efficacy is limited (Avouac *et al.*, 2007). Capsaicin causes localised burning pain, but as it takes a while for the body to synthesise, the capsaicin period of burning is followed by pain relief. Using the cream twice daily often means the burning sensation does not return after the first application.

Transcutaneous electrical nerve stimulation (TENS) and acupuncture have shown to be helpful in relieving pain (Itoh *et al.*, 2008) with anecdotal reports suggesting the application of *heat* or *cold* to joints to provide short-term pain relief. Heat can be applied by immersion in warm water, heat packs heated at home in the microwave, heat pads and wax. Cold is usually applied with an ice massage or by applying cold packs to the affected area. It is essential that a safe system for delivery is used to prevent any damage to the skin and surrounding tissues.

Most people with OA are managed in the primary care setting. However, if OA becomes severe with progressive limitation of functional and recreational activities, the opinion of an orthopaedic surgeon should be sought. Joint replacement is considered when conservative measures are unsuccessful and there is substantial impact on the person's quality of life (refer to Chapter 14 for elective care and arthroplasty of the hip, knee and shoulder).

Spondyloarthropathies

Spondyloarthropathies (SpA) are a group of common inflammatory rheumatic disorders, characterised by axial and/or peripheral arthritis associated with enthesitis, dactylitis and potential extra-articular manifestations, such as uveitis and skin rash. These conditions share a common genetic predisposition – the HLA-B27 gene. *Ankylosing spondylitis* (AS) *and psoriatic arthropathy* are the two most common forms; Table 13.1 lists additional arthropathies.

Ankylosing spondylitis (AS)

AS is a systemic, chronic inflammatory disease that affects the axial skeleton, causing inflammatory back pain, which can lead to structural and functional impairment. The condition has an insidious onset, often over a period of several years, and typically occurs before the age of 30; usually between the late teens and twenties with a male to female ratio of 3:1 (Sieper *et al.*, 2002). It affects men and women differently; women experience less severe disease with less involvement of the spine than men. However, women have more symptoms in the knees, wrists, ankles, hips and pelvis, whereas men most commonly experience involvement of the spine, pelvis, chest wall, hips, shoulders and feet (NASS, 2004). The cause is unknown. There are two central features: inflammation and new bone formation, especially in the spine. Although inflammation is assumed to trigger new bone formation, there is no close correlation between inflammation and **osteoproliferation**. The principle signs and symptoms include:

- Low back pain – of slow and gradual onset over several months and persistent in nature. Lower back pain in the lumbar spine and sacroiliac joints is often the initial complaint of approximately 90% of patients with the condition. Pain characteristically radiates to the buttocks or thighs, but never below the knee. Pain is worse in the morning or after a period of inactivity and may be relieved by mild physical exercise.
- Sacroiliitis (bi-lateral inflammation of the sacroiliac joints) – traumatic disease occurring at the point of attachment of skeletal muscles to bone, where recurring stress causes inflammation and often fibrosis and calcification.
- Stiffness – morning stiffness is a characteristic symptom, which may last for minutes to hours depending on disease severity and usually reduces during the day or is relieved by mild physical exercise.
- Enthesitis – inflammation at the point of attachment between skeletal muscles and bone.
- Peripheral arthritis – affecting about 10% of patients at presentation but eventually affects 40% of those with the condition. Peripheral arthritis is typically asymmetrical and predominantly affects the large joints of the appendicular skeletal system.
- Fatigue – some individuals may experience significant systemic symptoms including loss of weight during the early stages of disease, anaemia and depression.
- Acute anterior uveitis – inflammation of the eye occurs in 40% of patients on at least one occasion and 33% may experience recurring episodes which may lead to permanent damage and blindness if not treated promptly.
- Restricted spinal movement – occurs in all three planes (flexion, extension, rotation).
- Reduced costovertebral movement – results in reduced chest expansion and vital capacity.

Table 13.1 Other spondyloarthropathies

Reactive arthritis	Usually manifests itself as arthritis two to four weeks following a urogenital or enteric infection, often in patients bearing the HLA-B27 antigen. The risk of developing reactive arthritis has been shown to occur up to fifty times higher in this population, as opposed to the HLA-B27 negative population following exposure to a preceding infection.
Inflammatory bowel disease	Associated arthritis is usually a peripheral, large joint, lower limb, asymmetric oligoarthritis. It accompanies inflammatory bowel disease in about 10% of patients and occasionally pre-dates the onset of IBD. (Salvarani & Fries 2009)
Undifferentiated spondyloarthropathy or spondyloarthritis (uSpA)	This term is used to describe manifestations of spondyloarthritis in patients who do not meet criteria for any well-defined spondyloarthropathy. There is a female predominance of 1:3 and the clinical manifestations of this type of spondyloarthropathy are basically similar to all other spondyloarthropathies with fewer extra-articular manifestations.

- Invertible osteoporosis and associated spinal fractures.
- Aortic insufficiency.
- Atrial ventricle block.
- Pericarditis.
- Pulmonary fibrosis.

There are currently no specific diagnostic interventions; rather investigations may be used to exclude other potential diagnoses. Laboratory investigations include C-reactive protein (CRP) and erythrocyte sedimentation rate (ESR) which may be mildly elevated. Rheumatoid factor and antinuclear tests are negative with 95% of people with ankylosing spondylitis HLA-B27 positive. Although this is present in about 8% of the British population, most individuals will not have the condition although there is a strong familial tendency in people with ankylosing spondylitis. X-rays are diagnostic only in established cases with MRI imaging being a more helpful diagnostic tool.

Although AS is determined through clinical diagnosis, it is essential that alternative possible diagnoses are excluded, including mechanical back pain, infection, neoplasms and other inflammatory conditions. The British Society for Rheumatology (2004) advocates the use of the modified New York criteria (Geijer *et al.*, 2009) as a guide to diagnosis. The four-point grading reports grade 0 as normal; grade I with some blurring of the joint margins as suspicious; grade II as having minimal sclerosis with some erosion; grade III as definite sclerosis on both sides of joint/severe erosions with widening of joint space with or without ankylosis; and grade IV as complete ankylosis. Therefore a definitive diagnosis of ankylosing spondylitis requires radiological criteria:

- when sacro-iliitis is greater than grade I bilaterally or grade III or IV unilaterally
- plus at least one clinical criterion from either:
  - low back pain and stiffness for more than three months that improves with exercise but is not relieved by rest
  - limited motion of the lumbar spine in both sagittal and frontal planes or
  - limited chest expansion compared to normal values correlated for age and sex.

A key element of the overall management for all patients is new evidence-based recommendations produced by the International Assessment in Ankylosing Spondylitis Working Group in collaboration with the European League Against Rheumatism (IAAS 2006). Physiotherapy may be beneficial but the best option is unclear. Many patients find hydrotherapy particularly beneficial. NSAIDs appear to improve spinal and peripheral pain and function along with intra-articular or peri-articular corticosteroid injections to the sacroiliitis in small groups. Local corticosteroid injections for peripheral arthritis and enthesitis in ankylosing spondylitis are widely used to good effect. Intravenous methylprednisolone is occasionally used in severe unresponsive cases, but this use may decline with the ability to use new medications like tumour necrosis factor inhibitors.

Drugs that inhibit tumour necrosis factor (TNF) have revolutionised the treatment of ankylosing spondylitis. Four different drugs are currently available:

- etanercept – a recombinant TNF receptor
- infliximab – a chimeric monoclonal antibody given by intravenous infusion
- adalimumab and golimumab – both humanised monoclonal antibody to TNF given subcutaneously.

These drugs have rapid and substantial clinical effects, in significantly reducing spinal inflammation. The British Society of Rheumatology (2004) and NICE (2008b) have produced guidelines for the use of TNF inhibitors.

A large proportion of patients with AS develop hip arthritis. Hip replacements should be considered in patients with refractory pain or disability and with radiographic evidence of structural damage, independent of age. Spinal surgery may be of value in selected patients and is performed for a variety of reasons, including fusion procedures for segmental instability and wedge lumbar osteotomy for fixed kyphotic deformity. Patients with severe ankylosing spondylitis present anaesthetic difficulties and the risk and benefits of surgery need to be carefully considered.

Psoriatic arthritis (PA)

PA is an inflammatory arthritis associated with the skin disorder psoriasis. The exact aetiology is unknown, although more than 40% of people with the cutaneous disease of psoriasis are estimated to also have joint involvement. Although some patients with psoriasis may have coincidental osteoarthritis or rheumatoid arthritis, it is important to remember that psoriatic arthritis is prevalent in individuals with psoriasis. Psoriasis is believed to affect 1–3% of the population and psoriatic arthritis is believed to affect 1% and affects more than 7–42% of patients with psoriasis. The risk of psoriatic arthritis increases with a family history of spondyloarthropathy or nail pitting and the onset usually occurs between 30 and 55 years of age, affecting men and women equally. Psoriatic arthritis is considered a separate entity from rheumatoid arthritis because of the sero-negativity of rheumatoid factor and its tendency for asymmetrical involvement.

The exact aetiology has yet to be discovered. As with almost all autoimmune diseases, genetic, immunological and environmental factors are believed to play a part in the expression of psoriatic arthritis. Psoriatic arthritis is an inflammatory disease that manifests in both articular and extra-articular features. The disease can present with an arthritis affecting several joints of the hands or feet that is frequently symmetrical. This mimics the pattern of rheumatoid arthritis. Unlike individuals affected by rheumatoid arthritis, those with psoriatic arthritis often experience inflammation of the distal interphalangeal joints. Individuals affected may also present with inflammation of the spine and sacroiliitis. The disease can also present with a dactylitis: sausage-like digit or digits. Individuals with psoriatic arthritis can have arthritis of less than four joints, commonly of one large joint and three digits, or an arthritis affecting one joint, usually a large joint. Uncommonly, psoriatic arthritis can be an extremely aggressive and mutilating arthritis, resulting in joint destruction. Extra-articular features include psoriasis, iritis, mouth ulcers, colitis and aortic valve disease.

There is no single blood test to diagnose psoriatic arthritis, but it is recognised that individuals affected are usually rheumatoid factor negative and do not develop rheumatoid nodules. Markers of inflammation may be elevated in active psoriatic arthritis.

The medical management of psoriatic arthritis is similar to other inflammatory arthritides (see management of RA below). Jones *et al.* (2003) concluded that parenteral high dose methotrexate and sulphasalazine are two medications that showed demonstrable efficacy in psoriatic arthritis. Sulphasalazine alters bowel flora, inhibits folate metabolism and is generally well tolerated. It is considered effective, particularly in treating persistent peripheral arthritis.

Rheumatoid arthritis

Rheumatoid arthritis (RA) is a complex, chronic inflammatory condition, which has both articular and extra-articular effects. It is the most common inflammatory arthropathy and has the potential to cause a significant impact on quality of life. The predominant features of the condition are pain, swelling, stiffness of joints, reduced levels of function, fatigue and anaemia.

RA is a polyarthropathy and affects both sides of the body symmetrically with a fluctuating disease pattern and episodic disease flares. It commonly affects the small joints of the hands and feet, although larger joints can also be affected. RA has a prevalence of 1% in the population. Although people of any age can be affected, the peak age range for onset is 40–60 years and it affects women more frequently: 3:1 ratio. RA has a significant impact on life and can affect roles, relationships and levels of independence as the disease progresses.

The pathophysiology of rheumatoid arthritis is not fully understood and the initial trigger is unknown. It is an autoimmune condition where pro-inflammatory cytokines are known to have an important role in the pathogenesis causing chronic inflammation. Inflammation is the body's normal response to tissue injury, whether caused by bacteria, trauma, chemicals, heat or other phenomenon. Inflammation usually subsides when its task is completed, but maintenance of the inflammation in RA is thought to be caused by an autoimmune reaction in inflammatory arthritis. Inflammation of the synovial membrane surrounding the joint capsules and tendon sheaths is called synovitis. The synovial membrane is the inner membrane of tissue that lines a joint and secretes synovial fluid. The main function of this fluid is to lubricate the joint. It has been suggested that pathological changes caused by synovitis occur in three stages (Hill and Ryan 2000):

1. ***Cellular stage*** – joint becomes warm, swollen and tender causing stiffness and restricted movement.
2. ***Inflammatory stage*** – granulocytes accumulate in the synovial fluid before their destruction during the inflammatory process causes the release of enzymes.
3. ***Destructive stage*** – primarily affects the hyaline cartilage as vascular granulation tissue or "pannus" starts to erode the outer cartilage around the joint.

The symptoms of inflammation are redness, pain, heat, swelling and possibly loss of function of the affected joint. The clinical presentation of RA is often pain, persistent synovitis and early morning stiffness. Initial presentation is usually of symmetrical joint involvement with pain and inflammation of the metacarpal phalangeal (MCP), proximal interphalangeal (PIP) and metatarsal phalangeal (MTP) joints, although this may progress to other joints. Affected joints are often described as stiff, as if trying to move them against a resistant force. There are also extra-articular features of rheumatoid arthritis and these include fever, weight loss, fatigue, anaemia, ocular problems (scleritis, episcleritis and keratoconjunctivitis sicca), cardiac (pericarditis, endocarditis, pulmonary pleural effusions, and fibrosing alveolitis) and osteoporosis. The American College of Rheumatology (ACR) proposed in 1987 a set of classification criteria. These criteria, were initially meant for the enrolment of patients in clinical trials, but in some cases were used for diagnosis, they have shown unsatisfactory performance recently in the setting of early arthritis. In 2010 the ACR and the European League Against Rheumatism (EULAR) jointly developed new classification criteria, aiming to allow earlier patient classification, treatment and inclusion in clinical trials. The 2010 criteria include tender and swollen joint count, acute phase reactants, anti-cyclic citrullinated peptide antibodies (ACPA) or rheumatoid factor (RF) and symptom duration. These clinical and laboratory data are combined into a score ranging from 0 to 10.

NICE (2009a) recommends that people with suspected persistent synovitis are referred for specialist rheumatologist opinion with diagnosis based on clinical findings. Urgent referral should be made for patients who present with the small joints of the hands or feet affected, more than one joint affected and if there is a delay of three months or longer from the onset of symptoms.

A number of key blood tests assist in the diagnosis and monitoring of RA. These are full blood count, liver function and biochemistry tests, ESR and CRP. Immunological tests include rheumatoid factor, anti-nuclear antibody and anti-cyclic citrulline peptide. These are measures of autoantibodies, which are groups of immunoproteins produced by the immune system that mistakenly target and damage specific tissues and organs. Rheumatoid factor is an important immunological investigation as it determines whether RA is seropositive or seronegative. The significance of this is that seropositive RA may progress to a more aggressive form of the condition. Approximately 80% of people with RA are rheumatoid factor positive but a positive result alone does not mean a diagnosis of RA as it is thought that up to 5% of the population are rheumatoid factor positive without having rheumatoid arthritis. Anti-CCP helps to determine the prognosis of RA and is predictive of joint damage. It is a relatively new test and, therefore, not performed as a standard investigation in all centres.

X-ray remains a useful investigation for monitoring joint deterioration where bone erosions clearly appear. The use of ultrasound scanning is becoming standard practice in assessing and measuring the degree of synovitis in joints and soft tissue. It can also ascertain early erosions and tendon ruptures (Kane *et al.*, 2004).

Management

Management of RA should include early detection and treatment to control symptoms and complications, thus delaying disease progression, but parallel to regular monitoring of drug treatments. NICE has developed a clinical guideline on the management and treatment of RA in adults (2009a). Medication is recommended to control inflammation and pain, reduce disease progression, joint damage, disability and loss of function, achieve remission and improve quality of life. Drug therapy relies on various combinations of:

- analgesics
- NSAIDs
- corticosteroids
- DMARD (disease-modifying anti-rheumatic drugs)
- biologic therapies

Analgesics are used to reduce pain with anti-inflammatories reducing pain and stiffness caused by inflammation. NSAIDs are usually taken on a regular basis with disease-modifying anti-rheumatic drugs. Corticosteroids reduce inflammation, but are associated with significant long-term side effects such as hypertension, diabetes, osteoporosis and muscle wasting and are, therefore, mainly only used to provide temporary symptom relief. These drugs can be administered orally, intra-muscularly, intra-articularly or intravenously. Disease-modifying anti-rheumatic drugs (DMARDS) are the main second line treatment for patients with RA. They are used to suppress disease activity, often in combination with first line treatments and are recommended in the early stages of RA development. They can prevent the development of erosions and deformities. There are a number of different DMARDs with different modes of action, special precautions, indications, side effects and monitoring requirements. DMARDs can be used as monotherapy or in combination. Some of these include:

- **Methotrexate:** 7.5 mg once weekly to a maximum dose of 25 mg weekly. This is an immunosuppressant that can slow down the progression of arthritis making significant improvement in general wellbeing. It is usually taken orally in weekly doses, but can also be given by weekly injection. It is probably the most effective of the conventional disease-modifying drugs for moderate to severe rheumatoid arthritis
- **Sulphasalazine**: 500 mg daily to a maximum dose of 2–3 grams daily
- **Combination of antibiotic and anti-inflammatory:** it is usually commenced at 500 mg daily and increased weekly to a maximum tolerated dose of 2–3 grams daily
- **Leflunomide:** 10–20 mg daily
- **Hydroxychloroquine:** initially 400 mg daily, then typically reduced to 200 mg daily. This is an antimalarial compound that has been shown to suppress the immune system in a non-specific way. A rare side effect is accumulation of the drug at the back of the eye so patients must have periodic eye tests.

The DMARDs, penicillamine (for patients allergic to penicillin) and gold (used since the 1920s) have similar actions but are less commonly selected now as the time for onset of benefit can take up to six months.

Other management options

The development of monoclonal antibodies and molecules targeted at TNF has improved the management of patients with rheumatoid arthritis, offering a therapeutic option for highly active disease, uncontrolled by traditional DMARD therapies. This option improves function and reduces pain, early morning stiffness, swollen joints and fatigue and induces and maintains remission (Anderson, 2004). There are number of biologic therapies licensed for use in RA all of which block cytokines, reducing inflammation. Anti-TNF-alpha therapies may vary in their mode of administration, indications, dosing and side effects (Table 13.2).

Table 13.2 Biologic therapies and licensing indications

Drug Name	Structure	Delivery	Indications
Abatacept	Reduced T-cell activity	IV infusion SC injection	RA†
Adalimumab	mAb* to TNF	SC injection	RA, PsA‡, AS§
Certolizumab Pegol	PEGylated antibody fragment to TNF	SC injection	RA
Etanercept	Soluble fusion TNF receptor	SC injection	RA, PsA, AS
Golimumab	mAb to TNF	SC injection	RA, PsA, AS
Infliximab	mAb to TNF	IV infusion	RA, PsA, AS
Rituximab	Depletes B-cells	IV infusion	RA
Tocilizumab	mAb to IL6 receptor	SC injection	RA

*Monoclonal antibody
† Rheumatoid arthritis
‡Psoriatic arthritis
§ Ankylosing spondylitis

As RA has a considerable psychosocial impact on the patient with reports of depression, low self-esteem and isolation, a multi-disciplinary approach is recommended, including access to specialist physiotherapy, occupational therapy, podiatry and nurses (NICE 2009). Specialist physiotherapy aims to promote general fitness and exercise, as well as teaching specific exercises for joint flexibility, muscle strengthening and managing functional impairments. Hydrotherapy may be offered. This can also help to control pain and referral in the early stages of the disease can help prevent malalignment. Most patients also obtain relief from heat aids, and some using TENS.

Specialist occupational therapy facilitates independence. Problems with hand function are evaluated and appropriate management advice given. Aids to assist with daily living may include gadgets to help with washing and dressing. Specialist podiatrists provide advice with regard to footwear and foot care. The feet are often affected by RA causing mechanical damage and pain. Insoles and suitable footwear can be discussed. Specialist nurses are involved in monitoring and advising people about how to manage their disease to enable optimal physical, psychological and social functions. There are a number of specific specialist monitoring tools used by the expert nurse, for example disease activity (DA): DAS28 score alongside blood tests i.e. inflammatory markers ESR and CRP; daily function: health assessment score (HAQ); and general wellbeing: arthritis impact measurement scale. The specialist disease monitoring tools highlighted here are unlikely to be used by the orthopaedic nurse. Important facets of the role include patient education, facilitating self-management of symptoms, support at diagnosis and throughout the disease process, drug counselling and monitoring and the coordination of care within the multidisciplinary team. The rheumatology nurse specialist can also provide telephone support and review. Nurses within the hospital environment may be familiar with caring for patients during disease flares or advising patients with regard to elective procedures.

Osteoporosis

Metabolic bone disease is the term used to describe a range of conditions inclusive of osteoporosis, Paget's disease, osteomalacia and osteogenesis imperfecta (OI) (see Chapter 22 for further information regarding OI) that affect the quality of bone and are characterised by pain, deformity and fracture. This chapter will only discuss the most common of these; osteoporosis. The World Health Organization (WHO 1994, p. 12) define osteoporosis as

> (a progressive systemic skeletal disease characterized by low bone mass and micro-architectural deterioration of bone tissue, with a consequent increase in bone fragility and susceptibility to fracture.)

One in two women and one in five men over the age of 50 in the UK will fracture a bone mainly because of osteoporosis, with an estimated three million people in the UK alone suffering from the condition (www.nos.org.uk). Although fractures can occur in different parts of the body, the wrist, hip and spine are most commonly affected. Each year the numbers of people with osteoporosis in the UK rise as the population ages, resulting in over 70 000 hip fractures, 50 000 wrist fractures and 120 000 spinal fractures. Johnell and Kanis (2006) report the condition leading to nearly nine million fractures annually worldwide. Direct medical costs from fragility fractures to the UK healthcare economy were estimated at £1.8 billion in 2000, with the potential to increase to £2.2 billion by 2025, and with most of these costs relating to hip fracture care (see Chapter 18 for further exploration of fragility fractures relating to osteoporosis).

Prevention may not be totally attainable but the risk and severity can be reduced. For example, childhood through to young adulthood is the time to 'bank' good quality bone through diet and weight bearing activities as bone loses density with age. Consequently, as we age we are more at risk of a fragility fracture. From our mid-20s onwards our bodies constantly repair and renew bone, with whole parts of our skeletons reproduced every four to seven years. This process, known as 'bone remodelling', takes place on the bone's surface thanks to two sets of cells – osteoclasts and osteoblasts. Then from around the age of 40, the osteoclasts become more active and the osteoblasts less active; so more bone is removed and less is formed. This is known as 'age-related bone loss' which can lead to osteoporosis, particularly for those whose bones preexist with low density. By the age of 60 approximately 15% of all women have osteoporosis and this figure increases to over 25% by the age of 80 (NICE 2008b). Because of increased bone loss after the menopause in women and age-related bone loss in both women and men, the prevalence of osteoporosis increases markedly with age:

> (...because of increased bone loss after the menopause in women, and age-related bone loss in both women and men, the prevalence of osteoporosis increases markedly with age, from 2% at 50 years to more than 25% at 80 years, 52% in women. As the longevity of the population increases, so will the incidence of osteoporosis and fragility fracture.) (NICE 2012)

Education is therefore fundamental in the prevention and control of osteoporosis and in raising awareness, especially for primary and secondary prevention in post-menopausal women. The practitioner must identify what the patient knows already, identify risk factors, and inform of treatments and associated side effects of drug interventions. Box 13.1 provides examples of appropriate educational information.

Healthy bones have a shell of solid bone and an internal honeycombed network of spongy bone (see chapter 4). When osteoporosis is present, bones lose a certain amount of both structures. This is caused by age-related bone loss but other risk factors also have an impact. Risk factors include (Tanna 2009):

- *Genetic* – role in regulating bone, skeletal geometry and bone turnover density
- *Hormonal* – post menopausal women are at higher risk
- *Alcohol* – heavy alcohol consumption is associated with reduction in bone density
- *Nutritional* – important for bone health
- *Smoking* – associated with increased risk of fracture
- *Corticosteroids* – prolonged use is the most common cause of secondary osteoporosis
- *Physical inactivity/falls* – low bone density
- *Low body weight/weight loss – associated with greater bone loss and increased risk of fracture.*

Box 13.1 Patient education on osteoporosis

- Outline in simple terms what osteoporosis is
- Outline the causes and consequences of osteoporosis
- Emphasise how maintaining a healthy lifestyle can minimise the problem
- Explore patients' dietary habits – ensuring that they are eating meals that incorporate a wide variety of foods from the four main groups – fruit and vegetables, carbohydrates, dairy products and protein – natural way of providing minerals, vitamins and energy
- Identify the patient's knowledge of what foods contain calcium and their daily intake
- Emphasise that the minimal calcium intake should be 700 mg daily and in some cases 1000–12000 mg a day and is vital for healthy bones – gives examples to achieve this intake
- Outline what foods are rich in calcium and that low fat or fat free dairy products often have more calcium than full fat versions
- Discuss the importance of vitamin D to help the body absorb calcium: 15–20 minutes sun exposure to the face and arms 3–4 times weekly during the summer should provide with enough vitamin D for the year
- GP may prescribe a calcium and vitamin D supplement and or bisphosphonate, reinforce why it is important to comply with this and take as prescribed
- Identify if the patient smokes – explain how smoking impacts on the bone and construction and the need to avoid smoking
- Assess alcohol intake: risk factor if excessive – daily intake should be no more than 2–3 units daily for women – explains what a unit is
- Identify the degree of activity and exercise routine – outlines the value of weight bearing exercise – walking, swimming, golf
- Maintaining a safe environment – raise awareness of need to minimise risk of falls e.g. use of footwear, turn on the light at night to go to toilet
- Encourage questions and give accurate information
- Use available leaflets to illustrate and reinforce important points
- Ask some questions to check patient's understanding, record in notes

Diagnosis

Osteoporosis is usually diagnosed from a bone scan post-fracture or at an osteoporosis clinic. The Dual Energy X-ray Absorptiometry (DXA) scan is currently the most accurate and reliable means of assessing bone density and associated risk of fracture. It is a simple, painless procedure that routinely uses very low doses of radiation to scan the spine/hips, wrist or heel using T and Z scores as markers (Tanna 2009). The WHO (1994) define criteria generated the *T* score to imply the number of standard deviations (SD) which separate the patient from the mean value of a healthy young population. A *Z* score is the number of SD which separate the patient from an age-matched health population. In reality, osteopenia (bone mineral density lower than normal) has a T score between –1 and –2.5 SD, with osteoporosis a T score of –2.5 SD or below and progressively more severe osteoporosis; a T score of –2.5 SD or below with one or more associated fractures.

Drug treatments

Bisphosphonates are non-hormonal drugs that help maintain bone strength and reduce fracture rates. They inhibit osteoclast action and slow down the rate of bone resorption to maintain the patient's current bone mineral density (BMD) level and reduce the risk of fracture. The drugs have poor rates of absorption and potential gastrointestinal side effects and compliance is reported to be poor. Guidance on taking the drug is fundamental to patient compliance and outcome; it should be swallowed on an empty stomach, with a glass of water, while standing, then to remain upright and fasting for 30 minutes. The main drugs in this range are alendronic acid or alendronate (Fosamax), cyclical etidronate (Didronel PMO), ibandronate (Bonviva), risedronate (Actonel) and zoledronic acid (Aclasta). These have been shown to reduce the risk of fractures in the spine and, in some cases, the hip. NICE (2012) recommend Alendronate as a treatment option for the primary prevention of osteoporotic fragility fractures in the following groups:

- Women aged 70 years or older who have an independent clinical risk factor for fracture or an indicator of low BMD and who are confirmed to have osteoporosis. In women aged 75 years or older who have two or more independent clinical risk factors for fracture or indicators of low BMD. A DXA scan may not be required if the responsible clinician considers it to be clinically inappropriate or unfeasible.
- Women aged 65–69 years who have an independent clinical risk factor for fracture and who are confirmed to have osteoporosis.
- Postmenopausal women younger than 65 years who have an independent clinical risk factor for fracture (see below) and at least one additional

indicator of low BMD and who are confirmed to have osteoporosis.

- When the decision has been made to initiate treatment with Alendronate, the preparation prescribed should be chosen on the basis of the lowest acquisition cost available.

Alternative therapies include:

- *Hormone replacement therapy (HRT)* – oestrogen replacement for women at the menopause stage of their life, which helps maintain bone strength and reduces fracture rates.
- *Selective oestrogen receptor modulators (SERMs)* drugs act in a similar way to oestrogen on the bone, helping to maintain bone strength and reduce fracture rates, especially in the spine.
- *Testosterone therapy* is testosterone replacement for men with low testosterone levels to help maintain bone strength, calcium and vitamin D.

Osteomyelitis

Osteomyelitis is an acute or chronic infection of bone and its structures. The most common organism responsible is *staphylococcus aureus* (Lew and Waldvogel 2004). It is a progressive condition and associated inflammation leads to necrotic destruction of bone that can lead to an acute infection becoming chronic. It is relatively uncommon because bone is resistant to infection so it tends to occur in patients with significant risk factors such as diabetes that reduce their resistance or make their bone more vulnerable through trauma or surgery. Its severity and progression can depend on the source of infection, the virulence of the organism involved and the general health of the patient (Brady *et al.*, 2006). It is often a devastating problem for patients as it is very difficult to treat because of necrosis and disruption to blood supply to bone which means that systemic and local antibiotic therapy is unsuccessful. Many years of pain and disability are often the result sometimes with suppurating sinus wounds. The prevention of osteomyelitis following injury and surgery is a major driver for good infection prevention and control practice throughout the patient's care journey. It is also one of the reasons that prophylactic antibiotic therapy is often given following open fracture and orthopaedic surgery. Gosselin *et al.* (2009) found antibiotics to reduce the incidence of early infections in open fractures of the limbs.

There are several different classifications of osteomyelitis depending on the source of infection:

Endogenous (haematogenous) osteomyelitis

occurs when pathogens are carried in the blood from sites of infection elsewhere in the body – a process sometimes known as remote 'seeding'. The infection spreads from bone to adjacent soft tissues or remote infections such as urinary tract infection. The prevention of such infections is, therefore, central to orthopaedic care. This includes, for example, the avoidance of urinary catheterisation.

Endogenous osteomyelitis is more common in infants, children and older people. Before puberty bacteria can gain access to a child's bone, often accumulating in the metaphyseal region (growth area of the bone). The bacteria proliferate and trigger an initial inflammatory response. Once inflammation is initiated the small vessels in bone thrombose. The build-up of pressure in the bone causes the inflammatory exudate to move to the bone cortex separating the periosteum from underlying bone and resulting in a painful subperiosteal abscess. The white cells cannot remove the infected material, resulting in accumulation of infected and ischaemic tissue and the eventual necrosis of underlying bone tissue (sequestrum) which is radiologically visible. Lifting of the periosteum also stimulates an intense osteoblastic response and new bone is laid down partially or completely surrounding the infected bone (involucrum). Openings in the involucrum allow the exudate to escape into surrounding tissues and ultimately the skin through a sinus tract.

Exogenous osteomyelitis

is a key route of transmission; the infection enters through open fractures, penetrating wounds and surgical procedures.

Acute osteomyelitis in adults (sudden onset)

is usually haematogenous in origin but may be due to trauma in the femur, tibia humerus and thoracolumbar spine. Spinal osteomyelitis is more common in adults past middle age and can result in a spinal cord compression. Clinical presentation often includes (Chihara and Segreti 2010):

- a history of injury 2–3 months previously
- abrupt onset of high pyrexia
- generally feeling unwell

- restriction of movement of affected bone
- pain and tenderness including on-bone palpation
- local signs of inflammation including swelling, redness, heat and localised pain.

It is important that the symptoms are not confused with cellulitis, acute septic arthritis, acute rheumatism or a sickle cell crisis.

Investigations include:

- history and clinical examination
- blood counts
- microbiological culture of blood, wound swabs
- aspiration of material from the site of infection for microbiological analysis
- X-ray
- bone scan/CT/MRI.

Imaging will show soft-tissue swelling, narrowing or widening of joint spaces, bone destruction, and periosteal reaction. Bone destruction, however, is not apparent until after 10–21 days of infection (Lew and Waldvogel 2004).

Treatment options
include measures to support the limb or spine with a view to reducing pain. This might include traction, splintage or application of a cast. Intravenous antibiotic therapy is used initially and to cover any surgical period up to two weeks post-surgery. The switch to oral therapy may happen once the clinical condition stabilises and microbiology results suggest infection is resolved. Treatment for acute infection is usually for 4–6 weeks. Chronic infection is considered below. High doses of antibiotics are required to achieve suitable bone penetration in high enough concentrations in necrotic avascular bone (Lew and Waldgovel 2004)

Chronic osteomyelitis (slower onset)
is a severe, persistent and sometimes incapacitating infection of bone and bone marrow which is on the increase due to predisposing conditions such as diabetes mellitus and peripheral vascular disease (Hatzenbuehler and Pulling 2011). Aetiology includes inadequately treated acute osteomyelitis, post open fracture or surgery, infection with TB and syphilis, joint replacement/internal fixation of open fractures and contiguous spread from soft tissue infection. The inflammatory reaction to infection in bone continues over time, leading to sclerosis and deformity with presence of sequestrum, involucrum, local bone loss and persistent drainage and/or sinus tract formation. The most common organisms are *staph. aureus, streptococci, pneumococci* and *myobacterium tuberculosis* (Kneale and Davis 2005). Clinical presentation includes:

- previous history of acute infection/osteomyelitis
- chronic bone pain
- sinus formation and purulent drainage
- low grade or absent pyrexia
- if a sinus tract becomes obstructed the patient can present with a localised abscess, soft tissue infection or both
- persistently feeling unwell.

Treatment includes antibiotic therapy (IV/Oral) for a minimum of 6–12 weeks. Surgery is almost always necessary with chronic osteomyelitis as necrotic and dead bone needs to be debrided. Management might also include 'Papineau technique'/vacuum assisted closure (VAC) (Archdeacon and Messerschmitt 2006) with flaps, antibiotic impregnated beads, bone grafting, soft tissue management and stabilisation. This may often involve the removal of previous metalwork and instability caused by bone damage or loss may require external fixation. Prognosis is dependent on the patient's general health status. Outcomes are improved if treatment is started 3–5 days after the onset of the infection.

Timely diagnosis and intervention in an otherwise well patient can lead to full recovery, although follow-up over several months is needed to monitor for relapse. The condition can have a psychological impact on the patient if recovery is slow and pain severe.

Back pain

Back pain is a complex series of conditions with considerable variability in pathology and outcome. Most patients with new episodes recover within a few weeks but recurrence is common and individuals with chronic, long-standing back pain tend to show a more persistent course. Most back pain, fortunately, responds to a set of non-surgical interventions that facilitate a gradual return to normal activity for the patient. Patients need to be encouraged to move despite the presence of pain to aid recovery. Progressively intense range of movement and strengthening exercises offer improved stability of the lumbar spine under the guidance of a physiotherapist, while drugs facilitate increased movement and recommencement of normal activities. Drug regimens may include simple analgesics, NSAIDs and muscle relaxants, which can hasten a return to function. When back pain becomes chronic additional health professionals may become involved. The chronic pain service is often pivotal in developing a personalised plan with a variety of approaches to manage the differing types of pain, e.g. stronger opioids for escalating nociceptive type pain, additional medication for neuropathic pain and acupuncture, whilst psychology may better support a reduction in patient's mood /depression with antidepressants and alternative interventions such as cognitive behavioural therapy as chronic pain does appear to increase the risk of depression in some patients.

Low back pain (LBP) is the most common condition within the spectrum with many people experiencing it at some point in their life. Most low back pain episodes are mild and rarely disabling, with only a small proportion of individuals seeking intervention. LBP can impact upon the person's quality of life due to reduced mobility and pain and differential diagnosis is desirable to establish a probable cause, diagnosis and suitable treatments. A general practitioner (GP) most often makes the referral to an orthopaedic consultant which leads to a more in-depth history taking and physical examination using the 'look, feel and move' in conjunction with radiological evidence e.g. X-ray, MRI and CT in an attempt to ascertain a diagnosis which is not always attainable. '*Listening*' to the patient and family gives the practitioner the best opportunity to find the cause of low back pain. Treatment and care needs to consider the patients' individual needs and preferences. Good communication the provision of information is central in facilitating patient involvement in their care. NICE (2009b) offers specific guidance for the early management of low back pain and these are summarised in Box 13.2.

In 70% of cases, low back pain has no obvious aetiology or pathogenesis as most back pain is muscular or ligamentous in origin rather than skeletal. The soft tissue structures are located deep inside the body, so although radiography including MRI and CT scans can pinpoint anatomic anomalies in skeletal structures, such investigations cannot identify the specific causes of pain (Borenstein and Calin 2012). The presence of any of the 'red flags'; fever or weight loss, pain with recumbency, prolonged morning stiffness, acute fracture and viscerogenic pain related to a non-musculoskeletal organ system (e.g. genitourinary) might suggest systemic conditions (i.e. possible fracture, tumour or infection, cauda equina syndrome and spondyloarthropathy). Any red flag should be noted at the initial assessment, as they will influence the subsequent assessment and management of the patient.

Treatment should ideally involve a MDT approach to develop a patient-centred plan of care. A wide range of professionals can help the patient address challenges in both quality of life and the ability to undertake normal activities of daily living. Subsequently chronic back pain often leads to financial and relationship difficulties which may lead to depression. Spinal surgery is considered in Chapter 14.

Box 13.2 Evidence digest. Reproduced with permission from NICE

NICE Guideline (NICE 2009b): Low back pain: early management of persistent non-specific low back pain

Based on reviews of the evidence NICE Clinical Guideline 88 (2009) covers the early treatment and management of persistent or recurrent low back pain, defined as non-specific low back pain that has lasted for more than 6 weeks, but for less than 12 months. The guideline recommends the following principles of management:

- Keep the diagnosis under review at all times.
- Promote self-management; advise people with low back pain to exercise, to be physically active and to carry on with normal activities as far as possible.
- Offer drug treatments as appropriate to manage pain and to help people to keep active.
- Offer one of the following treatments, taking patient preference into account:
  - exercise programme
  - course of manual therapy
  - course of acupuncture.
- Consider offering another of these options if the chosen treatment does not result in satisfactory improvement.

Scoliosis

The spine has gentle curves that develop as a child grows, but within such natural curves three key deformities can develop; scoliosis, kyphosis and lordosis. Only scoliosis, the type most commonly met by the practitioner, will be discussed here. Scoliosis refers to a side-to-side curvature of the spine that affects a small percentage of the population, approximately 2% in women and less than half a percent of men. The condition has familial tendencies and the majority of scoliosis is 'idiopathic', (of no known cause) usually starting in the early teens or pre-teens and gradually progressing in severity of the curvature as growth occurs. Once the rapid growth of puberty is over, mild curves often do not change whilst severe curves nearly always develop further. Although scoliosis can occur in children with cerebral palsy, muscular dystrophy, spina bifida and other miscellaneous conditions, most scoliosis is found in otherwise healthy young people. Therefore, parents should watch for the following 'signs' of scoliosis beginning when their child is about eight years of age, with any one sign warranting investigation:

- uneven shoulders
- prominent shoulder blade or shoulder blades
- uneven waist
- elevated hips
- leaning to one side.

Adult scoliosis may represent the progression of a condition that began in childhood and was not diagnosed or treated during growth. What might have started out as a slight or moderate curve could have progressed in the absence of treatment. If allowed to progress, in severe cases adult scoliosis can lead to chronic severe back pain, deformity, and difficulty in breathing.

Cobb's angle is the measurement used for the evaluation of curves in scoliosis on an AP radiographic image of the spine using a protractor. A line is drawn along the superior end plate of the superior end vertebra involved in the curve and a second line drawn along the inferior end plate of the inferior end vertebra. If the end plates are indistinct, the line may be drawn through the pedicles. The angle between these two lines (or lines drawn perpendicular to them) is measured as the Cobb angle. Shaw *et al.* (2012) reported upon the use of smart phone technology to offer an equivalent Cobb measurement tool equal to the manual protractor. In S-shaped scoliosis, where there are two contiguous curves, the lower end vertebra of the upper curve will represent the upper end vertebra of the lower curve. Because the Cobb angle reflects curvature only in a single plane and fails to account for vertebral rotation it may not accurately demonstrate the severity of three dimensional spinal deformities. As a general rule a Cobb angle of 10 is regarded as a minimum angulation to define scoliosis.

Treatment options include:

- Doing nothing, which may be reasonable depending on the age of the person and the predicted outcome. Doing nothing in the teen years though may be disastrous.
- Bracing has been shown to be an effective method to prevent curves from getting more progressive. However this treatment is reserved for children and young people in whom a rapid increase in the curve needs to be thwarted. A brace worn 16 or more hours per day has been shown to be effective in preventing 90% or more of the curves from getting worse. Unfortunately, a brace worn 23 hours per day and worn properly does not guarantee that the curve will not continue to increase. Yet, in curves that are mild i.e. between 20 and 35 degrees, a brace may be quite effective. However, bracing cannot "hold" curves greater than 40 degrees. The brace may feel hot, hard and uncomfortable while it normally can't be seen under the clothes and can make a young person more self-conscious about their body image (http://www.scoliosisrx.com/).
- For those who already have a significant curve and deformity, surgery can reduce the curve and significantly reduce the deformity.

Surgery is usually offered to teen and pre-teens who already have a curve of around 40 degrees or more. Surgery can commence around 40 degrees while there are many excellent surgeons who defer to 45 or 50 degrees. In the adult the reasons for surgery include increasing discomfort or pain with an increasing curve. For many women the combination of a deformity in the hip line and the increasing discomfort make surgery a reasonable option. Others note the increasing deformity in the chest coupled with an increase in the rib hump. However for those persons surgery can (not always and certainly not guaranteed) reduce the deformity and the discomfort or pain.

Common surgical intervention includes anterior and posterior spinal fusion. Posterior spinal infusion only (Matusz *et al.*, 2005) with posterior spinal fusion (PSF) with spinal instrumentation has been the mainstay of surgical treatment since the late 1960s. Thoracoscopic anterior instrumentation is an alternative as instead of a long open thoracotomy to obtain exposure of the anterior spine, small incisions are made to allow introduction of a thoracoscope and working instruments. The advantages are less post-operative pain in the chest wall, better long-term cosmetics and equal release when compared to open discectomy plus alternative growth rod instrumentation (Ember and Noordeen 2005).

Spinal stenosis

Spinal stenosis refers to narrowing of the central spinal canal. Although narrowing does not always result in nerve compression, it can create pressure on the nerves, often resulting in pain or numbness in the region impacted by the compressed nerve or nerves. There are many causes including tumours, congenital defects, physical injury and bone disease. However the most prevalent causes are the ageing effects of intervertebral disc degeneration, bone overgrowth and ligament thickening. Lumbar and cervical areas are most commonly affected and both lead to significant pain, disability and impact on quality of life. Lumbar spinal stenosis has become the most common indication for spinal decompression surgery in older patients.

Intervertebral disc disease

Age-related changes in the intervertebral disc can lead to degeneration and increased likelihood of a clinical problem. A prolapsed intervertebral disc (often termed '*slipped disc*') commonly occurs in the lumbar and cervical areas which have more mobility which puts the discs at high risk of damage (Smith 2005). The primary symptom is pain of varying severity and frequency. Depending on the site of the disc prolapse and the nerve involvement, the patient will typically have intense radicular (nerve root) pain. The pressure that the disc puts on the nerve roots often causes neurological symptoms in addition to the pain, with some patients developing motor weakness.

The management of back pain is usually treated conservatively initially with MDT involvement and discussion with patients regarding realistic options (Murray, 2011). Medication, exercises and/or a local steroid injection via epidural may benefit patients. Surgery is indicated if the following indicators are present:

- unrelenting leg pain
- neural damage
- cauda equina syndrome

A central disc prolapse constitutes a medical emergency however. An immediate MRI scan is required. Decompression within 24 hours of the onset of symptoms is needed as the disc presses on the cauda equina, causing the following motor and sensory problems:

- loss of perianal sensation known as 'saddle anaesthesia'
- bilateral motor weakness in the legs
- sphincter disturbance to the bowel and bladder.

Summary

All key orthopaedic conditions discussed here continue to challenge patients and the nurse practitioners who care for them. With significant development of professional roles and increasing autonomy for nurses along with heightened engagement in evidence based practice and national guidance such as that from NICE the way in which care is delivered can ensure optimum outcomes whether treatment is conservative, pharmacological or surgical.

Recommended further reading

Brady, R.A., Leid, J.G., Costerton, J.W. and Shirtliff, M.E. (2006) Osteomyelitis: clinical overview and mechanisms of infection. *Clinical Microbiology Newsletter*, **28**(9), 65–72.

Hatzenbuehler, J. and Pulling, T.J. (2011) Diagnosis and management of osteomyelitis. *American Family Physician*, **1:84** (9),1027–1033.

Murray, M.M. (2011) Reflections on the development of nurse-led back pain triage clinics in the UK. *International Journal of Orthopaedic and Trauma Nursing*, **15**(3), 113–120.

National Institute for Clinical Evidence (NICE) (2009a) *Rheumatoid Arthritis – Full Guideline Rheumatoid Arthritis: National Clinical Guideline for Management and Treatment in Adults.* NICE, London.

Tanna, N. (2009) Osteoporosis and fragility fractures: identifying those at risk and raising public awareness. *Nursing Times*, **105**(38), 28–31.

References

Adam, W.R. (2011) Non-steroidal anti-inflammatory drugs and the risks of acute renal failure: number needed to harm. *Nephrology*, **16**(2), 154–155.

Anderson D.L. (2004) TNF Inhibitors: a new age in rheumatoid arthritis treatment. *American Journal of Nursing*, **104**(2), 60–68.

Archdeacon, M.T. and Messerschmitt, P. (2006) Modern Papineau technique with vacuum-assisted closure. *Journal of Orthopaedic Trauma*, **20**(2), 134–137.

Arthritis Research Campaign (2002) *Arthritis: The Big Picture*. Arthritis Research Campaign, Derbyshire, UK. Available at: http://www.ipsos-mori.com/Assets/Docs/Archive/Polls/arthritis.pdf (accessed 22 April 2014).

Arthritis Research UK (2011) *Arthritis in the UK: Key Facts*. Available at: www.arthritisresearchuk.org/pdf/Arthritis Key Facts.pdf (accessed May 2013).

Avouac, J., Gossec, L., Dougados M. *et al.* (2007) Efficacy and safety of opioids for osteoarthritis: a meta-analysis of randomized controlled trials. *Osteoarthritis and Cartilage*, **15**(8), 957–965.

Blackman, R (2011) *Scoliosis Treatment*. Scoliosis Research Institute. Available at: http://www.scoliosisrx.com/ (accessed November 2013).

Borenstein, D. and Calin, A. (2012) *Fast Facts: Low Back Pain* 2nd edn. Health Press, Oxford.

Brady, R.A. Leid, J.G., Costerton, J.W. and Shirtliff, M.E. (2006) Osteomyelitis: clinical overview and mechanisms of infection. *Clinical Microbiology Newsletter*, **28**(9), 65–72.

British Society for Rheumatology (BSR) (2004) *BSR Guidelines for Prescribing TNF α- Blockers in Adults with Ankylosing Spondylitis*. BSR, London.

Chihara, S. and Segreti, J. (2010) *Osteomyelitis. Disease-a-Month*, **56**(1), 66.

Doherty, M., Lanyon, P. and Ralston, S. (2006) Musculoskeletal disorders, in *Davidson's Principles & Practice of Medicine* (eds N. Boon, N. Colledge, B. Walker, et al.), Churchill Livingstone, London.

Ember, T., Noordeen, H. (2005) Growth rod spinal instrumentation to control progressive early onset scoliosis. *The Spinal Journal*, **5**(340), S125.

Fransen,M., McConnell, G., Herandez-Molina, G. and Reichenbach, S. (2010) Does land based exercise reduce pain and disability associated with hip osteoarthritis? A meta-analysis of randomized controlled trial. *Osteoarthritis Cartilage*, **18**(5), 13–20.

Geijer M., Gadeholt Göthlin G. and Göthlin J.H. (2009) The validity of the New York radiological grading criteria in diagnosing sacroiliitis by computed tomography. *Acta Radiologica*, **50**(6), 664–673. DOI:10.1080/02841850902914099.

Gosselin, R., Roberts, I. and Gillespie, W. (2009) Antibiotics for Preventing Infection in Open Limb Fractures. *Cochrane Database of Systematic Reviews* **1** (Art. No.: CD003764). DOI: 10.1002/14651858.CD003764.pub2.

Hill, J. and Ryan, S. (2000) *Rheumatology: A Handbook for Community Nurses*. Whurr Publishers, London.

Hill, S., Dziedzi, K. and Ong, B. (2010) The functional and psychological impact of hand osteoarthritis. *Chronic Illness*, **6** (2), 101–110.

Hurley, M., Walsh, N., Mitchell, H. *et al.* (2007) Clinical effectiveness of a rehabilitation program integrating exercise, self-management, and active coping strategies for chronic knee pain: a cluster randomized trial. *Arthritis and Rheumatism*, **57**(7), 1211–1219.

International Assessment in Ankylosing Spondylitis Working/European League Against Rheumatism (IAAS) (2006) Recommendations for the management of ankylosing spondylitis. *Annals of Rheumatic Diseases*, **65**, 442–452.

Itoh, K., Hirota, S., Katsumi, Y., Ochi, H. and Kitakoji, H. (2008) A pilot study on using acupuncture and transcutaneous electrical nerve stimulation (TENS) to treat knee osteoarthritis. *Chinese Medicine*, **3**: 2.

Johnell, O. and Kanis, J.A. (2006) An estimate of the worldwide prevalence and disability associated with osteoporotic fractures. *Osteoporosis International*, **17**, 1726–1733.

Jones, G., Crotty, M. and Brooks, P. (2000) Interventions for Treating Psoriatic Arthritis. *Cochrane Database of Systematic Reviews* **3** (Art. No.: CD000212). DOI: 10.1002/14651858.CD000212.

Kneale, J. and Davis, P. (eds.) (2005) *Orthopaedic and Trauma Nursing*, 2nd edn. Churchill Livingstone, Edinburgh.

Kosuwon, W., Sirichatiwapee, W., Wisanuyotin, T., Jeeravipoolvarn, P. and Laupattarakasem, W. (2010) Efficacy of symptomatic control of knee osteoarthritis with 0.0125% of capsaicin versus placebo. *Journal of Medical Association Thailand*, **93**(10), 1188–1195.

Lew, D.P. and Waldvogel, F.A. (2004) Osteomyelitis. *Lancet*, **364**, 369–379.

Matusz, D., Perez, O., Pateder, D., Kostuik, J. and Kebaish, K. (2005) Posterior only vs. combined anterior and posterior approaches to lumbar scoliosis in adults: a radiological comparison. *The Spinal Journal*, **5**(120), S162.

Murray, M.M. (2011) Reflections on the development of nurse-led back pain triage clinics in the UK. *International Journal of Orthopaedic and Trauma Nursing*, **15**(3), 113–120.

National Ankylosing Spondylitis Society (NASS) (2004) *Guidebook for Patients*. NASS, Mayfield East Sussex.

National Institute for Health and Clinical Excellence (NICE) (2008) Adalimumab, Etanercept and Infliximab for ankylosing spondylitis. NICE technology Appraisal Guidance 143. NICE, London.

NICE (2008a) *Clinical Guidelines for the Management of Osteoarthritis*. NICE, London.

NICE (2008b) TA160 Alendronate, Etidronate, Risedronate, Raloxifene and strontium ranelate for the primary prevention of osteoporatic fragility fractures in postmenopausal women. NICE, London.

NICE (2009a) *Rheumatoid Arthritis – Full Guideline. Rheumatoid Arthritis: National Clinical Guideline for Management and Treatment in Adults*. NICE, London.

NICE (2009b) *CG 88 Low Back pain: Early Management of Persistent Non-specific Low Back Pain*. NICE, London.

NICE (2012) *CG146 Osteoporosis: Assessing the Risk of Fragility Fracture*. NICE, London.

Salvarani, C. and Fries, W. (2009) Clinical features and epidemiology of spondyloarthritides associated with inflammatory bowel disease. *World Journal of Gastroenterology*, **15**(20), 2449–2455.

Shaw, M., Adam, C.J., Izatt, M.T., Licina, P. and Askin, G.N. (2012) Use of the iPhone for Cobb angle measurement in scoliosis. *European Spine Journal*, **21**(6), 1062–1068.

Sieper, J., Braun, J., Rudwaleit, M., Boonen, A. and Zink, A. (2002) Ankylosing spondylitis: an overview. *Annals of Rheumatic Diseases*, **61** Suppl 3, iii8 – iii18.

Smith, M. (2005) Care of patients with spinal conditions and injuries, in *Orthopaedic and Trauma Nursing* (eds J. Kneale, and P. Davis), Chapter 18. Churchill Livingstone, London.

Tanna, N. (2009) Osteoporosis and fragility fractures: identifying those at risk and raising public awareness. *Nursing Times*, **105**(38), 28–31.

WHO (1994) *Assessment of Fracture Risk and its Application to Screening for Postmenopausal Women*. WHO, Gevena.

Zhang, W., Nuki, G., Moskowitz, R.W. *et al.* (2010) OARSI recommendations for the management of hip and knee osteoarthritis: part III: changes in evidence following systematic cumulative update of research published through January 2009. *Osteoarthritis and Cartilage*, **18**(4), 476–499.

CHAPTER 14

Elective orthopaedic surgery

Brian Lucas[1], Mary Drozd[2], Sandra Flynn[3] and Vanessa Blair[4]

[1] *Queen Elizabeth Hospital, Kings Lynn, UK*
[2] *University of Wolverhampton, Walsall, West Midlands, UK*
[3] *Countess of Chester Hospital, Chester, UK*
[4] *Musgrave Park Hospital, Belfast, Northern Ireland, UK*

Introduction

The aim of this chapter is to provide an overview of the evidence base for the practice of orthopaedic elective surgical care. Planned, or elective surgery – in particular joint replacement (arthroplasty) – is the main focus of orthopaedic work. Elective surgery is a major life event for patients and they have high expectations of a successful operation and recovery. Orthopaedic practitioners play a key role in ensuring that patients are fully prepared for surgery and that they are supported during the perioperative and post-operative recovery period. Such surgery is resource intensive in terms of healthcare delivery and achieving the best outcomes as well as the best possible experience for patients is central.

Principles of care

The focus of care provision and the key care principles of elective surgery are firmly rooted in the ethos of safe and high quality service delivery as these are central in ensuring positive outcomes. The recent introduction of *enhanced recovery programmes* (ECPs), also referred to as *rapid recovery*, aims to optimise outcomes and improve patient experience through evidence-based pathways of care. A key element is striving to empower patients so that they become partners in their care (Driver *et al.*, 2012). There are four working principles of enhanced recovery:

1 Every patient is included in a pathway designed to enhance their recovery.
2 Preoperative preparation places the patient in the best possible condition for their surgery, helps to identify risks and instigates rehabilitation either before admission or soon after.
3 Patient management is pro-active and is evident across the whole pathway.
4 Patients play an active role and take responsibility for enhancing their recovery (DOH 2011).

In elective orthopaedic surgery settings, enhanced recovery pathways have been developed particularly for patients undergoing total hip replacement (THR) or total knee replacement (TKR) surgery. The main focusses are patient preparation and identifying and minimising risk. Patient empowerment is central to this and is promoted through:

- good communication
- shared decision making
- education and information
- support for patients/family members/carers
- advice resources
- clinician engagement
- patient engagement.

Communication

Communication is a vital tool for the delivery of safe and quality care and is a key priority for the multidisciplinary team. Effective communication helps to develop partnerships between service providers and service users. Patients must be kept informed about their treatment and be involved in decisions about their care. Good communication helps to manage patient expectations and make the care pathway less stressful,

Orthopaedic and Trauma Nursing: An Evidence-based Approach to Musculoskeletal Care, First Edition. Edited by Sonya Clarke and Julie Santy-Tomlinson.

helping to promote a sense of control so the patient is more able to participate in the recovery process.

Shared decision making

Shared decision making has become a prominent feature in the drive to achieve good healthcare outcomes. Decisions relating to treatment have traditionally been undertaken by clinicians although this practice is gradually evolving to include patient involvement in partnership with clinicians (Slover *et al.*, 2012). Collaboration between patient and clinician aims to:

- improve health outcomes
- empower the patient
- improve knowledge
- increase awareness of the benefits of treatment
- adjust unrealistic expectations
- alert patients to the degree of acceptable risks
- improve compliance with treatment
- improve satisfaction with care.

Within elective orthopaedic surgery shared decision making models have emerged in which clinicians and patients work together to decide on the best treatment option. This is seen as an important approach to joint replacement surgery (O'Neill *et al.*, 2007). There are three important components of shared decision-making:

- **Clinical assessment and evaluation** – help the clinician to present information based upon clinical findings about treatment options.
- **Patient perception** – every patient has a perception of their condition that is unique; everything they hear, see or experience is specific to them. It is important that the healthcare professional appreciates the patient's viewpoint, decision and subsequent physical, psychological and social affect that any treatment may have upon them.
- **Decision aids** – offer evidence-based impartial information about the treatment options for specific conditions (Fung *et al.*, 2008), particularly in circumstances where there may be uncertainty about the best treatment option. They present the patient with the risks and benefits of each option to help them to understand the benefits and risks.

Other important aspects of care provision include:

Education and Information

Education and the provision of information are key to ensuring that patients are prepared physically and psychologically for their surgery. This is considered in more detail in the section on preoperative preparation.

Support and advice

Involving and encouraging family member or carer participation can play a significant role in reinforcing the principles of enhanced recovery by helping to instil confidence prior to admission and following discharge from hospital and providing a means of support when the patient is no longer in direct contact with members of their healthcare team. Some hospitals provide peer support groups where patients can meet and chat with others who have had similar surgery. Additional support can also be provided by dedicated contact points at the unit where surgery will or has taken place. Information concerning advice and who to contact should be provided to all patients during every stage of their care pathway and on discharge from hospital.

Clinician engagement

Engaging clinical staff is critical to the success of enhanced recovery pathways and involves factors such as:

- team work – including collaborative working between primary and secondary care staff
- staff education and training
- developing and working to agreed protocols i.e. standardising anaesthetic or surgical practice
- identifying clinical champions and leaders
- recognising that patients are partners in their care
- audit of pathways and feedback to clinicians

Patient engagement

Without patient engagement enhanced recovery pathways cannot succeed, and involving them in planning, implementing and evaluating their pathway of care is crucial. Patients need to be encouraged to take ownership of their decision to proceed with surgery emphasising the active role the patient needs to adopt to feel empowered, in control and able to participate actively in their own recovery.

Preoperative care

The preoperative phase of elective surgery includes the journey from preoperative assessment, education, admission and discharge planning as well as all the components required in preparation for the surgery itself.

If effective, this phase of care can be as instrumental as good surgical technique in positive post-operative outcomes.

Preoperative assessment

As demands for shorter hospital stays increase – driven by cost reductions within healthcare systems – good preoperative assessment is imperative. It ensures that the patient is fully informed about the procedure and the post-operative recovery plan, is in optimum health and has made arrangements for admission, discharge and post-operative care at home.

Patients are graded relating to severity of their surgery:

Grade 1 – (minor) e.g. excision of lesion, joint injection

Grade 2 – e.g. knee arthroscopy

Grade 3 – e.g. lumbar discectomy, anterior cruciate ligament reconstruction

Grade 4 – (major) e.g. total joint replacement, joint revision.

The patient's medical/surgical history is assessed using the ASA (American Society of Anesthesiologists) which grades the patient using a scale in relation to their fitness for undergoing an anaesthetic (adapted from NICE 2003):

- ASA Grade 1 – a normal healthy patient, without any clinically important co-morbidity or clinically significant past/present medical history
- ASA Grade 2 – a patient with mild systemic disease, e.g. well controlled hypertension/diabetes/asthma
- ASA Grade 3 – a patient with severe systemic disease, e.g. angina/hypertension/diabetes/COAD/COPD all not well controlled
- ASA Grade 4 – a patient with severe systemic disease that is a constant threat to life
- ASA Grade 5 – a moribund patient who is not expected to survive without the operation
- ASA Grade 6 – a patient declared brain-dead and their organs are being harvested for donor purposes.

NICE (2003) make evidence-based recommendations regarding clinical investigations required prior to elective surgery, dependent upon the ASA and surgery grades. The recommendations are formulated into traffic light colour coded tables for uncomplicated decision making (Table 14.1).

Other important aspects to be considered are:

- baseline clinical observations
- weight and height for drug dosage calculations
- calculation of body mass index (BMI)

Table 14.1 Example of investigations required for patient ASA Grade 3: adults with co-morbidity from cardiovascular disease undergoing Grade 4 surgery e.g. total hip/knee replacement (adapted from NICE 2003). Reproduced with permission from NICE

Test	Investigations
Chest X-ray	Required
ECG	Required
Full blood count and group and save	Consider
Haemostasis – prothrombin time, INR	Required
Renal function	Required
Random glucose	Not required unless relevant history
Urine analysis/MSU	Required for orthopaedic surgery
Blood gases	Consider if relevant history
Lung function	Not required unless relevant history

- list of current medications
- any allergies or drug sensitivities
- methicillin resistant staphylococcus aureus (MRSA) screening of nose, axilla, groin and any wounds
- Skin integrity and potential for peri- and/or post-surgery skin breakdown
- oral/dental checks for decay or disease.

Preoperative education

Preoperative education can be provided at the same time as preoperative assessment or in a separate individual or group education session prior to surgery. This has been shown to be more effective than post-admission teaching in terms of patients' knowledge and retention (Stern and Lockwood 2005; JBI 2010a). The aim is to provide the foundations for effective decision making enabling informed consent, information regarding the procedure itself and post-operative expectations, care and rehabilitation. The knowledge gained can affect the perception of patients' preparedness for surgery and their ability to control post-operative pain, which therefore improves the patients overall stay (Kearney *et al.*, 2011).

Education can be delivered via one-to-one instruction, group sessions, printed information (i.e. booklet, pamphlet, and information sheet), learning package, audio-visual presentation, and lectures or a combination of these methods (Stern and Lockwood 2005; JBI 2010a).

Some surgeons now offer structured online courses regarding surgery, whilst other patients choose their own online searches (Kearney *et al.*, 2011). With recent technological initiatives, surgical teams need to cater for the change in trend and provide information via differing mediums, to assess the effectiveness of this teaching tool. Involvement of the multi-disciplinary team (MDT) enables each member of the team to contribute to the patient's care and prevents duplication.

Discharge planning

The aim of discharge planning is to reduce hospital length of stay, prevent unplanned readmissions and improve the co-ordination of services following discharge from hospital using the discharge plan tailored to the individual patient (Shepperd *et al.*, 2010). Addressing the physical, psychological and social needs of the patient (and their parent or carer) pre-operatively enables discharge to be considered early in the care process with any referrals to MDT or other agencies made early to prevent delays in discharge.

Admission

Admission is dependent upon practice at institution level or surgeon/anaesthetist preference. Patients can be admitted on the day of surgery or one to two days prior if there is significant medical history and high anaesthetic risk; e.g. a patient with emphysema can be admitted up to two days prior to surgery to ensure medical fitness. Admission nursing assessment should focus on the patient's overall health status and nursing care plans are based on mutually established realistic, client-centred, measurable, clear and concise goals (JBI 2010a). The admission process requires nurses with specialised knowledge in orthopaedics to ensure that the patient is safely prepared for the operation and provide support as hospital admissions can be traumatic and stressful events (Lucas 2008).

Skin preparation

Antiseptic body wash was historically used as a strategy for the prevention of surgical site infections (SSIs) but there is conflicting evidence surrounding this (JBI 2011a). NICE (2008) clinical guidelines, the Joanna Briggs Institute (JBI 2011b) and a Cochrane review (Webster and Osborne 2007) all found no clear evidence that the use of chlorhexidine solution before surgery was beneficial, indicating it may not be cost-effective in comparison to detergent or a bar of soap. The recommendation is for patients to shower or bath using soap either the day before or on the day of surgery to clean the skin surface and therefore reduce microbial load. Neither does hair removal reduce the risk of surgical site infection (NICE 2008), although the presence of hair can interfere with the exposure of the incision and subsequent wound, the suturing of the incision and application of adhesive drapes and wound dressings (JBI 2011a). Three methods of hair removal are currently used: shaving, clipping and chemical depilation, and both JBI (2011a) and NICE (2008) recommend the use of electric clippers with a disposable head, ideally on the day of surgery, as shaving can compromise skin integrity and depilation can irritate skin. Hair removal should be completed on the ward rather than operating theatre as loose hair may contaminate the sterile surgical field (Tanner *et al.*, 2006).

Fasting

The principle of fasting from fluids and solids prior to surgery is to reduce the risk of vomiting and aspiration of stomach contents at the induction of general anaesthetic (GA) (Kohyratty *et al.*, 2010). Patients are rarely aware of the rationale for fasting, so this should be included in preoperative education to reduce anxiety. This is considered in more detail in Chapter 10.

Pre-medication

Premedications are given to reduce preoperative anxiety although a sedative pre-medication is not compulsory. A Cochrane systematic review (Smith and Pittaway 2002) found that premedication did not improve the length of stay and the sedated patient may require closer attention for safety and closer monitoring while awaiting surgery. The JBI (2010b) note an absence of clear research findings surrounding the use of anxiolytic premedication in adult patients undergoing day surgery under general anaesthetic, so this should be based on clinical judgement. Patients should take their routine medications prior to surgery unless otherwise advised by the anaesthetist, and surgeons should ask that anti-coagulant medications such as warfarin, aspirin and clopiderol be stopped for at least five days prior to surgery and sometimes replaced with low molecular weight heparin (LMWH) dependent upon the patient's medical history and risk of thromboembolism (Chapter 9).

Consent

Informed consent is legally required, and should be obtained prior to all nursing and medical procedures (Cohn and Larson 2007). Patients must have full understanding of the procedure, the risks and any alternatives that are available and have made the decision of their own free will, without coercion and are legally able to make the decision.

Safety checklist

In 2008, the World Health Organization (Haynes *et al.*, 2009) published guidelines that recommended practices to ensure the safety of surgical patients worldwide. The Surgical Safety Checklist is intended for use by clinicians to improve the safety of operations and reduce unnecessary surgical deaths and complications. The safety checks begin on the ward and once the checklist and documentation is complete, the patient is transferred to the operating department where the perioperative phase commences. See Box 14.1 and Figure 14.1.

Box 14.1 Evidence summary Improving clinical outcomes through implementation of the WHO Surgical Safety Checklist (Haynes *et al.*, 2009). Reproduced with permission from Massachusetts Medical Society

This large-scale study was conducted in eight hospitals in eight cities (including London, England), representing a variety of economic circumstances and diverse patient populations. The hospitals participated in the WHO's Safe Surgery Saves Lives programme and implemented a 19-item checklist designed to improve team communication and consistency of care. They hypothesized that this would reduce complications and deaths relating to surgery.

The study prospectively studied pre-intervention and post-intervention periods at the participating sites. The checklist was introduced via lectures, written materials or written guidance. Patients were followed up prospectively until discharge or for 30 days, whichever came first, for death and complications such as myocardial infarction, wound infection or sepsis. 3733 patients were enrolled during the baseline period and 3955 patients after the post-implementation phase. There were no significant differences between the patients in the two phases of the study. The in-hospital death rate was shown to decrease from 1.5% to 0.8%, and serious complications from 11% to 7% after introduction of the checklist. The overall rates of surgical site infection and unplanned reoperation also declined significantly.

The authors acknowledged that the combined effects of team building and cultural changes may also have played a part in the positive results, rather than the checklist on its own.

Perioperative care

The care of patients in the operating theatre, from arrival in the anaesthetic room to leaving the recovery area requires staff that are skilled and knowledgeable in both orthopaedic and theatre care. While dealing predominantly with surgery requiring inpatient care, the principles are also applicable to day case orthopaedic surgery.

Anaesthetic preparation

The approach to anaesthesia is carefully planned by the anaesthetic team prior to surgery, taking into consideration the patient's general health status. The patient will also have been informed of these intentions. Anaesthesia allows surgery to take place by rendering the patient insensible to pain and sensation, together with loss of consciousness if a general anaesthetic is used (Woodhead and Wicker 2005). Depending on the type of surgery and the patient characteristics, anaesthesia may be:

- **Local** – only the immediate area is anaesthetised; e.g. a block to allow carpal tunnel surgery to be performed.
- **Regional** – axillary block for hand or forearm surgery (Wing Wai and Irwin 2012) or spinal anaesthetic for lower limb surgery (Royal College of Anaesthetists 2008).
- **General** – the patient is unconscious for the operation. This can be used for all operative procedures in patients who are fit for a general anaesthesia.

For pain relief an epidural anaesthetic or a nerve block may be used in addition to a spinal or general anaesthetic; for example a femoral nerve block for analgesia in total hip replacement surgery.

Intraoperative period

Along with general surgical considerations, effective operating department procedures include ensuring the correct positioning of the patient to allow surgical and anaesthetic access while at the same time maintaining patient dignity and managing risk from harm; for example, shoulder surgery patients can be positioned in an upright/beach chair or supine position (Dutta 2011), resulting in different pressure points. The maintenance of patient safety, temperature, correct patient moving/handling and infection control measures must also be considered.

SIGN IN (to be read out loud)

Before induction on anaesthesia

Has the patient confirmed his/her identity, site, procedure and consent?
- ☐ Yes

Is the surgical site marked?
- ☐ Yes/not applicable

Is the anaesthesia machine and medication check complete?
- ☐ Yes

Does the patient have a:

Known allergy?
- ☐ No
- ☐ Yes

Difficult airway/aspiration risk?
- ☐ No
- ☐ Yes, and equipment/assistance available

Risk of >500 ml blood loss (7 ml/kg in children)?
- ☐ No
- ☐ Yes, and adequate IV access/fluids planned

TIME OUT (to be read out load)

Before start of surgical intervention
for example, skin incision

Have all team members introduced themselves by name and role?
- ☐ Yes

Surgeon, Anaesthetist and Registered Practitioner verbally confirm:
- ☐ What is the patient's name?
- ☐ What procedure, site and position are planned?

Anticipated critical events

Surgeon:
- ☐ How much blood loss is anticipated?
- ☐ Are there are specific equipment requirements or special investigations?
- ☐ Are there any critical or unexpected steps you want the team to know about?

Anaesthetist:
- ☐ Are there any patient specific concerns?
- ☐ What is the patient's ASA grade?
- ☐ What monitoring equipment and other specific levels of support are required, for example blood?

Nurse/ODP:
- ☐ Has the sterility of the instrumentation been confirmed (including indicator results)?
- ☐ Are there are equipment issues or concerns?

Has the surgical site infection (SSI) bundle been undertaken?
- ☐ Yes/not applicable
  - o Antibiotic prophylaxis within the last 60 minutes
  - o Patient warming
  - o Hair removal
  - o Glycaemic control

Has VTE prophylaxis been undertaken?
- ☐ Yes/not applicable

Is essential imaging displayed?
- ☐ Yes/not applicable

Name:	
Signature of Registered Practitioner:	

SIGN OUT (to be read out loud)

Before any member of the team leaves the operating room

Registered Practitioner verbally confirms with the team:
- ☐ Has the name of the procedure been recorded?
- ☐ Has it been confirmed that instruments, swabs and sharp counts are complete (or not applicable)?
- ☐ Have the specimens been labeled (including patient name)?
- ☐ Have any equipment problems been identified that need to be addressed?

Surgeon, Anaesthetist and Registered Practitioner:
- ☐ What are the key concerns for recovery and management of this patient?

Name:	
Signature of Registered Practitioner:	

PATIENT DETAILS

Last name:	
First name:	
Date of birth:	
NHS Number*:	
Procedure:	

*If the NHS Number is not immediately available, a temporary number should be used until it is

Figure 14.1 Surgical checklist

There are a plethora of roles within the operating theatre which vary according to the way in which operating department practice has developed locally and nationally. Advanced roles in the operating department now include practitioners who have received additional training and education and may assist with retaining retractors, dissect soft tissue/bone, prepare ligament grafts, place intraoperative drains, close wounds and safely transfer the patient from operating table to bed post-surgery (Jones *et al.*, 2012). All practitioners who work within the sterile field need not only to attend to the technical aspects of surgery but also to non-technical skills (Mitchell *et al.*, 2011) including 'situation awareness' (watching and anticipating the next stage of the procedure), communication (verbal and non-verbal cues), teamwork (coordinating activities), task management and coping with stress and fatigue (their own and other members of the team). An important consideration for patients having regional anaesthesia is communication during the surgery as they have two overarching needs: wanting to have control (knowledge) and trust in staff (Bergman *et al.*, 2012).

Recovery

After surgery patients should be fully conscious and clinically stable before they return to the ward or are discharged. Transfer of the patient from the operating theatre to the recovery room is an important consideration as transfers from one surface to another involve risk such as dislocation of a hip prosthesis following joint arthroplasty and appropriate equipment such as abduction wedges or pillows may need to be in place to maintain the correct position. The recovery staff will assume responsibility for the patient and care for them according to a model such as ABCDE (Hatfield and Tronson 2009):

- A – airway
- B – breathing
- C – circulation
- D – drips, drains and drugs
- E – extras.

'Extra' considerations may include elevation of a limb and care of a cast or a back slab (Chapter 8). Peripheral neurovascular observations are necessary following limb surgery and where casts/traction are being used (Chapters 8 and 9).

Recovery occurs in stages and can be characterised as Stages 1–3 (Hatfield and Tronson, 2009):

Stage 1 – patients have just left the theatre and are expected to stay in the recovery room for one hour following general anaesthesia and half an hour after local anaesthesia. Vital signs, nausea/pain, conscious level and output from drains or bleeding from wound sites should be monitored and any abnormalities reported to the anaesthetist and/or surgeon. Operations performed under tourniquet such as limb surgery may result in up to one litre of blood loss in the recovery room, requiring careful monitoring along with checking of vacuum drains. Thirty minutes should elapse before the last dose of opioid analgesia and discharge from the recovery room.

Stage 2 – relates to transfer of patients to the ward once vital signs are stable, the patient is conscious, pain is controlled and there is no excessive wound drainage or bleeding. Transfer should take place with portable suction, oxygen and other emergency equipment available. Some elective orthopaedic patients will be transferred to the Intensive Care Unit (ICU) for extended Stage 1 recovery. A review of 22 000 primary and revision THR patients found that 130 were admitted to ICU and that independent risk factors were smoking, cemented arthroplasty, general anaesthesia, allogeneic transfusion, higher C-reactive protein, lower haemoglobin level, higher body mass index and older age (AbdelSalam *et al.*, 2012). Whatever the transfer destination, it is important that the receiving staff have a comprehensive handover including operation performed, surgeon's instructions, intraoperative details such as blood loss, anaesthetic type, condition in recovery and checking of the wound dressing, drains and any other drains or infusions by the receiving staff (Woodhead and Wicker 2005).

Stage 3 – discharge home and longer-term follow up. For day case procedures this happens when vital signs have been stable for at least one hour, pain is adequately controlled, there is an absence of nausea/vomiting and the patient is able to drink, eat and pass urine.

Post-operative care

The drive for shorter hospitalisation post-surgery means that patients more frequently return directly to the ward environment instead of an ICU or High Dependency Unit (HDU). This enables continuity of care as the nursing staff can monitor the patient through regular observation and, if the patient is physically fit, haemodynamically stable and spinal anaesthetic or nerve blocks have worn off, they can commence mobilisation on the day of surgery (day 0). This enables the patient to use the new joint, reducing risk of VTE and chest infection as the patient is not lying supine in bed. Effective post-operative care involves:

- monitoring of clinical observations in accordance with policy and appropriately recorded onto EWS/ MEWS chart (Chapter 16)
- assessment of neurovascular status bilaterally (Chapter 9)
- management of pain (Chapter 11)
- monitoring of input (oral and IV)/output (vomitus, urinary and blood loss) via fluid balance chart, especially in the first 24 hours (Chapter 10)
- assessment and management of wound/dressings/ drains (Chapter 12)
- encourage deep breathing exercises and initiate chest physiotherapy if required to prevent chest infection
- encourage leg exercises to reduce risk of DVT, and administer VTE prophylaxis (Chapter 9)
- initiate mobilisation and rehabilitation.

Blood replacement

Blood loss during orthopaedic surgery is unavoidable, particularly during THR and transfusion of blood is sometimes required. There are currently three techniques available for transfusing blood within the orthopaedic setting:

- allogeneic; blood from an unrelated donor
- cell salvage; collecting blood from the patient during surgery for transfusion during or after surgery
- perioperative autologous donation (PAD) – the collection of patients' own blood prior to surgery for transfusion if required (Carless *et al.*, 2010).

Allogeneic blood transfusion in elective orthopaedic surgery is risky and best avoided. PAD is justified in patients who have developed immune responses because of repeated transfusions or in situations where there is doubt about the safety of the blood supply. It is also believed to reduce the need for transfusions of donor blood and is safer than receiving an allogeneic transfusion (Carless *et al.*, 2010; Henry *et al.*, 2001; JBI 2010c). A Cochrane review suggested that cell salvage reduces the need for allogeneic red cell transfusion and did not appear to impact adversely on clinical outcomes (Carless *et al.*, 2010). Many alternative strategies are currently being employed to reduce the number of transfusions required including anti-fibrinolytic compounds such as aminocaproic acid and tranexamic acid. Tranexamic acid is an antifibrinolytic agent, which effectively blocks this fibrinolytic activity, causing a marked reduction in post-operative bleeding (Sepah *et al.*, 2011).

Discharge planning/rehabilitation

There is increasing pressure for discharge from hospital as early as possible. Nurses are in the key position of coordinating discharges in collaboration with the MDT, patient and family. Planning commences in the preoperative phase as delayed discharges and prolonged hospitalisation can place the patient at additional risk and there are financial and efficiency implications for the service. Good practice requires units to develop standards, protocols and audit tools in order to monitor the quality of discharges. Such criteria relate to physical, psychological and social benchmarks (RCN 2013):

Physical criteria

- conscious level and orientation should be consistent with preoperative state
- haemodynamically stable or similar to preoperative status
- tolerating food and fluids orally, nausea and vomiting should be minimal
- urinary catheter removed and micturition has occurred
- pain under control and patient given sufficient oral analgesia for discharge
- minimal surgical site bleeding. Patient should be given instructions on wound care or appropriate referral to community nursing teams or GP surgery to follow-up
- mobility using appropriate aids to a level dependent upon surgery and physiotherapy goals achieved
- X-rays reviewed by surgical team confirming correct placement of prosthesis.

Psychological criteria

- Provide information regarding recovery at home – both verbal and written.
- Follow-up appointment instructions should be given to the patient or their parent/carer, e.g. removal of sutures or clips, outpatient physiotherapy and consultant review.

- Check appropriate discharge medication has been provided; patient/carer may need support and guidance on administration. Pay particular attention to VTE prophylaxis and highlight importance.
- Contact telephone numbers should be given to the patient or their parent/carer both for emergency and continuing care.
- General practitioner (GP) letter should be given to the patient/carer or posted depending on unit policy.
- Next-day visit from a community nurse or telephone call either from the community team or as an extended role of the hospital-based team.

Social criteria

- Suitable transport home – not public transport.
- Home environment suitable for the patient following the procedure/surgery undertaken, equipment in place prior to time of discharge if possible.
- Parent/carer/support network arrangements made for taking time off work or arranging care of children and even pets to reduce initial stress during recovery period.

Patient education/health promotion

Patients are expected to continue care at home following discharge so they and significant others must understand and remember the health and treatment information provided (Johnson *et al.*, 2003). The patient is expected to continue exercises and progress mobility although timescales will differ for each individual. Other issues include:

- Hip replacement dislocation precautions – avoid bending >90 degrees; avoid adduction (crossing operative leg over midline); avoid internal/external rotation or twisting.
- Knee replacement – elevate the leg and apply ice to knee to relieve swelling. Kneeling can be problematic due to numbness.
- Inform dentist of prosthetic joint as antibiotic cover is required for any procedures lasting >30 minutes due to risk of bacterial infection.
- Metal detectors have varying sensitivity and can alarm, therefore a medic alert card indicating an artificial joint provided by hospital or surgical team.
- Details of implant size and type is provided to National Joint Register with the patient's consent.

There are some significant problems that may arise and require urgent treatment. Patients and carers should be aware of these and the resulting consequences if not reported or acted upon:

- It is common to have a low-grade fever after surgery and it is important to ascertain infective source, ensuring it is not related to the surgery.
- Swelling is normal for the first three to six months after surgery, but severe lower limb pain accompanied by swelling should be reported due to increased risk of DVT.
- Chest pain or shortness of breath are signs of a pulmonary embolism.

Common types of orthopaedic surgery

The decision to undertake surgery may have taken place after many months or years of conservative measures such as physiotherapy and various medications prior to agreeing to elective surgical intervention. Much orthopaedic surgery is conducted for joint arthropathies such as osteoarthritis (Chapter 13) and bone, joint and soft tissue deformities and conditions. While there are many types of orthopaedic surgery the elective orthopaedic procedures discussed in this chapter will focus on the principles of care following surgery and on the most commonly performed procedures: joint replacement surgery and spinal decompression.

Arthroplasty or total joint replacement (TJR)

Arthroplasty refers to the surgical refashioning of a joint. It aims to relieve pain and to retain or restore movement, is considered to be one of the most successful operations in orthopaedic surgery and is well established. Arthroplasty surgery has become available for almost every joint with the hip and knee being the joint most frequently replaced. People are living longer and consequently the incidence of osteoarthritis is increasing. It is a debilitating condition that negatively affects quality of life. The aim of arthroplasty is to resolve pain and disability by removing diseased components of joints and replacing them with dynamically stable material such as metal, plastic or ceramics. Over many years replacement of most joints has become possible, but the most commonly performed surgery is total hip and total knee replacement.

It is anticipated that a hip or knee replacement should last for 10–15 years. National Joint Registries provide a central database for hip, knee, elbow, shoulder and ankle replacements which provide statistics related to patient outcomes and complications in a '... *continuous drive to improve the quality of outcomes and ensure the quality and cost-effectiveness of joint replacement surgery.'* (NJR 2012 p. 15). Annual reports enable sharing of important data and clinical evidence with clinicians, helping surgeons to choose the best implants for their patients as well as understand joint replacement survivorship (how long a device lasts before it needs replacing or modifying).

Different types of arthroplasty include:

- **Excision arthroplasty** – the bone surfaces are removed and the space between them is allowed to fill with fibrous tissues. It is the simplest and sometimes most satisfactory arthroplasty but leaves an unstable joint. An excision arthroplasty of the hip is called a Girdlestone's procedure. It is most often used as a salvage procedure for a failed total hip replacement. The patient's leg will be shorter as a result of this surgery.
- **Replacement hemiarthroplasty** – only one surface of the joint is replaced with an artificial material such as metal. An example is a Thompson's hemiarthroplasty used for some patients with a hip fracture (Chapter 18).
- **Arthroplasty or total joint replacement (TJR)** – usually performed to relieve pain, improve function and reduce the degree of disability for a patient suffering with a degenerative, inflammatory or traumatic condition. TJR is the surgical treatment of choice when conservative treatments are not successful in managing the pain (Schoen 2009). Articular bone ends are replaced by prosthetic implants. Prostheses are made from a variety of materials including:
  - stainless steel
  - chrome/cobalt
  - titanium alloy
  - high density polyethylene.

Prostheses can either be cemented or uncemented into position. In the case of THR, new generations of total hip prostheses are currently being tested including metal-on-metal, ceramic-on-ceramic and metal-on-ceramic in the hope that they have the potential to improve outcomes for longer periods of time, but their efficacy currently remains uncertain (Pivec *et al.*, 2012).

Hip surgery – THR and hip resurfacing

A total hip replacement is the most commonly performed elective orthopaedic procedure. Its primary functions are to treat hip pain and disability caused by diseases such as osteoarthritis or rheumatoid arthritis. It is occasionally performed for patient with a hip fracture (Chapter 18).

THR surgery involves the dislocation of the hip joint so that the femoral head and any damaged cartilage in the acetabulum can be removed. This is achieved through a 20–30 cm surgical incision allowing dissection of soft tissue, muscle and joint capsule. Incisions may be lateral, antero-lateral or posterior. A lateral or antero-lateral approach preserves the posterior part of the joint capsule thus reducing the risk of posterior dislocation of the prosthesis post-operatively. However these approaches necessitate the splitting of the abductor muscles which can lead to an increased incidence of postoperative limp and muscle weakness. A posterior approach weakens the posterior joint capsule with a greater risk of dislocation but the abductor muscles are not split.

Minimally invasive total hip replacement aims to avoid damage to the muscles and tendons around the hip joint. A single or double incision of 10 cm or less in length is made. Division of muscles is less extensive than in standard approaches and specially designed retractors and customised instruments are used. However, longer-term results of surgery using a smaller incision are not yet available and there are concerns about increased prosthesis malpositioning and transient lateral femoral cutaneous nerve palsy due to reduced visibility of the joint during surgery.

Regardless of surgical technique the joint is prepared and the prosthesis inserted in a similar way. After removal of the femoral head the femur is prepared by reaming a hole down its medullary canal so that the femoral component can be fitted; this may be cemented in place or be cementless (press-fit). The acetabular socket is prepared to receive the cup in which the femoral component rotates; this may also be cemented or cementless. The surgeon aims to achieve equal leg length but on occasions there is a leg length discrepancy, either a shorter or longer operated leg, because of the extent of bone loss due to disease or because of the need to ensure a stable joint. Patients should be made aware of this possibility prior to surgery. After insertion of the femoral and acetabular components the hip joint is then put through the full range of movement in order to test for stability before the joint capsule and overlying muscles are sewn up.

The total hip replacement may need revision after 10–15 years due to aseptic loosening of the prosthetic joint and/or cement cracking although for many patients the prosthesis may last much longer. Occasionally a revision is needed earlier due to infection or aseptic loosening of the prosthesis causing pain and discomfort.

Revision surgery is more complex than the primary THR and is usually performed by specialist surgeons. The procedure involves opening the joint, removing the prosthetic components and any bone cement followed by a reconstruction of the joint using new prosthetic components. Bone grafting may be indicated. For an infected prosthesis surgery is conducted in two stages; the first stage is removal of the infected prosthesis and treatment with antibiotics, usually intravenously. Once it has been established that the infection has been eradicated the second stage is carried out: insertion of the new prosthesis.

Hip resurfacing involves the resurfacing of the femoral head with a titanium shell. A long incision, often longer than a traditional THR incision, is required because although the hip is dislocated in order to expose the femoral head, this is not removed but rather smoothed to fit the shell on top so it is not as easy to visualise the acetabulum, which is reamed and fitted with a metal cup. This procedure is used for younger patients with osteoarthritis who may need a THR in the future as it aims to reduce pain, restore function and delay the need for a THR for some years. Hip resurfacing and large-diameter metal-on-metal THR reduce the risk of dislocation because the contact area between the components is greater. They also have less debris due to wear.

There is some emerging evidence that hip resurfacing and metal-on-metal THRs have a higher revision rate than conventional THR and that metallic debris may cause periprosthetic soft tissue reactions leading to prosthesis failure. There are also concerns that the metal debris may cause elevated metal ions systemically leading to metal toxicity and possibly cancer, though the evidence is not conclusive. The fears have led to a decline in the use of metal-on-metal prostheses, especially in women of childbearing years as there some evidence that metal ions can cross the placenta.

Specific post-operative nursing care after THR or hip resurfacing is related to reducing the risk of dislocation, mobilisation and psychological recovery. The prevalence of dislocation varies but is around 4% (Smith *et al.*, 2012). It tends to occur either in the first three months, due to component malposition or abductor deficiency, or many years postoperatively secondary to prosthesis wear. A triangular shaped abduction wedge, often known as a Charnley wedge, is used in some centres to prevent abnormal hip movements for the first few days after surgery. To reduce the risk of dislocation patients are taught:

- not to flex their hip joint more than ninety degrees,
- to avoid excessive adduction of the leg and
- to avoid twisting on the leg when turning.

They are often advised to sleep on their back for the first six weeks and are provided with a raise for their bed and chair as well as a raised toilet seat to prevent hip flexion greater than ninety degrees. There is some evidence to suggest that such precautions may not be necessary and that patients should be allowed more freedom of movement, especially following an anterior or antero-lateral surgical approach (Restrepo *et al.*, 2011).

Within enhanced recovery programmes early mobilisation is encouraged and in some centres the physiotherapists will get the patient out of bed in the recovery room. The point at which a patient is mobilised is tailored to the individual and influenced by additional factors such as spinal anesthesia and pain management modality. The majority of patients are allowed to fully weight bear immediately, although if there is any potential instability a period of 6–12 weeks non- or partial-weight bearing may be ordered. Patients initially mobilise with a walking frame or sticks for up to six weeks, although in some centres patients may stop using them earlier. Physiotherapy is rarely needed after discharge from acute care but postoperative exercises should be performed by patients up to three times per day for at least six weeks.

THR surgery is a major life event and preoperative education should have prepared patients for the extended recovery period, which may be 3–6 months. This may need reinforcing after surgery as patients experience the reality of initial restricted mobility and discomfort from the surgery.

Total knee replacement (TKR) surgery

The most common indication for a total knee replacement is osteoarthritis of the knee joint. The most commonly used incision is midline with a medial parapatellar approach, with the patella and extensor mechanism everted to gain access to the joint. The mini-incision total knee replacement involves an incision 10 to 12 cm long over the knee, compared with the conventional total knee replacement which requires an incision 20 to 30 cm long. The same prostheses are inserted using specially designed instruments (NICE, 2010). The tibial plateaux and the distal femoral joint surfaces are resected and holes are then drilled in the bones so that the prostheses can be inserted. The tibial joint surface is replaced by a polyethylene bearing, usually attached to a metal base prosthesis and the distal femur with a metal prosthesis. Any arthritis on the patella surface may be removed and a plastic component, like a button, inserted although this is not always performed. The patella is then flipped back into position and the incision closed. As with THR, aseptic loosening of the knee prosthesis may require revision surgery after 10–15 years, or earlier due to infection.

For some individuals only part of the knee may be affected by arthritis and a partial or unicompartmental knee replacement may be indicated. This can be performed for younger patients who do not wish to undergo a more invasive TKR. However there is a risk that the patient may develop arthritic changes in the remaining aspects of the knee requiring a conversion to a total knee replacement. Unicondylar knee replacements were around five times more likely to be revised for pain than were cemented total knee replacements (NJR, 2012). Another reason for revision of unicondylar knee replacements is loosening of the prosthesis.

After TKR or unicondylar knee replacement it is important that the knee joint is mobilised so that flexion and extension can be maximised. For the majority of patients this can be achieved with exercises supervised by physiotherapy and nursing staff but for others a continuous passive movement (CPM) machine may be used. The leg is secured to the CPM machine on the bed which slowly flexes and extends the knee joint. The evidence suggests that there is little advantage in the medium or long term of using a CPM machine for the majority of patients and that its use should be restricted to patients with poor preoperative knee movement who may find it difficult to flex and extend the knee post-operatively.

Patients can normally fully weight bear immediately after surgery unless there is any instability in the joint, which may necessitate a period of partial weight bearing and/or the wearing of a removable splint. The use of crutches or a stick for the first 4–6 weeks may be helpful in providing support, although not all centres advocate this. Optimum recovery may take up to 12 months but at that stage 10–15% of patients are not satisfied with the results of surgery, often because of unrealistic expectations such as being able to kneel on the prosthesis.

Shoulder arthroplasty

A shoulder replacement is indicated for patients with a painful shoulder and destruction of the glenohumeral joint. Glenohumeral arthroplasty is performed for degenerative joint disease such as rheumatoid arthritis or other inflammatory arthropathy, osteoarthritis or fractures of the proximal humerus. Other reasons may be due to avascular necrosis of the humeral head, mal- or non-union of a proximal humeral fracture and chronic deficiency of the rotator cuff (Lucas 2005). The procedure can be successful at reducing the pain from arthritis, but due to the complexity of the shoulder joint, function and mobility are not as successful as with a THR or TKR at this time.

There are different types of shoulder replacement surgery. A total shoulder replacement (TSR) involves replacing the arthritic joint surfaces with a humeral component consisting of a metal ball with a stem fixed into the humerus and a plastic glenoid component. The humeral component may be cemented or uncemented; the glenoid component is generally cemented. A shoulder hemiarthroplasty consists of a stemmed humeral component articulating on the natural glenoid cavity and is suitable for patients with a healthy glenoid cavity. Surface replacement arthroplasty in the form of a small metal cap placed over the humeral head is gaining popularity as it is less invasive and can be used for patients with earlier stages of shoulder joint degeneration. The aim of shoulder resurfacing arthroplasty is to replace only the damaged joint surfaces, with minimal bone resection. A reverse TSR is used for patients who have a torn rotator cuff, severe arthritis and a torn rotator cuff or a previous failed TSR. The metal ball is attached to the glenoid cavity and the plastic socket to the humerus. This allows the patient to move the arm using the deltoid muscle rather than the torn rotator cuff. This is a relatively new type of procedure and long-term results are not therefore available. In the short term there are higher complication rates than a conventional TSR due to loosening and dislocation.

For these types of surgery a deltopectoral or anterosuperior surgical approach is used. The deltoid muscle is split to expose the shoulder joint. Depending on the exact nature of the surgery the glenoid and humerus are prepared, which may involve a hole being drilled in the bone. Post-operatively there is a risk of dislocation as the shoulder joint is shallow and the articulating surfaces do not fit as closely as in the hip joint. It remains important to maintain the mobility of the joint so exercises are usually started the day after surgery. Initially these are passive – the physiotherapist, nurse or patient (using their other hand) move the joint gently through its range of movement and the patient bends forward and allows the arm to dangle down and swing at ninety degrees without any local muscle activity. Functional hand use at table height is also usually allowed. Patients would normally wear a sling to support the arm between periods of exercise. After approximately six weeks more active exercises can be introduced to strengthen the muscles surrounding the prosthesis.

Spinal surgery

Musculoskeletal injuries and conditions affecting the spine are amongst the most debilitating of all health care events (Smith 2005). Many spinal conditions can progress to requiring surgical intervention. Spinal stenosis may result in spinal decompression being indicated and intervertebral disc disease may lead to a spinal decompression.

Spinal decompression

There are different techniques used to perform spinal decompression. The goal is to ensure a careful freeing of the affected nerves by removal of bone, disc and facet capsule causing the narrowing of the canal. Options include (Smith 2005):

- discectomy: for a herniated disc
- laminotomy: to open up more space posteriorly in the spinal canal by partial removal of the posterior part of the vertebral bone
- laminectomy: removal of posterior part of vertebral bone
- foraminotomy: widening of the opening where the nerve roots leave the spinal canal
- spinal fusion: fusing of adjacent vertebra using bone grafting or screws/rods/plates. Often necessary when multi-level laminectomy is carried out in order to provide spinal stability.

Following a spinal decompression, Smith (2005) recommends the patient may be nursed in a flat position with one pillow under the head and neck unless otherwise indicated by the medical team. An alternative position is to lie on their side, with knees bent and a pillow between the legs. A pillow may also be placed under the knees for support when sleeping supine. The patient should however avoid sleeping in the prone position (Smith 2005). The patient will be assessed pre-operatively for the risk of venous thromboembolism and appropriate actions must be implemented to minimise the risk post–operatively (NICE 2010). Nursing actions may include the measuring and fitting of thromboembolitic deterrent stockings (TEDS) for the patient, ensuring an adequate fluid intake, foot, ankle and breathing exercises along with early mobilisation. The medical team will consider the pharmacological anticoagulation medication required.

Analgesia will be prescribed and administered regularly following an individual patient pain assessment and the pain management must be reviewed with the patient and the medical team regularly (Smith and Roberts 2011). Patients are mobilised once the effects of the anaesthetic have disappeared and the patient has been assessed as able to mobilise with support from the healthcare team initially. Pressure ulcer assessment and prevention is ongoing to reduce any untoward pressure ulcers from forming (NICE 2005). When getting up from the bed, the patient should turn to the side, using their arms to push up while the legs should swing over the side of the bed. Any movements that will twist the neck or lower spine should be avoided (Smith 2005).

Fluids and diet will be encouraged once the patient feels able to tolerate them. Following any surgery to the body, nourishment is required to aid the healing of the surgical wound. The wound usually has a simple post-operative dressing and must be checked regularly for any leakage. The patient's fluid input and output must be monitored closely and documented. Attention to the patient's bowel action following surgery is also required. Alongside this all vital signs will be undertaken, documented and any abnormalities must be reported promptly to senior nursing and/or medical staff (Smith and Roberts 2011). Neurovascular observations of the limbs is undertaken and documented (Judge 2007, Department of Health 2010, NMC 2011).

Depending on the complexity of the surgery, the patient may be well enough to leave hospital 1–10 days later. The patient will need to avoid strenuous activities for around six weeks. Most people can return to work after this time (NHS Choices 2013).

Summary

Elective orthopaedic surgery encompasses a range of procedures from day case surgery such as knee arthroscopy to joint replacements requiring in-patient stay. However the principles of care remain the same. Patients benefit from surgery if they are involved in the decision to operate and are fully prepared for what will happen to them along the patient pathway. Orthopaedic nurses can play a key role in ensuring systems are in place, such as Joint Schools, to allow this preparation to occur. Fitness for surgery and anaesthesia also needs to be established and can be achieved through nurse-led preoperative assessment. Orthopaedic theatre staff require skills and knowledge not only in perioperative nursing but also in orthopaedic care if they are to play a full part in maximising the benefits of surgery for the patient. Key orthopaedic principles such as correct moving and handling and early detection of potential complications such as peripheral neurovascular deficit are vital skills for theatre staff. In the recovery phase of elective orthopaedic surgery patients require skilled care from orthopaedic nurses who are knowledgeable about the normal recovery pathway and can act if any abnormalities occur.

Recommended further reading

Kehlet, H. (2011) Fast-track surgery: an update on physiological care principles to enhanced recovery. *Langenbecks Archives of Surgery*, **396**, 585–590.

National Institute for Clinical Excellence (NICE) (2014) *Total Hip Replacement and Resurfacing Arthroplasty for End-stage Arthritis of the Hip* (review of Technology Appraisal Guidance 2 and 44) G304. NICE, London.

Pivec, R., Johnson, A.J., Mears, S.C. and Mont, M.A. (2012) Hip arthroplasty. *The Lancet*, **380**(9855), 1768–1777.

Royal College of Nursing (2013) *Right blood, right patient, right time: RCN guidance for improving transfusion practice*. RCN, London. Available at: http://www.rcn.org.uk/__data/assets/pdf_file/0009/78615/002306.pdf. (accessed 17 April 2014)

Wainwright, T. and Middleton, R. (2010) An orthopaedic enhanced recovery pathway. *Current Anaesthesia and Critical Care*, **21**(3), 114–120.

References

AbdelSalam, H., Restrepo, C., Tarity, T.D., Sangster, W. and Parvizi, J. (2012) Predictors of intensive care unit admission after total joint arthroplasty. *The Journal of Arthroplasty*, **27** (5), 720–725.

Bergman,M., Stenudd, M. and Engström, A. (2012) The experience of being awake during orthopaedic surgery under regional anaesthesia. *International Journal of Orthopaedic and Trauma Nursing*, **16**(2), 88–96.

Carless, P.A., Henry, D.A., Moxey, A.J. *et al.* (2010) Cell salvage for minimising perioperative allogeneic blood transfusion. *Cochrane Database of Systematic Reviews* **4**(Art. No.: CD001888). DOI: 10.1002/14651858.CD001888.pub4.

Cohn, E. and Larson, E. (2007) Improving participant comprehension in the informed consent process. *Journal of Nursing Scholarship*, **39**(3), 273–280.

Department of Health (DoH) (2010) *Essence of Care*. DoH, London.

Department of Health (2011) *Enhanced Recovery Partnership Programme*. DoH, London.

Department of Health (2012) *Liberating the NHS: No Decision About Me, Without Me*. DoH, London. www.dh.gov.uk (gateway 16942).

Driver, A., Lewis, W., Haward-Sampson, P. and Dashfield, E. (2012) How enhanced recovery can boost patient outcomes. *Nursing Times*, **108**(16), 18–20.

Dutta, A.K. (2011) Positioning in upper-extremity surgery. *Operative Techniques in Sports Medicine*, **19**(4), 231–237.

Fung, C.H., Lim, Y.W., Mattke, S., Damberg, C. and Shekelle, P.G. (2008) Systematic review: the evidence that publishing patient care performance data improves quality of care. *Annals of Internal Medicine*, **148**, 111–123.

Hatfield, A. and Tronson, M. (2009) *The Complete Recovery Room Book*. Oxford University Press, Oxford.

Haynes, A.B., Weiser, T.G., Berry, W.R. *et al.* (2009) A surgical safety checklist to reduce morbidity and mortality in a global population. *The New England Journal of Medicine*, **360**(5), 491–499.

Henry, D.A., Carless, P.A., Moxey, A.J. *et al.* (2001) Preoperative autologous donation for minimising perioperative allogeneic blood transfusion. *Cochrane Database of Systematic Reviews* **4** (Art. No.: CD003602). DOI: 10.1002/14651858.CD003602.

Joanna Briggs Institute (JBI) (2010a) *Preoperative Care: Management*, Evidence Summaries. Available at:http://search.proquest.com/docview/921766970?accountid=26447 (accessed 11 August 2013).

Joanna Briggs Institute (JBI) (2010b) *Day Surgery (Adults): Premedication for Anxiety* Evidence Summaries. Available at:http://search.proquest.com/docview/921809269?accountid=26447 (accessed 11 August 2013).

Joanna Briggs Institute (JBI) (2010c) *Blood Transfusion: Auto-Transfusion*, Evidence Summaries. Available at:http://search.proquest.com/docview/921809237?accountid=26447 (accessed 11 August 2013).

Joanna Briggs Institute (JBI) (2011a) *Preoperative Skin Preparation: Hair Removal*, Evidence Summaries. Available at:http://search.proquest.com/docview/922251316?accountid=26447 (accessed 11 August 2013).

Joanna Briggs Institute (JBI) (2011b) *Surgical Wound Infections (Postoperative): Preoperative Skin Antiseptics*. Evidence Summaries. Available at:http://search.proquest.com/docview/921817168?accountid=26447 (accessed 11 August 2013).

Johnson, A., Sandford, J. and Tyndall, J. (2003) Written and verbal information versus verbal information only for patients being discharged from acute hospital settings to home. *Cochrane Database of Systematic Reviews* **4**(Art. No.: CD003716). DOI: 10.1002/14651858.CD003716.

Jones, A., Arshad, H. and Nolan, J. (2012) Surgical care practitioner practice: one team's journey explored. *Journal of Perioperative Practice*, **22**(1), 19–23.

Judge, N. (2007) Neurovascular assessment. *Nursing Standard*, **21**(45), 39–44. Available at: http://www.snjourney.com/ClinicalInfo/Systems/PDF/NeuroVas%20Assessment.pdf (accessed 18 November 2013).

Kearney, M., Jennrich, M. K., Lyons, S., Robinson, R. and Berger, B. (2011) Effects of preoperative education on patients outcomes after joint replacement surgery. *Orthopaedic Nursing*, **30**(6), 391–396.

Khoyratty, S., Modi, B.N. and Ravichandran, D. (2010) Preoperative starvation in elective general surgery. *Journal of Perioperative Practice*, **20**(3), 100–102.

Lucas, B. (2005) Care of patients with upper limb injuries and conditions, in *Orthopaedic and Trauma Nursing* (eds J. Kneale and P. Davis) (2005). Churchill Livingstone, London, Chapter 21.

Lucas, B. (2008) Total hip and total knee replacement: preoperative nursing management. *British Journal of Nursing*, **17**(21), 1346–1351.

Mitchell, L., Flin, R., Yule, S. *et al.* (2011) Thinking ahead of the patient. *International Journal of Nursing Studies*, **48**(7), 818–828.

Murray, M.M. (2011) Reflections on the development of nurse-led back pain triage clinics in the UK. *International Journal of Orthopaedic and Trauma Nursing*, **15**(3), 113–120.

National Joint Registry for England and Wales (NJR) (2012) *9th Annual Report 2012*. Available at: www.njrcentre.org.uk (accessed 5 October 2012).

NHS Choices (2013) *Lumbar Decompression Surgery*. Available at: http://www.nhs.uk/conditions/Lumbardecompressivesurgery/Pages/Whatisitpage.aspx (accessed 18 November 2013).

National Institute for Clinical Excellence (NICE) (2003) *Preoperative Tests. The Use of Routine Preoperative Tests for Elective Surgery*. NICE, London. Available at: http://www.nice.org.uk/nicemedia/pdf/preop_fullguideline.pdf (accessed 18 November 2013).

NICE (2005) Pressure Ulcers- prevention and treatment. Available at: http://www.nice.org.uk/nicemedia/live/10972/29887/29887.pdf (accessed 18 November 2013).

NICE (2007) *Competencies for Recognising and Responding to Acutely Ill Patients in Hospital*. NICE, London. Available at: http://www.nice.org.uk/nicemedia/live/11810/58247/58247.pdf (accessed 18 November 2013).

NICE (2008) *Surgical Site Infection Prevention and Treatment of Surgical Site Infection*. NICE, London. Available at:http://www.nice.org.uk/nicemedia/live/11743/42379/42379.pdf (accessed 1 May 2014).

NICE (2010) *Reducing the Risk of Venous Thromboembolism (Deep Vein Thrombosis and Pulmonary Embolism) in Patients Admitted to Hospital*. Available at: http://guidance.nice.org.uk/CG92 (accessed 18 November 2013).

NICE (2010) *Mini-incision Surgery for Total Knee Replacement*. NICE, London.

Nursing and Midwifery Council (NMC) (2011) *Record Keeping Guidance for Nurses and Midwives*. NMC, London. Available at: http://www.nmc-uk.org/Documents/NMC-Publications/NMC-Record-Keeping-Guidance.pdf (accessed 8 November 2013).

O'Neill, T., Jinks, C. and Ong, B.N. (2007) Decision-making regarding total knee replacement surgery: a qualitative meta-synthesis. *BMC Health Services Research*, **7**, 52. DOI:10.1186/1472-6963-7-52. Available at: http://www.biomedcentral.com/1472-6963/7/52 (accessed 17 April 2014)

Pivec, R., Johnson, A.J., Mears, S.C. and Mont, M.A. (2012) Hip arthroplasty. *The Lancet*, **380**(9855), 1768–1777.

Restrepo, C., Mortazavi, S.M., Brothers, J., Parvizi, J., and Rothman, R.H. (2011) Hip dislocation: are hip precautions necessary in anterior approaches. *Clinical Orthopaedics and Related Research*, **469**(2), 417–422.

Royal College of Anaesthetists (2008) *Anaesthetic Choices for Hip or Knee Replacement*. Royal College of Anaesthetists, London.

Royal College of Nursing (RCN) (2013) *Day Surgery Information: Discharge Planning*. Sheet 4. RCN, London. Available at: http://www.rcn.org.uk/__data/assets/pdf_file/0011/78509/004_465.pdf (accessed 22 April 2014).

Schoen, D. (2009) Hip and knee arthroplasties. *Orthopaedic Nursing*, **28**(6), 323–327.

Sepah, Y.J., Umer, M., Ahmad, T. *et al.* (2011) Use of tranexamic acid is a cost effective method in preventing blood loss during and after total knee replacement. *Journal of Orthopaedic Surgery and Research*, **6**, 22.

Shepperd, S., McClaran, J., Phillips, C.O. *et al.* (2010) Discharge planning from hospital to home. *Cochrane Database of Systematic Reviews* **1**. See update 2013, **1** (Art. No.: CD000313). DOI: 10.1002/14651858.CD000313.pub4

Slover, J., Shue, J. and Koenig, K. (2012) Shared decision-making in orthopaedic surgery. *Clinical Orthopaedics and Related Research*, **470**(4), 1046–1053.

Smith, A.F. and Pittaway, A.J. (2002) Premedication for anxiety in adult day surgery. *Cochrane Database of Systematic Reviews* **3**.

See update Walker KJ, Smith AF. Premedication for anxiety in adult day surgery. *Cochrane Database of Systematic Reviews* 2009, **4**(Art. No.: CD002192). DOI: 10.1002/14651858. CD002192.pub2.

Smith, J. and Roberts, R. (2011) *Vital Signs for Nurses. An introduction to Clinical Observations.* Wiley Blackwell, Chichester.

Smith, A.J., Dieppe, P., Vernon, K., Porter, M. and Blom, A.W. (2012) Failure rates of stemmed mental-on-metal hip replacements: analysis of data from the National Joint Registry of England and Wales. *The Lancet*, **379**(9822), 1199–1204.

Smith, M. (2005) Care of patients with spinal conditions and injuries, in *Orthopaedic and Trauma Nursing* (eds J. Kneale and P. Davis), Churchill Livingstone, London, Chapter 18.

Stern, C. and Lockwood, C. (2005) Knowledge retention from preoperative patient information. *International Journal of Evidence-Based Health Care* **3**(3): 45–63.

Tanner, J., Woodings, D. and Moncaster, K. (2006) Preoperative hair removal to reduce surgical site infection. *Cochrane Database of Systematic Reviews* **2**. See update Tanner J, Norrie P, Melen K. Preoperative hair removal to reduce surgical site infection. *Cochrane Database of Systematic Reviews* 2011, **11** (Art. No.: CD004122). DOI: 10.1002/14651858.CD004122. pub4.

Webster, J. and Osborne, S. (2007) Preoperative bathing or showering with skin antiseptics to prevent surgical site infection. *Cochrane Database of Systematic Reviews* **2**. See update Webster J, Osborne S. Preoperative bathing or showering with skin antiseptics to prevent surgical site infection. Cochrane Database of Systematic Reviews 2012, **9**(Art. No.: CD004985). DOI: 10.1002/14651858.CD004985. pub4.

Wing Wai, C.L. and Irwin, M.G. (2012). Regional blocks in orthopaedics. *Anaesthesia and Intensive Care Medicine*, **13**(3), 89–93.

Woodhead, K. and Wicker, P. (2005) *A Textbook of Perioperative Care.* Elsevier, Edinburgh.

CHAPTER 15
Musculoskeletal oncology over the lifespan

Helen Stradling
Nuffield Orthopaedic Centre, Oxford, UK

Introduction

Sarcoma is a rare form of cancer which affects all age groups and all parts of the body. There are approximately 3200 new diagnoses in the United Kingdom (UK) each year (Sarcoma UK 2012). It affects connective tissue of the body including bone, muscle, nerve, fat and blood vessel cells. A sarcoma is often described as either 'bone' or 'soft tissue' as although it usually affects bone it can also be found extra-skeletally. Conversely sarcoma that primarily affects soft tissue can also be found in bone. Sarcoma is a primary cancer which originates from one of the cells of connective tissue. Bone cancer can also be metastatic in instances where a primary cancer, for example lung or breast, has spread to the bone. This is treated very differently to sarcoma and so practitioners need to be aware of the differences.

Bone sarcoma is more prevalent in younger age groups whereas soft tissue sarcoma is more likely in older age, although this does not make either exclusive to these age groups and there is currently no definitive evidence to show any reason for this. Sarcoma has a slightly higher incidence in males than females but the reason for this is also unclear. The importance of a prompt diagnosis cannot be overstated as this has a direct effect on prognosis, especially if the delay leads to the patient presenting with metastatic disease. The signs and symptoms of sarcoma can be as simple as a non-painful soft tissue swelling or as severe as a pathological fracture of bone. Figure 15.1 shows a soft tissue sarcoma of the upper arm. Figure 15.2 shows a pathological fracture of the distal femur.

Patients do not tend to become systemically unwell with sarcoma at an early stage and this can be a deterrent to diagnosis as a painful limb could have many differential diagnoses, of which sarcoma does not rank highly in the minds of many practitioners. It is suggested that a general practitioner (GP) will only encounter an average of one sarcoma diagnosis in their career. It is important for practitioners to not only be aware of sarcoma, but to have a knowledge base that will support them well when coming into contact with these patients and their families. Due to the rare nature of this cancer type is it unlikely that a person newly diagnosed with sarcoma would have heard of it before, or know of someone who has been given the diagnosis previously. This can make the diagnosis even more daunting than a diagnosis of a more common cancer type. For them to be cared for by a practitioner who is also unaware of the implications of their diagnosis and treatment can lead to a very disjointed, misinformed care pathway in which the patient and family feel unsupported.

The majority of sarcoma will be treated surgically in an orthopaedic setting but, due to the fact that sarcoma can be diagnosed in any anatomical site, practitioners could come into contact with sarcoma in any setting. It is therefore of paramount importance for sarcoma education to be included in orthopaedic as well as oncology texts.

Bone sarcoma

Bone sarcoma occurs in the younger age group under the age of 30 years. There is one type of bone cancer, chondrosarcoma, that originates from cartilage cells that has greater prevalence in the older age range of 50 years plus. The two most common types of bone sarcoma in the younger population are Ewing's sarcoma and osteosarcoma. Bone sarcoma can occur in any skeletal bone but remains more prevalent in the long bones of the limbs

Orthopaedic and Trauma Nursing: An Evidence-based Approach to Musculoskeletal Care, First Edition. Edited by Sonya Clarke and Julie Santy-Tomlinson.

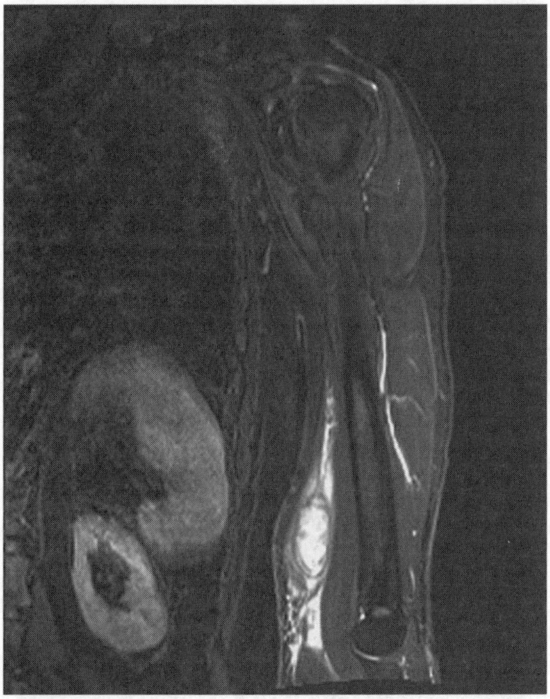

Figure 15.1 MRI scan showing soft tissue sarcoma of the upper arm

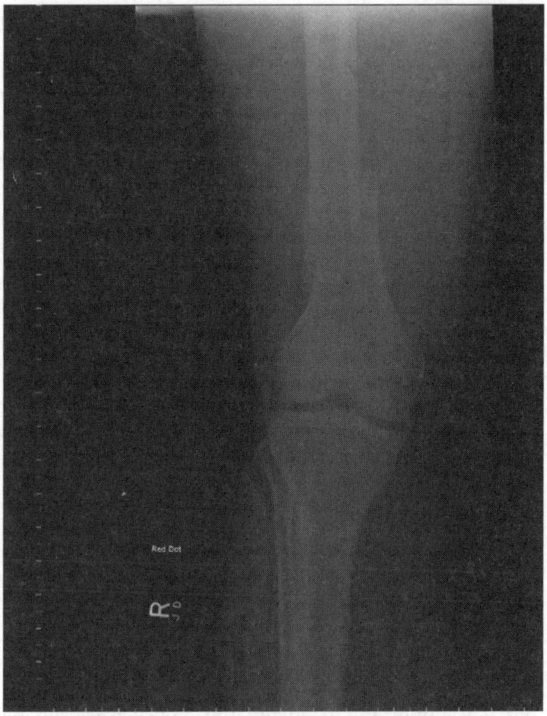

Figure 15.2 X-ray showing pathological fracture of the distal femur

and the pelvis. They often occur around joints which may be a reason for them being misdiagnosed as the differential diagnoses can be seen as a more likely diagnosis.

Signs and symptoms

The most common symptom of bone sarcoma is pain in the affected area. This pain can be more of an issue at night and can wake a person from their sleep due to its intensity. In some cases the bone tumour can break through the cortex of the bone involved and invade soft tissue, resulting in a noticeable soft tissue mass unlike tumors that are contained within bone. Bone tumours can also weaken bone and this can lead to the first symptom presenting as a pathological fracture. Although pathological fractures are associated with older patients, they can occur in patients of all ages with bone tumors. Although the majority of patients with a primary bone sarcoma do not feel systemically unwell, patients with Ewing's sarcoma can suffer from fever and a general malaise.

Diagnosis

Bone sarcoma cannot always be detected on X-ray and therefore the need for further investigation where bone pain cannot be explained is very important. Diagnosis of bone sarcoma should never be given without a proven histological diagnosis. This ensures the type of sarcoma is established and the correct treatment regimen is administered from the outset. It is vital that the diagnosis is made correctly in the first instance to reduce delays in treatment and therefore to improve outcomes. Any patient with a suspected bone sarcoma should be referred to a specialist centre. Specialist centres ensure that patients are cared for by clinicians and specialist staff who regularly care for patients and families with this rare group of cancers. Any lesion that is suspicious of a primary malignant bone tumour should have a biopsy in a specialist centre (Hogendoorn *et al.*, 2010). The biopsy can be undertaken in a number of ways: either under image guidance, be it ultrasound, fluoroscopy or computed tomography (CT), or as an open procedure in the operating theatre (the preferred option for children). The decision relating to how the biopsy should be performed will be discussed within the specialist multidisciplinary team (MDT) and will depend on the size, location and histological subtype of the

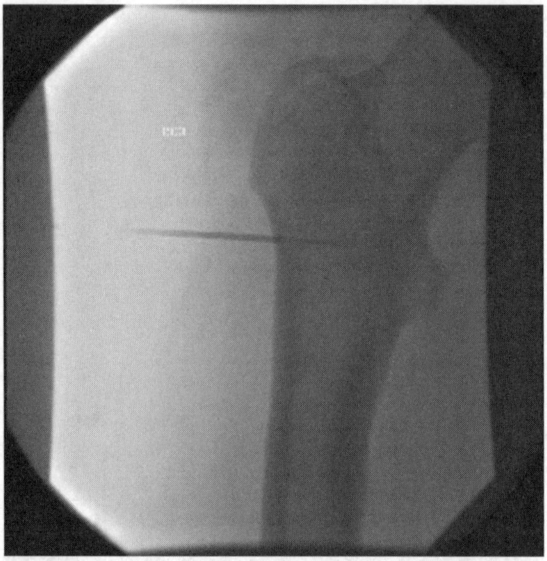

Figure 15.3 Fluoroscopic guided biopsy of a chondrosarcoma of the distal humerus

tumour. Biopsies need to be undertaken by specialists and it is important to ensure the biopsy tract can be removed as part of the plan. Caution is needed for patients who are taking anticoagulation therapy as this may lead to a delay in the biopsy whilst the medication is temporarily withdrawn in order for clotting assessment to be made. Figure 15.3 shows a fluoroscopic guided biopsy of a chondrosarcoma of the right femur.

Impact of delayed diagnosis

Delays in diagnosis of bone sarcoma are common in all parts of the pathway mainly due to lack of awareness of the potential for a malignant diagnosis (Grimer *et al.*, 2010). The longer a patient has to wait for a diagnosis, especially with high-grade bone sarcoma, the more likely it will be that they may have metastases at diagnosis. This is a factor in a poorer prognosis and it is therefore vital to gain a diagnosis and commence treatment as soon as possible. See Box 15.1 for discussion of evidence underpinning early diagnosis.

Staging

Staging of sarcoma should be undertaken once a definite diagnosis has been given. Staging should include a CT scan or, more commonly, a PET scan; these give the treating clinician information relating to whether metastatic disease is present. This is important when deciding on the treatment plan for patients; for example, it would be less likely for a surgeon to offer an amputation as a surgical option if the patient already has lung metastases.

Box 15.1 Evidence digest. Reproduced with permission from The Royal College of Surgeons of England

Study of sarcoma size at presentation (Grimer 2006)

This study looked at a total of 1460 patients who had been diagnosed with sarcoma and who had received three years of post-operative follow-up. The patients had been cared for at one hospital and the aim of the study was to look at whether the size of sarcoma at presentation had a bearing on the patient's outcome. The NICE (2005) guidelines for sarcoma state that any patient with a soft tissue mass of over 5 cm should be referred to a sarcoma specialist and presumed to be a sarcoma until proven otherwise. The study took the size of sarcoma at time of diagnosis and this information was gained from the medical notes of all the patients. It showed that the mean size of soft tissue sarcoma at presentation was 10 cm which is double the recommended size for referral. Bone sarcoma had an average of 11.3 cm and there seemed to be little difference with changes in patient age or type of sarcoma diagnosis. The detection of metastatic disease at presentation had a direct link to the size of sarcoma at diagnosis. The prognosis for all patients without metastatic disease worsened with the increase in size of tumour. The outcome of the study was to increase the awareness of sarcoma to try to reduce the size of these tumours at diagnosis. The hope is that with smaller tumours being diagnosed the patient's overall outcomes and prognoses will improve.

Treatments

The treatment for a sarcoma will depend on the histological diagnosis of each lesion. Treatments including surgery, chemotherapy and radiotherapy are options that will be determined by the results of histology. Some patients receive surgery alone, where others may need to have a combination of surgery, chemotherapy and radiotherapy.

Surgery can vary considerably for both bone and soft tissue sarcoma removal. For soft tissue sarcoma it can be as simple as wide local excision of the lesion or there could be extensive excision of the tumour and surrounding soft tissue that necessitates subsequent plastic surgery reconstruction. For bone sarcoma, the surgery can be as straightforward as an excision of a bone tumour with no reconstruction needed, to surgery including amputation of a limb or limb lengthening using external fixation and bone transport (Chapter 8). Surgery for bone sarcoma of a limb now focuses much more upon limb salvage, whereas in the past amputation would have been the preferred surgical option. Limb salvage is the preferred choice due to the advances in limb salvage surgery. This includes the improvement of the type of prostheses that are available to be used and also the new techniques available to orthopaedic surgeons, for example bone transport. Orthopaedic nurses are therefore very involved in the surgical care of bone sarcoma patients. Children now have the option of a non-invasive growing prosthesis which enables lengthening of the prosthesis as a day case non-operative procedure rather than having to undergo a number of operations to extend the prosthesis which was the previous method. Patients with chondroma of the sacrum may require a total sacrectomy, this can be very invasive surgery which can lead to the loss of nerves, potentially leaving the patient incontinent and in need of stoma reconstruction. Surgery with a curative intent aims to be much more radical than surgery for a palliative intent. The surgery for sarcoma should be discussed with the patient who should be supported by the multidisciplinary team.

Radiotherapy for primary bone sarcoma is usually undertaken on a daily basis, Monday–Friday for a period of up to six weeks.

Chemotherapy for primary bone sarcoma will also depend on the histological diagnosis, but can be given in the day care setting or as an inpatient for up to four to five days depending on the treatment regimen. This means that the length of treatment for primary bone sarcoma can last as long as nine to 12 months. This is a factor that needs to be taken into account when the patients are often of an age where they are at school, attending university or in the early stages of employment. A number of the chemotherapy agents used to treat bone sarcoma can cause infertility. This is an issue for teenagers and young adults and needs to be discussed in detail with them. Patients with issues relating to fertility should be counselled suitably and referred to fertility centres when appropriate. The type of chemotherapy used is extremely toxic and the team need to ensure that patients are fit enough to tolerate it. Many centres do not offer the high dose chemotherapy to patients over the age of 40. Due to the toxic nature of the treatments used, patients over the age of 40 will have the option of high dose chemotherapy discussed with them on an individual basis. From experience many people over the age of 40 who do start high dose chemotherapy are unable to finish the course of treatment due to the high incidence of side effects which become intolerable for them

The types of treatments used will be discussed in more detail with each subtype of sarcoma and also in the evidence digest. The most common types of bone sarcoma will now be further explored. See Box 15.2 for a discussion of clinical practice guidelines.

Box 15.2 Evidence digest. Reproduced with permission from OUP

Clinical practice guidelines: Bone sarcomas: ESMO Clinical Practice Guidelines for diagnosis, treatment and follow-up (Hogendoorn 2010).

Soft Tissue Sarcomas: ESMO Clinical guidelines for Diagnosis, treatment and follow-up (Casali *et al.*, 2008).

A number of leading specialists have worked together to produce European guidelines for the diagnosis, treatment and follow-up of these tumours.

The guidelines clearly define the pathway for which any patients with suspected sarcoma should follow, this includes:

- referral to a specialist sarcoma service
- biopsy to ONLY be undertaken by a member of the specialist sarcoma MDT
- treatment plans to be discussed by the sarcoma MDT and decided on an individual basis
- follow-up to include regular scanning for disease recurrence and metastatic disease.

These guidelines are intended to ensure the early diagnosis and correct treatment for sarcoma patients. It is, however, identified that all patients should be taken on an individual basis when it comes to treatment planning, taking into account size, grade and location of tumour, along with age and co-morbidities of the patient and the presence or not of metastatic disease.

Osteosarcoma

Osteosarcoma is a disease which is still not fully understood. It was first described in 1805 by French surgeon Alexis Boyer who found that these lesions were a very different type of disease to other bone lesions (Peltier

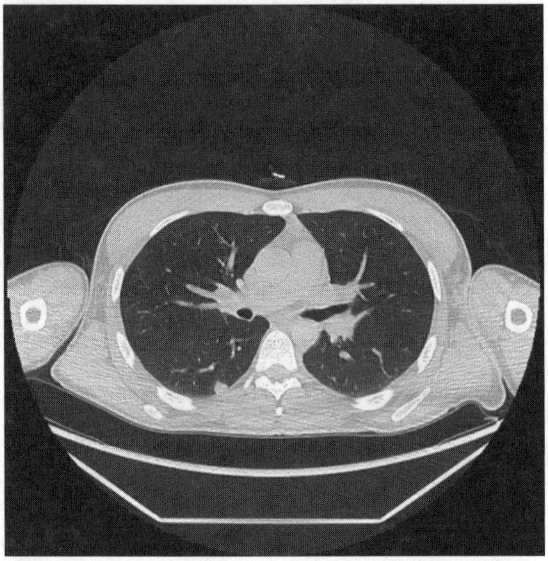

Figure 15.4 CT scan of the chest showing metastatic osteosarcoma

1993). Osteosarcoma is the most common type of bone sarcoma and in the UK, for example, it accounts for approximately 131 new diagnoses each year (NCIN 2012). Osteosarcoma has its highest incidence between the ages of five and 20 years. It is very uncommon in the under fives, although not unreported, and increases in incidence with age throughout the teenage years. It has a higher incidence in males than females although there is no apparent reason for this.

Osteosarcoma becomes a life threatening condition once metastatic disease is present. Once a diagnosis of osteosarcoma has been made the need for staging scans, usually CT scan of the chest or PET CT, is of paramount importance. Metastatic disease can be undetectable very early on in the disease process but it is reported that approximately 80% of patients with a high-grade osteosarcoma diagnosis will present with metastatic disease (Kim and Helman 2010). Figure 15.4 shows metastatic chest disease of a 32-year-old osteosarcoma patient.

Treatment for osteosarcoma depends, as with all sarcomas, on the histological subtype. A low-grade parosteal osteosarcoma can be treated with surgery alone to remove the tumour. A high grade osteosarcoma of bone is treated with a combination of chemotherapy and surgery. The chemotherapy is given neo-adjuvantly and again adjuvantly depending on response rate. The chemotherapy regime used most often is MAP chemotherapy, a combination of doxorubicin, cisplatin and methotrexate. Although there is still no worldwide census on the best chemotherapy regimens for osteosarcoma, a review by Anninga *et al.* (2011) shows that drug regimens using three drugs, such as MAP, are the most effective. This chapter does not expand upon MAP as this is an orthopaedic text and it is hoped to focus the nurse on the orthopaedic treatments for these patients. Links for the chemotherapy treatments are however included for further reading.

When caring for patients in the orthopaedic setting who have received chemotherapy as part of their treatment it is important to be aware of the side effects which may affect their health. Surgery is usually planned in the 'window' between chemotherapy cycles to take advantage of reduced risk from the side effects. Neutropenic sepsis is the most important side effect to be considered and is due to cytotoxic chemotherapy agents causing myelosuppression and immunosuppression. If neutropenic sepsis occurs it can be life threatening and all cancer centres have guidelines for practitioners to follow when this is suspected. Patients require intravenous antibiotics within a certain timescale and this has been described as 'door to needle in 60 minutes'. Signs to look for are:

- temperature of >38 °C
- flu-like symptoms
- dehydration.

If these occur an urgent blood test is required to assess the patient's neutrophil count. An absolute neutrophil count (ANC) of <1.0 × 109/L is diagnostic of neutropenia.

Nausea and vomiting are side effects of chemotherapy which can often be avoided with the use of anti-emetic agents. Unfortunately hair loss is a side effect which cannot be avoided in most cases as the drugs affect rapidly dividing cells such as the hair.

In 2011 NICE licensed the use of mifamutide (Mepact) in the treatment of patients with fully resected, non-metastatic osteosarcoma between the ages of two and 30 years. Mepact is an immunomodulator and is the first real advance in drug treatment for osteosarcoma in 20 years. Its precise mode of working in osteosarcoma is not known, but is thought to cause white blood cells to release chemicals which kill the cancer cells. It is used alongside conventional surgery and chemotherapy. The drug is given as an IV infusion over one hour, twice a week for the first 12 weeks and once a week for the following 24 weeks. It is a very expensive treatment option, but has been shown to produce an increase in overall survival (Kager *et al.*, 2010).

Ewing's sarcoma

Ewing's sarcoma was first described in 1921 by James R Ewing who noted that the histology in a bone tumour that had been thought to be an osteosarcoma looked different in that it had 'round cells' which looked like blood vessels and initially he termed it 'endothelioma of bone'. He first discussed a patient who was thought to have osteosarcoma of bone, who for some reason had not received the usual treatment of surgery at that time but had been treated with other modalities including radiation. Osteosarcoma was known to not be radiosensitive and so when his patient had a complete response to the radiation treatment, Ewing knew that he was dealing with something different. Unfortunately the patient then went on to have a recurrence of the tumour and it was decided that biopsy was required to settle the conundrum. It was here that Ewing found the different histological appearances and a little while later James Codman termed it Ewing's sarcoma. Surgery and radiotherapy were initially the only treatments used to treat Ewing's sarcoma until the 1960s when it was found to be responsive to certain chemotherapy agents (Samuels and Howe 1967; Cupps *et al.*, 1969). In the 1980s the genetic diagnosis of Ewing's sarcoma became possible with the identification of the chromosomal translocation between chromosomes 22 and 11, t (11;22). This defect can be found only in Ewing's cancer cells, is not inherited and is found in approximately 90% of Ewing's sarcomas. This has helped with the histological diagnosis and subsequent treatment.

As with osteosarcoma, patients diagnosed with Ewing's sarcoma have systemic staging undertaken prior to commencement of treatments. Ewing's can be treated successfully with chemotherapy and radiotherapy, but in certain cases surgery is also part of the treatment regime. Chemotherapy for Ewings sarcoma has also become streamlined over the years and patients are often treated in line with the Euro-E.W.I.N.G 99 trial protocol which includes vincristine, ifosfamide, etoposide and doxorubicin. These drugs are given in combination and usually on a three-weekly cycle, as an inpatient for a maximum of six cycles. Again, due to the nature of the toxicity of the drugs patients require echocardiogram and EDTA creatinine clearance tests prior to the commencement of the regime. As discussed in the osteosarcoma section, patients who are having these toxic drug regimens need to have attention paid to their general health in order to diagnose any potential problems as soon as they occur.

Chondrosarcoma

Chondrosarcoma is the bone sarcoma which tends to affect those in the older age group but, as with all sarcomas, they are seen in all ages. The chance of being diagnosed with a chondrosarcoma increases with age and has no known definite cause. Chondrosarcoma is most common in the humerus and distal femur and has only a slightly higher incidence in males than females. Chondrosarcoma accounts for approximately 25% of malignant bone tumours and has a diverse behaviour pattern from the low-grade local tumour to the high-grade metastasising tumour (Fleming and Murphey 2000). Chondrosarcoma arises from the cartilage cells and certain conditions increase the chance of benign bone tumours differentiating into a chondrosarcoma including enchondroma, osteochondroma, multiple exostosis, Ollier's disease and Malfucci's syndrome (Unni and Inwards 2010). Patients with a diagnosis of chondrosarcoma require full staging as with all sarcoma patients and this is usually in the form of a bone scan and CT scan of the chest. The majority of chondrosarcoma are low-grade localised tumours that require only surgical excision. This can be anything from a curettage and cementation to an endoprosthetic replacement. Figure 15.5 is of an X-ray showing chondrosarcoma of the proximal humerus.

Patients receiving surgery for excision of chondrosarcoma are cared for very similarly to any orthopaedic patient but it needs to be remembered that they have been given a cancer diagnosis and therefore will require psychological support. Very few patients have a diagnosis of dedifferentiated chondrosarcoma and they will need to discuss their treatment options with an experienced sarcoma oncologist who may or may not offer chemotherapy as a treatment option depending on the extent of disease and the patient's age. Most chondrosarcoma are resistant to

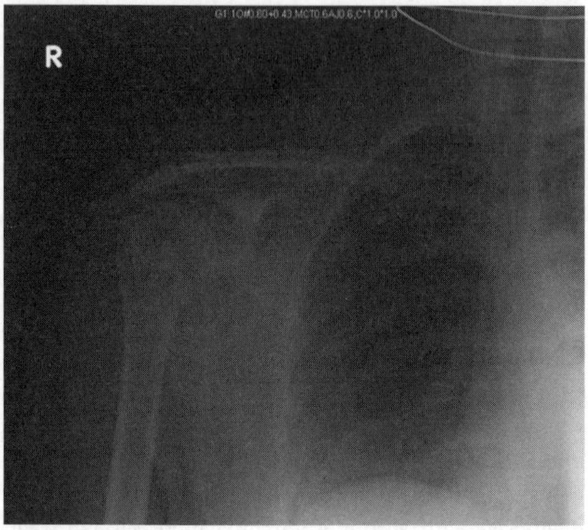

Figure 15.5 X-ray showing chondrosarcoma of the proximal humerus

radiotherapy treatment and so this is not a preferred treatment option.

Other bone sarcoma diagnoses are less common and are beyond the scope of this chapter, but need to be assessed and treated on an individual basis.

Soft tissue sarcoma

Soft tissue sarcoma is more common than bone sarcoma and can affect all age groups and all anatomical sites of the body. There are many more subtypes of soft tissue sarcoma than bone sarcoma. From clinical experience liposarcoma appears to be the most common subtype and the thigh appears to be the most common anatomical site.

Signs and symptoms

Soft tissue sarcomas usually present as a soft tissue mass which can be either painful or pain free and can cause symptoms or be asymptomatic. The fact that the signs and symptoms can vary so drastically could also be a reason for them to be misdiagnosed. Soft tissue sarcomas are often difficult to locate on plain X-ray but ultrasound and MRI are much more useful to describe the size, site and positioning of the tumour in relation to other anatomical structures. As with bone sarcoma, patients do not usually become systemically unwell.

Diagnosis

The pathway for soft tissue sarcoma diagnosis is not as clearly defined as that of Bone sarcoma but it is advised that patients with suspected soft tissue sarcoma are seen within services which have experience in dealing with these tumours (Grimer *et al.*, 2010). MRI can show suspicious features of a soft tissue mass but again the histological diagnosis is crucial to treatment decisions. Suspected soft tissue sarcoma is mainly biopsied under ultrasound guidance, although in some cases the soft tissue biopsies are undertaken by clinicians in the outpatient clinic setting. Again consideration and caution may need to be taken for patients receiving anticoagulation therapy. Grimer (2006) undertook a study which showed that the size of soft tissue sarcoma at diagnosis has an impact on prognosis. This study reviewed the cases of over 3000 patients who had been diagnosed with soft tissue sarcoma over a 20-year time period. It was shown that the average size of soft tissue sarcoma at diagnosis was 10.7 cm and this had not significantly reduced in the last 20 years. It also showed that the size of tumour at diagnosis had a direct effect on whether the patient could receive limb salvage surgery against amputation, and the incidence of metastatic disease at presentation. The UK guidance on sarcoma is currently that any soft tissue mass of 5 cm or over should be treated as a soft tissue sarcoma until proven otherwise (National Institute of Clinical Excellence 2005).

Treatments

As with bone sarcoma, the treatments offered to soft tissue sarcoma patients also depends on the histological subtype. The main treatment options for soft tissue sarcoma without metastatic disease are surgery and radiotherapy. Chemotherapy is usually used more when the disease is metastatic.

The most common subtypes of soft tissue sarcoma will now be considered in more detail.

Liposarcoma

Liposarcoma is the most common type of soft tissue sarcoma in adults. It was first described in the 1860s as a malignant tumour of fat by Rudolph Virchow. Liposarcoma can arise in any part of the body and is currently subtyped as follows:

- well differentiated
- dedifferentiated

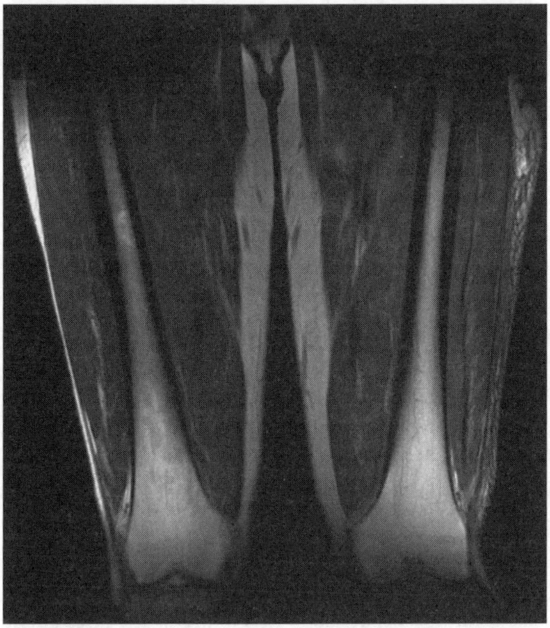

Figure 15.6 MRI scan of liposarcoma of the thigh

- myxoid
- round cell
- pleomorphic.

The most common sites of presentation are:

- Well differentiated liposarcoma tends to arise in the limb and retroperitoneum.
- Myxoid and/or round cell as well as pleomorphic arise in the limbs.
- Dedifferentiated liposarcoma mainly arises in the retroperitoneum

Liposarcoma is more common in the older population and rare in children (Vocks *et al.*, 2000), and has a slightly higher incidence in males than females. Figure 15.6 shows an MRI scan of Liposarcoma of the thigh.

The presentation of liposarcoma, as with most soft tissue sarcoma, usually includes:

- soft tissue swelling
- pain
- reduced range of movement
- numbness.

However, patients with liposarcoma of the retroperitoneal cavity often complain of:

- abdominal pain
- weight loss
- nausea
- vomiting.

The treatment for liposarcoma is usually surgical excision although radiotherapy is now being used more frequently as a neo-adjuvant treatment for myxoid liposarcoma of the limb and trunk. It allows less radiation to be used than in the adjuvant setting and clinically does not appear to cause any adverse complications for surgery. Chemotherapy is not routinely used for liposarcoma in the primary diagnosis setting but can be used in the presentation of high grade tumours and metastatic liposarcoma (Dalal *et al.*, 2008). This would be discussed with each individual patient after presentation at a specialist sarcoma MDT and remains, at this time, experimental.

Synovial sarcoma

Synovial sarcoma is another common type of soft tissue sarcoma and is more prevalent in the younger age groups, especially within the first two decades of life (Vargas 2012). Synovial sarcoma does not, as its name suggests, arise in synovial joints but is named due to its similarity of cells to those of primitive synoviocytes. The most common anatomical sites for these tumours are around the knee but they can also be found often in the hands and feet. Synovial sarcoma has a specific chromosomal translocation which makes its diagnosis more specific as this is present in 90% of confirmed cases. The chromosomal translocation occurs at t(X;18) (p11.2;q11.2) (Knösel *et al.*, 2010). This means that the X18 chromosome is affected and the p11:q11 are the points on the chromosome where the translocation takes place. Surgery is the main treatment option in this group of tumours. Although there have been discussions relating to the use of neo-adjuvant chemotherapy, it has been show to date that this does not increase overall survival and so remains controversial (Vargas 2012).

As with all tumour removal surgery the ultimate aim is to gain local control and therefore a wide local excision is recommended; an excision margin of 1–3 cm is appropriate. The ability to gain this much clearance during surgery will depend on the location of the tumour and radiotherapy may be used adjuvantly if there is concern about clear margins. Synovial sarcoma has a high incidence of metastatic spread (Stefanovski *et al.*, 2002) and patients with this disease should have very careful follow-up, as with all sarcoma patients.

Leiomyosarcoma

Leiomyosarcoma is a soft tissue sarcoma which originates in smooth muscle cells and can appear at any site of the body. For the purpose of this text leiomyosarcoma of the trunk and limbs will be the focus, however these tumours are common gynaecological tumours. Leiomyosarcoma tends to arise most commonly in adults and is one of the few soft tissue sarcomas that is more common in women, possibly related to the fact that they are most common in the gynaecological setting (Shah *et al.*, 2005). Leiomyosarcoma accounts for approximately 10% of all soft tissue sarcomas (Schwartz 2007). Those that arise within venous walls have a poorer prognosis due to their ability to spread through the venous system leading to a higher incidence of metastatic disease. In the limb, leiomyosarcoma is most commonly treated with surgery to remove the tumour, the extent depending on its location, size and the patient's general health. Radiotherapy and chemotherapy can be used in the treatment of high grade tumours and metastatic disease and this would be discussed with each individual patient as required.

Malignant peripheral nerve sheath tumour (MPNST)

Malignant peripheral nerve sheath tumours arise from peripheral nerves or cells related to nerve sheath; for example, Schwann cells, perineural cells or fibroblasts. The term MPNST is now used to cover tumours which were previously named malignant schwannoma, neurofibrosarcoma and neurogenic sarcoma (Weiss and Goldburn 2001). MPNST is most commonly seen in adults, but has been noted in babies as young as 11 months (Ellison *et al.*, 2005). It is seen most commonly in conjunction with large peripheral nerves such as the sacral nerve, brachial plexus and sacral plexus.

Treatment for MPNST is again surgically focused. The completion of surgery gaining wide (negative) margins is the intended outcome as this has been shown to reduce the likelihood of recurrence and metastatic disease (Geller and Gerbhardt 2006). The use of radiotherapy and chemotherapy in this tumour type is also controversial and needs to be discussed with each patient on an individual basis to weigh up the potential benefits against potential costs in terms of side effects which may be long-term.

Epithelioid sarcoma

Epithelioid sarcoma is the most common sarcoma of the hand and is a disease which is often found in the younger age group. These tumours are aggressive in nature and although they tend to be slow growing are known to often cause ulceration (Schwartz 2007). Epithelioid sarcoma often spreads along tendon sheaths and to lymph nodes associated with a high rate of recurrence and metastatic disease. It is suggested that an aggressive wide local excision should be used in the first instance (Scwartz 2007). Due to the aggressive nature of this disease radiotherapy is often used in the neo-adjuvant setting and chemotherapy is used on an individual basis.

Rhabdomyosarcoma

Rhabdomyosarcoma accounts for approximately 20% of all soft tissue sarcoma. The embryonal and alveolar types are common in children and are the most common sarcoma in children whereas the pleomorphic type affects adults. A clear histological definition of rhabdomyosarcoma was available in 1946 when these tumours were found to have a distinct morphology of rhabdomyoblasts (Stout 1946). Due to the nature of this disease and its occurrence in children, the treatment consists of a combination of surgery, radiotherapy and chemotherapy. The survival rate for these children has greatly improved for localised disease with an 80% five year survival (Punyko *et al.*, 2005). In patients with metastatic disease however, the survival rate has not really improved with a disease free survival rate at five years of only 30% (Oberlin *et al.*, 2008).

Metastatic bone disease

Metastatic bone tumours are becoming more common now that treatments for cancer are improving. These tumours occur when a primary cancer of another origin spreads to bone. The most common of these are breast, lung, renal and prostate and usually present with the following symptoms:

- pain in affected bone
- loss of mobility
- very often pathological fracture.

Figure 15.7 Shows metastatic renal cell carcinoma of the proximal humerus

If these tumors are solitary they can be treated successfully with surgery and adjuvant treatment as deemed necessary by the oncologist treating their primary cancer site. It is important for the orthopaedic surgeon planning to operate on these patients to discuss their prognosis with the relevant oncologist. It would be more

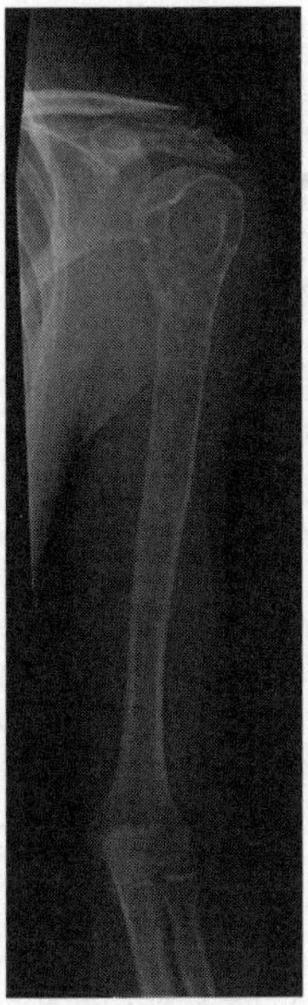

Figure 15.7 Metastatic renal cell carcinoma of the proximal humerus

appropriate to offer an endoprosthetic replacement to a patient who had a relatively good prognosis than to someone who may only have weeks or months to live. This can sometimes be a very difficult decision to make so honest discussion relating to prognosis with all of the parties involved, including the patient and family, is key to ensuing the surgery is in the best interest of the patient.

Patients who are inpatients in the orthopaedic setting for surgery for metastatic bone disease often have more complex needs due to their primary cancer diagnosis, especially if they are still receiving oncology treatments. To have links to the patient's specialist nurse/keyworker and oncology teams during this time will enable the practitioner caring for them to discuss any needs that may arise which are oncological rather than orthopaedic. The following provides good practice recommendations for the management of metastatic bone disease:

http://www.boa.ac.uk/publications/documents/metastatic_bone_disease.pdf.

Clinical trials

Clinical trials for sarcoma take place in various centres. The location of these depends on the nature of the trial and the services needed to undertake the clinical trial. Bone sarcoma, due to its rarity, does not have a large number of trails open at any one time and it is the responsibility of the lead clinician to ensure the patient and family are aware of any clinical trials which they may be eligible to enter, even if it means they will receive their treatment in a different treatment centre. The problem with clinical trials in this group of patients is the fact that the number of patients diagnosed each year is low and therefore recruitment into clinical trials is small. The importance of clinical trials cannot be reiterated enough in a disease process where the development of treatments is slow to progress.

Nursing and psychological care

The nursing care of patients who have a diagnosis of primary bone sarcoma will depend very much on the treatments they receive. Surgery is usually undertaken in an orthopaedic setting under the care of an orthopaedic surgeon but frequently in collaboration with a plastic surgeon. The plastic surgery component of sarcoma treatment allows reconstruction of defects following the initial tumour removal. This is often done at the time of initial surgery but can also be undertaken at a later date if necessary. The age of the patient will also determine if the surgery is undertaken within the paediatric or adult setting. Depending on the nature of the surgery performed, patients can have a short hospital stay, for example, for a straightforward excision of bone tumour, or a longer hospital stay for amputation, complex endoprosthetic replacement or limb lengthening with Ilizarov technology. Patients receiving chemotherapy will usually do so as an inpatient and within the oncology setting. Orthopaedic practitioners need to be aware of the common side effects of chemotherapy treatments, especially when surgery is an integral part of the treatment regimen and often within a very tight timescale between chemotherapy cycles.

Psychological support for patients and families with cancer is of paramount importance (Macmillan Cancer Support 2011). The diagnosis of cancer in itself is frightening; however, when you are then given a diagnosis that you have probably never heard of, or known anyone with the same, it can be even more challenging. The Internet is a growing resource for information and can be very useful, but can also be extremely confusing and frightening for patients and their families. If a patient searches 'sarcoma' the result will be several million hits and the information available is not always in a format that meets the patient's needs. It is therefore important for appropriate information to be given regarding the disease and a treatment plan in a carefully considered and timely fashion with specialist nursing support. Sarcoma support groups are also available for patients and their families, although this is a personal choice and not all patients are happy to take part. General psychological support for cancer patients is available in cancer centres, but this service is not always easily accessible so specialist nurses and other sarcoma professionals are crucial to the provision of the appropriate psychological support of sarcoma patients.

The role of specialist nursing

Specialist nursing in cancer care has been found to be of great benefit to both patients and families (National Cancer Action Team 2010). These roles allow a continuity of care to patients at a time when they may feel very 'out of control' following a cancer diagnosis. The roles are mainly supportive and advisory; however some of the roles do include hands-on care also, especially in a chemotherapy setting. Specialist nursing roles can be health service funded or funded by cancer charities, for example Macmillan Cancer Support or Marie Curie in the UK. See Box 15.3 for discussion of the value of specialist roles.

These roles enable the patient and their family access to:

- specialist support prior to diagnosis
- specialist support and information at the time of diagnosis and throughout the treatment pathway
- a 'constant' in the many number of different health professionals that they encounter throughout their journey
- a point of support that can refer the patient and family onto other services as required, including benefits advice, dietician and palliative care for example.

Sarcoma follow-up

Sarcoma follow-up, as with most cancer follow-up regimes, is a regular process of having scans and X-rays undertaken to assess for recurrent/metastatic disease and a clinical examination. The following shows a typical follow-up pathway for patients who have had surgery and/or radiotherapy for sarcoma:

- 2-week following surgery histology and wound check review
- 3-month follow-up with baseline MRI and chest X-ray and clinical examination
- 3-monthly reviews up to year two with chest X-ray and clinical examination at each appointment

Box 15.3 Evidence digest

The patient's perspective: a patient narrative written by a sarcoma patient who had access to specialist nurses

'In October 2010 I was diagnosed with a sarcoma in my left calf, a very rare cancerous tumour which was high grade and aggressive. I was immediately faced with the likelihood that I was about to undergo surgery which could result in part amputation of my left leg. Upon visiting the [hospital where my treatment would take place] beforehand, my family and I met Sarah, a specialist Macmillan Nurse. We were all touched by Sarah's incredibly positive, sensitive nature straight away, and we knew that we were in good hands. She gave us her contact details during the first meeting, and told us to contact her with any query or problem, at any time.

Sarah, together with Jane (Sarah's colleague), provided a high level of support during the process of diagnosis, hospital admittance and after care. Whenever we were in need of advice and help in any way, Sarah and Jane would always reply to our calls or emails and gave 110% to resolve every issue every time. Their help and guidance helped to speed up my recovery after surgery and radiotherapy.

Following the dedication and world class expertise of everyone in the Sarcoma Unit, we are now living life normally again. Thankfully, my leg is completely intact, after undergoing 5 hours of intensive surgery last October, although I was told afterwards that the margins were very narrow. I have now carefully resumed my favourite sport of mountain biking.

My family and I have felt so fortunate to have such a compassionate and professional team to support us with my fight against this cruel and indiscriminate illness. We would like to thank Sarah, Jane and everybody in the [hospital] for everything that they have done for us, and for their continued care.' James (age 37)

Note: names have been changed to protect confidentiality

- 6-monthly reviews up to year five with chest X-ray and clinical examination at each appointment
- Annual review with chest X-ray and clinical examination at each appointment up to year ten.

Patients who are receiving, or have received, chemotherapy may have a slightly increased rate of follow-up. If at any point during the follow-up plan the patient should have signs of recurrent or metastatic disease they should automatically have MRI/CT scan undertaken and if disease is confirmed they would be treated accordingly. Patients with high grade disease at presentation are more likely to go on to develop disease recurrence or metastatic disease; it cannot be ruled out for any sarcoma patient, hence the need for regular follow up.

A diagnosis of recurrent or metastatic disease can be as devastating for a patient and family as their original diagnosis was. The support needed by them can be much more intense than previously and professionals may find that patients given a subsequent diagnosis become even more anxious. Treatment for recurrent or metastatic disease is decided on an individual basis, taking into account the amount of disease present, its anatomical site and the age of the patient. It is in the metastatic setting that more chemotherapy may be used than in the initial primary treatment, especially for soft tissue sarcoma, and is discussed on an individual basis. In some cases the specialist teams will need to discuss with some patients and families that treatment is no longer an option and this is where specialist palliative care teams are involved to ensure the patient and family receive the supportive care they require.

Palliative care

Palliative care for bone sarcoma patients will be needed when there is no cure for the disease and patients begin to suffer symptoms. The input from palliative care providers is crucial to ensure end of life care needs are met. Often, palliative care services are happy to be contacted prior to the patient needing any input so that contact can be made and the start of a relationship can be sought. Palliative care can be undertaken in a number of settings:

- In the hospital setting palliative care can be provided by the ward staff with or without the input from specialist hospital palliative care nurses. This sometimes has to be undertaken when a patient deteriorates very quickly and it becomes very difficult to transfer them to a hospice or home.
- In the hospice setting palliative care is undertaken by specialist palliative care staff in a more relaxed, appropriate setting.
- At home palliative care can be undertaken by family with support from community staff, both general and specialist palliative care.

Hospices can very often provide support prior to any interventional palliative care input being needed. This can include relaxation treatments, music therapy and other services. It is important to discuss with patients and families the value of services which hospices can provide. Some find it very difficult to attend a hospice for supportive care as they feel they 'only go to a hospice to die'. It is therefore essential to explain the nature of the services that can be provided which other NHS settings are unable to offer.

The preferred place of palliative care should be the decision of the patient and family. When patients have had to travel a large distance to have their sarcoma treatment it is often more appropriate for them to receive palliative care in a setting which is closer to home. This allows them to have visits from all family and friends who may not be able to travel. It also allows patients and families to move away from what may have been a time of very intense treatment.

Summary

It will now be obvious that sarcoma care is not straightforward. The need for definite histological diagnosis is key to ensuring the patients receive the correct treatments for their disease, be it surgery, radiotherapy, chemotherapy or a combination of all three. Due to the fact that sarcoma can affect all age groups and all anatomical sites the need for knowledge about this disease in the general orthopaedic community is high. Care of these patients has to be within the realms of a specialist MDT and be undertaken by specialist teams who are experienced in sarcoma care (Grimer *et al.*, 2010). The importance of early diagnosis cannot be stressed enough. Prognosis depends very much on a diagnosis that is made before metastatic disease has a chance to present. Hopefully by raising awareness of this disease everyone can work towards a common goal of earlier diagnosis.

Practitioners working in the specialty of orthopaedics will inevitably care for sarcoma patients or suspected

Box 15.4 Sarcoma related websites

- http://www.sarcoma.org.uk/ (accessed September 26th 2012)
- http://www.bcrt.org.uk/ (accessed September 26th 2012)
- http://www.macmillan.org.uk/Cancerinformation/Cancertypes/Bone/Bonecancer.aspx (accessed October 5th 2012)
- http://www.macmillan.org.uk/Cancerinformation/Cancertypes/Softtissuesarcomas/Softtissuesarcomas.aspx (accessed October 5th 2012)
- http://www.cancer.gov/cancertopics/pdq/treatment/adult-soft-tissue-sarcoma/HealthProfessional/page3 (accessed September 24th 2012)
- http://www.boa.ac.uk/publications/documents/metastatic_bone_disease.pdf (accessed October 12th 2012)

sarcoma patients during their working time. It is important to remember that even though this is a rare disease there are health professionals specialising in sarcoma who are happy to share their knowledge in order to help raise awareness and make the patient pathway a smooth and informed one. See Box 15.4 for further online resources to find out more about sarcoma care and musculoskeletal oncology.

Recommended further reading

Anninga, J.K., Gelderblom, H., Fiocco, M. *et al.* (2011) Chemotherapeutic adjuvant treatment for osteosarcoma: where do we stand? *European Journal of Cancer,* **47**(16), 2431–2445.

Grimer, R.J., Mottard, S. and Briggs, T. (2010). Focus on earlier diagnosis of bone and soft-tissue tumours. *Journal of Bone and Joint Surgery,* **92-B**(11), 1489–1492. Available at: http://www.bjj.boneandjoint.org.uk/content/92-B/11/1489.abstract (accessed 13 July 2012).

National Institute of Clinical Excellence (NICE) (2006) *Improving outcomes guidance for people with sarcoma.* Available at: http://www.nice.org.uk/nicemedia/live/10903/28934/28934.pdf (accessed 24 April 2014).

Sewell, M., Neophytou, D., Sewell, T., Hanna, S. and Briggs, T. (2012) *Management of metastatic bone disease.* Available at: http://www.gmjournal.co.uk/uploadedFiles/Redbox/Pavilion_Content/Our_Content/Social_Care_and_Health/GM_Archive/2012/April/GMApr2012p33.pdf (accessed 24 April 2014).

References

Anninga, J.K., Gelderblom, H., Fiocco, M. *et al.* (2011) Chemotherapeutic adjuvant treatment for osteosarcoma: where do we stand? *European Journal of Cancer,* **47**(16), 2431–2445.

Casali, P.G., Jost, L., Verweii, J. and Blay, J.Y. (2008) Soft tissue sarcomas: ESMO clinical recommendations for diagnosis, treatment and follow-up. *Annals of Oncololgy,* **19**(Suppl. 2), ii89–93.

Cupps, R.E., Ahmann, D.L. and Soule, E.H. (1969) Treatment of pulmonary metastatic disease with radiation therapy and adjuvant actinomycin D. Preliminary observations. *Cancer,* **24**(4), 719–723.

Dalal, K.M., Antonescu, C.R. and Singer, S. (2008) Diagnosis and management of lipomatous tumors. *Journal of Surgical Oncology,* **97**(4), 298–313.

Ellison, D.A., Parham, D.M. and Jackson, R.J. (2005) Malignant triton tumor presenting as a rectal mass in an 11-month-old. *Pediatric Developmental Pathology,* **8**(2), 235–239.

Flemming, D.J. and Murphey, M.D. (2000) Enchondroma and chondrosarcoma. *Seminars in Musculoskeletal Radiology,* **4**(1), 59–71.

Geller, D. and Gerbhardt, M. (2006) *Malignant Peripheral Nerve Sheath Tumours* (MPNST). Available at: http:/sarcomahelp.org/mpnst.html (accessed 12 October 2012).

Grimer, R. (2006) Size matters for Sarcoma. *Annals of the Royal College of Surgeons England,* **88**(6), 519–524.

Grimer, R.J., Mottard, S. and Briggs, T. (2010) Focus on earlier diagnosis of bone and soft-tissue tumours. *Journal of Bone and Joint Surgery,* **92**(11), 1489–1492.

Hogendoorn, P.C., ESMO/EUROBONEL Working group (2010) Bone sarcoma: ESMO Clinical Practice Guidelines for diagnosis, treatment and follow up. *Annals of Oncology,* **21**(Suppl. 5), 204–213.

Kager, L., Potschger, U. and Bielack, S. (2010) Review of Mifamurtide in patients with Osteosarcoma. *Therapeutics and Clinical Risk Management.* Available at: http://www.ncbi.nlm.nih.gov/pmc/articles/PMC2893760/ (accessed 12 September 2012).

Kim, S.Y. and Helman, L.J. (2010) Strategies to explore new approaches in the investigation and treatment of osteosarcoma. *Cancer Treatment and Research,* **152**, 517–528.

Knösel, T., Heretsch, S., Altendorf-Hofmann, A. *et al.* (2010) TLE1 is a robust diagnostic biomarker for synovial sarcomas and correlates with t(X;18): analysis of 319 cases. *European Journal of Cancer,* **46**(6), 1170–1176.

Macmillan Cancer Support (2011) Psychological and emotional support provided by Macmillan Professionals: An evidence review. Available at: http://www.macmillan.org.uk/Documents/AboutUs/Commissioners/PsychologicalandEmotionalSupportProvidedbyMacmillanProfessionalsEvidenceReviewJuly2011.pdf (accessed 23 July 2012).

Mastrangelo, G., Fadda, E., Cegolon, L. et al. (2010) A European project on incidence, treatment and outcome of sarcoma. *BMC Public Health* **10**: 188. Available at: http://www.biomedcentral.com/content/pdf/1471-2458-10-188.pdf (accessed 3 May 14).

National Cancer Action Team (NCAT) (2010) *Quality in Nursing Excellence in Cancer Care: The Contribution of the Clinical Nurse Specialist.* Available at: http://www.ncat.nhs.uk/sites/default/

files/Excellence%20in%20Cancer%20Care.pdf. (accessed 17 August 2012).

National Cancer Intelligence Network (NCIN) (2012) *Bone Sarcomas: Incidence and Survival Rates in England*. Available at: http://www.ncin.org.uk/publications/data_briefings/bone_sarcomas_incidence_and_survival.aspx (accessed 13 July 2012).

National Institute of Clinical Excellence (NICE) (2005) *Referral Guidelines for Suspected Cancer.* Available at: http://www.nice.org.uk/nicemedia/pdf/CG027quickrefguide.pdf (accessed 15 August 2012).

Oberlin, O., Rey, A., Lyden, E. *et al.* (2008) Prognostic factors in metastatic rhabdomyosarcomas: results of a pooled analysis from United States and European cooperative groups. *Journal of Clinical Oncology*, **26**(14), 2384–2389.

Peltier, L.F. (1993) *Orthopedics: A History and Iconography*. Norman Publishing, San Francisco, CA, USA.

Punyko, J.A., Mertens, A.C., Baker, K.S. *et al.* (2005) Long-term survival probabilities for childhood rhabdomyosarcoma. A population-based evaluation. *Cancer*, **103**(7), 1475–1483.

Samuels, M.L., and Howe, C.D. (1967) Cyclophosphamide in the management of Ewing's Sarcoma. *Cancer*, **20**(6), 961–966.

Sarcoma UK (2012) http://www.sarcoma.org.uk/what-is-sarcoma (accessed 9 August 2012).

Schwartz, H. (2007) *Orthopaedic Knowledge Update: Musculoskeletal Tumors 2*. American Academy of Orthopaedic Surgeons, Rosemont, IL, USA.

Shah, H., Bhurgri, Y., and Pervez, S. (2005) Malignant smooth muscle tumours of soft tissue – a demographic and clinicopathological study at a tertiary care hospital. *Journal of the Pakistan Medical Association*, **55**(4), 138–143.

Stout, A.P. (1946) Rhabdomyosarcoma of the skeletal muscles. *Annals of Surgery*, **123**, 447–472.

Stefanovski, P.D., Bidoli, E., De Paoli, A. *et al.* (2002) Prognostic factors in soft tissue sarcomas: a study of 359 patients. *European Journal of Surgical Oncology*, **28**, 153–164.

Unni, K.K. and Inwards, C.Y. (2010) *Dahlin's Bone Tumours*, 2nd edn. Lippincott Williams and Wilkins, Philadelphia.

Vocks, E., Worret, W.I. and Burgdorf, W.H. (2000) Myxoid liposarcoma in a 12-year-old girl. *Pediatric Dermatology*, **17**(2), 129–132.

Vargas, B. (2012) *Synovial Cell Sarcoma*. Available at: http://emedicine.medscape.com/article/1257131-overview (Accessed 08 August 2012).

Weiss, S.W. and Goldburn, J.R. (eds) (2001) *Enzinger and Weiss's Soft Tissue Tumors*, 4th edn. Mosby, St. Louis.

PART IV
Musculoskeletal trauma care

CHAPTER 16
Principles of trauma care

Fiona Heaney[1] and Julie Santy-Tomlinson[2]
[1] *University College Hospital Galway, Galway, Ireland*
[2] *University of Hull, Hull, UK*

Introduction

Trauma is a major cause of death and disability worldwide and is the primary cause of mortality in the first four decades of life (Henning *et al.*, 2011). Those who survive physical trauma are often left with significant long-term or permanent life changing disabilities resulting particularly from head, spine and limb threatening injuries. Several reports suggest that management of the patient sustaining trauma is often sub-optimal (NCEPOD 2007). This chapter will discuss the priorities of care in the assessment, management and treatment of individuals suffering musculoskeletal trauma whilst considering the impact of injury to other tissue besides bone on care needs. In emergency and initial care of the patient following trauma the practitioner works as part of a multidisciplinary team with the aim of preserving life and preventing death and then with the aim of preventing complications and facilitating recovery and prevention of disability.

Pre-hospital care

Pre-hospital management of the patient sustaining trauma has a major impact on overall outcome and care. Management at the scene and during transfer to hospital consists of (Soloman *et al.*, 2005):

- maintenance of airway
- protection of the spine
- ensuring and supporting ventilation and perfusion
- controlling bleeding
- initiating IV and fluid replacement and managing shock
- pain management
- immobilisation of fractures and soft tissue injury
- safe transfer to hospital.

Mechanism of injury

Traumatic injury results from the transfer of energy from the environment to human tissue. It can be subdivided into blunt and penetrating trauma. Penetrating trauma involves tissue directly affected by an object which enters tissue, while blunt trauma may affect other tissue further away from the site of impact during energy transfer. Assessment of the patient following blunt trauma can be more difficult as the extent of the injury may not be externally obvious at first. Understanding the potential effects of the mechanism of injury is useful in patient triage as well as in predicting morbidity and mortality (Haider *et al.*, 2009) although there is some uncertainty about validity (Boyle *et al.*, 2008). The mechanism of injury can have a predictive value for diagnosing a subsequent injury. For example, the classic presentation of a patient who fell from a height and sustained bilateral calcaneal fractures should also instigate investigation for vertebral injury as this type of mechanism often involves a transfer of energy/trauma to the spine. Although the mechanism of injury can raise suspicion as to the presence of certain injuries, Richards (2005) warns that the presence of other injuries cannot predict presence of spinal injury or vice versa and that each patient requires an individual full examination as soon as possible after the injuring event.

Primary survey

On arrival at the emergency department (ED) trauma patients are assessed and treated based on the ATLS (Advanced Trauma Life Support) Protocol (American College of Surgeons 2004). This offers a globally standardised approach to trauma resuscitation that is understood by the whole team and enables a focus on

Orthopaedic and Trauma Nursing: An Evidence-based Approach to Musculoskeletal Care, First Edition. Edited by Sonya Clarke and Julie Santy-Tomlinson.

the life threatening aspects of injury as a priority rather than the injury which is most obvious. This means that musculoskeletal injury may not be an early priority. The primary survey is performed by the emergency/trauma care team simultaneously with resuscitation and consists of the following (mnemonic: A B C D E):

Airway (with spinal precautions)
Breathing
Circulation
Disability
Exposure/Environment Control

The primary survey should be repeated whenever there is a change in the patients' status. It is followed by a more definitive secondary survey where a head-to-toe examination is performed to identify all injuries and formulate a plan of care.

Airway with spinal precautions

Airway management is one of the core priorities in caring for trauma patients. It has been suggested that loss of a patent airway is second only to complete cardiopulmonary arrest as the most significant cause of death following trauma (WHO 2004). The airway is the gateway to the chain of oxygen delivery (Figure 16.1) without which all other links in the chain will fail, leading to organ dysfunction and death.

Assessment of the airway involves observing for causes of obstruction such as foreign bodies, tongue, teeth, oedema, blood and other secretions. Obstructions should be cautiously removed and excess secretions controlled by suctioning. A 'blind sweep' should never be performed to remove a foreign body as it may push the obstruction further down the pharynx. The simplest method of assessing a patient's airway is to ask them "Are you OK?". A logical response in a normal voice

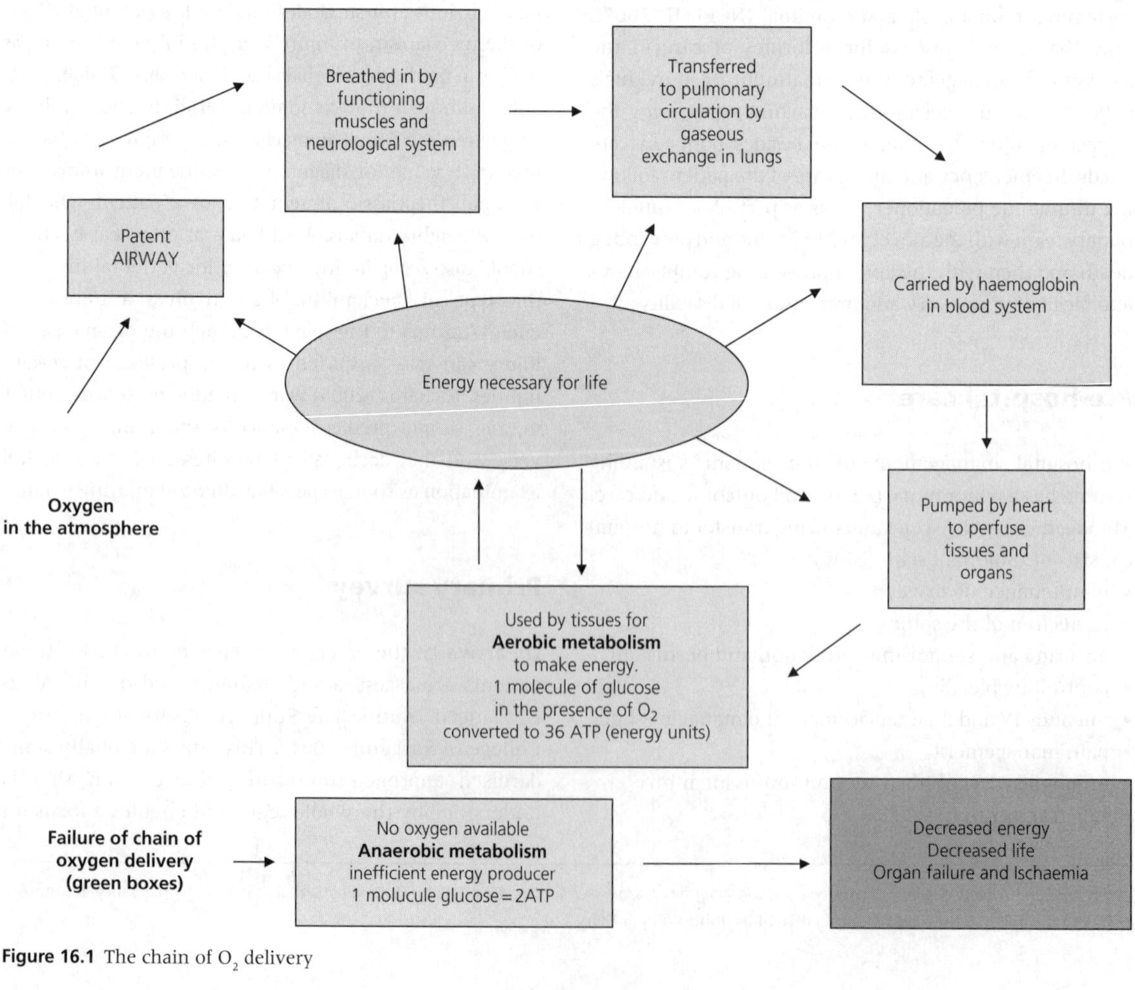

Figure 16.1 The chain of O_2 delivery

indicates the patient not only has a patent airway, but also that the brain is adequately perfused with oxygen. In the unconscious patient the airway can be maintained by insertion of an oropharyngeal airway (Figure 16.2).

An intact gag reflex indicates that the patient can maintain their own airway and the insertion of an airway device could lead to vomiting, cervical movement or raised intracranial pressure and must be avoided. Potential threats to the airway should also be assessed such as the presence of fractures, soft tissue injuries and burns. The victim of trauma is at risk for spinal injury and spinal immobilisation is maintained by placing the patient on a spinal board with immobilisation of the cervical region with sandbags or a 'head hugger' until any potential spinal injury can be ruled out. The head tilt/chin lift and jaw thrust positions are the standard manoeuvres for maintaining a patent airway (Figure 16.3).

Breathing

The patient should be assessed for the presence of injuries that may impede breathing. These include those that would affect the muscular act of breathing such as injuries to the lungs, chest wall and diaphragm along with those impeding the neurological response such as brain and spinal nerve injuries. Significant potential chest injuries in the trauma patient include:

- **Tension pneumothorax** occurs when a pleural tear allows air into the pleural cavity during inspiration but prevents it from exiting on expiration. Emergency treatment involves the insertion of a large bore cannula into the pleural cavity to allow the air to escape, followed by a chest drain.
- **Open pneumothorax** occurs when there is a significant wound to the chest wall which allows air to move freely into the pleural cavity. Treatment involves insertion of a chest drain.
- **Haemothorax** occurs when a laceration leads to accumulation of blood in the pleural cavity, leading to compression of the lung and impaired breathing. Treatment involves draining the pleural cavity of blood, although this is done cautiously in the case of a massive haemothorax as rapid blood loss may lead to circulatory collapse.
- **Flail chest** this occurs when more than one rib is fractured at multiple sites and seriously affects breathing. Emergency treatment involves intubation and ventilation.
- **Cardiac tamponade:** a wound which penetrates the heart results in bleeding into the pericardial sac. This reduces the volume of blood entering the ventricles prior to systole which reduces cardiac output and affects the delivery of oxygen and perfusion of tissues and vital organs. Emergency treatment consists of removing the blood from the pericardial sac by pericardiocentesis or thoracotomy.

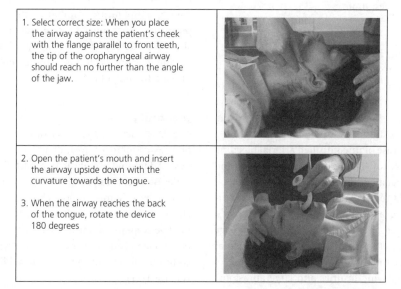

1. Select correct size: When you place the airway against the patient's cheek with the flange parallel to front teeth, the tip of the oropharyngeal airway should reach no further than the angle of the jaw.	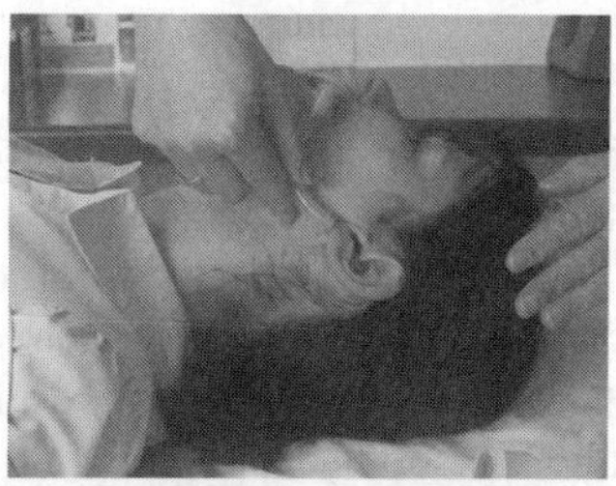
2. Open the patient's mouth and insert the airway upside down with the curvature towards the tongue. 3. When the airway reaches the back of the tongue, rotate the device 180 degrees	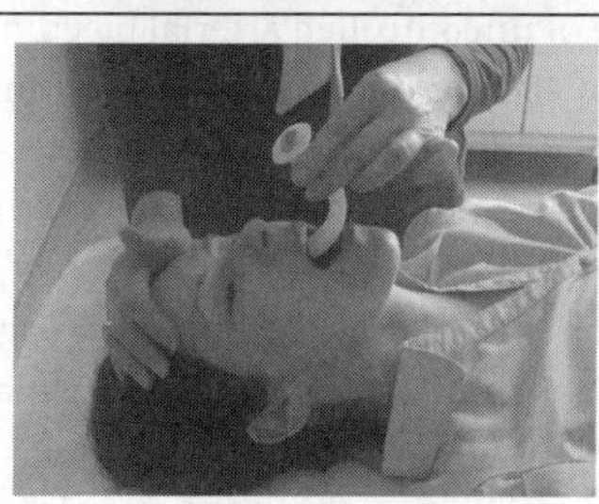

Figure 16.2 Insertion of a Guedal airway

Head tilt/chin lift One hand is placed over patient's forehead and firm backward pressure is applied with the palm to tilt the head back. Fingers of the other hand are placed under the bony portion of the lower jaw near the chin to bring the chin forward	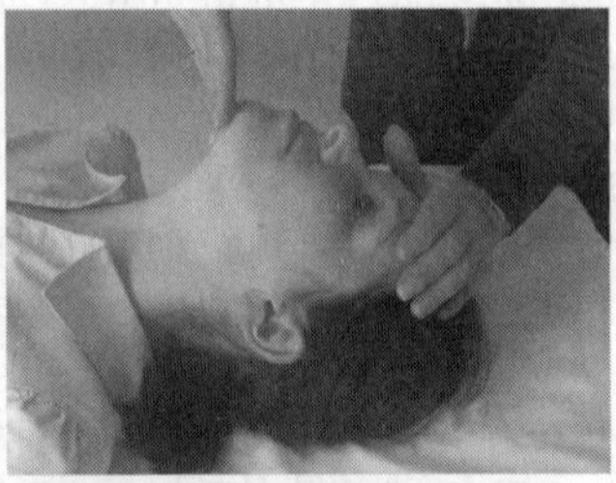
Jaw thrust (where spinal injury suspected) Place the four fingers of both hands on each side of the lower jaw. Once in place, the jaws are tilted upward making sure that the head and neck remain in position.	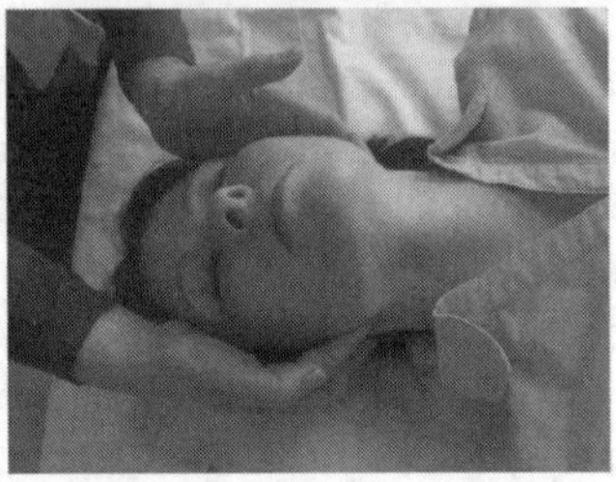

Figure 16.3 Maintaining an airway

Nursing/clinical assessment involves a full set of vital signs, paying particular attention to respiration. Observing the thoracic region for bruising and lacerations can help identify the presence of soft tissue injury. Supplemental oxygen should be considered. In all trauma patients the goal is to achieve an inspired oxygen concentration of 100% (Gwinnutt and Driscoll, 2003). Treatment of trauma patients with significant chest injuries often involves the insertion of a chest drain. Hence practitioners should be competent in the care of the patient with a chest drain.

Circulation

Hypotension occurs as a result of haemorrhage in the trauma victim and should be assumed until proven otherwise (Duncan and Moran 2009). Control of bleeding is the first priority by application of direct pressure where possible at the site of bleeding using pressure bandages/dressings or by application of a tourniquet in the case of uncontrolled arterial bleeding (Roissant *et al.*, 2010). Perfusion of vital organs and tissues with oxygenated blood is dependent on blood volume and rapid replacement of lost volume is crucial in preventing a break in the chain of oxygen delivery (Figure 16.1). In addition to blood seepage from wounds and other injuries, loss of extracellular fluid from wounds involving a large surface area of the body (e.g. degloving injuries and large abrasions) should be considered when estimating volume loss. Assessment must involve observing the patient's colour, temperature, capillary refill and degree of diaphoresis (sweating). The rate and quality of the pulse should be determined manually. IV access should be obtained, chosen fluids administered and wounds dressed to control bleeding.

Box 16.1 The AVPU System

A Alert
V Only responding to verbal stimulus
P Only responding to pain
U Unresponsive to any stimulus

Disability

The AVPU score (Box 16.1) can be used to perform a brief assessment of an individual's level of consciousness. Additional use of the more detailed Glasgow coma scale (Box 16.4) can give a clearer picture of the patient's neurological status. Blood glucose should always be checked in the unconscious patient as hypoglycaemia may be responsible for the loss of consciousness as aerobic metabolism in the neurological system is reliant on sufficient levels of glucose in addition to oxygen (Figure 16.1)

Exposure/environment control

In order to make a comprehensive assessment it is imperative that all clothing be removed from trauma patients whilst making every effort to maintain dignity and privacy. Wet clothing can have the added effect of reducing body temperature. Clothing is often removed with the use of scissors to ensure minimal movement of patients with suspected spinal injury. If alert, the patient's permission should be sought and the practitioner must be mindful of preserving the individual's dignity and the rapid loss of body heat related to exposure. To prevent sudden hypotension some garments may be left on the patient with gross hypovolaemia until adequate fluid resuscitation is ensured (Gwinnutt and Driscoll 2003) as clothing can provide pressure.

Secondary survey

The secondary survey is performed by the team after the primary survey has been completed and any immediate threats to life have been treated. A head-to-toe assessment is performed to determine any undiagnosed injuries or fractures.

Haemorrhage control and acute coagulopathy

Uncontrolled post-traumatic bleeding is one of the leading causes of potentially preventable death in trauma patients; so much so that the ABC approach to trauma may be changed to CABC to take account of catastrophic haemorrhage control as the initial priority (Henning 2011). Significant blood loss is affected by both direct injury and trauma related coagulopathy. Early identification of the bleeding source with timely efforts to minimise bleeding, restore tissue perfusion and haemodynamic stability are key in the management of patients with massive bleeding (Rossaint *et al.*, 2010). The coagulation process in haemorrhaging patients is adversely affected by exhaustion of the coagulation system, dilution from fluid resuscitation and physical factors such as acidosis and hypothermia that further compromise coagulation function (Spahn and Ganter 2010). This change in coagulopathy in conjunction with hypothermia and acidosis are interlinked and have been termed the 'lethal triad' (Figure 16.4). The haemorrhaging patient is at an acute risk for development of hypovolaemic shock. For more information on the physiology and management of shock consult Chapter 9.

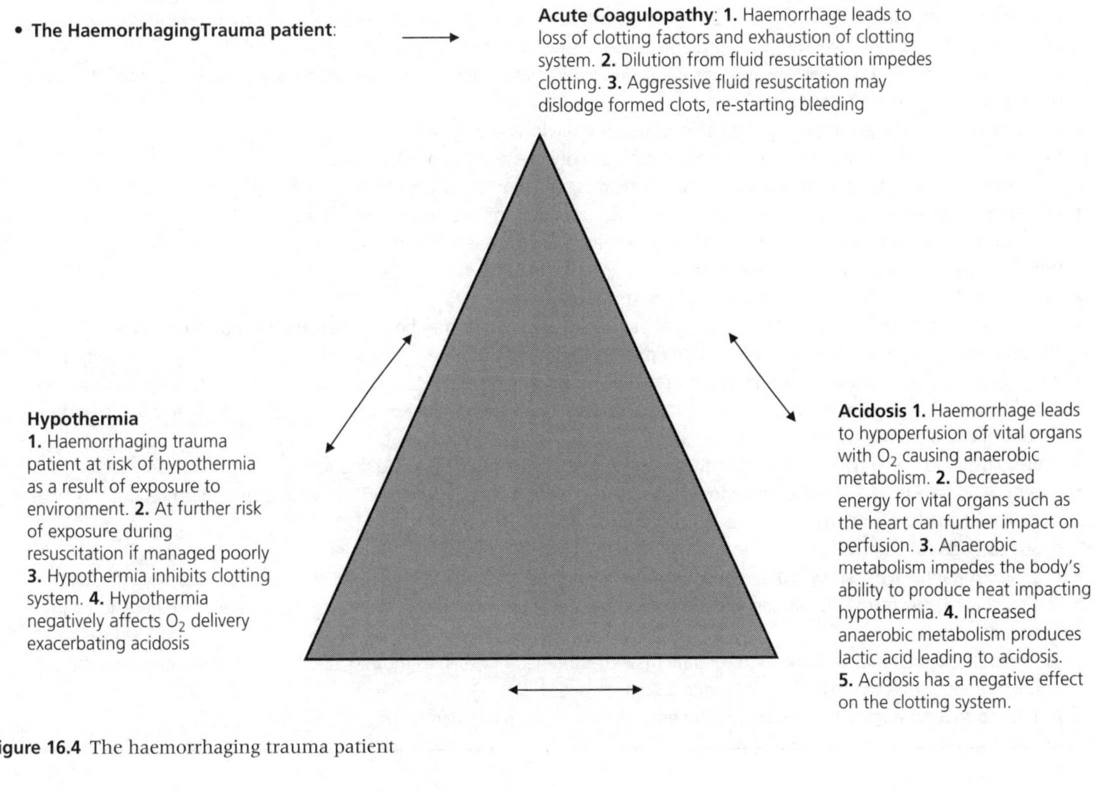

• The HaemorrhagingTrauma patient:
Acute Coagulopathy: 1. Haemorrhage leads to loss of clotting factors and exhaustion of clotting system. 2. Dilution from fluid resuscitation impedes clotting. 3. Aggressive fluid resuscitation may dislodge formed clots, re-starting bleeding
Hypothermia
1. Haemorrhaging trauma patient at risk of hypothermia as a result of exposure to environment. 2. At further risk of exposure during resuscitation if managed poorly 3. Hypothermia inhibits clotting system. 4. Hypothermia negatively affects O2 delivery exacerbating acidosis
Acidosis 1. Haemorrhage leads to hypoperfusion of vital organs with O2 causing anaerobic metabolism. 2. Decreased energy for vital organs such as the heart can further impact on perfusion. 3. Anaerobic metabolism impedes the body's ability to produce heat impacting hypothermia. 4. Increased anaerobic metabolism produces lactic acid leading to acidosis. 5. Acidosis has a negative effect on the clotting system.

Figure 16.4 The haemorrhaging trauma patient

Wound management

Controlling bleeding is the primary concern in the initial management of an acute wound. Inspection and exploration of a wound in a well-lit environment can help facilitate identification and management of the source of bleeding. Early transfer to surgery for haemorrhage control has been associated with increased survival (Roissant *et al.*, 2010). Box 16.2 considers best practice in the management of acute traumatic wounds.

Spinal precautions

Spinal precautions is a term used to describe strict immobilisation of the spine. Wherever a spinal injury is diagnosed or suspected the whole spine should be immobilised. Spinal immobilisation signifies the maintenance of spinal alignment, which should take into account the normal alignment of the individual's spine and pre-existing conditions such as ankylosing spondylitis. Cervical immobilisation can be attained by application of a cervical collar and a 'head-hugger' or sandbags. A recent Cochrane review (Kwan *et al.*, 2009) raised concern that cervical spine immobilisation may be associated with a higher morbidity and mortality than non-immobilisation and highlighted the paucity of evidence on the effectiveness of spinal immobilisation strategies. Although further robust evidence is required on the efficacy of cervical collars, current recommendations are summarised in Box 16.3.

Cervical collars are designed to restrict neck flexion, extension, lateral tilt and rotation, and do not restrict axial loading. In choosing a collar for a patient it is important to follow manufacturers' instructions regarding sizing to ensure a proper fit. The patient's chin should rest

Box 16.2 Evidence digest

Acute wound management: revisiting the approach to assessment, irrigation, and closure considerations (Nicks *et al.*, 2010)

An evidence-based approach must be adopted in the assessment and management of acute traumatic wounds. The objectives are to attain a functional closure, decrease risk for infection and minimise scar formation. Although every wound must be assessed and managed individually, Nicks *et al.'s* (2010) systematic review of the evidence gives the following general recommendations:

- Assessment of the wound including location, length, width, depth, tissue type, neurovascular and functional status, of surrounding structures, presence of debris and contaminants and range of motion.
- Patient assessment including history of injury, infection/contamination risk, medication history and allergies, tetanus cover and comorbidities that may affect wound healing.
- Assessment and management of wound pain through topical, local or regional anaesthesia.
- Decontamination of the wound including brushing off any dry chemicals prior to irrigation.
- Cleansing of the wound through application of a compress, irrigation or soaking as appropriate.
- All wound surfaces should be irrigated, paying particular attention to flaps and wound edges.
- Avoid unnecessary and excessive irrigation of clean wounds in highly vascularised areas.
- Wounds appearing dry, gangrenous and/or ischaemic are non-healable due to ischemia.
- Debridement may be necessary to remove devitalised tissue.
- In the absence of intrinsic, extrinsic or mechanical damage acute wounds may be debrided and closed immediately.
- Heavily contaminated wounds may need delayed primary closure to decrease infection risk.
- Wounds that are left to heal by secondary intention need follow-up assessment and possible secondary debridement.
- Dependent on wound severity, all patients with an unknown vaccination history or who have received fewer than three doses should receive a tetanus diphtheria vaccine (Td).
- Inadequately vaccinated patients (excluding those with a clean, minor wound) should also receive tetanus immune globulin (TIG).
- Patients who have received three or more tetanus vaccines prior to the injury only need Td vaccination if their previous dose was:
  - >10 years ago for clean, minor wounds
  - >5 years ago for other wounds.
- The need for antibiotic therapy is determined by wound type and method of closure, patient characteristics and infection risk.
- The most predictive factors for wound infection are wound location, wound age, depth, configuration, contamination and patient age.
- Antibiotic therapy should be considered for patients at heightened risk such as those with prosthetic joints, on corticosteroids, at risk of endocarditis or those that are immunocompromised.
- A dressing that provides a warm moist healing environment is recommended.

Box 16.3 Evidence digest. Reproduced with permission from College of Emergency Medicine

The initial management of alert adult patients with a potential cervical spine injury (College of Emergency Medicine 2010)

The practice of adopting spinal precautions in a patient following neck trauma has been widely adopted through fear of exacerbating or inadvertently causing a spinal injury. This guideline reviews the evidence for the management of patients with a suspected or actual spinal injury. Recommendations on neck immobilisation are as follows (for further recommendations on decision making, timing and type of imaging required see full guideline):

Neck immobilisation/cervical collars

- Patients at risk of cervical spine injuries should have their neck immobilised.
- The use of a collar to immobilise the neck is not compulsory in patients with pre-existing spinal anatomical abnormalities, as it may force the neck into an unnatural position with detrimental consequences.
- Cervical spine immobilisation should be continued until a full clinical and risk assessment is performed which indicates that the collar can be safely removed.
- Cervical collars should only be removed by staff who have undergone training in the use of a validated cervical spine clinical decision rule.
- Nurses can safely apply clinical decision making rules for cervical spine clearance following specific training, although further study and more rigorous evidence is recommended in this area.
- Further evidence in the form of randomised controlled trials is warranted in the area of efficacy of cervical collar application.

centrally on the chin rest and not slide down inside or protrude out over the chin rest. The collar is designed to fit snugly and not constrict the patient's ability to breathe, cough, swallow or vomit (Webber-Jones *et al.*, 2002). Once the collar is fitted the patient should be regularly assessed to ensure the following:

- The collar fits the patient correctly.
- Assess neurological status before and after any interventions involving changing the collar.
- Skin care is performed at least daily. When the collar is removed to perform skin care manual in-line stabilisation of the patient's head and neck should be ensured by adopting the correct head hold. One part of the collar is removed at a time and the back of the patient's head can be inspected during the log roll. *Always follow the immobilisation directions documented in the patient's chart.*
- The skin is assessed for evidence of breakdown particularly the occiput, chin, ears, mandible ridge, shoulders, sternum and laryngeal prominence.
- The collar itself should be cleaned daily and inside padding changed/cleaned as per manufacturers' instructions.

Thoracic and lumbar spine immobilisation can be achieved by placing the patient on a spinal board for transfer and on a firm mattress surface. Access to the patient's posterior surface can be achieved by performing a log roll. A log roll is a manual handling procedure whereby a patient is rolled from lying on one aspect of the body to lying on another, whilst maintaining correct vertebral alignment. It may be required for inserting or removing a spinal board, examination, providing specific nursing care or for the purpose of relieving pressure (Harrison 2000). A guide to performing a safe log roll is provided in Figure 16.5.

Neurological assessment should take into account any motor or sensory deficits that may indicate a spinal cord injury. On arrival to the Emergency Department patients are assessed for their risk of spinal injury. Decision making tools such as the NEXUS score (Hoffman *et al.*, 2000) and Canadian c-spine rule (Stiell *et al.*, 2001) can assist in determining which patients can be cleared from suspected cervical spine injury without imaging. These scores apply to conscious patients and a difficulty arises when attempts are made to clear the spine of an unconscious patient. Richards (2005) suggests that decision making tools with the aid of imaging technology also have a place in diagnosing spinal clearance of unconscious patients and recommends extending the CT of the brain to include the cervical spine in at-risk unconscious trauma patients.

Musculoskeletal assessment

All limbs and joints are palpated and examined for signs of fracture, soft tissue injury or neurovascular compromise. It is important that a baseline neurovascular assessment is performed to determine limb perfusion and motor and sensory function. Any deficit or change in neurovascular status needs further medical consultation and investigation. Affected limbs may be manipulated and splinted to maintain optimal alignment and stability. Open limb fractures should be managed prior to attending to closed fractures as there is an increased risk of chronic infection if treatment is delayed. See Chapter 7 for guidance on performing a thorough musculoskeletal assessment.

Wherever the injury suggests the possibility of spinal injury, the whole spine should be immobilized during any transfers between surfaces (Harrisson, 2000)

Preparation

1. Ensure all equipment required is at hand considering the reason for rolling the patient.
2. Ensure the availability of the correct number of staff. As a rule a minimum of five people are required (Harrisson 2000), more may be required depending on the size of the patient and manual handling assessment. This consists of team leader, 3 assistants and the remaining person to insert a spinal board or provide required nursing care. The team leader is the most experienced person.
3. The area must be free from clutter and the head of the bed shouldbe removed.
4. The bed should be adjusted to the height of the leader who is in control of the cervical region. Ensure the brakes are on.
5. Wash hands as per local policy.

Performing the roll

6. The leader approaches the patient in the patient's line of vision, explains the procedure and gains verbal consent.
7. The patient's motor and sensory function is assessed and recorded by the team leader.
8. If a cervical collar is in situ, do not remove it for the log rolling procedure.
9. The leader takes position at the head of the bed and takes control of the patient's head
10. Traction should never be applied
11. If head blocks are in situ, the leader places a hand on the lateral aspects of the block.
12. As an assistant removes a block, the leader replaces their hand on the side of the patients head and carefully slides hands one at a time into the head hold position.
13. The assistant staff assume position: The tallest at the patient's shoulders, the next at the patient's hips and the other at the patient's legs. The patient's arms are placed across their chest.

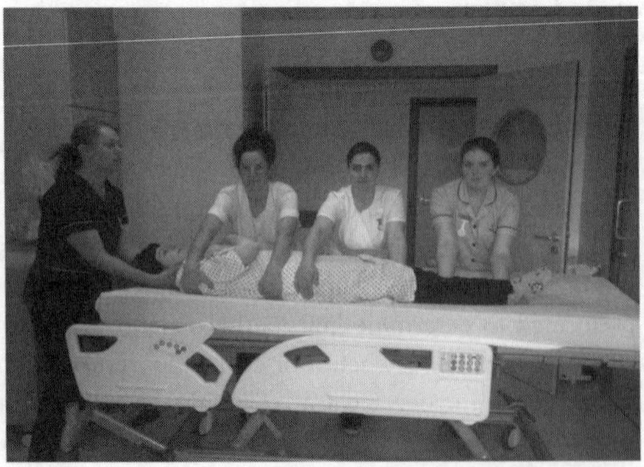

14. The command for rolling the patient is given. For example **"Ready Steady Roll"**. When the command for **"roll"** is issued the patient is rolled in a smooth controlled manner, as a unit, towards the assistants.
15. As the patient is rolled towards staff, their weight is transferred from the front to the back leg while remaining forward facing.

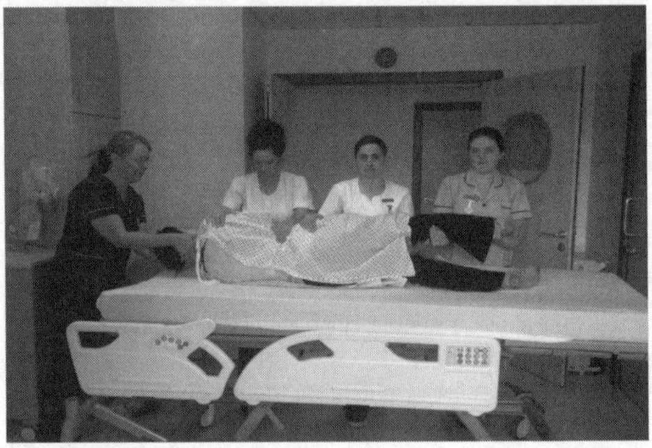

16. The staff and patient remain in this position until the appropriate nursing care or examination is complete.
17. The leader monitors patient alignment continually to keep the spine in line. In a healthy patient without pre-existing spinal disease, spinal alignment implies that the patient's nose should be in line with his/her umbilicus. If the patient has evidence of pre-existing spinal disease such as ankylosing spondylitis, keeping the spine in line implies that the **spine should be kept in the line that is normal for the patient before the injury (Wardrope *et al.*, 2004).** Difficulties may arise when maintaining spinal alignment in children, due to the disproportionate size of the child's head compared to their body. Therefore, before rolling the child back into the supine position ensure an appropriate level of padding is placed in situ below the level of the child's shoulders (Harrison,2000). An appropriate sized neck roll should be inserted to support the cervical curve and a thin pad positioned beneath the occiput to relieve pressure. (Harrison, 2000).
18. The patient is returned onto their back as follows: The leader issues the command to roll back as in step 14
19. As the patient is rolled away from staff, their weight is transferred from the back to the front leg while remaining face forward.
20. On return to the supine position, the team members must remain in position until released by the leader, who first ensures that torso, pelvis and legs are in alignment.
21. As the blocks are being replaced the leader carefully slides hands out from position, one at a time.
22. The team leader re-examines and records the patient's motor and sensory function. It is crucial that the same person undertakes both pre and post transfer examinations (Harrisson, 2000). Any changes in sensory/ motor function should be reported to a senior member of the medical staff and documented clearly.
23. Wash hands as per hospital policy
24. Document care as appropriate.

Figure 16.5 Performing a safe log roll

Severe injury and polytrauma

Once the primary and secondary surveys have taken place there is a need to plan the definitive care of any skeletal injuries. The existence of more than one injury (be it skeletal, soft tissue or organ) indicates, however, that not only has the patient sustained significant high energy trauma, but that there is a greater likelihood of an extreme physiological response to tissue damage which can result in severe life-threatening complications such as extreme inflammatory responses, metabolic dysfunction, severe immunosuppressive responses and coagulopathy (clotting disorders) which can lead to multiorgan failure and potential death (Keel and Trentz 2005). It is essential, therefore, that all injuries are identified at the time of the secondary survey so that their existence can be included as part of the overall management plan. The severity of these injuries is sometimes assessed using a trauma scoring system designed to help practitioners to identify care and management priorities and to ascertain risks to life. Such scoring systems can be useful when there is an isolated injury, but tend to be less accurate where more than one injury is involved. They categorise injuries of the respiratory, cardiovascular, nervous systems and abdomen, extremities and skin as minor to critical and take into account any existing complications. Their main purpose is to provide an alert for the need for prompt assessment and treatment as well as a way of prioritising injuries (Pape *et al.*, 2010).

Multiple trauma (often termed polytrauma) can include, in addition to skeletal injury, injuries to the head, face, neck, spine, chest, trunk and abdomen and their underlying organs and structures including major blood vessels and nerves along with severe traumatic skin wounds. The physiological assault of a complex pattern of injury often requires care in an intensive/critical care unit where the patient's condition can be carefully monitored from a respiratory and cardiovascular perspective and mechanical ventilation and other therapies can be provided.

Injuries to the pelvis, head and spine are those injuries which are the most likely to lead to death. Hence these are often the focus of emergency care and in the period immediately after resuscitation and stabilisation and following admission. Where there are several injuries and where there is no reason to suspect vascular damage (with potential for severe bleeding) the principles of 'damage control orthopaedics' are usually employed. This acknowledges a need to focus on stabilising those injuries most likely to threaten life before undertaking definitive final orthopaedic surgery to stabilise limb fractures, for example. This often, initially, involves temporary splintage or external fixation of long bone fractures of the limbs and conservative management of major wounds until such time as other injuries are stabilised and the patient is physiologically able to cope with major orthopaedic surgery (McRae and Esser 2008). This provides specific challenges for the care of the patient in both the critical care and ward settings.

Pelvic fractures

The pelvis is a large bowl-shaped ring made up of several bony components and strong ligaments which provides protection for the pelvic organs and transfers weight from the upper to lower body. As such it is an extremely stable structure, requiring significant trauma to disrupt it. Most commonly the pelvic ring suffers major injury through the crushing of the lower abdomen. Examples of mechanisms of injury include a motor vehicle or industrial accident or disasters such as earthquakes and blasts where parts of buildings trap victims. A significant amount of force is needed to disrupt the pelvic ring and this can result in two significant effects:

1. That the mechanism of injury involved significant force. This warns the clinical team that any resultant injury to the area is likely to be severe
2. That there is potential for severe damage to structures contained within the pelvis such as major blood vessels and nerves, the bladder, urethra, bowel and genitalia.

Because the pelvis forms a ring, it is often the case that crushing it involves 'breaking' it in two places (either by bony fracture or disruption to ligaments and joints) and may also involve severe disruption of the ligaments that contribute to pelvic stability at the symphisis pubis and sacroiliac joints. This can result in an unstable injury in which two parts of the pelvis become capable of moving separately, potentially resulting in further severe damage to the structures within the pelvis. Bleeding from damaged major blood vessels within or around the pelvis is a major cause of death in the trauma patient and requires careful fluid replacement and haemodynamic stabilisation. This bleeding may not always be obvious at first as the retroperitoneum has the capacity to hold up to four litres in the adult. Therefore careful assessment and monitoring of vital signs is paramount in diagnosing haemorrhage. The individual's normal blood pressure and previous diagnosis of hypertension should be considered in this assessment. Severely displaced fractures of the pelvis can be stabilised using pelvic binding or temporary external fixation while the patient is stabilised physiologically (Chapter 8). Signs of injury to the bladder and urethra must be carefully observed including assessment of urinary output and any signs of blood at the urethral meatus. Any suspicion of urethral trauma suggests urethral catheterisation is contraindicated and a supra-pubic catheter should be inserted. Injury to the bowel is also a concern and observation should include an assessment for the presence of any lower abdominal pain, distension and absence of bowel sounds.

Minimally displaced stable fractures of the pelvic ring can often be treated conservatively. These can be very painful and the patient requires careful support and pain management while healing and remobilisation commence gradually.

Head injury

Skeletal trauma is often associated with head injury – a major cause of death and long-term disability following traumatic injury – which may be associated with other skeletal and soft tissue injuries. Head injury is defined as (SIGN 2009, p. 2):

> (a history of a blow to the head or the presence of a scalp wound or those with evidence of altered consciousness after relevant injury.)

The level of consciousness according to the Glasgow Coma Scale (GCS) (Box 16.6) is usually used to categorise the severity of a head injury as follows (SIGN 2009):

- mild 13–15
- moderate 9–12
- severe <8.

Injury is usually the result of blunt trauma to the head and includes injury to the skull and may or may not include injury to the brain. Fractures of the skull can include both closed and compound fractures and are usually linear or depressed. Depressed fractures are most likely to cause associated brain injury due to damage caused by the bone being pushed in towards the brain.

There are a number of different types of brain injury with potential intracranial complications that might lead to death or disability:

- contusion or bruising of brain tissue
- cerebral laceration
- focal injuries localised to specific areas

Box 16.4 The Glasgow Coma Scale. Reproduced with permission from Elsevier

Eyes open	
Spontaneously	4
To speech	3
To pain	2
None	1
Best verbal response	
Orientated	5
Confused	4
Inappropriate words	3
Incomprehensible sounds	2
None	1
Best motor response	
Obey commands	6
Localise pain	5
Withdraw to pain	4
Decorticate	3
Decerebrate	2
No response	1
(Teasdale and Jennett 1974)	

- intracerebral haemorrhage
- vascular damage including:
  - extradural haematoma
  - subdural haematoma.

Minor head injury (e.g. GCS >13) requires careful observation using the GCS and identification of any deteriorating parameters. Apparent minor head injury can lead to significant cerebral damage and physical effects and it is therefore essential that the practitioner recognises any need for immediate medical attention. Frequent neurological observation using the GCS are essential in all patients who meet the definition of head injury defined above until the patient is deemed stable neurologically. It is essential that the GCS is recorded clearly and it is recommended that the three individual components of the scale (eye-opening, verbal response and motor responses) are described separately in all verbal and written communications and records so that the information always accompanies the total score. NICE (2007b) also recommend that in all head injured patients it is essential that pain is managed effectively (especially if there are other skeletal injuries) as unmanaged pain can lead to a rise in intracranial pressure and increased risk of haemorrhage.

Detecting early neurological deterioration can expedite neurosurgical interventions that can prevent permanent disability or death from the deteriorating brain injury. Although the majority of head injuries are minor, they can be associated with other skeletal injuries or other trauma and the mechanism of injury may mean that in some hospitalised trauma patients severe head injury is more likely. It may also be masked by a focus on other more obvious injuries in the early stages of management of the multiply injured patient.

The following are indications of significant brain injury (NICE 2007b) and should instigate medical referral and urgent CT scan of the brain:

- GCS <13 when first assessed in the ED
- GCS <15 when assessed in ED two hours after injury
- suspected open or depressed skull fracture
- sign of fracture at skull base (blood in the ear, 'panda' eyes/periorbital ecchymosis, cerebrospinal fluid leakage from ears or nose, Battle's sign/bruising over the mastoid process)
- post-traumatic seizure
- focal neurological deficit
- more than one episode of vomiting
- increased amnesia of events more than 30 minutes before trauma.

In addition it is recommended that a neurosurgeon is involved if the patient is on a non-neurosurgical unit if any of the following occur:

- persistent coma
- unexplained confusion for more than four hours
- deterioration in GCS (especially in motor response)
- progressive focal neurological signs
- seizure without full recovery.

It is always careful frequent assessment and recording of these parameters that can detect the patient in need of intervention and the practitioner is central to this.

Major wounds, crush Injuries and traumatic amputations

Injury can be associated with major wounds due to both blunt and sharp trauma. Mechanisms of injury that involve the 'crushing' of a part of the body between two hard surfaces occur most commonly in motor vehicle and industrial accidents as well as in incidents where blasts, collapsed buildings or multiple passenger transport systems are involved. Underlying tissues are compressed and surrounding tissue and organs may be severely damaged. An underlying fracture associated with significant tissue damage presents a major challenge to the trauma team for four main reasons:

1 A high possibility of severe infection, not only of damaged soft tissue, but of underlying skeletal tissue (see Chapter 17 for further discussion the management of compound fractures).
2 Damage to the blood vessels supplying tissue leading to ischaemia and necrosis of tissue and a risk of anaerobic infection.
3 Such severe damage to neurovascular structures that the limb (or part of a limb) has no viable circulation and damage is so severe that amputation is the only possible course of action. In some incidents the limb or part of limb may have been traumatically amputated at the time of the injury. In this instance it is important to consider the care of the severed body part when attending to wound care, taking into account X-rays, ischaemic time and asepsis.
4 The physiological impact of a large amount of tissue damage may result in a patient who is critically ill as discussed above.

Patients with significant wounds may require resuscitation and need careful monitoring for signs of vascular instability and sepsis along with judicious intravenous hydration and pain management. Significant wounds require meticulous asepsis and their management needs to be considered using a team approach which involves orthopaedic trauma surgery as well as plastic surgery teams. The decision to amputate or salvage an injured limb is based on multiple factors such as location of injured part, age and pre-existing conditions, type of injury, ischaemic time and presence of infection, and generally a consensus from two experts is required prior to amputation. Scoring systems can be helpful in making the decision between primary amputation and limb salvage (Shanmuganthan 2008). Long-term care focuses on rehabilitation (Chapter 6) and wound care (Chapter 12) paying particular attention to debridement of devitalised tissue, shaping of the stump, psychological care, pain assessment and relief of phantom sensations, and promoting optimal function and mobility.

Rhabdomyolysis

Skeletal injury, particularly where significant soft tissue and muscle is involved, can release the contents of muscle cells into the circulation releasing the muscle protein myoglobin into the blood stream. This can result in a relatively uncommon but serious condition known as 'crush syndrome' or *rhabdomyolysis*. Because of the size and toxicity of the myoglobulin, it can affect the glomerular filtration rate of the kidney and result in acute renal failure. The patient becomes seriously ill. Although rhabdomyolysis may be largely without symptoms, the practitioner should assess renal function by observing the volume of urine output as well as for red or 'cola' coloured urine, the patient may also complain of generalised muscle pain and weakness. Any concerns should be immediately reported to medical staff. Diagnosis is confirmed by detecting the level of muscle enzymes in the blood and treatment centres on flushing the myoglobulin out of the system through dialysis. Rhabdomyolysis can often coincide with compartment syndrome (Chapter 9) and a high suspicion of its development should be maintained when caring for patients following crush injuries.

Monitoring, deterioration and early warning scores

Patients with severe or multiple injury can be physiologically unstable for several days or weeks following admission and even following transfer from the intensive care setting to a general hospital trauma ward. It is essential, therefore, that the patient's physiological status is carefully monitored until complete stability is assured. Even some weeks after the injury and subsequent surgery patients remain at risk of significant complications (see Chapter 9 for further discussion of these).

A common and widely recommended approach to monitoring patients following injury is the use of an early warning score with the aim of detecting clinical deterioration in the patient as early as possible so that active measures can be taken to prevent further deterioration and intensive care unit admission. This recognises the link between physiological observations and adverse clinical outcomes. A variety of different early warning score methods are in use internationally depending on local policy, but the principles remain the same. Early warning scores involve calculating a score derived from regular observations of the following parameters:

- mental response
- pulse rate
- BP
- respiratory rate
- temperature and
- urinary output.

Of these respiratory rate is considered to be the most important in identifying a change in the patient's condition and some systems do not include urinary output although there are numerous reasons why this should be included in standard monitoring practice. Careful and frequent (as often as every 30 minutes if the practitioner has reason to suspect the patient may be at risk of deterioration) recordings are made on a specialised chart which enables the practitioner to identify any changes immediately. The score will often have a threshold of deterioration in the physiological parameters at which the practitioner needs to take action. This action initially involves seeking immediate medical attention, referral to a senior medical practitioner if necessary and possible referral to the intensive/critical care team. Many hospitals now provide an intensive care outreach service or similar where ward staff can seek the support of an critical care practitioner in monitoring the patient, making decisions and identifying action needed. Research is increasingly indicating that early warning scores are an effective way to recognise the deteriorating patient in need of intervention with potential to decrease the number of patients who require emergency resuscitation and some are now being developed for specific populations such as children.

Early warning scores and the deteriorating patient

The ability to identify a deteriorating patient and act appropriately is fundamental to quality orthopaedic nursing care in all settings, especially in the trauma setting. Odell *et al.* (2009) suggest that inexperience, lack of skill and excessive workloads greatly impedes the ward nurse's ability to detect and manage these patients. The use of Early Warning Scores (EWS) also known as Patient at Risk Scores (PARS) or Modified Early Warning Scores (MEWS) have become increasingly popular for the identification and monitoring of critically ill patients with their use being recommended in the care of all patients admitted to an acute hospital setting (NICE 2007a). In the United Kingdom EWS are commonly used for the assessment of ill patients (Rees 2003). Their use has been a more recent development in Ireland which was the first country to adopt a national early warning system (HSE 2011).

EWS are calculated from simple physiological parameters that are routinely monitored at the patients' bedside (Figure 16.6). Depending on the observations made, the patient is given a score which helps quantify

Feidhmeannacht na Seirbhíse Sláinte
Health Service Executive

Tús Áite do Shábháilteacht Othar
Patient Safety First

Hospital Name:

....

Document Number during this Admission ☐

Patient Name:
Date of Birth:
Healthcare Record No:
Addressograph

NATIONAL EARLY WARNING SCORE
ADULT PATIENT OBSERVATION CHART

Escalation Protocol Flow Chvart

Total Score	Minimum Observation Frequency	ALERT	RESPONSE
1	12 Hourly	Nurse in charge	Nurse in charge to review if new score1
2	6 Hourly	Nurse in charge	Nurse in charge to review
3	4 Hourly	Nurse in charge & Team/On-call SHO	1. SHO to review within 1 hour
4-6	1 Hourly	Nurse in charge & Team/On-call SHO	1. SHO to review within ½ hour 2. If no response to treatment within 1 hour contact Registrar 3. Consider continuous patient monitoring 4. Consider transfer to higher level of care
≥7	½ Hourly	Nurse in charge & Team/On-Call Registrar Inform Team/On-Call Consultant	1. Registrar to review immediately 2. Continuous patient monitoring recommended 3. Plan to transfer to higher level of care 4. Activate Emergency Response System (ERS) *(as appropriate to hospital model)*
Note: Single score triggers			
Score of 2 HR ≤ 40 (Bradycardia)	½ Hourly	Nurse in charge & Team/On-call SHO	1. SHO to review immediately
*Score of 3 in any single parameter	½ Hourly or as indicated by patient's condition	Nurse in charge & Team/On-call SHO	1. SHO to review immediately 2. If no response to treatment or still concerned contact Registrar 3. Consider activating ERS

*In certain circumstances a score of 3 in a single parameter may not require ½ hourly observations i.e. some patients on O_2.

- When communicating patients score inform relevant personnel if patient is charted for supplemental oxygen e.g. post-op.
- Document all communication and management plans at each escalation point in medical and nursing notes.
- Escalation protocol may be stepped down as appropriate and documented in management plan.

IMPORTANT:
1. If response is not carried out as above CNM/Nurse in charge must contact the Registrar or Consultant.
2. If you are concerned about a patient escalate care regardless of score.

Adapted from CYMRU chart

CONSIDER SEPSIS

Sepsis = Known or Suspected Infection & Systemic Inflammatory Response Syndrome (SIRS)

Defined as the presence of 2 or more of the following

Temperature > 38°C or < 36°C
Respiratory Rate > 20 breaths per min
$PaCO_2$ < 4.3 kPa
Heart Rate > 90 beats per min
White Cell Count > 12 or < 4

Diagnosed Sepsis →

Intervention:
Action within One Hour
COMPLETE SEPSIS SIX

1. **High Flow Oxygen**
2. **Lactate Check**
3. **Fluid Challenge**
4. **Urine Monitoring**
5. **Cultures***
6. **Antimicrobial Therapy**

(* blood, wounds, invasive line sites, sputum, urine etc as appropriate)

Adapted from CYMRU chart

Version 3 December 2011

Figure 16.6 Example of an early warning score assessment sheet. Reproduced with permission from Health Service Executive

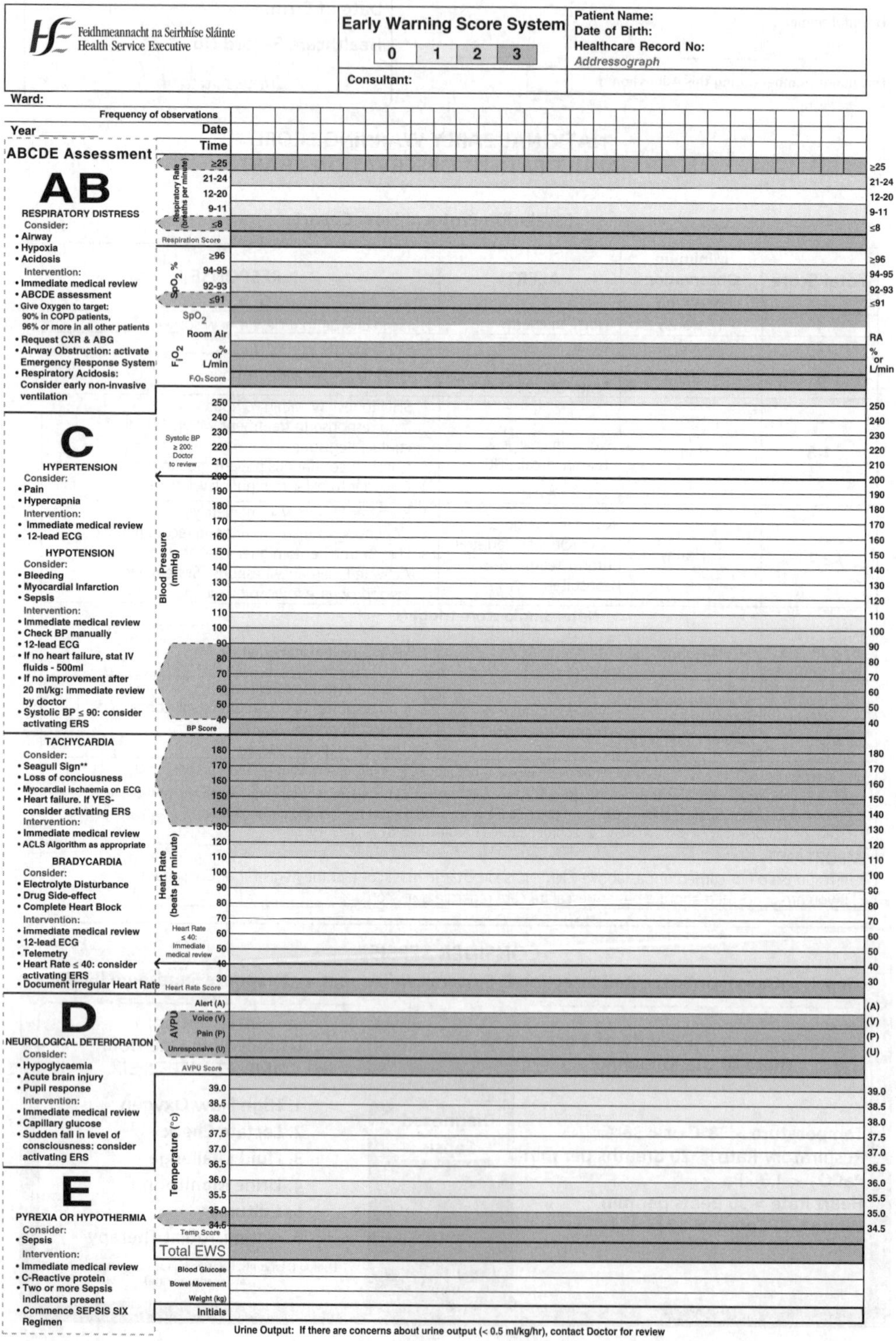

Feidhmeannacht na Seirbhíse Sláinte
Health Service Executive

Early Warning Score System

0	1	2	3

Consultant:

Patient Name:
Date of Birth:
Healthcare Record No:
Addressograph

Ward:

Frequency of observations
Year ______ Date
Time

ABCDE Assessment

AB

RESPIRATORY DISTRESS
Consider:
- Airway
- Hypoxia
- Acidosis

Intervention:
- Immediate medical review
- ABCDE assessment
- Give Oxygen to target: 90% in COPD patients, 96% or more in all other patients
- Request CXR & ABG
- Airway Obstruction: activate Emergency Response System
- Respiratory Acidosis: Consider early non-invasive ventilation

Respiratory Rate (breaths per minute): ≥25, 21-24, 12-20, 9-11, ≤8
Respiration Score

SpO_2 %: ≥96, 94-95, 92-93, ≤91

SpO_2
Room Air (RA)
F_iO_2: % or L/min
F_iO_2 Score

C

HYPERTENSION
Consider:
- Pain
- Hypercapnia

Intervention:
- Immediate medical review
- 12-lead ECG

HYPOTENSION
Consider:
- Bleeding
- Myocardial Infarction
- Sepsis

Intervention:
- Immediate medical review
- Check BP manually
- 12-lead ECG
- If no heart failure, stat IV fluids - 500ml
- If no improvement after 20 ml/kg: immediate review by doctor
- Systolic BP ≤ 90: consider activating ERS

Systolic BP ≥ 200: Doctor to review

Blood Pressure (mmHg): 250, 240, 230, 220, 210, 200, 190, 180, 170, 160, 150, 140, 130, 120, 110, 100, 90, 80, 70, 60, 50, 40
BP Score

TACHYCARDIA
Consider:
- Seagull Sign**
- Loss of conciousness
- Myocardial ischaemia on ECG
- Heart failure. If YES- consider activating ERS

Intervention:
- Immediate medical review
- ACLS Algorithm as appropriate

BRADYCARDIA
Consider:
- Electrolyte Disturbance
- Drug Side-effect
- Complete Heart Block

Intervention:
- Immediate medical review
- 12-lead ECG
- Telemetry
- Heart Rate ≤ 40: consider activating ERS
- Document irregular Heart Rate

Heart Rate ≤ 40: Immediate medical review

Heart Rate (beats per minute): 180, 170, 160, 150, 140, 130, 120, 110, 100, 90, 80, 70, 60, 50, 40, 30
Heart Rate Score

D

NEUROLOGICAL DETERIORATION
Consider:
- Hypoglycaemia
- Acute brain injury
- Pupil response

Intervention:
- Immediate medical review
- Capillary glucose
- Sudden fall in level of consciousness: consider activating ERS

AVPU: Alert (A), Voice (V), Pain (P), Unresponsive (U)
AVPU Score

E

PYREXIA OR HYPOTHERMIA
Consider:
- Sepsis

Intervention:
- Immediate medical review
- C-Reactive protein
- Two or more Sepsis indicators present
- Commence SEPSIS SIX Regimen

Temperature (°c): 39.0, 38.5, 38.0, 37.5, 37.0, 36.5, 36.0, 35.5, 35.0, 34.5
Temp Score

Total EWS
Blood Glucose
Bowel Movement
Weight (kg)
Initials

Urine Output: If there are concerns about urine output (< 0.5 ml/kg/hr), contact Doctor for review

Figure 16.6 *(Continued)*

National Early Warning Score Key (ViEWS)

SCORE	3	2	1	0	1	2	3
Respiratory Rate (bpm)	≤ 8		9 - 11	12 - 20		21 - 24	≥ 25
SpO_2 (%)	≤ 91	92 - 93	94 - 95	≥ 96			
Inspired O_2 (FiO_2)				Air			Any O_2
Systolic BP (mmHg)	≤ 90	91 - 100	101 - 110	111 - 249	≥ 250		
Heart Rate (BPM)		≤ 40	41 - 50	51 - 90	91 - 110	111 - 130	≥ 131
AVPU/CNS Response				Alert (A)			Voice (V), Pain (P), Unresponsive (U)
Temp (°C)	≤ 35.0		35.1 - 36.0	36.1 - 38.0	38.1 - 39.0	≥ 39.1	

Note: Where systolic blood pressure is ≥ 200 mmHg, request Doctor to review.

This Section is for reference only. Where Glasgow Coma Score is required, please use separate sheet.

Glasgow Coma Scale

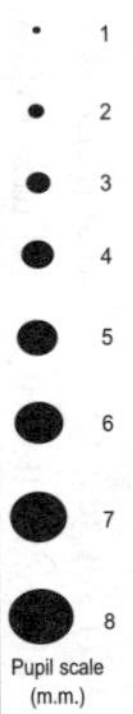

		Date: / Time:	GCS						
COMA SCALE		Spontaneously	4						
	Eyes open	To Speech	3						Eyes closed by swelling = C
		To Pain	2						
		None	1						
	Best verbal response	Orientated	5						Endotracheal tube or tracheostomy =T
		Confused	4						
		Inappropriate words	3						
		Incomprehensible sounds	2						
		None	1						
	Best motor response	Obey commands	6						Usually record the best arm response
		Localize Pain	5						
		Flexion to Pain	4						
		Abnormal Flexion	3						
		Extension to Pain	2						
		No Response	1						
		Total G.C.S.							
PUPILS	right	Size							+ reacts – no reaction C eyes closed
		Reaction							
	left	Size							
		Reaction							
LIMB MOVEMENT	ARMS	Normal power							Record right (R) and left (L) separately if there is a difference between the two sides
		Mild weakness							
		Severe weakness							
		Spastic flexion							
		Extension							
		No response							
	LEGS	Normal power							
		Mild weakness							
		Severe weakness							
		Extension							
		No response							
		Initials							

With kind permission of Beaumont Hospital

Patient Name:

Date of Birth:

Healthcare Record No:

Addressograph

Please use this space for additional monitoring charts, e.g. Pain Score Chart

**** Seagull Sign: This is when the Heart Rate is above the Systolic Blood Pressure**

Note: The National Early Warning Score has adopted the VitalPAC™ Early Warning Score (ViEWS) parameters.

Acknowledgements: A modified version of the CYMRU Vital Signs Record was reproduced with permission from its developers. Support and advice was provided by the Health Directorate, ACT Government, Australia.

Figure 16.6 (*Continued*)

Box 16.5 Evidence digest: the evidence for early warning scores to date

> In 1997 Morgan *et al.* (1997) first reported the use of an EWS in the detection of seriously ill deteriorating patients (Morgan *et al.*, 1997) and their use on both medical and surgical wards is now well established (Fullerton *et al.*, 2012). Several studies suggest that the presence of critically abnormal vital signs can be a good predictor of patient deterioration and mortality risk (Bleyer *et al.*, 2011; Fullerton *et al.*, 2012; Garcea *et al.*, 2010). This implies that monitoring and rapid response to abnormal vital signs may positively influence mortality rates. Although there has been a mass acceptance of EWS use, they have yet to be rigorously validated. A recent Cochrane review suggests there is minimal evidence to support the adoption of EWS in the identification and management of critically ill patients and that further research in this area is warranted (McGaughy *et al.*, 2007). Considering the massive uptake of EWS use, it can be presumed that it is only a matter of time before more rigorous evidence is accumulated.

their health status and risk for critical illness. This score highlights the need for clinical intervention and/or admission to an intensive care facility. It is anticipated that early warning scores taking into account all physiological parameters can more readily identify deteriorating patients than waiting for more obvious changes such as a marked drop in systolic blood pressure which is often a pre-terminal event (Rees 2003). Once the patient's score indicates they are at risk for further deterioration or a critical event, a response system is enacted depending on the individual hospital's policy. In general a score of three indicates the need for a medical review. Box 16.5 considers the evidence base for EWS.

The use of early warning scores in conjunction with clinical judgment has been found to be more effective at identifying patients at risk of adverse clinical outcomes than clinical judgment alone in pre-hospital admitted patients (Fullerton *et al.*, 2012). There have been many advances and expansions on the role of the orthopaedic nurse. Nursing decision making and intuition is linked to clinical experience and is thought to improve over time as the nurse progresses to expert level (Banning 2007). It is often the nurses' intuitive judgment that alerts them to deterioration in patient condition and vital signs are then performed to confirm these findings (Odell *et al.*, 2009). Conversely, Thompson *et al.* (2007) suggest that clinical experience is not a predictor of high quality decision making in recognising patients at risk of a critical event, with nurses overestimating the need to intervene and recommends a more structured approach. EWS are designed as an assistive tool in identifying the critically ill or deteriorating patient; however they should not overrule clinical judgment with many institutions recommending an escalation of care regardless of score if the nurse is concerned (HSE 2011).

Once a patient is identified as at risk for a critical incident, fast intervention and review is imperative. Some nurses may find it hard to articulate their clinical concerns about a patient to their medical colleagues, resulting in a delayed response and acknowledgement of the gravity of these concerns, which can be frustrating for both parties (Odell *et al.*, 2009). In the same manner junior nurses may lack the confidence to alert senior medics to their concerns. EWS afford nurses the means to insist on a medical review and to refer upwards to more senior clinicians, as indicated by the patient's EWS score, (Rees 2003) assisting them in their role as patient advocates.

A set of vital signs usually includes the patient's temperature, pulse, respirations, blood pressure and, more recently, oxygen saturations. It is a core tool in performing a nursing assessment performed routinely as part of a patient's care and more often dependent on the individual's condition and treatment (e.g. performed more regularly in post-operative care). In the ritual of performing vital signs their importance can sometimes be overlooked and they are a task that is often delegated to student nurses or healthcare assistants. Many healthcare institutions have abandoned vital signs monitors in preference for the traditional sphygmomanometers and nursing assessments of look, listen and feel, believing that it encourages a more accurate assessment of patient condition (Raynor 2010).

Respirations

Respiratory rate is the most important observation for assessing a patient's clinical status, yet it is often the one that is least recorded (Parkes 2011). When assessing respirations consider rate, rhythm and depth. The rhythm indicates the pattern of breaths a minute. One of the most common breathing abnormalities, Cheyne Strokes, involves a pattern of breaths followed by apnoeic episodes. Abnormalities of depth are mainly hypopnea and hyperpnoea. Hypopnea involves shallow respirations usually indicative of impending respiratory failure (Massey and Meredith 2010). Hyperpnoea is characterised by rapid and deep respirations (Kussmals) indicative of the body's compensatory mechanism. Hyperventilation occurs in the effort to dispose of excess carbon dioxide (Massey and Meredith 2010). The normal respiratory rate for an adult is 14–20 breaths a minute. The rate is assessed by observing the chest wall (rise and fall) for a full minute. Bradypnoea indicates a respiratory rate <8 breaths a minute and is seen in depression of the respiratory centre, for example a narcotic overdose. Tachypnoea indicates a respiratory rate >20 breaths a minute and it can indicate either a drop in arterial blood oxygen saturation or compensation in the presence of metabolic acidosis. Rates above 27 breaths a minute are an important predictor of cardiac arrest (Smith *et al.*, 2011). Some reasons for tachypnoea in the orthopaedic patient include:

- fat embolism
- pulmonary embolism
- respiratory tract infection
- airway trauma/obstruction
- haemothorax/pneumothorax
- sepsis
- haemorrhage
- rhabdomyolysis
- pulmonary oedema
- pneumonia
- bone metastases related hypercalcaemia
- cervical/thoracic spinal cord injury.

Oxygen saturation

Pulse oximetry indicates a patient's arterial oxygenation levels and, in conjunction with respiratory rate, can give a clearer clinical picture of pulmonary status. However it is important not to be too reliant on oxygen saturation as there can be falling oxygen delivery despite normal arterial oxygen saturation; metabolic acidosis can increase the respiratory rate even though the arterial oxygen saturation may be normal. Hence, a normal SPO^2 does not rule out acute respiratory distress. In addition pulse oximetry can be affected by other variables such as movement, the presence of unusual haemoglobin varieties, a cold environment, poor perfusion, arrhythmias and the presence of nail varnish (ACT Health 2007). Some reasons for decreased oxygen saturations in the orthopaedic patient include:

- fat embolism
- pulmonary embolism
- respiratory tract infection
- airway trauma/obstruction
- haemothorax pneumothorax
- sepsis
- hypovolaemia
- rhabdomyolysis
- pulmonary oedema
- pneumonia.

Temperature

A raised temperature often indicates the presence of infection. However sepsis should also be considered in a patient with a "normal" temperature. Septic patients often present as hypothermic as an overwhelmed immune system may lack the ability to generate a response. For more information on septic shock see Chapter 9. Some reasons for altered temperature in the orthopaedic patient include:

- Infection or sepsis,
- exposure
- autonomic dysreflexia (refer to Chapter 19).

Pulse

The heart rate is an important aspect of the chain of oxygen delivery (Figure 16.1). In simple terms when there is a deficiency in oxygen delivery the heart beats faster to try and compensate. Cardiac output is the amount of blood pumped out by each ventricle in one minute. Cardiac output is dependent on the heart rate and stroke volume which is the amount of blood pumped out by a ventricle with each contraction. When the blood volume is decreased or heart muscle damaged the stroke volume is decreased and the heart rate is increased in an effort to maintain cardiac output (tachycardia). Some common reasons for tachycardia in an orthopaedic patient include:

- hypovolaemia
- sepsis
- fat embolism
- pulmonary embolism
- electrolyte imbalance
- substance abuse.

Blood pressure

Blood Pressure = Cardiac Output × Peripheral Resistance

A decrease in blood pressure suggests a decrease in cardiac output and may result in delayed or insufficient oxygenation of tissues. Early warning scores focus on the systolic measurement and hypotension, as a falling blood pressure is a key indicator of a critical event. This is not to say that a hypertensive patient doesn't warrant review, and clinical judgment should be used at all times.

Common causes of hypertension in the orthopaedic patient include:

- pain
- autonomic dysreflexia
- bone metastases related hypercalcaemia.

Common causes of hypotension in the orthopaedic patient include:

- hypovolaemia
- sepsis
- cardiogenic shock
- neurogenic shock
- dehydration.

The patient in spinal shock or with a spinal cord injury will have a lower pulse rate and blood pressure due to unopposed vagal nerve activity (Chapter 19).

Mental status

A depressed level of consciousness or sudden onset of confusion is a clear sign of a deteriorating patient and may be as a result of intracranial disease, inadequate oxygen delivery or metabolic abnormalities (e.g. hypoglycaemia). The patient with a head injury or sudden altered consciousness level requires more in-depth monitoring than that provided by EWS such as the Glasgow coma scale. Some reasons for a depressed level of consciousness in the orthopaedic patient include:

- head trauma/injury
- cerebrovascular disease/haemorrhage
- encephalitis
- delirium
- hypoglycaemia
- electrolyte imbalances
- substance abuse
- hypoxia related (e.g. fat embolism, pulmonary embolism, sepsis).

Urinary output

Urinary output is not routinely recorded as part of an EWS but some institutions have adopted it as a 6th parameter where patients are catheterised. A decreased urine output is an indicator of patient deterioration and is often one of the earliest signs of decline. The expected output for an adult is >0.5 ml/kg per hour. For example a patient weighing 60 kg should produce 30 mls/hr. Some reasons for a low urinary output in the orthopaedic patient include:

- dehydration
- hypovolaemia
- shock
- urinary obstruction/trauma
- renal failure
- low output cola-coloured urine consider rhabdomyolysis.

Summary

Significant traumatic injury can be life threatening. Care systems are in place which are designed to prevent death at each stage of care. Knowledge of the effects of trauma and careful assessment and observation of the patient following trauma is the main feature of successful care and of preventing and recognising life threatening deterioration and potential for significant life changing disability.

Recommended further reading

Duncan, N.S. and Moran, C. (2009) Initial resuscitation of the trauma victim. *Orthopaedics and Trauma*, **24**(1), 1–8.

Gwinnutt, C.L. and Driscoll, P.A. (eds) (2003) *Trauma Resuscitation: The Team Approach*. Taylor and Francis, London.

NCEPOD (2007) *Trauma: Who Cares? A Report of the National Confidential Enquiry Into Patient Outcome and Death*. Available at: http://www.ncepod.org.uk/2007report2/Downloads/SIP_report.pdf (Accessed 1 August 2012).

O'Shea, R.A. (2005) *Principles and Practice of Trauma Nursing*. Churchill Livingstone, Edinburgh.

Skinner, D.V. and Driscoll, P.A. (2013) *ABC of Major Trauma*, 4th edn. Wiley Blackwell, Oxford.

References

ACT Health (2007) *Early Recognition of the Deteriorating Patient Program*. Available at: http://health.act.gov.au/professionals/general-information/compass/login/adult-program/ (accessed 1 July 2012).

American College of Surgeons (2004) *ATLS Advanced Trauma Life Support Program for Doctors*, 7th edn. American College of Surgeons, Chicago.

Banning, M. (2007) A review of clinical decision making: models and current research. *Journal of Clinical Nursing*, **17**(2), 187–195.

Bleyer, A.J., Vidya, S., Russel, G.B. *et al.* (2011) Longitudinal analysis of one million vital signs in patients in an academic medical center. *Resuscitation*, **82**(11), 1387–1392.

Boyle, M.J., Smith, E.C. and Archer, F. (2008) Is mechanism of injury alone a useful predictor of major trauma? *International Journal of the Care of the Injured*, **39**(9), 986–992.

College of Emergency Medicine (2010) *Guidelines on the Management of Alert, Adult Patients with Potential Cervical Spine Injury in the Emergency Department*. College of Emergency Medicine, London.

Driscoll, P., Bates, D. and Lomas, G. (2003) Resuscitation and stabilization of the severely injured patient, in *Trauma Resuscitation: The Team Approach* (eds C.L. Gwinutt and P.A. Driscoll), Taylor and Francis, London, pp. 1–24.

Duncan, N.S. and Moran, C. (2009) Initial resuscitation of the trauma victim. *Orthopaedics and Trauma*, **24**(1), 1–8.

Fullerton, J.N., Price, C.L., Silvey, N.E., Brace, S.J. and Perkins, G.D. (2012) Is the Modified Early Warning Score (MEWS) superior to clinical judgment in detecting critical illness in the pre-hospital environment? *Resuscitation*, **83**(5), 557–562.

Garcea, G., Ganga, R., Neal, C.P. *et al.* (2010) Preoperative early warning scores can predict in-hospital mortality and critical care admission following emergency surgery. *Journal of Surgical Research*, **159**, 729–734.

Gwinnutt, C.L. and Driscoll, P.A. (eds) (2003) *Trauma Resuscitation: The Team Approach*. Taylor and Francis, London.

Haider, A.H., Chang, D.C., Haut, E.R., Cornwell, E.E. and Efron, D.T. (2009) Mechanism of injury predicts patient mortality and impairment after blunt trauma. *Journal of Surgical Research* **153**(1), 138–142.

Harrison, P. (2000) *Managing Spinal Injury: Critical Care*. Spinal Injuries Association, London,

Henning, J., Woods, K. and Howley, M. (2011) Management of major trauma. *Anaesthesia and Intensive Care Medicine*, **12**(9), 383–386.

Hoffman, J.R., Mower, W.R., Wolfson, A.B. *et al.* (2000) Validity of a set of clinical criteria to rule out injury to the cervical spine in patients with blunt trauma. National Emergency X-Radiography Utilization Study Group. *New England Journal of Medicine*, **343**(2), 94–99.

Health Service Executive (HSE) (2011) *National Policy and Procedure for the Use of the Modified Early Warning Score System to Recognise and Respond to Clinical Deterioration*. HSE, Dublin.

Keel, M. and Trentz, O. (2005) Pathophysiology of polytrauma. *Injury*, **36**(6), 691–709.

Kwan, I., Bunn, F., Roberts, I. on behalf of the WHO Pre-Hospital Trauma Care Steering Committee (2009) Spinal immobilisation for trauma patients. *Cochrane Database of Systematic Reviews* **2** (Art. No.: CD002803). DOI: 10.1002/14651858.CD002803.

Mann, S. and Bowler, M. (2008) Using an early warning score tool in community nursing. *Nursing Times*, **104**(20), 30–31.

Massey, D. and Meredith, T. (2010) Respiratory Assessment 1: Why do it and how to do it? *British Journal of Cardiac Nursing*, **5**(11), 537–541.

McGaughy, J., Alderdice, F., Fowler, R. *et al.* (2007) Outreach and early warning systems (EWS) for the prevention of intensive care admission and death of critically ill adult patients on general hospital wards. *Cochrane Database of Systematic Reviews* **3**(Art No.:CD005529). DOI:10.1002/14651858.CD005529.PUB.2.

McRae, R. and Esser, M. (2008) *Practical Fracture Treatment*, 5th edn. Churchill Livingstone, Edinburgh.

Morgan, R.J., Williams, F. and Wright, M.M. (1997) An early warning scoring system for detecting developing critical illness. *Clinical Intensive Care*, **8**, 100.

National Institute for Health and Clinical Excellence (NICE) (2007) *Acutely Ill Patients in Hospital: Recognition of and Response to Acute Illness in Adults in Hospital*. NICE, London.

National Institute for Health and Clinical Excellence (2007) *Head Injury. Triage, Assessment, Investigation and Early Management of Head Injury in Infants, Children and Adults*. CG56. NICE, London. Available at: http://www.nice.org.uk/nicemedia/pdf/CG56QuickRedGuide.pdf (accessed 22 April 2014).

NCEPOD (2007) Trauma: Who Cares? A Report of the National Confidential Enquiry Into Patient Outcome and Death. Available at: http://www.ncepod.org.uk/2007report2/Downloads/SIP_report.pdf (accessed 1 August 2012).

Nicks, B.A., Ayello, E.A., Woo, K., Nitziki-George, D. and Sibbald, R.G. (2010) Acute wound management: revisiting the approach to assessment, irrigation, and closure considerations. *International Journal of Emergency Medicine*, **3**(4), 399–407.

Odell, M., Victor, C. and Oliver, D. (2009) Nurses' role in detecting deterioration in ward patients: systematic literature review. *Journal of Advanced Nursing*, **65**(10), 1992–2006.

Pape, H., Pietzman, A.B., Schwab, C.W. and Giannoudis, P.V. (eds) (2010) *Damage Control Management in the Polytrauma Patient*. Springer, New York.

Parkes, R. (2011) Rate of respiration: the forgotten vital sign. *Emergency Nurse*, **19**(2), 12–17.

Raynor, F.K. (2010) Trust brings back manual checks of vital signs to enhance patient safety. *Nursing Standard*, **24** (30), 8.

Rees, J.E. (2003) Early warning scores. *Update in Anaesthesia*, **17** (10), 30–33.

Teasdale, G. and Jennett, B. (1974) Assessment of coma and impaired consciousness. A practical scale. *Lancet*, **2**(7872), 81–84.

Richards, P.J. (2005) Cervical spine clearance: a review. *International Journal of the Care of the Injured*, **36**(2), 248–269.

Roissant, R., Bouillon, B., Cerny, V. *et al.* (2010) Management of bleeding following major trauma: an updated European guideline. *Critical Care*, **14**(2), 1–29.

Shanmuganthan, R. (2008) The utility of scores in the decision to salvage or amputate in severely injured limbs. *Indian Journal of Orthopaedics*, **42**(4), 368–376.

Scottish Intercollegiate Guidelines Network (SIGN) (2009) Early *Management of Patients with a Head Injury*. National

Clinical Guideline 110. Available at: http://www.sign.ac.uk/pdf/sign110.pdf (accessed 3 January 2013).

Smith, I., Mackay, J. and Fahrid, N. (2011) Respiratory rate measurement: a comparison of methods. *British Journal of Healthcare Assistants*, **5**(11), 18–23.

Soloman, L., Warwick, D.J. and Nayagam, S. (2005) Management of major injuries, in *Apleys Concise System of Orthopaedics and Fractures* (eds L. Soloman, D.J. Warwick and S. Nayagam), 3rd edn, Hodder Arnold, London, pp. 257–265.

Spahn, D.R. and Ganter, M.T. (2010) Towards early individual goal-directed coagulation management in trauma patients. *British Journal of Anaesthesia*, **105**(2), 103–105.

Stiell, I.G., Wells, A.G., Vandemheen, K.L. *et al.* (2001) The Canadian C-spine rule for radiography in alert and stable trauma patients. *Journal of the American Medical Association*, **286**(15), 1841–1848.

Thompson, C., Bucknall, T., Estabrookes, C.A. *et al.* (2007) Nurses' critical event risk assessments: a judgment analysis. *Journal of Clinical Nursing*, **18**, 601–612.

Webber-Jones, J.E., Thomas, C.A. and Bordeaux, R.A. (2002) The management and prevention of rigid cervical collar complications. *Orthopaedic Nursing*, **21**(4), 19–25.

World Health Organization (WHO) (2004) *Guidelines for Essential Trauma Care*. WHO, Geneva.

CHAPTER 17

Principles of fracture management

Sonya Clarke[1], Julie Santy-Tomlinson[2], Sinead McDonald[3] and Pamela Moore[4]

[1] *Queen's University Belfast, Belfast, UK*
[2] *University of Hull, Hull, UK*
[3] *Royal Victoria Hospital, Belfast, UK*
[4] *Royal Victoria Hospital, Belfast, UK*

Introduction

Resulting from a variety of mechanisms of injury, fractures form the bulk of orthopaedic work in the trauma setting. The care of patients with fractures demands an understanding of how injury affects bone and the surrounding soft tissue and how the process of bone repair can be facilitated through effective management and care. In spite of the relatively severe forces required to fracture a bone, skeletal injuries are extremely common and are a major reason for attending the emergency department. Fracture clinics are often the largest and busiest outpatients' settings in any acute general hospital and sustaining a fracture is a significant reason for admission to hospital. The incidence of fracture in the general population in England, as one example, has been estimated to be as high as 3.6 fractures per 100 people per year. This represents a significant public health burden and significant cost to society (Donaldson *et al.*, 2008). The highest incidence of fracture is found in young males from 16 to 24 years of age, often due to high energy trauma and frequently involving long bones. Conversely, those aged 65 or older primarily suffer a fracture due to falls following which the most common injuries include those occurring as fragility fractures in the wrist, proximal femur, upper humerus, vertebrae and pelvis/pubic rami as these sites are most often affected by osteoporosis. Of all musculoskeletal injuries fractures are the most serious, contributing to approximately 40% of fatalities due to trauma and associated complications. See Chapter 16 for further general information about the care and management of the patient following trauma. The present chapter mainly focuses on the principles of fracture management and care in the adult although many such principles can be applied to the care of the child and young adult. Chapters 23 and 24 specifically consider fractures in children.

Causes and types of fractures

Fractures involve a loss of continuity in the substance of bone. They are usually the result of different types and magnitude of blunt force. The force required to result in a fracture of the shaft of femur in a healthy person aged 25, for example, is significant and is also considerably greater than that needed to result in the fracture of a hip in the older person with osteoporotic bone. An assessment and understanding of the 'mechanism of injury' can provide essential information that can assist with differential diagnosis and subsequent management of fractures. This can also help identify non-accidental injury in vulnerable patients such as children (Chapter 21), adults with a learning disability, those with mental health conditions such as dementia and those with complex physical or cognitive impairment.

There are five blunt forces that commonly result in fracture:

Shearing

occurs when one end of a bone is motionless while the other end is bowed or bent. When a shearing force is applied, a transverse or linear fracture occurs in

Orthopaedic and Trauma Nursing: An Evidence-based Approach to Musculoskeletal Care, First Edition. Edited by Sonya Clarke and Julie Santy-Tomlinson.

which one section of bone moves away from the other. This is often the result of a person attempting to stop themselves falling by putting out a hand to 'save' themselves; known as a 'fall on an outstretched hand' or FOOSH. Shearing forces are also created by a direct blow from a large instrument or object and can be significant in injures to the epiphyseal plate in children and young adults.

Compression

is a force that pushes inward from the end of a bone. This often causes multiple fracture lines that are wide-reaching and which tend to radiate from the point of impact. This type of force is most often applied to the skull or vertebral bodies. The shape of the displaced bone often reflects the instrument that has created the fracture. This mechanism is also common in fragility fractures of osteoporotic bone.

Bending

is the most common type of force. The force is delivered at a right angle, causing a triangular fracture, usually through its cross-section. This tends to cause fracture lines at the point of impact or on the side opposite to the break. A common fracture caused by a bending force is a 'Parry fracture' of the ulna, occurring when a person holds out their arms in self-defence and the impact causes inward displacement of the bone.

Torsion

involves twisting forces; one end of bone is held motionless while the other end is twisted, often resulting in a spiral fracture. This can occur in sporting injuries such as football and skiing and can be the result of non-accidental injury in children and babies.

Tension

is a force that pulls on the long axis of a bone which may cause a fracture, but more often causes dislocation of the joint. When the force is strong enough, a section of healthy bone may be pulled away by a ligament under tension; this is known as an avulsion fracture.

Describing fractures

Fractures are described according to several criteria, often in combination:

- the force involved in the fracture (mechanism of injury) e.g. compression, impacted, burst (of vertebral body), depressed (fracture of skull)
- the severity of the fracture ; simple, complex, comminuted (several fragments)
- the direction, appearance shape or position of the fracture line e.g. oblique, transverse, spiral, linear
- the anatomical site of the fracture e.g. intertrochanteric (proximal femur), mid-shaft (femur), supracondylar (distal femur) and any articular surface involvement
- special features of the fracture ; e.g. compound (open) or closed, incomplete (or 'greenstick'), avulsion, rotation, shortening, angulation or fragmentation.

Some fractures are also named after the surgeon who first described them, for example Potts fracture of the ankle, Colles fracture of the wrist. Figure 17.1 shows a few examples of types of fractures (see also Figure 23.3).

The mechanism of injury determines the fracture pattern. Sudden or direct trauma, for example, typically results in a complete fracture in adults with an oblique/transverse pattern. In children this can sometimes result in an incomplete/buckled 'Greenstick' fracture (Chapter 24). Indirect forces away from fracture site often produce a spiral pattern. Repetitive force on a bone causes mechanical strain and fatigue, resulting in a 'stress' fracture.

It is important for the nurse/practitioner to understand the terms used to describe fractures as this is the language that is used in team discussions when planning and reviewing fracture management options.

Fracture repair

The process of fracture repair is a remarkable physiological process that results in a healed structure that, providing the conditions are right, will be as mechanically sound post-healing as prior to the fracture. It is essential that the practitioner has an understanding of the physiology of fracture healing as this has a direct bearing on the decision making and planning processes for fracture management. Each of the stages and events in the bone healing process is central to decision making regarding treatment and management options as well as influencing the care of the patient.

The process of bone healing can be broken down into several phases (Figure 17.2), but usually occurs in a seamless sequence of events. The timing of these events

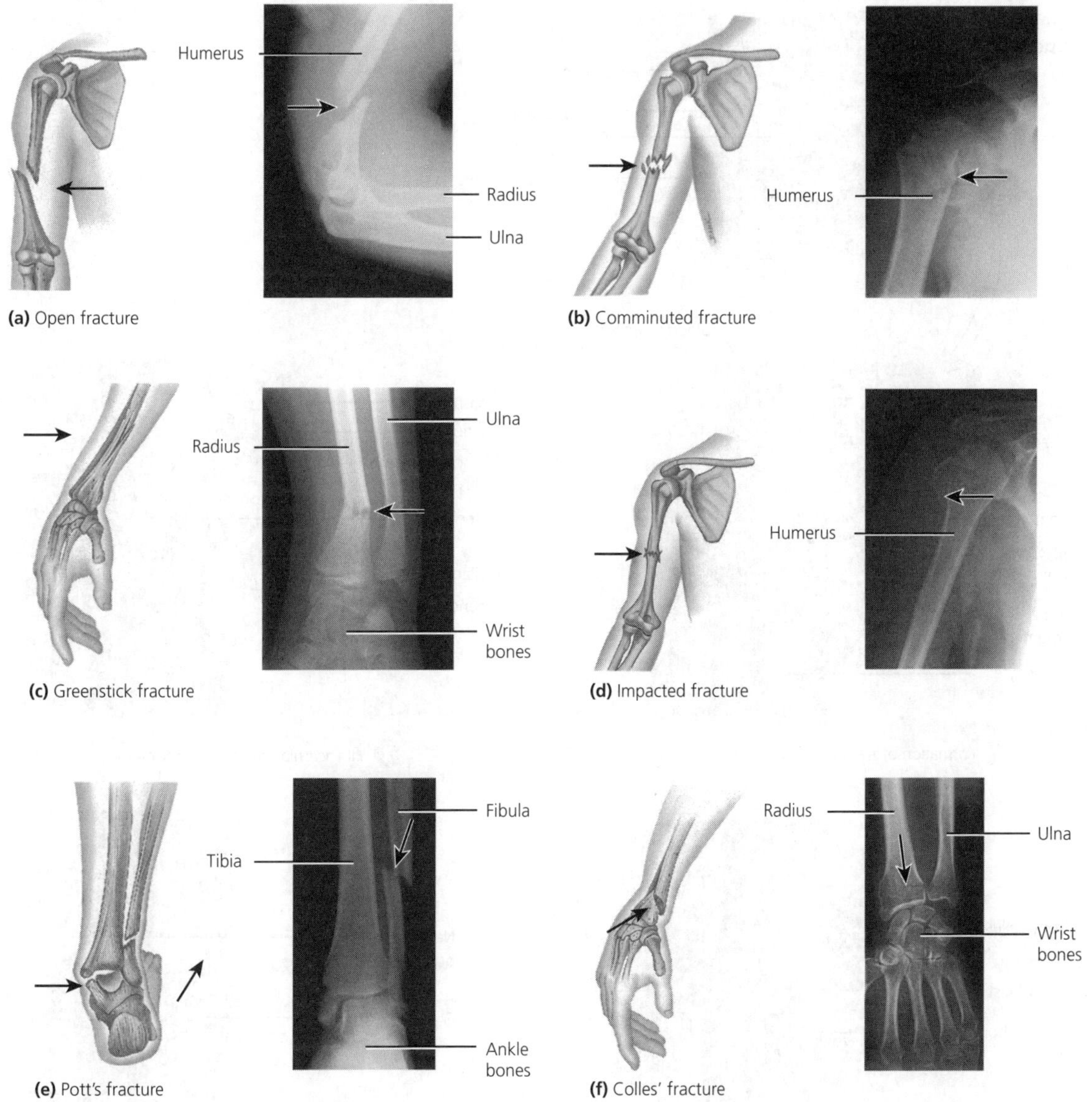

Figure 17.1 Examples of types of fractures. Kuntzman, A.J. and Tortora, G.J. *Anatomy and physiology for the manual therapies*. 2010, Wiley. This material is reproduced with permission of John Wiley & Sons, Inc.

will vary according to the nature of the bone fractured, the type of fracture and other factors such as blood supply and the state of health of the patient. Fracture healing times are shortest, for example, in young children with incomplete fractures; sometimes as little as two or three weeks. Flat bones such as the clavicle and scapula that do not bear any weight can often heal in around six weeks. A long bone fracture (e.g. femur) in a healthy adult takes on average 12 weeks to heal, but this time is extended considerably in older patients with concurrent medical conditions and with osteoporosis/fragility fracture. Some bones have a poorer blood supply than others and this has a significant impact on healing. Tibial fractures may take up to 24 weeks to heal even in a healthy adult.

1. Haematoma and inflammation

In the early weeks following injury fracture healing is much like that of any other tissue. Bone is highly

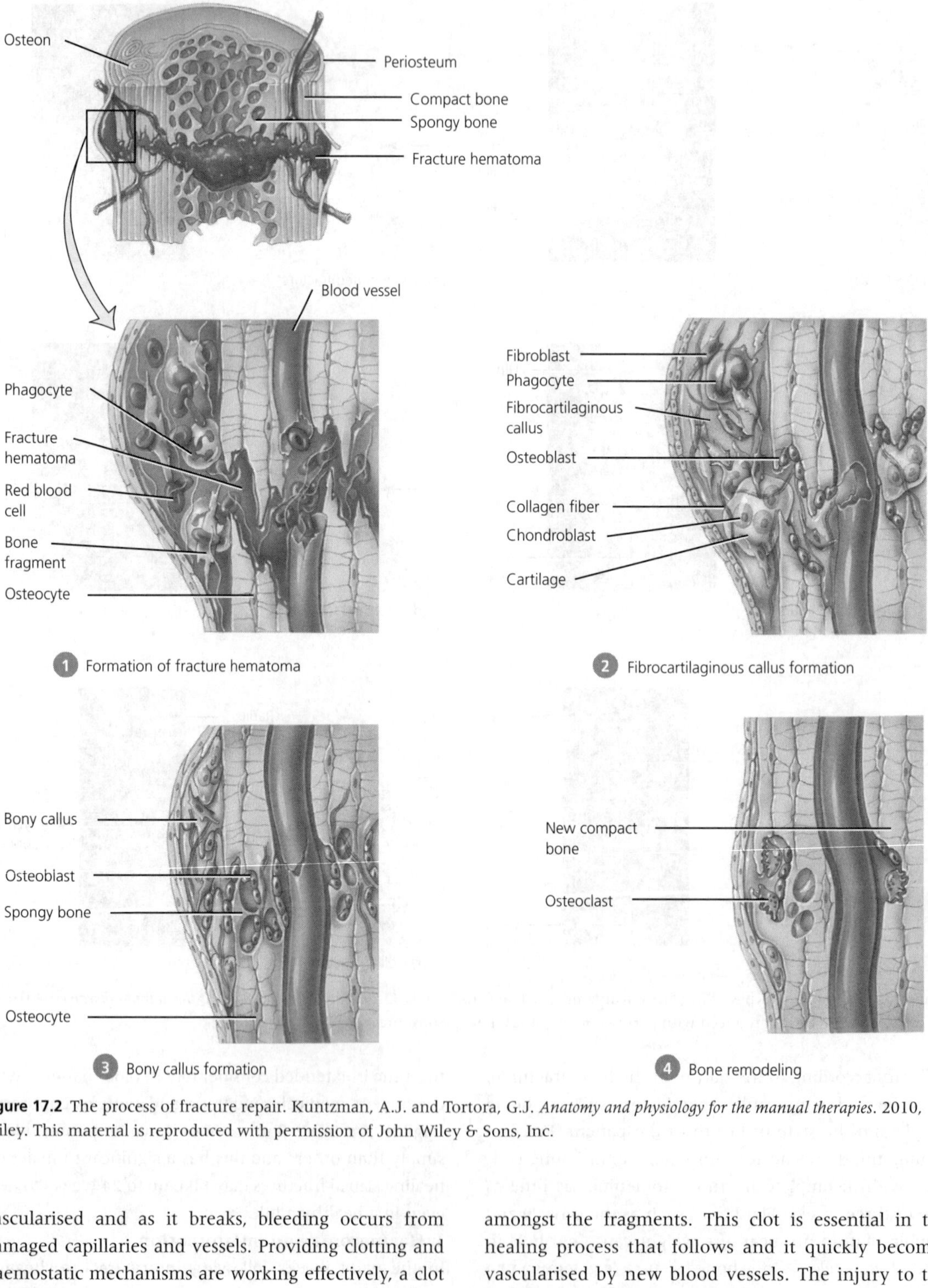

Figure 17.2 The process of fracture repair. Kuntzman, A.J. and Tortora, G.J. *Anatomy and physiology for the manual therapies*. 2010, Wiley. This material is reproduced with permission of John Wiley & Sons, Inc.

vascularised and as it breaks, bleeding occurs from damaged capillaries and vessels. Providing clotting and haemostatic mechanisms are working effectively, a clot rapidly forms between the two bone ends and/or amongst the fragments. This clot is essential in the healing process that follows and it quickly becomes vascularised by new blood vessels. The injury to the bone and surrounding tissue results in an initial acute inflammatory response which stimulates the migration of macrophages to the site of injury. These are central in the phagocytosis of the clot and necrotic tissue debris. Disturbance of this inflammatory process can adversely affect healing.

There are two types of specialised cells that are central to bone healing:

Osteoblasts: lay down new bone matrices

Osteoclasts: resorb bone enabling bone remodelling to take place.

2. Granulation

Gradually collagen fibres are laid down within the clot as it is absorbed by the macrophages. Mineral salts, including calcium, are deposited within the new framework. During the first few weeks after the fracture, the blood clot is invaded by macrophages and osteoclasts and the sharp bone edges are removed (Dandy and Edwards 2009).

3. Primary callus

Cells begin to proliferate and lay down new woven bone with collagen arranged in short bundles of fibres. This stage relies greatly on a good blood supply to the fracture site. A cuff of woven bone gradually forms, initially under the periosteum and at the ends of the bone. This brings the bone ends together externally but does not yet bridge the gap between them centrally. This stage lacks the lamellar arrangement of mature bone and as yet has little strength (Woolf 2000).

4. Bridging callus

Gradually the gap between the bone ends is bridged by granulation tissue and osteoblasts. Collars of subperiosteal bone begin to advance across the fracture gap. Reaching a stage where bone has formed enough bridging callus takes between 6 and 12 weeks in healthy adults, although there are differences in timing in the developing and ageing musculoskeletal system.

5. Remodelling

Once union has taken place and weight bearing has begun to occur, the bone is gradually reshaped and smoothed through a process of resorption. This can take up to a year. This process enables any minor displacement of bone to be rectified as the bone develops a structure that reflects the mechanical forces placed upon it. For this reason, fracture healing is greatly enhanced by weight bearing (axial loading) once bridging callus has formed and this is considered when making treatment decisions.

Assessment and emergency care

A full holistic assessment of the patient is an essential part of providing care for patients with fractures rather than focusing entirely on the suspected fracture. In addition to the general care and management of the traumatically injured patient described in Chapter 16, there are a number of specific considerations in relation to the patient with a fracture in the first hours following the injury.

A full history that includes the mechanism of injury should comprise:

- description of events
- time since injury
- pain and inability to weight bear at the time of injury and since.

Holistic assessment of the patient and injury should include:

- swelling
- visible deformity of the limb
- assessment for any associated numbness or paraesthesia
- assessment for any signs of compromised blood supply
- observation for any wounds over or close to the fracture site.

The main symptom of fracture is pain. It is often this that sends the patient for treatment within minutes or hours after the initial injury. On the whole this pain is severe but there are some types of fractures (impacted fractures of the proximal femur for example) that produce less pain and may lead the patient to delay seeking treatment. Effective pain management should be provided as discussed in Chapter 11 prior to any detailed assessment of the injury. Other symptoms include swelling and reduced mobility of the affected limb/joint. There may also be a tendency to protect the limb due to tenderness and discomfort over the affected area and the patient will be reluctant to allow the practitioner to touch the limb. Loss of power, deformity of the limb and irregularity of the contour of the limb may also be noted. Crepitus (bony grating) may be also heard or felt and movement at the fracture site may have been noted by the patient at the time of injury but during examination this should not be tested for as movement at the fracture site should be avoided.

All patients with a suspected fracture require a radiographic examination. X-ray images taken from two or more angles provide the team with a detailed view of the fracture that can be used in planning treatment.

A number of 'decision rules' are in use in the emergency department (ED) to help the practitioner decide if a patient requires an X-ray. The most common of these are the Ottawa Ankle Rules (Stiell *et al.*, 1994) and Ottawa Knee Rules (Stiell *et al.*, 1997), which provide assessment criteria that have been shown by research to be predictive of fracture or otherwise and help to reduce the number of unnecessary X-rays.

While assessment and definitive treatment planning is taking place, care needs to focus on ensuring minimum mobility at the fracture site. Any movement of the fracture can lead to further soft tissue and neurovascular damage. This can, in turn, lead to increased blood loss (for this reason all patients with major long bone fractures require intravenous access and fluid replacement). The limb or body part should be carefully but firmly splinted to prevent undue movement of the fracture while the patient is being moved and assessed. No attempt should be made to change the position of the limb or 'manipulate' the fracture at this time. The type of splinting used will vary according to the site of the fracture. In the limbs splints should include the joint above and below the fracture. In upper limb injuries a sling can often be used to support the arm. If an unstable pelvic fracture is suspected 'pelvic binding' (e.g. wrapping a folder sheet around the pelvis) can be applied in order to reduce the contents of the pelvis and providing pressure to any sites of haemorrhage. Suspected spinal fractures are immobilised using a spinal board initially along with head blocks to immobilise the neck. Splints and immobilising devices should only be applied temporarily until a full assessment can be conducted. The neurovascular status of the limb should be assessed both prior to and following application of any splint (Chapter 9).

An important consideration in the initial management of fractures at the scene of injury, during transfer and in early hospital management is the management of pain. Pain can vary but is often very severe and increased by any movement. In spite of this, pain management can often be neglected both at the scene of the injury and during emergency management (Chapter 11). Pre-hospital care practitioners are increasingly able to administer both systemic and regional analgesia at the scene and it is important that good pain assessment and analgesia practice is maintained throughout the early stages of care in order to facilitate patient comfort and reduced anxiety whilst assessment and planning take place. In the case of lower limb fractures, femoral nerve blocks are increasingly used. The advantages of this approach include better facilitation of assessment with less pain, faster and more effective pain relief and avoidance of the complications of systemic analgesics (Black *et al.*, 2012) which can be particularly important in the older person with a fracture.

It is particularly important to remember that the use of NSAIDs is contraindicated in patients with fractures as they have been shown to inhibit bone healing in a number of animal studies, although the voracity of the evidence is considered controversial (Hernandez *et al.*, 2012). This does, however, mean that an important group of analgesics is not generally available for this group of patients and so other options must be considered carefully.

The complications of fractures

The care of patients with fractures should take into account the fact that bony injuries have a high rate of complications and can be associated with a significant physiological response to trauma. The complications of fractures are seen more often in severe fractures of long bones and the bones of the axial skeleton such as the pelvis, spine, head and chest wall as these are usually associated with high impact mechanisms of injury and are frequently combined with other injuries such as multiple fractures and significant injury to soft tissue and visceral organs. The main complications of fractures include (see Chapter 9 for further detail):

- ***Haemorrhage*** – blood loss from a closed fracture of the mid shaft of the femur can, for example, amount to up to one litre and severe 'open book' fracture of the pelvis up to 3 litres (McRae and Esser 2008) amounting to life-threatening haemorrhage and shock.
- ***Fat Embolism*** and fat embolism syndrome, especially in fractures of the shaft of femur.
- ***Compartment Syndrome*** and other types of neurovascular injury.
- ***Infection*** – especially in compound fractures which can lead to osteomyelitis.
- ***Complications arising from immobility*** e.g. venous thromboembolism, pressure ulcers (Chapter 12), chest infection, urinary tract infection, muscle wasting, constipation.
- ***Complications arising from surgery*** e.g. haemorrhage and shock, haematoma, wound infection (Chapter 12), wound dehiscence.

Management of fractures

The primary goals of fracture management are to achieve fracture healing without deformity and to restore function so that the patient can resume normal daily life (McRae and Esser 2008). Five main aspects of fracture treatment and management are summarised as the 'five Rs':

- ***Resuscitation*** – Resuscitation of the patient following trauma is always a priority and is considered in detail in Chapter 16. Fracture and associated soft tissue trauma cause considerable bleeding and shock. First aid is fundamental when there is high suspicion of fracture (diagnosis) and immobilisation of the fracture is pivotal in preventing haemorrhage and further injury.
- ***Reduction*** – Some displacement of fractures can be accommodated by the healing (remodelling) process. Significant displacement, angulation or rotation need early closed reduction or open reduction with or without internal/external fixation depending on the stability of the fracture and the medical condition of the patient. Intra-articular fractures require anatomical reduction to ensure joint surfaces are maintained as much as possible.
- ***Restriction*** – Fractures require immobilisation to facilitate the healing process. This prevents mobility at the facture site and can take a variety of forms dictated by the initial fracture management plan.
- ***Restoration*** – a full understanding of the fracture gained from assessment will result in definitive management of fractures. Chapter 8 explores key musculoskeletal interventions commonly used to treat fractures. Principal approaches include one or a combination of the following:
  - External methods
    - casts, splints and orthotics
    - traction
    - external fixation
    - closed reduction
  - Internal methods
    - open reduction with or without internal or external fixation
    - internal fixation e.g. plates, screws and intramedullary nails
    - total or hemi-arthroplasty
    - K-wires.
- ***Rehabilitation*** – Following a significant period of immobilisation of several weeks or months, joints will become stiff and muscles are weakened by lack of use, even if the patient has exercised the joints not immobilised. The patient will need to gradually re-engage with movement of the limb, joints and muscles as strength and flexibility gradually improve. In some cases this journey will depend on a number of factors including the severity of the injury, the medical and general fitness of the patient and their motivation to reach their rehabilitation potential (see Chapter 7 for further discussion of the principles of rehabilitation). This may require a period of outpatient physiotherapy. Some patients may have residual disability following rehabilitation.

Facilitating fracture healing

An understanding of what encourages and inhibits fracture healing is helpful in understanding the conditions required for healing and those interventions likely to be most effective in supporting healing. Numerous factors may mean that fractures do not heal (non-union) or heal slowly (slow or delayed union) or do not heal in good/anatomic position (malunion).

Fracture healing is encouraged by:

- Firm (but not too tight) immobilisation of the fracture in the early stages of healing so that the gradually revascularised haematoma is not disrupted.
- Axial loading (weight bearing) once bridging callus has formed to enable new bone to be laid down along lines of stress.
- Good general health and diet which provides the protein, calories, calcium and other nutrients required to physiologically support healing.

Fracture healing is inhibited by:

- Movement at the fracture site during the earlier stages of healing as this disrupts newly forming capillaries.
- Poor circulation to the fracture site reducing the availability of oxygen and the nutrients required for healing.
- Diseased and weakened bone (e.g. osteoporosis) in which bone cells are less active.
- Joint involvement. Synovial fluid inhibits healing. Disruption of articular (hyaline) cartilage often leads to secondary osteoarthritis is later life.
- Large amounts of surrounding soft-tissue damage.
- Infection.

- Some drugs, especially NSAIDs, as these have been shown to inhibit healing because they dampen down the much needed inflammatory response.
- Poor general health and nutrition.
- Smoking.

These factors are taken into account when choosing methods for supporting fractures whilst they heal.

Open fractures

Open, or compound, fractures occur when there is a break in the skin, providing a conduit between the external environment and the fracture. There are two mechanisms by which this can occur:

1 ***From without in.*** External injury to the skin and soft tissues overlying the fracture opens a wound that connects with the fracture.
2 ***From within out.*** Sharp edges of the fracture lacerate overlying soft tissue and pierce the skin. This mechanism can also result in a fracture blister. Fluid of blood-filled blisters lie over the fracture and, although the skin might not be broken, should be treated as a compound fracture wound.

Open fractures are associated with significant soft tissue damage and, as a consequence, are at significant risk of infection. All open fractures must be assumed to be contaminated and the main aim of treatment is to prevent infection. In the emergency setting, the wound should be photographed so that repeated uncovering is avoided and then covered with a sterile dressing on presentation. Antibiotic prophylaxis should be administered and tetanus immunisation status evaluated. Open fractures require early operation and ideally this should be performed within six hours of injury. In the event that early surgery does not take place, stabilisation with external fixation is recommended (BOA/BAPRAS 2007: see Box 17.1). Aims of surgery are to:

- clean the wound
- remove devitalised tissue
- stabilise the fracture.

Small clean wounds can be sutured but large dirty wounds debrided and left open. Debrided wounds can be closed by delayed primary suture at five days. Postoperative wound management is a challenge and some centres now employ Negative Wound Pressure Therapy as a wound management strategy (Blum *et al.*, 2012). If there has been significant soft tissue loss, reconstruction will be required under the care of a plastic surgeon.

A 'Gustilo' (Gustilo *et al.*, 1984) classification system (Table 17.1) is commonly used to describe soft tissue injury associated with a compound fracture and is used to direct treatment. The use of a classification system is important as it facilitates communication among clinicians, as well as assisting clinicians in decision making, anticipating potential problems,

Box 17.1 Evidence digest: Management of open fractures (BOA/BAPRAS 2009)

Standards from BOA/BAPRAS (2009) offer an evidence-based approach to the management of patients with complex injuries of the lower limb that include a fracture and significant associated soft tissue injury – an open or compound fracture – which most often occur in the lower leg. It is based on guidelines developed by representatives of two specialist medical associations with an interest in these complex injuries which often result in disability and amputation. Although the guidelines were generated by a group of orthopaedic and plastic surgeons, they have great relevance to the entire trauma team including nurses and other practitioners.

The guidelines illustrate clearly how it is not always possible to base practice on 'higher' levels of evidence such as randomised trials when these are few or are conflicting, as is the case in this aspect of care. The authors have, however, been able to draw on other forms of evidence both in publications and clinical experience and expertise to put the evidence in context and offer clinicians a set of useful practical recommendations for 'best' practice. The document shows how 'evidence-based' does not always mean based on randomised controlled trials of interventions and how other forms of evidence can be central in ensuring effective care. In particular the recommendations focus on the need for a multidisciplinary approach to care that meets the needs of patients with these complex injuries and facilitates careful, expert management of both the skeletal and the soft tissue injury.

Practitioners need to take note, in particular, of their responsibilities for wound care, assessment for neurovascular complications and the rehabilitation and psychosocial support of the patient and family. What the document also illustrates is how important it is that nursing and other non-medical staff have an in-depth knowledge of treatment decisions and options so that the care they provide can take into account that knowledge and understanding, particularly in making sure that patients receive adequate support and information during their care journey.

Table 17.1 Gustilo classification system for compound fractures (Gustilo *et al.*, 1984). Reproduced with permission from LWW

Type I	An open fracture with a wound <1 cm long and clean
Type II	An open fracture with a laceration >1 cm long without excessive soft tissue damage, flaps, or avulsions
Type III	Massive soft tissue damage, compromised vascularity, severe wound contamination, and marked fracture instability
Type IIIA	Adequate soft tissue coverage of a fractured bone, despite extensive soft tissue laceration, flaps or high-energy trauma irrespective of the size of the wound
Type IIIB	Extensive soft tissue injury loss with periosteal stripping and bone exposure; usually associated with massive contamination

suggesting treatment options, predicting patient and surgical outcomes and documenting cases. However there are discussions regarding the inter-observer reliability of the Gustilo classification plus its ability to predict patient outcome. Other classifications systems include the Mangled Extremity Severity score (MESS) (Johansen *et al.*, 1990). Management of the open fracture depends on the site of injury and type of fracture. The wound is subsequently stabilised either temporarily or definitively. If soft-tissue coverage over the injury is inadequate, soft-tissue transfers or free flaps are performed when the wound is clean and the fracture is definitively treated. Closed reduction should be performed initially for any fracture that is displaced, shortened or angulated. This is achieved by applying traction to the long axis of the injured limb and then reversing the mechanism of injury/fracture, followed by subsequent immobilisation through casting or splinting. Splints and casts can be used with barriers to accomplish reduction including soft tissue interposition and hematoma formation that create tension in the soft tissues.

Management of common fracture types

This section of the chapter provides an overview of the common upper and lower limb fractures in adults. Spinal and hip fractures are further explored in Chapters 19 and 18 respectively with Chapters 23 and 24 dedicated to fractures in the infant, child and young person.

Lower limb fractures

The bones of the lower limb play an important role in standing and ambulation. Fractures in this region, therefore, have a significant impact on patient mobility and ability to carry out activities of daily living and employment. They also commonly require admission to hospital. The femur and tibia are major long bones which bear the most significant weight in standing and walking. They require significant force to fracture and are, therefore, likely to be associated with patterns of multiple injury and significant soft tissue damage and are the most prone to complications. Fractures around the ankle and foot have different mechanisms and patterns of injury but can also have a significant impact on patient independence.

Fractures involving the femur

Fractures can involve any part of the femur. Fractures at the proximal end of the femur between the femoral head and greater and lesser trochanters often occur as fragility fractures in older people. These are considered in detail in Chapter 18. Fractures of the diaphyseal shaft of the femur are classified in three sections:

- proximal third (subtrochanteric)
- middle third
- distal third and femoral condyles.

The emergency management of the patient with a fracture of the femur requires full consideration of the principles of resuscitation and advanced trauma life support as considered in Chapter 16.

Many fractures of the femur are often displaced, angulated or shortened because of the action of the large muscles of the thigh. The management of femoral shaft fractures is most often by open reduction and internal fixation with an intramedullary nail. If the fixation is stable it allows early mobilisation, reducing the risk of complications due to immobility. Conservative management of fractures is most common in children and older people who are unfit for anaesthetic. Fractures of the femoral component of the knee joint often involve the articular surface of the joint and are significantly displaced. They are difficult to internally fix because intramedullary nails have difficulty obtaining fixation of the bone so close to a major joint. Specifically designed plates, screws and wires are often used, but fixation can be unstable.

Fractures involving the tibia

Tibial fractures occur due to a major impact to the lower leg. The tibia is particularly vulnerable to twisting (torsion) forces and fractures are often spiral, sometimes involving the knee or ankle joint and X-ray images should include both joints. In this part of the leg the anterior tibial border lies very close to the surface and is covered by only a thin layer of skin and adipose tissue. This anatomy not only makes this bone very vulnerable to injury but means that open fractures are common. In addition the blood supply to both the bone and overlying soft tissue is problematic resulting in fractures that heal more slowly and with more complications than others. Swelling and neurovascular compromise are significant problems following tibial fractures. It is essential therefore that care includes elevation of the lower leg preferably using a Braun frame so that elevation can be achieved which raises the ankle above the level of the heart.

Tibial shaft fractures affect the region between the knee and ankle joint along the diaphysis of the tibia. It is the most common diaphyseal fracture and mechanisms of injury can include both low and high impact, torsional forces, repeated stress and minor trauma to pathologically weakened bone. It is most common in young adult males following road traffic trauma and sporting injuries. Undisplaced fractures can be treated conservatively with a long leg cast with a walking heel added once there is evidence of callus formation on X-rays. Displaced fractures often respond to closed reduction and a long leg cast. After 4–6 weeks a Sarmiento cast or functional cast brace may be applied. Definitive treatment of displaced unstable fractures requires either internal fixation with an intramedullary nail or external fixation with an circular frame.

Other fractures of the tibia, the ankle and in the foot are considered in Table 17.2 which provides an overview of lower limb fractures and some management options.

Upper limb fractures

Fractures of the upper limb are the most common site of injury. They are particularly common following a fall on an outstretched hand (FOOSH) in all age groups, especially in older people. Other common mechanisms include a blow to the arm and twisting injuries. Injuries often occur as a result of sport and leisure activities, workplace incidents and social violence. They can also be part of a pattern of multiple injuries following high energy trauma associated with other significant fractures of the lower limb, pelvis, chest, spine or head.

Injury and immobility of the upper limb can cause significant problems for the patient in carrying out activities of living such as personal hygiene and eating and drinking, especially if the dominant arm is affected. Elderly frail people, in particular, need significant support in coping during the period of immobilisation. Swelling is a significant issue in the upper limb. This can be managed by elevation of the limb using a sling or splint and encouraging the patient to regularly exercise those joints not included in the cast or splint following medical and physiotherapy guidance. 'Neighbour' strapping is often used to immobilise the fracture in finger injuries. It is essential, like all strapping, that this is not too tight and that the neurovascular status of the fingers is regularly checked, especially if swelling is a feature. Re-strapping may be required if swelling increases as well as when it subsides.

Treatment depends on the specific injury pattern, associated injuries, bone quality and the patient's functional status/physical demands. Like all fractures, those in the upper limb can be classified as simple or complex. Simple fractures without associated ligamentous disruption include isolated fracture of the radius or ulna, or both, and often occur as a result of direct trauma. They may be open or closed, displaced or un-displaced, comminuted or displaced, impacted and angulated. Complex fractures with ligamentous disruption disrupt either the proximal/distal or both radio-ulnar articulations, and part or all of the interosseous membrane.

Complications of fractures in the upper limb and their management include neurovascular compromise, damage to tendons and compartment syndrome. Late complications include carpal tunnel syndrome, malunion, post traumatic arthritis and residual stiffness of the elbow, wrist and fingers.

Table 17.3 provides an overview of upper limb fractures and some management options.

Table 17.2 Summary of common fractures of the lower limb and their management (McRae and Esser 2008). Reproduced with permission from Elsevier

Description	Specific # name	Epidemiology/ usual MOI	Conservative management	Surgical management	Special issues & considerations
Fractures of the tibia around the knee					
Tibial Plateau #	'Bumper' fracture	High energy, compressive force e.g. motor vehicle collision (MVC) or fall. A blow from the side of the knee	If stable and minimally displaced – functional cast brace for 6–8 weeks	If unstable ORIF using cannulated screws, plate and screws, wires or external fixation	Often comminuted. Commonly associated with haemarthrosis of the knee on presentation. Disruption of the knee joint is a significant problem with rupture of cruciate and collateral ligaments and menisci. The greater the disruption of knee joint surfaces the more likely the development of secondary osteoarthritis
Fractures around the ankle (includes fractures of any section of the mortice joint of the ankle involving the talus, distal fibula (medial malleolus) and distal tibia (lateral malleolus)					
Ankle fractures "Potts'" fracture classifications:	One malleolus # = First degree Two malleoli # = Second degree (bimalleoloar) Bimalleolar + fracture of articular surfaces of tibia (trimalleolar)	Rotational forces, inversion and eversion of the foot at the ankle. Most injuries occur during walking or running	Stable injuries with minimal swelling in below knee cast for 6 weeks; NWB for first few days then add walking heel	Unstable injuries with marked swelling & bruising on both sides of ankle: ORIF with wires, screws plates followed by back slab or removable cast/splint to prevent foot drop. NWB for 6 weeks	Associated with significant swelling and risk of neurovascular compromise. Soft tissue of the ankle is very complex. Injury associated with significant tendon and ligament injury Severe injuries require lengthy rehabilitation
Fractures of the foot					
Talus #s		Foot on the pedal in motor vehicle accidents or fall from a height	Undisplaced #s: Below knee cast with 'toe' platform and NWB for 3 months. Displaced #s: closed reduction, plantar flexion of the foot and cast as above	Unstable and displaced #s ORIF with K wires, screw or pin	Blood supply to talus is poor and avascular necrosis common. Secondary osteoarthritis Is also common
Calcaneal #s		Fall from height onto the heels	If subtalar joint not involved: wool bandage, elevation with heel free of pressure (preferably with Braun frame) and NWB until pain subsides	Most displaced and unstable fractures require ORIF with screw followed by below knee cast for 6 weeks	MOI often associated with spinal fractures Fractures often avulsion (from Achilles tendon and calf muscles) Swelling and bruising are significant and must be managed carefully with elevation Chronic heel pain may occur following healing
Metatarsal #s		Crushing or heavy object dropped on foot	Wool and crepe bandage of below knee cast for 6–7 weeks	Unstable and comminuted #s associated with multiple fractures may require ORIF with K-wire	Associated soft tissue injury may be severe. May be stress/fatigue #s e.g. "March" Fracture

(Note: provided as an illustration only. Decisions depend on the fracture characteristics and surgeon preference – examples only provided. Not all fractures are considered, only the most common)

Abbreviations: # = fracture, MOI = Mechanisms of injury ORIF = open reduction and internal fixation NWB = non-weight bearing

Table 17.3 Summary of common fractures of the upper limb and their management

Description	Specific # name	Epidemiology/ Usual MOI	Conservative management	Common surgical management	Special issues & considerations
Upper arm					
Proximal, humerus # (surgical neck & anatomical neck (rare), tuberosities)	Described by number of parts of #	Pathological/fragility fracture in the elderly following FOOSH or onto side. High energy trauma in younger adult/child Excessive arm rotation/twisting. Direct violence	Minimally displaced #s treated with external support from broad arm sling or collar and cuff. Body bandages reduce rotational forces. Closed reduction with traction in line with the humerus	Severely displaced and angulated #s require ORIF or external fixation	Often with significant bruising down the arm Healing problems common in elderly fragility #s
Humeral shaft # (mid-shaft or distal)		FOOSH or direct violence pathological/fragility fracture in the elderly High energy in younger adult/child	U-slab/Hanging Cast with collar/cuff (weight of arm/cast reduces #). Functional bracing an option after 2–3 weeks	ORIF with plates/screws or intramedullary nail. External fixation	Fracture often displaced by action of pectoralis muscles. Significant risk of neurovascular compromise especially radial nerve palsy. X-rays should include shoulder and elbow and shoulder. Extensive bruising common
Forearm and wrist fractures					
Isolated radial or ulnar #		Both radius and ulna often fractured. FOOSH or other indirect force. Direct violence (less common)	Treatment depends on injury pattern, associated injuries, bone quality & patient's functional status/physical demands. MUA if angulated. Back slab with broad arm sling. Non-displaced initially treated with long arm cast. Ulna #s option of change to functional brace	External fixation an option. If displaced & < 10 degrees angulation or < than 50% shaft displacement open reduction and internal fixation (ORIF) with plate and screw required. Combined radius/ulna #, plate and screw are best option. Above elbow cast	Commonly includes dislocation of radial head with ulna # (see below Monteggia #)
Proximal ulna with dislocation of radial head	Monteggia fracture	Forced pronation. High energy trauma or violent fall/blow to the arm	Usually requires ORIF as # is unstable	Reduction most successfully achieved through ORIF followed by above elbow cast and sling	Classification (BADO 1967): Bado type 1: radial head displaced anteriorly (59%) Bado type 2: radial head displaced posteriorly (5%) Bado type 3: radial head displaced laterally (26%) Bado type 4: injuries with an associated # radial shaft have been designated Bado type 4 (1%)

Distal 1/3 of radial shaft with disruption of the distal radio ulnar joint (DRUJ)	Galeazzi fracture	Forced pronation (FOOSH)	Unstable fracture so requires surgery to prevent late slipping	ORIF with plating & closed reduction of the DRUJ; some require open reduction of DRUJ as interposition of extensor carpi ulnaris with long arm (LA) plaster cast in supination 6 weeks	
Metaphyseal # of distal radius within 2.5cm of articular surface (dorsal displacement)	Colles fracture	FOOSH Peak ages 5–14 yrs (3:1 boys : girls) & 60–69 yrs (4:1 female : male)	If undisplaced: immobilised in short arm cast 5–6 weeks If displaced fracture then a closed reduction is carried out by longitudinal traction with volar pressure then cast in palmar flexion and ulnar deviation for 5–6 weeks in a short arm cast. If position slips then further reduction may be required	If reduction unsuccessful open reduction and internal fixation. Comminuted #s may require K wires with / without ORIF for complex #s and external fixation for intra-articular #s	"dinner fork deformity" of distal radius Important to rule out median nerve injury & rupture of tendon
Distal radial # with volar displacement (reverse Colles #)	Smiths fracture	FOOSH	displaced # commonly involves reduction then POP with wrist in supination for 3–4 weeks	often requires ORIF with a buttress plate and screws or external fixator	Comminuted displaced intra–articular #s are difficult to manage
Scaphoid #		very common Fall on extended arm with dorsiflexed wrist or punching	Treatment of stable #s with short arm cast with /without thumb incorporated for 8–11 weeks (95% achieving union after 11 weeks)	K wire fixation when closed reduction unsuccessful. Cast should be applied for 8 weeks with follow up X-rays at 3, 6, and 12 months.	Pain on direct palpation of bone over 'anatomical snuff box'. May not show on xray until the # line separates. Poor blood supply and poor healing potential. Avascular necrosis and non-union common
Hand fractures					
Metacarpal #s - head, neck, shaft and base	Include: 'Boxers' # neck of 5th metacarpal	36% fractures of the hand Clenched fist striking a solid object (punching)	Neighbour strapping for 3–4 weeks	Only angulation > 45 degrees requires ORIF	Lacerations caused by impact with teeth – irrigate, explore & consider tetanus/antibiotic
# dislocation at base of Carpometacarpal (CMC) joint of the thumb	Bennets #	CMC joint subluxation; adduction/compression/ through shaft producing shearing force e.g. basketball/skiing	Reduced with traction, abduction and pronation in cast to tip of thumb X-ray weekly / Cast is on 4 weeks when pins then removed	Percutaneous pinning if unstable or reduction unsuccessful.	Can be intra-articular
Phalangeal #s (base, shaft, neck or tuft)		Sports, machinery or falls in the older person. Crush injury	Neighbour strapping	Unstable displaced injuries may require ORIF with screws and/or plate or wires	Frequent review of neighbour strapping and swelling required

(Note: provided as an illustration only. Decisions depend on the fracture characteristics and surgeon preference – examples only provided. Not all fractures are considered, only the most common)
Abbreviations: # = Fracture, FOOSH = Fall on outstretched hand, ORIF = open reduction and internal fixation, MUA = manipulation under anaesthetic, DRUJ = distal radio ulnar joint

Evidence-based practice in fracture care and outcomes

Ensuring that practice is evidence-based through both conduct and use of research and audit is essential in setting standards for improving quality of care for patients and ensuring that their fracture has the best possible healing outcome. There is a large body of medical research that considers various aspects of the management of fractures. Research projects around the world are constantly comparing fracture treatment methods against others using randomised controlled trial and other robust research methods. Examples of such trials might include comparing the use of intramedullary nailing versus the use of external fixation or the use of BMP2 (Bone morphogenetic protein 2) to stimulate the production of bone. There is also a good deal of research that has considered the role of physiotherapy in recovery and rehabilitation following skeletal injury. Research for nursing practice is often focussed on general aspects of fracture care considered in more detail in other chapters of this book, such as wound and pain management, the prevention of complications and rehabilitation. The care of the patient following a fragility fracture of the hip is particularly well researched (Chapter 18).

Many health care providers are now engaged in audit of data about fracture outcomes. Such systems aim to produce valid, accurate, consistent and timely data focusing on fracture management options and measuring performance to facilitate evidence-based practice through audit and research. Audit is a quality improvement process that aims to improve patient care and outcomes through systemically reviewing care against explicit criteria. It is often followed by the implementation of change and practice development. The key component of clinical audit is that the performance is reviewed (or audited) to ensure that what should be done is being done and, if not, that it provides a framework to enable improvements to be made. Information is gathered regarding different types of fractures, their classifications, their treatment and the outcomes of that treatment. This provides information about the effectiveness of fracture management in a given unit, but also enables the sharing of good practice between units through benchmarking. Audit data captured should include demographic data, accident dates and times, dates and times of presentation to health service, admission to fracture units, time to surgery and discharge dates and times as well as discharge destinations and information about fracture management. A particularly successful example of this is provided by the National Hip Fracture Database in the UK (with many equivalents elsewhere in the world), described in more detail in Chapter 18. This has enabled the use of audit data to drive improvements in care for this specific group of patients.

Summary

In summary this chapter informs the reader on fracture healing, types and description of fracture, plus epidemiology and fracture outcomes. The value of history taking, using classification systems and importance of identifying mechanism of injury are also considered prior to providing the reader with examples of common fractures that present in the adult and their associated complications.

Recommended further reading

Note: the following texts provide the practitioner with detailed information regarding the care and management of patients with specific types of fractures:

Jester, R., Santy, J. and Rogers, J. (2011) *Oxford Handbook of Orthopaedic and Trauma Nursing*. Oxford University Press, Oxford.

McRae, R. and Esser, M. (2008) *Practical Fracture Treatment*, 5th edn. Churchill Livingstone, Edinburgh.

References

Bado, J.L. (1967) The Monteggia lesion. *Clinical Orthopedic Related Research*, **50**, 71–86.

Black, K.J., Murphy, N.G., Thompson, K., Bevan, C.A. and Howard, J.J. (2012) Nerve blocks for initial pain management of femoral shaft fractures in children. *Cochrane Database of Systematic Reviews*. Issue **1** (Art. No.: CD009587). DOI: 10.1002/14651858.CD009587.

Blum, M.L., Esser, M., Richardson, M., Eldho, P. and Rosenfeldt, F.L. (2012) Negative pressure wound therapy reduces deep infection rate in open tibial fractures. *Journal of Orthopaedic Trauma*, **26**(9), 499–505.

British Orthopaedic Association/British Association of Plastic Reconstructive and Aesthetic Surgeons (2009) *Standards for the Management of Open Fractures of the Lower Limb. A Short Guide.* BOA/BAPRAS, London. Available at:http://www.bapras.org.uk/downloaddoc.asp?id=141 (accessed 15 June 2013).

Dandy. D.J. and Edwards, D.J. (2009) *Essential Orthopaedics and Trauma,* 5th edn. Churchill Livingstone/Elsevier, Edinburgh.

Donaldson, L.J., Reckless, I.P., Scholes, S., Mindell, J.S. and Shelton, N.J. (2008) The epidemiology of fractures in England. *Journal of Epidemiology and Community Health,* **62**(2), 174–180.

Gustilo, R.B., Mendoza, R.M. and Williams, D.N. (1984) Problems in the management of type III (severe) open fractures: A new classification of type III open fractures. *Journal of Trauma,* **24**, 742–746.

Hernandez, R.K., Do, T.P., Critchlow, C.W., Dent, R.E. and Jick, S.S. (2012) Patient-related risk factors for fracture-healing complications in the United Kingdom general practice research database. *Acta Orthopaedica,* **83**(6), 653–660.

Johansen, K., Daines, M., Howey, T., Helfet, D. and Hansen S.T. (1990) Objective criteria accurately predict amputation following lower extremity trauma. *Journal of Trauma,* **30**, 568–572.

Kuntzman, A.J. and Tortora, G.J. (2010) *Anatomy and Physiology for the Manual Therapies.* Wiley, New Jersey.

McRae, R. and Esser, M. (2008) *Practical Fracture Treatment,* 5th edn. Churchill Livingstone, Edinburgh.

Stiell, I.G., McKnight, R., Greenberg, G.H. *et al.* (1994) Implementation of the Ottawa Ankle Rules. *Journal of the American Medical Association,* **271**(11), 827–832.

Stiell, I.G., Wells, G.A., Hoag, R.H. *et al.* (1997) Implementation of the Ottawa Knee Rule for the Use of Radiography in Acute Knee Injuries. *Journal of the American Medical Association,* **278** (23), 2075–2079.

Woolf, N. (2000) *Cell, Tissue and Disease. The Basis of Pathology.* W.B. Saunders, Edinburgh.

CHAPTER 18

Fractures in the older person

Karen Hertz[1] and Julie Santy-Tomlinson[2]

[1] *University Hospital of North Staffordshire, Stoke-on-Trent, UK*

[2] *University of Hull, Hull, UK*

Introduction

As the world's population ages, musculoskeletal trauma in the older person presents a growing challenge to healthcare systems. Although management of older people following trauma needs to follow the general considerations described in Chapter 17, there are also some differences and specific considerations which must be taken into account when caring for the older patient.

There are several different mechanisms of injury of trauma in older people including many of those to which younger patients are subjected. The most common cause of injury in older people, however, is a fall and it will be fall-related trauma which is the focus of this chapter. The care of older trauma patients requires highly skilled, specialised care whatever the cause. The practitioner also needs to be aware of the issues surrounding patients being admitted as a result of elder abuse and ensure that local policies for reporting are followed in order to protect vulnerable older people from further harm (see Chapter 1).

The global development of orthogeriatric models of care, particularly in the management of patients with a hip fracture, has become a key feature of improvements in care delivery over the last few decades. This chapter aims to provide an overview of evidence-based fracture management, care and rehabilitation for older people, focusing specifically on fragility fractures. The intention is to assist the practitioner in providing skilled, high quality, age-sensitive care. Such care must consider the specific needs of older people and minimise the complications of injury, hospitalisation and surgery whilst facilitating the restoration of functional ability.

Fragility fracture

Older people with fractures normally present as a result of a fragility fracture. It is estimated that there is one fragility fracture worldwide every three seconds, equating to 25 000 per day (International Osteoporosis Foundation 2012). Almost all result in attendance at an emergency department (ED), admission to hospital or a general practitioner visit. 'Fragility' fracture is defined as a fracture that results from 'low energy' trauma and is caused by mechanical forces that would not ordinarily result in a fracture. The World Health Organization (WHO) has noted that the injury results from a fall from a standing height or less affecting an older person with osteoporosis or osteopoenia (Kanis *et al.*, 2001). Osteoporosis is a chronic disease that weakens bone strength and is characterised by low bone mass and structural deterioration of bone tissue, with a consequent increase in bone fragility leading to susceptibility to fracture (Chapter 13). The onset is often asymptomatic and may only be recognised after a person falls and sustains a fracture. The annual numbers of fragility fractures in most developed countries are very high and considered to be a major challenge for health services. According to the National Osteoporosis Society almost half of all women and one in six men will experience an osteoporotic fracture during their lifetime. It is expected that incidence will continue to increase as the population ages. Osteoporosis already affects one in three women and one in 12 men aged over 50, particularly post-menopausal women. The incidence in both sexes is known to rise rapidly with age due to increased bone loss after the menopause in women and age-related bone loss in both women and men. The prevalence of osteoporosis increases markedly with age: from 2% at

Orthopaedic and Trauma Nursing: An Evidence-based Approach to Musculoskeletal Care, First Edition. Edited by Sonya Clarke and Julie Santy-Tomlinson.

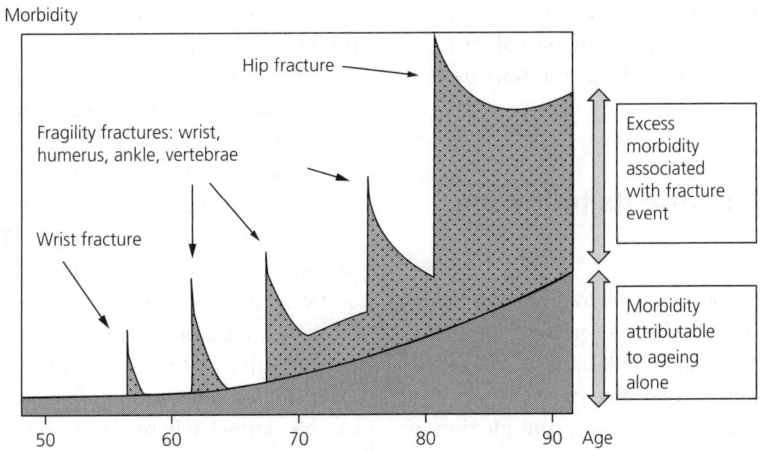

Figure 18.1 Fracture morbidity. Adapted from BOA/BGS 2007 with permission

50 years to more than 25% at 80 years in women. As the longevity of the population increases, so will the incidence of osteoporosis and associated fragility fractures (NICE, 2012). Individuals may have a life expectancy of up to forty years after their first fragility fracture potentially resulting in a need for long-term management of the issues and associated risks.

Fragility fractures occur most commonly in the spine (vertebrae), hip (proximal femur) and wrist (distal radius) and less often in the arm (humerus), pelvis, ribs and other bones. They result in significant pain and severe disability, often leading to a reduced quality of life. Hip and vertebral fractures are also associated with decreased life expectancy. Every fragility fracture signals an increased risk of future fractures – at least doubling the risk of further fractures as well as risk of premature mortality. Figure 18.1 demonstrates how the progress of osteoporotic fractures occurs across the lifetime. At its worst, the individual's experience of osteoporosis can be one of remorseless progression: from Colles' fracture and minor (and perhaps minimally symptomatic) vertebral fractures to the major distress, dependency and disability of hip fracture.

The usual care people receive after fragility fracture can be inadequate. There is frequently a failure to recognise osteoporosis as the cause of the fracture and to initiate long-term management of the condition. Problems with coordinating the key elements of care including: case-finding those at high risk; providing falls prevention; bone protection; fracture surgery and rehabilitation, can result in sub-optimal care and associated poor outcomes for patients. Recent thinking, however, acknowledges that *'optimal care is cheaper than suboptimal care'* (DOH, 2009) on the basis that better care results in better outcomes as well as reduced complications and length of stay with a greater chance of return to independent living. Focusing on high quality, optimal care is, therefore, an essential aim of service/practice development.

Several studies have shown that a previous fracture at any site is associated with a doubling of risk of further fracture (McLellan *et al.*, 2004, Kanis *et al.*, 2004) highlighting the need to identify (or 'case-find') those who have sustained such a fracture in order to initiate early clinical assessment, investigation and treatment. For patients aged over 50 proactive case-finding in acute hospitals by fracture liaison services involves identification, by a specialist practitioner, of any patients presenting with a fragility fracture either through emergency care, fracture clinics or orthopaedic wards or by identification of vertebral fractures on X-rays performed for the specific purpose or other reasons. The following steps are recommended:

- investigate bone density
- commence drug treatment according to national guidelines/local policy (Chapter 13)
- referral to falls services
- monitor and support medication compliance.

As many as half of post-menopausal women who have had a prior fragility fracture, will go on to sustain a hip fracture. Targeting these at risk groups in primary care and through fracture liaison in acute services provides ready access to those at greatest risk of hip fractures and offers some chance of reducing the numbers of fractures in the future and treatment reduces the fracture risk by 50% (DoH 2009).

Caring for older patients following trauma

Looking after older people following trauma must follow the same principles for trauma management for all age groups as discussed in Chapter 16. It must be recognised, however, that the normal and abnormal changes that occur with ageing, relating to anatomy and physiology, and compounded by past medical history and active co-morbidities, mean that mortality increases in older people as a result of morbidity and that the normal physiological responses will be different to those of a younger adult. Specific considerations relating to ageing include:

- ***Airway*** – ageing can cause degeneration of the physiological airway and musculoskeletal pathology such as osteoarthritis. It can also reduce neck and spine flexibility, making airway management difficult.
- ***Breathing*** – loss of respiratory resilience, particularly with chronic obstructive pulmonary disease, means that patients can hypoventilate when supplemental oxygen is considered. They still need oxygen therapy, but require closer monitoring in recognition of this. Older people are also more at risk of respiratory failure because of the increased work of breathing.
- ***Circulation*** – reduction in cardiopulmonary reserve means that there is an increased risk of fluid overload when administering intravenous fluids (particularly colloids), requiring closer monitoring. Normal heart rate and blood pressure are not a guarantee of normal cardiac output and the use of beta blockers and anti-hypertensive agents can mask the signs of deterioration. In the event of cardiac arrest, beta blockers and antiplatelet medications will negatively influence outcome.
- ***Disability*** – prolonged inactivity and disuse often limits ultimate functional outcome and impacts on survival.
- ***Exposure*** – skin and connective tissue undergo extensive changes in the ageing process, resulting in diminished thermoregulation, increased risk of infection, poor wound healing and increased susceptibility to hypothermia.

It is important to consider older people following trauma as individuals and make sure that a full and comprehensive history is obtained that includes relevant co-morbidities and medication history along with an overview of previous functional ability and personal and social history. Assessment and subsequent care is best provided and managed by effective teams working to sound orthogeriatric principles. These include treating the fracture while considering the causes of the fall and any unstable co-morbidities as well as initiating effective rehabilitation while assessing and treating bone health with the aim of preventing further fractures. Over the last few years, hospital mortality has reduced in care settings where orthogeriatric input is available. In addition to the principles of fracture management described in Chapter 17, there are a number of specific considerations when managing fractures in older people. Osteoporosis, for example, not only makes fracture more likely, it also means that fractures are more likely to be comminuted – making anatomical reduction of the fracture problematic. The condition slows fracture healing and makes achieving sound internal fixation more difficult, meaning that fixation needs to be more robust and durable.

Hip fracture

Hip fracture is the plain English term for a proximal femoral fracture (or PFF). It refers to a fracture occurring in the area between the edge of the femoral head and 5 cm below the lesser trochanter (Figure 18.2). Such fractures are mostly fragility fractures occurring in older people. Half of all patients admitted with a hip fracture have had a previous fragility fracture – a 'signal' fracture that gives health care providers the opportunity to commence treatment to reduce the likelihood of hip fracture occurring. It is important to stress that identifying those patients at risk of this is central to decreasing the number of patients sustaining a hip fracture in the future.

Hip fracture is the commonest reason for admission to an orthopaedic unit, accounting for more than 20% of orthopaedic bed occupancy. In women over 45 years hip fractures can account for a higher proportion of hospital bed occupancy than other common conditions (DoH 2009), making the injury a major challenge as a common serious injury which is predominantly a

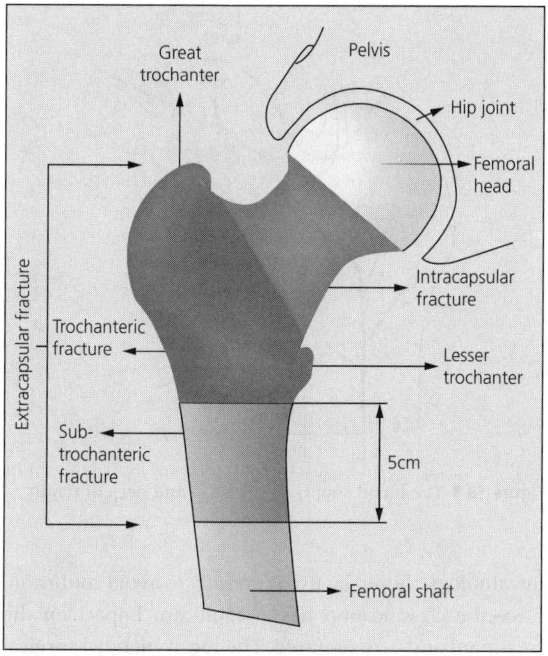

Classification of hip fractures. Fractures in the blue area are intracapsular and those in the red and orange areas are extracapsular

Figure 18.2 Classification of hip fracture. From Parker and Johanssen 2006 with permission

phenomenon of later life. The average age of a person with a hip fracture is 83 years for men and 84 years for women. In the UK, for example, about 70–75 000 hip fractures occur annually and the total annual cost (including medical and social care) for all UK cases is estimated to be about £2 billion (NHFD, 2010). A similar picture is reported in many other developed nations such as Australia, Canada and Sweden (Kanis *et al.*, 2012) although statistics suggest that rates are beginning to decline in some areas (Leslie *et al.*, 2009, Pasco *et al.*, 2011). The majority of expenditure is accounted for by hospital bed days and by health and social aftercare costs. It is predicted that by 2020 the number of people experiencing hip fracture in the UK will be in the region of 101 000 (BOA/BGS 2007).

For many previously fit patients, sustaining a hip fracture means loss of mobility and, for some of the frailer patients, the permanent loss of their ability to live at home. At present about a quarter of patients admitted to hospital following hip fracture come from institutional care and around 10–20% of those admitted from home ultimately move to institutional care.

It is widely documented that mortality at one year following hip fracture is approximately 30% (Parker and Anand 1991, SIGN 2009, BOA/BGS 2007). However, fewer than half of deaths are attributable to the fracture itself, reflecting the frailty of the patients and associated high prevalence of co-morbidities and complications. It is often the occurrence of a fall and consequent fracture that signals underlying ill health. Hence, hip fracture is by no means an exclusively surgical concern. Its effective management requires the coordinated application of nursing, medical, surgical, anaesthetic and multidisciplinary rehabilitation skills and a comprehensive approach covering the entire journey from emergency care to discharge. Increasingly the approach of an orthogeriatric model has been adopted in caring for patients following hip fracture – demonstrating significant improvements in care and patient outcomes along with reduced mortality.

Diagnosis

Patients with a hip fracture typically present to emergency services unable to walk and may exhibit shortening and external rotation of the affected limb. Frequently, but not exclusively, they give a history of trauma and have hip pain. In some instances patients may complain only of vague pain in their buttocks, knees, thighs, groin or back and their ability to walk may be unaffected. The majority of hip fractures are easily identified using plain X-rays, but an apparently normal X-ray does not necessarily exclude a fractured hip. Where there is doubt regarding the diagnosis (for example, a radiologically normal hip X-ray in a patient who remains symptomatic) and where the radiographs have been reviewed by a radiologist, alternative imaging should be performed. Magnetic resonance imaging (MRI) should be offered where hip fracture is suspected despite negative anteroposterior pelvis and lateral hip X-rays. If MRI is not available within 24 hours, or is contraindicated, computed tomography (CT) should be undertaken (NICE 2011).

Management

Surgical intervention is the treatment of choice for almost all patients following hip fracture. Exceptions are those in whom the fracture is already healing in a satisfactory alignment and those whose expected survival is, for reasons unrelated to hip fracture, very short. The NHFD report (2012) identified that less than 3% of

Box 18.1 Evidence digest: Timing of hip fracture surgery

Timing of surgery is known to have a significant effect on patient outcomes and early surgery is recommended for most patients, preferably on the day of or the day following admission and at the very least within 48 hours. This supports the target introduced by Best Practice Tariff in April 2010 for England and Wales that advocates that patients are operated on within 36 hours of admission to hospital. It is known that every 7.85 hours of delay in surgery after the initial 48 hours equates to an extra day in hospital (Bottle and Ayling 2006). AAGBI (2011) reviewed the meta analysis of Shiga *et al.* (2008) and Khan *et al.* (2009) and identified that delaying surgery beyond 48 hours from admission is associated with prolonged inpatient stay, increased morbidity (pressure ulcers, pneumonia and venous thromboembolism) and, where delay is prolonged, increased mortality. There is no evidence to suggest that outcome is improved by delaying surgery to allow pre-operative physiological stabilisation. However, the benefits of prompt surgery must be balanced against the risks of certain untreated conditions and NICE (2011) recommend that correctable co-morbidities should be identified and treated immediately so that surgery is not delayed by:

- anaemia
- anticoagulation
- volume depletion
- electrolyte imbalance
- uncontrolled diabetes
- uncontrolled heart failure
- correctable cardiac arrhythmia or ischaemia
- acute chest infection
- exacerbation of chronic chest condition.

patients did not have surgery. The timing of surgery has been shown to be important and this is discussed in Box 18.1.

Hip fractures are divided into two main groups depending on their relationship to the capsule of the hip joint (Figures 18.2 and 18.3). Those within the joint capsule are termed *intracapsular* or *femoral neck* fractures. Those below the insertion are *extracapsular*. The extracapsular group is then further sub-classified into *trochanteric* and *subtrochanteric* fractures. There is a practical basis to the division into intracapsular and extracapsular fractures relating to both the blood supply of the femoral head and the mechanics of fixation (Figures 18.3 and 18.4a and b). It is, therefore, inaccurate to classify all hip fractures as fractures of the neck of the femur as this region is involved only in some fractures and the

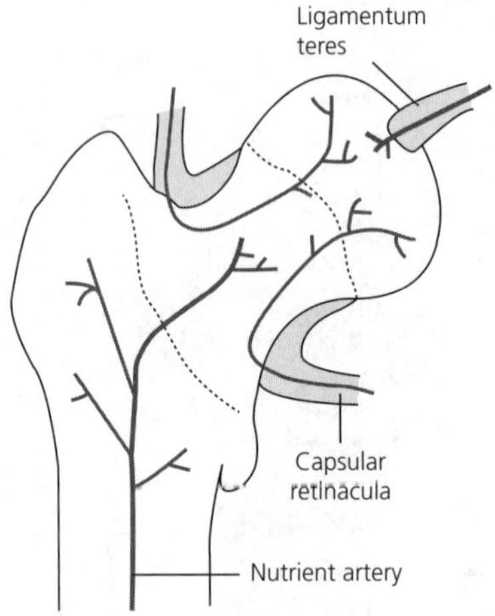

Figure 18.3 The blood supply to the head and neck of femur

terminology should be used carefully to avoid confusion, since the classification has a significant impact on the treatment and care required. The recommended surgical procedure for the different fracture groups is as follows:

Undisplaced intracapsular fractures

Surgical treatment is almost mandatory. Some impacted fractures may be difficult to diagnose but prognosis for impacted or undisplaced fractures is good following internal fixation conducted with a widely used method that is familiar to the surgeon such as cancellous bone screws (Mak *et al.*, 2010).

Displaced intracapsular fractures

Surgical treatment is almost mandatory for displaced intracapsular fractures as they will not unite without fixation or replacement. Replacement arthroplasty is used in patients with a displaced intracapsular fracture (e.g. hemi-arthroplasty or total hip replacement) because of the risk of avascular necrosis of the femoral head as a result of disruption to local blood supply resulting from displacement of the fracture. The femoral head derives its blood supply from three sources (Figures 18.3 and 18.4): the nutrient artery and vessels from the joint capsule and the ligament teres. When the femoral head is displaced the blood supply from all but the ligament teres is disrupted and this may be severe enough to cause ischaemia, resulting in bone death (avascular necrosis) and subsequent collapse of the femoral head. This leads to destruction of the joint,

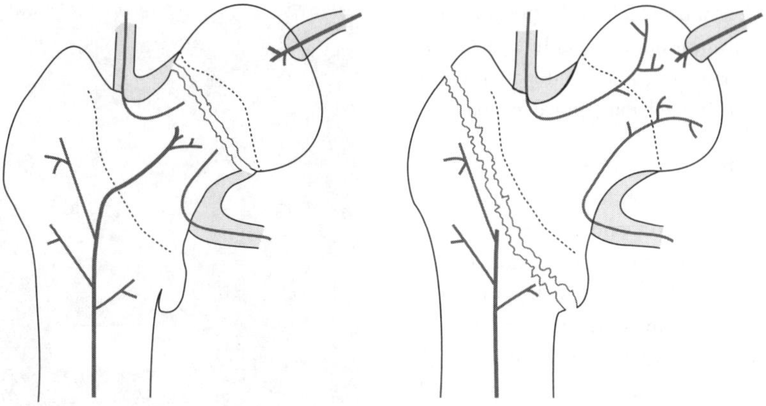

Figure 18.4 a and b Examples of disruption of the blood supply to the head and neck of femur following fracture a) Minimal disruption of the blood supply following extracapsular fracture e.g. intertrochanteric fracture, and b) Significant disruption of the blood supply following intracapsular fracture e.g. subcapital fracture

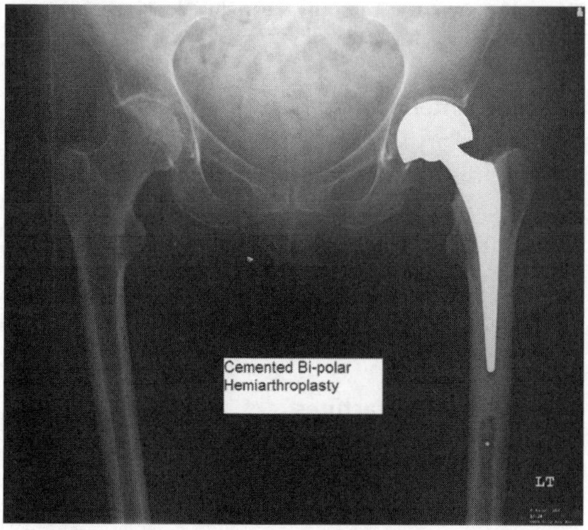

Figure 18.5 Hemiarthroplasty. Reproduced with permission from Mr Philip John Roberts

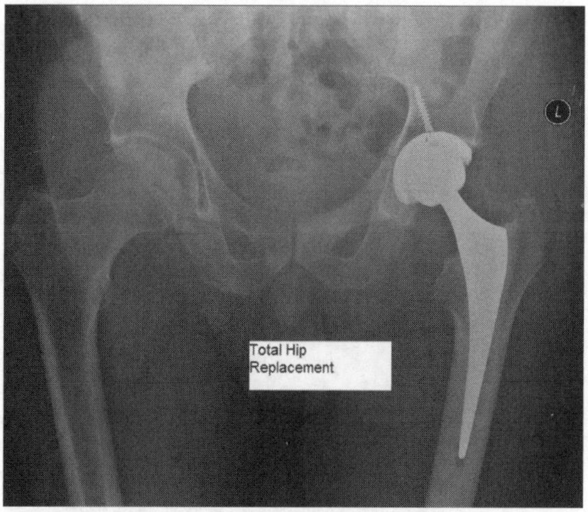

Figure 18.6 Total hip replacement. Reproduced with permission from Mr Philip John Roberts

causing ongoing pain and deformity. Hemi-arthroplasty (Figure 18.5) is commonly performed for displaced intra-capsular fractures. Compared to uncemented arthroplasty, cemented arthroplasty is said to improve hip function and is associated with lower residual pain post-operatively. Blood loss from an intracapsular fracture at the time of injury is minimal because of the poor vascular supply at the fracture site (AAGBI 2011).

There is an increasing body of evidence to support total hip replacement (THR) over hemi-arthroplasty in selected patients (Figure 18.6). This is recommended by NICE (2011) who suggest that total hip replacements are offered to patients with a displaced intracapsular fracture who prior to the fracture:

- were able to walk independently **and**
- are not cognitively impaired **and**
- are medically fit for anaesthesia and the procedure.

THR is recommended for active patients or those with pre-existing joint disease, rather than hemi-arthroplasty because of acetabular wear and inferior functional outcome experienced with a hemi-arthroplasty. THR is, however, unsuitable for patients with dementia due to their reduced ability to follow postoperative movement restrictions and a consequently higher dislocation rate. Patients need to be able to understand and follow the post-operative guidance to prevent dislocation, but if able to do so will achieve higher functional outcomes and patients with underlying joint destruction will experience less pain.

Extracapsular fractures

Management of extra capsular fractures should reflect the differences in presentation and symptoms. Blood loss from an extracapsular fracture is much greater than that from an intracapsular fracture; loss from the cancellous bone at this site may exceed one litre. The greater the degree of comminution and the larger the size of the bone fragments, the greater the blood loss. In addition, greater periosteal disruption causes extracapsular fractures to be considerably more painful than intracapsular fractures. They can be treated conservatively, healing after six to eight weeks of traction and bed rest, but such management is associated with greatly increased morbidity and mortality and a considerably reduced chance of the patient regaining independence and/or returning home (AAGBI 2011). Undisplaced extracapsular fractures are often treated with cannulated screws (Figure 18.7). Surgical intervention for other fractures is recommended as follows.

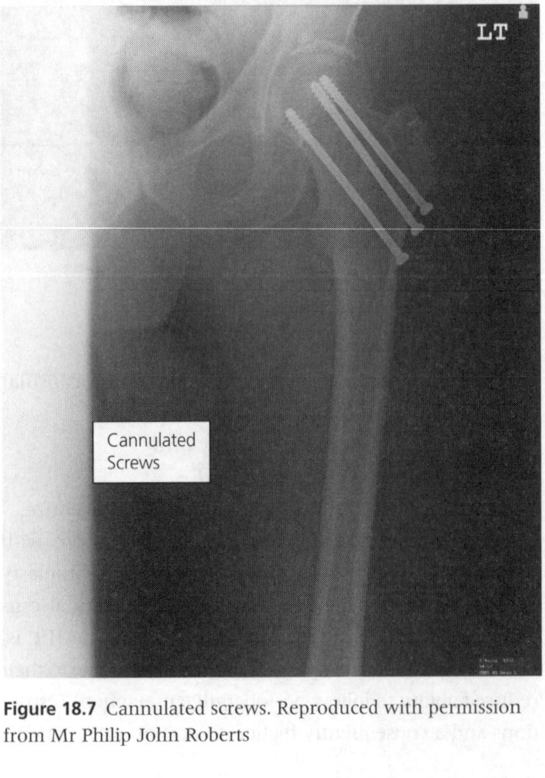

Figure 18.7 Cannulated screws. Reproduced with permission from Mr Philip John Roberts

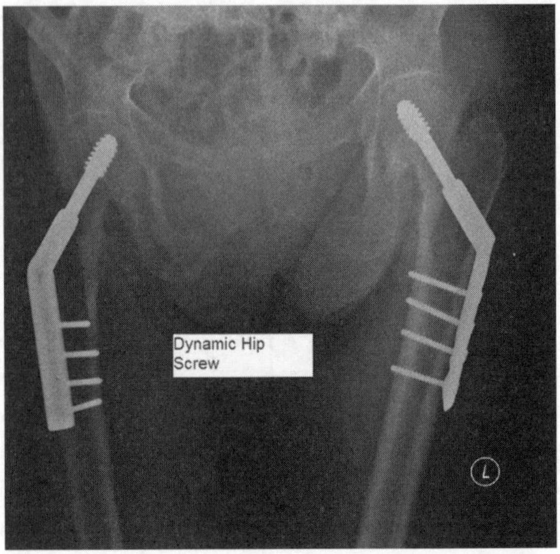

Figure 18.8 Dynamic hip screw. Reproduced with permission from Mr Philip John Roberts

Intertrochanteric fractures

Extra medullary implants such as a sliding hip screw are used in the fixation for patients with trochanteric fractures above and including the lesser trochanter (NICE 2011) (Figure 18.8). This stabilises the fracture, reduces pain and allows early mobility. The movement allowed by the implant in only one plane and axial loading of the fracture encourages bone healing.

Subtrochanteric fractures

These fractures are less common, accounting for about 5–10% of all hip fractures. They present a considerable challenge to the surgeon as the high mechanical forces in this region lead to an increased risk of fixation failure. NICE (2011) recommends the use of an intramedullary nail to treat patients with a subtrochanteric fracture such as the proximal femoral nail (Figure 18.9) which requires shorter duration of surgery and shorter hospital stay. It also results in fewer orthopaedic complications and there is less need for major re-operations than with other types of fixation (Mak *et al.*, 2010).

Ethical considerations in treatment of patients with hip fracture

Approximately 25% of hip fracture patients have moderate or severe cognitive impairment and a further 15–25% have mild cognitive impairment. In order for the patient to consent to, or refuse, hip fracture surgery, they must be

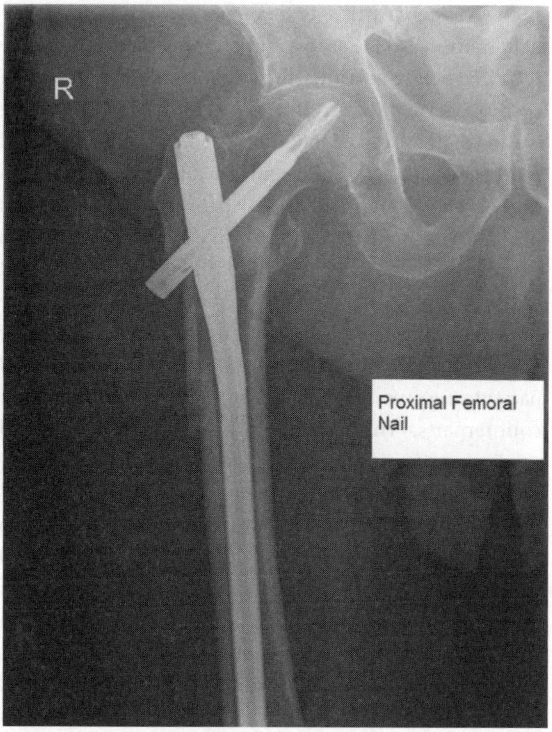

Figure 18.9 Proximal femoral nail. Reproduced with permission from Mr Philip John Roberts

able to give consent voluntarily, based on a decision made following presentation and understanding of information about the procedure. The patient must be judged as having capacity to make that decision: they must be able to understand the information, remember it and use it to reach a decision. In this age group, the ability to assimilate information and communicate decisions may be impaired by poor vision, hearing or speech and steps should be taken to overcome these problems (AAGBI 2011). In some circumstances the operating team may be unable to satisfy themselves that the patient can give consent. If the patient does not have an advocate with a legal responsibility for decision making on their behalf an alternative approach needs to be found. Depending on national law and guidance and following close liaison with family or carers surgery may progress if two surgeons agree that it is in the patient's best interests.

Nursing management of patients with a hip fracture

Older adults with hip fracture represent a growing number of the patients cared for by orthopaedic nurses around the world. This group are at increased risk of the more familiar peri-operative complications such as venous thromboembolism, pneumonia and urinary tract infections. Normal age-related changes, the stress of fracture, hospitalisation and chronic medical conditions also predispose them to other serious problems including inappropriately managed pain, malnutrition, dehydration, constipation, pressure ulcers, delirium, functional decline and death (Koval and Zuckerman, 1995; Mak *et al.*, 2010). The majority of patients are admitted to an acute hospital where they are cared for by nurses who must also manage the care of patients with other traumatic injuries alongside the special care needs of the older adult. There are a number of guidelines related to best practice medical management strategies for this population but until recently there has been no guidance specific to the nursing care of older patients with hip fracture.

Care of the older adult is complex and best achieved by an interdisciplinary team approach. The concept of *orthogeriatrics* is well established in the medical and surgical care of this patient – care led by a collaborative orthopaedic and geriatric approach – but the concept has not yet become widely established in nursing care of this patient group. Even so, both skilled orthopaedic and elderly care nursing are vital in order to provide effective and appropriate care. Nurses are an integral contributor to the orthogeriatric team or, as described by NICE (2011) 'the hip fracture programme', as they are in an ideal position to co-ordinate care provision. The complex sharing of care between orthopaedic surgeons and orthogeriatricians could become fragmented and less effective if the care is not managed or coordinated effectively. The role of a specialist nurse or coordinator can vary according the size, culture and organisation of each individual unit, but such coordination is currently undertaken by a variety of nurses in different roles including; hip fracture nurse specialists, elderly care nurse specialists, trauma nurse coordinators and nurse practitioners. These advanced practitioners are well placed to ensure that the patient experience is positive, that they are appropriately prepared for surgery, placed early on a scheduled trauma surgery list, have a coordinated care and rehabilitation programme and are discharged to home or to an appropriate care setting.

Practitioners should be mindful of the complications that can occur in older patients and must monitor them closely at the same time as liaising with family and carers in order to promptly detect changes in patient condition. The most significant care issues relate to pain, malnutrition, dehydration, constipation, delirium, pressure ulcers and mobility/function. The quality of care being provided to the patient is reflected in these aspects of care and they are issues that respond to nursing management strategies, hence they can be referred to as *nurse sensitive quality indicators*. The following evidence-based principles of care following hip fracture have been identified in a set of international guidelines (Maher *et al.*, 2012, Maher *et al.*, 2013).

Pain

Hip fracture is painful and early fracture surgical fixation provides the most effective pain relief. Accurate pain assessment is the foundation for successful pain management because good pain control in the early stages of care will promote comfort and confidence. Later on, if pain is poorly controlled, mobilisation will be delayed – bringing with it the complications of prolonged bed rest and immobility leading to increased dependency and an associated rise in the risk of post-operative delirium.

A formalised analgesia protocol should be followed. Simple analgesics such as paracetamol should be prescribed and administered on a regular basis (unless contraindicated) and additional opioids or nerve blocks used in conjunction with the paracetamol to provide pain relief as required. NICE (2011) suggest that assessment of the patient is made immediately upon presentation at hospital and analgesia should be given routinely at that time. Within 30 minutes of administering initial analgesia, a further assessment of pain should be made, giving additional analgesia if required. Assessment and administration of analgesia should then occur hourly until the patient is settled and then regularly as part of routine care. The aim of analgesia should be to give sufficient pain relief to allow movements necessary for investigations, nursing care and rehabilitation.

Pain in older people is often under-reported by patients and undetected by practitioners. Cognitive impairment places patients at particularly high risk of this. Pain assessment scales alone do not provide the essential elements to guide treatment. It is extremely important to know the onset and duration, location, predisposing factors or influences and the type of pain. The acute pain of the fracture is often in conjunction with chronic pain which may be related to other co-morbid conditions such as osteoarthritis or malignancy. Visual analogue pain scores (VAPS), at rest and on movement, should be recorded before and after the administration of analgesia (RCP/BGS/Pain Society 2007). This form of self-reporting is the single most reliable measurement of pain. Verbal reports of pain are valid and reliable in patients with mild to moderate dementia or delirium. The diagnosis of pain in a patient with cognitive impairment due to dementia or delirium may be particularly difficult and requires familiarity with the patient and will require information from relatives or carers. Many studies have shown that cognitively impaired and acutely confused patients receive less analgesia than their unimpaired counterparts. This is generally because nursing and medical staff rely on self-reporting of pain and rarely consider pointers to the presence of pain such as moaning, sighing or holding a guarded posture, tachycardia and high blood pressure (BOA 2007). The use of a tool to tell staff about the individual needs of a person with dementia such as the 'This is Me' form available from the Alzheimer's Society, encourages relatives and carers to document individual patient information and personal behaviours. Working with families of patients with dementia or delirium to complete this document will support pain assessment. See Chapter 11 for further consideration of general issues related to pain management.

Malnutrition

Malnutrition is often associated with ageing and is characterised by diminished hunger and thirst, along with chronic illness patterns. There are many causes of malnutrition including:

- ***Reduced intake*** – poor appetite due to illness, food aversion, nausea or pain when eating, depression, anxiety, side effects of medication or drug addiction.
- ***Inability to eat*** – due to being fasted for investigations or surgery, reduced levels of consciousness, confusion, difficulty in feeding oneself due to weakness, arthritis or other conditions such as Parkinson's disease, dysphagia, vomiting, painful mouth conditions, poor oral hygiene or dentition and restrictions imposed by surgery or investigations.
- ***Lack of food availability*** – particularly prior to admission, due to poverty, poor quality diet at home, problems with shopping and cooking as well as issues with food availability in hospital or in care homes.

- ***Impaired absorption*** – due to medical and surgical problems affecting digestion; stomach, intestine, pancreas and liver/or absorption.
- ***Altered metabolism*** – increased or changed metabolic requirements related to illness or treatment e.g. cancer, surgery, organ dysfunction.
- ***Excess losses*** – vomiting, diarrhoea, nutrient fistulae, stomas, losses from nasogastric tube and other drains or skin exudates from wounds.

Up to 60% of hip fracture patients are clinically malnourished on admission to hospital. This can lead to serious consequences such as:

- increased risk of infections including surgical site infection and respiratory and urinary tract infection
- delayed wound healing and increased risk of pressure ulcer development
- impaired respiratory function
- muscle weakness and functional decline
- reduced cognitive function and depression.

Many older people do not eat and drink adequate amounts while in hospital, putting their health and recovery at risk and hospitalised hip fracture inpatients are thought to have only half their recommended daily energy, protein and other nutritional requirements (BOA 2007). Nutrition is an interdisciplinary concern, which requires effective liaison and communication between all members of the team. A number of approaches to nutritional support have been studied. The strongest evidence for the effectiveness of nutritional supplementation exists for oral protein and energy feeds, multi-nutrient feeds (providing energy, protein, vitamins and minerals), which may reduce the risk of death or complication and possibly the length of stay (BOA 2007; Duncan *et al.*, 2006). Patients' acceptance of supplement drinks is often poor. It is therefore crucial that all staff dealing with patients recovering from hip fracture understand the importance of adequate nutritional intake and that specific attention is given to helping people to eat at meal times. Simple practical measures such as providing additional carers or volunteers to assist in nutrition can be effective, as well as other strategies such as meal times protected from disturbance and systems that highlight patients at risk of malnutrition such as coloured trays. Routine nursing care must include an assessment of nutritional intake and, where appropriate, referral for dietetic advice. General issues related to nutrition and the orthopaedic patient are considered in more detail in Chapter 10.

Dehydration

Dehydration is highly prevalent among older orthopaedic patients and carries with it significant potential adverse consequences. Older adults admitted to hospital from home or other care facilities often present with dehydration for a variety of reasons. This can include pre-existing restricted fluid intakes which may relate to normal age-related changes, diminished thirst reflex and subsequent diminished fluid intake. Many patients who suffer from incontinence or frequency may self-regulate fluid intake to reduce the risk of incontinence and because of difficulty accessing toilet facilities. Diuretic use can result in altered fluid balance. A long post-fall lie on the floor can also result in reduced fluid intake.

Dehydration decreases circulatory volume, resulting in diminished perfusion to organs and tissues and is implicated in the development of delirium, acute kidney injury, pressure ulcers, falls, venous thromboembolism and urinary tract infections. Optimised perioperative fluid management helps to reduce the incidence of dehydration and therefore reduces morbidity and hospital stay (Price *et al.*, 2004). Every effort must be made to ensure that intravenous fluid is prescribed on admission and that it is administered over the correct time. Strict fluid balance monitoring along with shortest possible periods of pre-operative fasting also prevent or improve dehydration.

Electrolyte imbalances, particularly hyponatraemia and hypokalaemia, are common in the post-operative period and reflect limited renal reserve. The situation may be made worse by diuretics and inappropriate maintenance of intravenous fluids. This limited renal reserve is also reflected in the high risk of acute kidney injury (AKI) in hip fracture patients, which is estimated to be 16% (Bennet, 2010). Older patients admitted to hospital for emergency surgery are at increased risk of acute kidney injury and its associated pre- and post-operative complications. This can be because of pre-existing co-morbid conditions, age and complex polypharmacy, which often includes diuretics and nephrotoxic medication such as angiotensin-converting enzyme inhibitors (ACE inhibitors) used in the management of hypertension and heart failure and non-steroidal anti-inflammatory drugs

(NSAIDs) used for pain relief. Baseline renal function is a good predictor for AKI, but establishment of this may be difficult in hip fracture patients as they may be acutely dehydrated on admission with or without the presence of some chronic renal dysfunction. Close monitoring of fluid balance and blood biochemistry is essential to prevent or identify renal injury.

Constipation

Constipation is a significant risk for patients following hip fracture and prevention should be considered early in the care pathway. Use of opioid analgesics including codeine (even in low doses), dehydration, altered diet (particularly decreased fibre in the diet) and lack of mobility can all increase this risk (SIGN 2009). This is considered in more detail in Chapter 9.

Delirium

Delirium (sometimes called 'acute confusional state') is a clinical syndrome characterised by disturbed consciousness and altered cognitive function or perception. It has an acute onset and a fluctuating course (NICE 2010). It is a common, but serious and complex clinical syndrome associated with poor outcomes. As many as 65% of patients who have sustained a hip fracture may develop delirium. It is commonly categorised as being hypoactive or hyperactive, reflecting the nature of the behaviour seen in patients.

Delirium is independently associated with a variety of adverse outcomes including pressure ulcers, functional decline, longer hospital stay and institutionalisation. Prompt detection coupled with ongoing assessment and targeted nursing interventions have been proven to reduce the incidence and severity of symptoms of those suffering from delirium (NICE, 2010; Mak *et al.*, 2008). Assessment and the establishment of baseline cognition is a critical and often challenging first step in delirium detection and close communication between the nursing team and family or carers is essential. In addition to information from family members, undertaking an initial Abbreviated Mental Test Score is essential. Although this is not an assessment tool for delirium, it will provide baseline information relating to cognitive function. If there is any suspicion of delirium, tools such as the Short Confusion Assessment Method (shortCAM) are recommended by NICE (2010) for more comprehensive assessment, although training is required in order to undertake the assessment as it is often difficult to distinguish between delirium and dementia.

It is suggested that prevention of delirium is possible in up to 30% of cases (Inouye *et al.*, 1999, Marcantonio *et al.*, 2001). Early attention to risk factors, particularly in patients with underlying dementia, should be addressed early and good communication with patients, family and carers can help practitioners to recognise subtle changes. If delirium is evident it is important to identify and manage any possible underlying cause or combination of causes (BGS 2005) by:

- Seeking early comprehensive orthogeriatric review.
- Withdrawing or reducing culprit drugs such as opiates, where appropriate.
- Effective management of pain.
- Monitoring and screening for infection, while using universal precautions to prevent infection.
- Avoid use of devices that increase the risk of infection such as urinary catheters.
- Alcohol withdrawal increases the likelihood of patients developing delirium so management of withdrawal is key to avoiding delirium. Use of a protocol to manage chemical dependency withdrawal such as the Clinical Institute Withdrawal Assessment (CIWA) score can help ensure symptoms of withdrawal are identified and addressed early.
- Provide effective reassuring communication and reorientation (for example explaining where the person is, who you are and what your role is).
- Invite/encourage family, friends and carers to participate in care.
- If a person with delirium is distressed or considered a risk to themselves or others and verbal and non-verbal de-escalation techniques are ineffective or inappropriate, consider medication and other methods to maintain safety such as low beds and higher levels of supervision.

Pressure ulcers

Development of pressure ulcers is a frequent complication of hip fracture and surgery and up to one third of patients will develop a pressure ulcer (BOA 2007). Patients with pressure ulcers following hip fractures require significantly more nursing care, longer hospital stay, increased hospital costs and use more health care resources following discharge compared to patients without pressure ulcers (Chaves *et al.*, 2010). Given the very high risk, prevention and management of pressure ulcers in this group of patients is, therefore, central to effective, high quality care. Chapter 12 provides detailed evidence-based advice for both prevention and management of pressure ulcers which is equally applicable to a patient with a hip fracture.

Rehabilitation of the older person following fractures

Although a section of this book (Chapter 6) has considered rehabilitation for patients as a result of orthopaedic conditions, orthopaedic surgery or injury, it is important to consider rehabilitation specifically for patients following all types of fragility fracture, but particularly those following hip fracture. This group of patients is older and more likely to have co-morbid conditions which will adversely affect rehabilitation abilities and outcomes if not managed appropriately. The evidence available in the literature mainly considers rehabilitation following hip fracture, but these programmes can easily be transferred to any type of fragility fracture.

Currently orthopaedic rehabilitation models are fragmented and have not been well evaluated in terms of functional outcome when compared to length of hospital stay. There are, however, three main pathways for patients following hip fracture which are described by NICE (2011):

1 The traditional pathway of care is that a patient with hip fracture is admitted to a trauma ward where the orthopaedic surgical team lead both surgical care and subsequent rehabilitation. Geriatrician input to such wards is limited with referrals and medical queries being dealt with on a consultative basis by the on-call medical registrar or on occasional geriatrician visits, but without a proactive geriatrician lead to the multidisciplinary team.
2 A more collaborative model of care through formal 'orthogeriatric' care, with older trauma patients admitted to a trauma ward or specialised unit under the joint care of both geriatricians and orthopaedic surgeons.
3 Hip fracture programmes (HFP), with the orthogeriatric medical team contributing to joint preoperative patient assessment and increasingly taking the lead for post-operative medical care, multidisciplinary rehabilitation (MDR) and discharge planning, with ongoing governance for rehabilitation in hospital or as part of a community rehabilitation scheme as described below.

After initial surgical care and mobilisation in the first two models of care, early post-operative transfer to an orthogeriatric rehabilitation unit or mixed rehabilitation unit for ongoing treatment is another option. This may be additionally supported by community rehabilitation as **early supported discharge** (ESD) or **intermediate care** at home. Patients are discharged home from the acute trauma ward or, in some cases, a rehabilitation ward within the hospital supported with a 4–6 week rehabilitation package. This service may include patients living in care homes, but may be limited to patients returning to live independently in their own homes.

The evidence strongly supports the orthogeriatric approach to hip fracture management, and NICE (2011) recommend the development of hip fracture programmes. In this model management and care is undertaken by collaborative working between orthopaedic surgeons, orthogeriatricians, nurses and allied health professionals who have expertise in the care of older patients in surgical environments and associated specific needs. This represents a considerable change in the organisation of medical and surgical management of hip fracture patients. It requires a change in philosophy that needs to be embedded into trauma care as a whole and reflected in pre- and post-qualifying nurse education programmes for health professionals.

The ethos of effective hip fracture programmes is that the care should be provided by professionals interested in high quality care and achievement of best functional outcomes for this group of patients, wherever rehabilitation occurs. This includes discharge from the hip fracture programme when optimal physical, medical and functional ability have been achieved and means that patients are not discharged prematurely without achieving their potential. Programmes must be based on the premise that cost and quality are not in conflict. A review of the available literature and a cost-based analysis of such a programme confirmed that looking after hip fracture patients well (in terms of preventing complications, achieving better functional outcomes, preventing further falls, preventing readmission) was cheaper than looking after them badly (BOA 2007).

NICE (2011) clearly outline how such a programme may encompass all types of rehabilitation settings (e.g. acute hospital rehabilitation, geriatric orthopaedic unit rehabilitation or ESD programmes) as long as patients are selected appropriately for ESD and the hip fracture programme team retain governance for care. This approach needs to ensure the minimum number of transfers between care settings to ensure that consistency and continuity are maintained. Transfers between care settings not only lengthen stay, but also reduce the likelihood of final discharge home.

Nurses working in acute hospital trauma wards are central to the care of patients following hip fracture. They need to embrace the principles of excellent trauma nursing practice, but need to provide this in a manner that is focused clearly on the specific needs of older people. This involves consideration of the surgical post-operative complications of pain, dislocation and wound infection and the complications specific to older people such as delirium, dementia, malnutrition and pressure ulcer development. This must include working with patients, carers, therapists, community health or social care teams to promote safe and appropriate discharge home or to the care setting that best meets the patient's needs.

Consideration of palliative care for patients following hip fracture

Studies have shown that an estimated 18 to 28% of older hip fracture patients die within one year of fracture. Of those who survive, it is estimated that between 24 and 75% will not return to their pre-fracture level of independence (Koval *et al.*, 1994, Mak *et al.*, 2010). Although palliative care originally focused on patients with cancer, it is now well documented that consideration for a palliative care approach should be made for people at the end of their lives for non-malignant as well as malignant disease. Palliative care is defined by the World Health Organization (2011) as:

> ...an approach that improves the quality of life of patients and their families facing the problem associated with life threatening illness, through the prevention and relief of suffering by means of early identification and impeccable assessment and treatment of pain and other problems, physical, psychosocial and spiritual. Palliative care affirms life and regards dying as a normal process, and intends neither to hasten nor to prolong death. Using a team approach palliative care addresses the needs of patients and their families, including bereavement counselling if necessary.

This philosophy of care allows for physical, psychological, social and emotional care for patients, their families and carers when the patient with a hip fracture is frail and does not have the physical resilience to survive the trauma of the fracture. Effective models of care for patients with hip fracture actively lend themselves to the inclusion of patient-centred palliative care when appropriate. Typically, palliative care is provided by an interdisciplinary team who focus on the assessment and treatment of pain and other symptoms while ensuring that care is enhanced by patient-centred communication and decision-making across the continuum of care settings, from hospital to home.

Identifying patients for whom a palliative care approach is most appropriate is difficult. Many patients presenting with hip fracture also have multiple co-morbidities; in the 2011/12 NHFD report 67% of patients were graded at American Society of Anaesthesiologists (ASA) GRADE III or above (Chapter 14), identifying those who have severe systematic disease that limits activity or is life threatening. It could be suggested that these are the people for whom palliative care should be considered. However, many such patients recover well post-operatively, leave hospital and have a good functional outcome and ongoing quality of life. Appropriate models of end of life care are currently a matter of considerable discussion. Palliative care has not previously been a natural consideration in orthopaedic care so this is a matter for continuing debate and discussion rather than something that is currently integrated into practice.

It is the responsibility of the orthogeriatric or hip fracture team, through good communication with patients' families and carers, to identify those people who have been having the typical period of decline pre-fracture and for whom the physical insult of fall, fracture, surgery and hospitalisation leads to the hastening of end of life. It then becomes the responsibility of the team to prepare the patient and family not only physically, financially and emotionally, but also to ensure that ongoing care and treatment is appropriate to the patient's needs and this may or may not include surgical intervention. If a hip fracture complicates or precipitates a terminal illness, surgery should be considered as part of a palliative care approach in order to minimise pain and other symptoms, not necessarily to regain functional ability (NICE 2011). Surgery provides significant pain relief that will then not only allow nursing interventions to be undertaken more comfortably, but will facilitate transfer from an acute orthopaedic unit to either home or to another care setting in keeping with the patients and/or carers end of life wishes.

Hip fracture audit

Older people who sustain a hip fracture deserve to receive the best healthcare possible every time they present to a hospital, but there often remains a disparity in care that patients receive globally, nationally and locally. This is demonstrated year on year in hip fracture audit reports. Hip fracture care over the last few years has received considerable attention following national initiatives such as the National Hip Fracture Database (NHFD) in the UK. This audits the BOA/BGS (2007) six standards of care, the Royal College of Physicians' Audit of Falls and Bone Health, the Department of Health's Commissioning Toolkit and the development of NICE Clinical Guideline 124 on the management of hip fracture. Hip fracture audit was first undertaken in Sweden and similar ventures are in place in many other countries such as Australia, New Zealand, Canada and Ireland. In the UK, those units which provide evidence of high quality care (through NHFD audit) receive additional financial rewards. This provides an unprecedented opportunity for units to improve care and patient services.

Conclusion

The care of patients following hip fracture presents a major challenge for trauma, rehabilitation and community services and particularly to nurses. Increasing evidence for best practice is leading to improvements in care that are demonstrable through audit. The way in which services are organised will continue to have an impact on the outcomes of care and there remains a need for staff to be motivated to care for this vulnerable group of patients and to receive education that ensures they have the right knowledge and skills to do so.

Recommended further reading

British Orthopaedic Association/British Geriatric Society (BOA/BGS) (2007) *Care of Patients with Fragility Fractures*. London: BOA. Available at: http://www.bgs.org.uk/pdf_cms/pubs/Blue%20Book%20on%20fragility%20fracture%20care.pdf (accessed 19 November 13).

Maher, A.B., Meehan, A.J., Hertz, K. *et al.* (2012) Acute nursing care of the older adult with fragility hip fracture: An international perspective. Part 1. *International Journal of Orthopaedic and Trauma Nursing*, **16**(4), 177–194.

Maher, A.B., Meehan, A.J., Hertz, K. *et al.* (2013) Acute nursing care of the older adult with fragility hip fracture: An international perspective. Part 2. *International Journal of Orthopaedic and Trauma Nursing*, **17**(1), 4–18.

NICE (2011) *Hip Fracture: The Management of Hip Fracture in Adults*. NICE Clinical Guideline 124. NICE, London.

NICE (2012) *Osteoporosis: Assessing the Risk of Fragility Fracture*. NICE Short Guideline. NICE, London.

Parker, M. and Johansen, A. (2006) Hip fracture. *British Medical Journal*, **333**(7557), 27–30.

References

Association of Anaesthetists of Great Britain and Ireland (AAGBI) (2011) *Management of Proximal Femoral Fractures*. Available at:http://www.aagbi.org/sites/default/files/femoral%20fractures%202012_0.pdf (accessed 19 November 2013).

Bennet, S.J. (2010) Acute renal injury following hip fracture. *Injury*, **41**(4), 335–338.

Bottle, A. and Aylin, P. (2006) Mortality associated with delay in operation after hip fracture: observational study. *British Medical Journal*, **332**, 947–950.

British Geriatric Society (2005) *Guidelines for the Prevention, Diagnosis and Management of Delirium in Older People in Hospital*. Available at: http://www.bgs.org.uk/index.php/clinicalguides/170-clinguidedeliriumtreatment?showall=andlimitstart (accessed 19 November 2013).

British Orthopaedic Association (BOA) (2007) *Standards for Trauma (BOAST). BOAST 1: Hip Fracture in the Older Person*. BOA, London. Available at: http://www.boa.ac.uk/LIB/LIBPUB/Documents/BOAST%201%20-%20Hip%20Fracture%20in%20the%20Older%20Person%20Version%201%20-%202008.pdf (accessed 19 November 2013).

British Orthopaedic Association/British Geriatric Society (BOA/BGS) (2007) *Care of Patients with Fragility Fractures*. BOA, London. Available at: http://www.bgs.org.uk/pdf_cms/pubs/Blue%20Book%20on%20fragility%20fracture%20care.pdf (accessed 19 November 2013).

Chaves, L.M. Grypdonck, M. and DeFloor, T. (2010) Protocols for pressure ulcer prevention: are they evidence-based? *Journal of Advanced Nursing*, **66**(3), 562–572.

Department of Health (2009) *Fracture Prevention Services: Economic Evaluation*. DOH, London. Available at:http://www.cawt.com/Site/11/Documents/Publications/Population%20Health/Economics%20of%20Health%20Improvement/fractures.pdf (accessed 19 November 2013).

Duncan, D.G., Beck, S.J., Hood, K. and Johansen, A. (2006) Using dietetic assistants to improve the outcome of hip fracture: a randomised controlled trial of nutritional support in an acute trauma ward. *Age and Aging*, **35**(2), 148–153.

International Osteoporosis Foundation (2012) *Capture the Fracture Report*. Available at: http://www.iofbonehealth.org/capture-fracture-report-2012 (accessed 19 November 2013).

Inouye, S.K., Bogardus, S.T., Charpentier, P.A. *et al.* (1999) A multicomponent intervention to prevent delirium in hospitalized older people. *New England Journal of Medicine*, **340**(9), 669–676.

Kanis, J.A., Oden, A., Johnell, O. *et al.* (2001). The burden of osteoporotic fractures: a method for setting intervention thresholds. *Osteoporosis International*, **12**(5), 417–427.

Kanis, J.A., Johnell, O., De Laet, C. *et al.* (2004) A meta-analysis of previous fracture and subsequent fracture risk. *Bone* **35**(2): 375–382.

Khan, S.K., Kalra, S., Khanna, A., Thiruvengada, M.M. and Parker, M.J. (2009) Timing of surgery for hip fractures: A systematic review of 52 published studies involving 291,413 patients. *Injury*, **40**, 692–697.

Kanis, J.A., Oden, A., McCloskey, E.V. *et al.* (2012) A systematic review of hip fracture incidence and probability of fracture worldwide. *Osteoporosis International*, **23**(9), 2239–2256.

Koval, K.J. and Zuckerman J.D. (1994) Hip fractures: overview and evaluation and treatment of femoral neck fractures. *Journal of the American Academy of Orthopaedic Surgeons*, **2**(3), 141–149.

Leslie, W.D., O'Donnell, S., Jean, S. *et al.* (2009) Trends in hip fractures in Canada. *Journal of the American Medical Association*, **302**(8), 883–889.

Maher, A.B., Meehan, A.J., Hertz, K. *et al.* (2012) Acute nursing care of the older adult with fragility hip fracture: An international perspective. Part 1. *International Journal of Orthopaedic and Trauma Nursing*, **16**(4), 177–194.

Maher, A.B., Meehan, A.J., Hertz, K. *et al.* (2013) Acute nursing care of the older adult with fragility hip fracture: An international perspective. Part 2. *International Journal of Orthopaedic and Trauma Nursing*, **17**(1), 4–18.

Mak, J., Cameron, I. and March, L. (2010) Evidence-based guidelines for the management of hip fractures in older persons: An update. *Medical Journal of Australia*, **192**(1), 37–41.

Marcantonio, E., Flacker J., Wright, J. and Resnick, N., (2001) Reducing delirium after hip fracture: A randomized trial. *Journal of the American Geriatrics Society*, **49**: 516–522.

McLellan, A., Reid, D. and Forbes, K. (2004) *Effectiveness of Strategies for the Secondary Prevention of Osteoporotic Fractures in Scotland*. CEPS 99/03. NHS Quality Improvement Scotland, Edinburgh.

National Hip Fracture Database (NHFD) (2010) *The National Hip Fracture Database National Report 2010*. Available at: http://www.rcseng.ac.uk/news/docs/NHFD%20%28final%29.pdf (accessed 21 November 2013).

National Hip Fracture Database (NHFD) (2012) *The National Hip Fracture Database National Report 2012*. Available at: http://www.nhfd.co.uk/003/hipfractureR.nsf/0/da44e3a946a14e4180257a6f001eb4db/$FILE/NHFD%20National%20Report%202012%20Summary.pdf (accessed 21 November 2013).

National Osteoporosis Society http://www.nos.org.uk (accessed 4 April 2014).

National Institute for Health and Clinical Excellence (NICE) (2010) *Understanding NICE Guidance: Delirium* (103). NICE, London.

NICE (2011) *Hip Fracture: The Management of Hip Fracture in Adults*. NICE Clinical Guideline 124. NICE, London.

NICE (2012) *Osteoporosis: Assessing the Risk of Fragility Fracture*. NICE Short Guideline. NICE, London.

Parker, M. and Anand, J. (1991) What is the true mortality of hip fractures? *Public Health*, **105**(6), 443–446.

Parker, M. and Johansen, A. (2006) Hip fracture. *British Medical Journal*, **333**(7557), 27–30.

Pasco, J.A., Brennan, S.L., Henry, M.J. *et al.* (2011) Changes in hip fracture rates in south-eastern Australia spanning the period 1994–2007. *Journal of Bone Mineral Research*, **26**(7), 1648–1654.

Price, J.D., Sear, J.J.W. and Venn, R.R.M. (2004) Perioperative fluid volume optimization following proximal femoral fracture. *Cochrane Database of Systematic Reviews* **1** (Art. No.: CD003004). DOI:10.1002/14651858.CD003004.pub2.

Royal College of Physicians, British Geriatrics Society and the British Pain Society (2007) *The Assessment of Pain in Older People*. RCP/BGS/BPS, London. Available at: http://www.bgs.org.uk/Publications/pubdownlds/Sep2007PainAssessment.pdf (accessed 20 November 2013).

Scottish Intercollegiate Guidelines Network (SIGN) (2009) *Management of Hip Fracture in Older People*. National Clinical Guideline 111. Available at: http://www.sign.ac.uk/pdf/sign111.pdf (accessed 21 November 2013).

Shiga T., Wajima Z. and Ohe Y. (2008) Is operative delay associated with increased mortality of hip fracture patients? Systematic review, meta-analysis and meta-regression. *Canadian Journal of Anaesthesia*, **55**(3),146–154.

World Health Organization (2011) *Palliative Care for Older People: Better Practice*. WHO, Geneva. Available at: http://www.euro.who.int/__data/assets/pdf_file/0017/143153/e95052.pdf (accessed 22 April 2014).

CHAPTER 19

Spinal cord injury

Donna Poole and Pauline Robertson

Royal National Orthopaedic Hospital, Stanmore, Middlesex, UK

Introduction

The care of the individual following spinal cord injury (SCI) is complex and often provided by specialist practitioners. Sometimes, however, it is provided in general hospitals by practitioners who care for people with SCI rarely or intermittently. This chapter, therefore, aims to provide an overview of the care required from the time of injury and initial management, considering care needs through to rehabilitation and the planning for initial reintegration back into the community. The chapter will focus on the essential role of the nurse in this process as part of the wider multidisciplinary team (MDT) and will provide practitioners working in orthopaedic and musculoskeletal trauma settings with the evidence, guidance and knowledge required to underpin effective practice for the person with SCI.

Spinal cord injury

A **spinal injury** is often referred to as damage to the spinal column, the rigid support structure composed of the spinal vertebrae. There is also a risk that such a spinal injury can lead to damage to the cord and become a **spinal cord injury** (SCI). This is a life changing, catastrophic event that can result in partial or complete paralysis/neurological loss affecting the limbs and the autonomic nervous system.

Incidence, prevalence and demographics of SCI vary worldwide. There are said to be 40 000–60 000 people living with SCI in the UK (BASCIS 2006). Data collection varies internationally and incidence is usually estimated per million of the population. It is estimated that in the USA such injuries affect 40 per million of the population (National Spinal Cord Injury Statistics Centre, 2012) and approximately 15 per million in Australia (Norton 2009). It is relatively rare and has a reasonably good life expectancy as understanding and management of the condition grows. The financial, personal and societal costs of the complications of SCI, however, are considerable and initial trauma management, complication prevention and the care provided from the time of injury to reintegration into the community are central in ensuring the best outcomes for the patient and family. This presents significant challenges to practitioners.

Developments in the ways in which SCI care is organised locally around the world play an important part in how patient care is managed, enabling continued improvements in care through knowledge and skill development and the use of research, audit and monitoring of care pathways to ensure that care is provided at the point of need in a timely and effective manner to avoid complications. Care pathways for people with a new SCI are developed through consultation with the person, their families, carers and practitioners, enabling them to participate in designing their care. The development of trauma management systems has played a major role in providing the best resuscitation of the patient. In many areas it is a care standard for the injured person to be referred to a specialist spinal cord injury centre (SCIC) within four hours of arrival at hospital so that specialist care and advice can be sought from the outset. In many localities spinal outreach services (SOS) are now providing telephone support and advice, outreach visits for assessment and training and emotional support for patients, staff and relatives. Such services

Orthopaedic and Trauma Nursing: An Evidence-based Approach to Musculoskeletal Care, First Edition. Edited by Sonya Clarke and Julie Santy-Tomlinson.

work alongside patient groups and associations such as spinal injuries associations (SIA) and other organisations which support patients, carers and practitioners. Although the condition is rare, many aspects of care are fundamental. Even so, there are highly specialist aspects of care that are unfamiliar to many practitioners and it is crucial that more is known and understood to ensure the best outcomes possible for the injured person and their family.

Patterns of injury

SCI is not confined to any particular age group. Acute admissions to SCI centres in the UK, for example, ranged from 3 to 103 years in 2007–8, with 20% of new injuries occurring between 21 to 30 years of age (Barr 2009). Non-traumatic causes of injury such as infection, tumour and ischaemia account for approximately 28% of cases. Falls also account for an increasing proportion of traumatic SCI and the percentage of older people with SCI has been rising (BASCIS 2006). Children and older people sustaining SCI are more susceptible to the effects of severe polytrauma than other age groups (Harrison, 2007). This chapter will focus on traumatic causes of SCI, but the principles of and rationale for care will be applicable in all cases even if initial management of the injury may be different.

Traumatic SCI may be the result of both high and low velocity impacts and mechanisms of injury vary. These include; forced flexion of the spine, sudden vehicle deceleration, flexion rotation (e.g. fall off a motorcycle at speed or 'rolling' a vehicle), compression (diving or fall from a horse) and hyperextension (hitting the head or chin). Injury is often associated with unexpected sudden deceleration, impact or collision with or without associated loss of consciousness (LOC), localised pain or deformity of the spinal column or loss of sensation and or movement in upper and lower limbs. The speed of impact and the height of a fall are not indicators for severity of spinal cord injury; in fact, most falls resulting in SCI tend to be from a low height (from 1 metre or less). It is important to maintain a high index of suspicion of SCI after any trauma and always in the unconscious patient at the scene with initial management including early appropriate spinal column protective measures (ACS 2008).

Anatomical considerations

As discussed in Chapter 4, the spinal column comprises the bony elements from cervical vertebra (C1–7), thoracic vertebra (T1–12), lumbar vertebra (L1–5) and sacral vertebra (S1–5, fused in adults) and the coccyx (four fused). This surrounds the vertebral canal which, in turn, surrounds the spinal cord. Ligaments surround all the bony surfaces; the key ones being the anterior longitudinal ligament, the posterior longitudinal ligament and the ligamentum flavum. This creates a corset-like effect that stabilises the whole spinal structure.

The spinal cord is surrounded by cerebrospinal fluid (CSF) and enclosed by meninges, providing a flexible, protective system within a semi-rigid frame that allows movement of the spine while protecting the cord and spinal nerves. Most movement occurs at the cranio-cervical, cervico-thoracic or thoraco-lumbar junction where the most rigid part of the structure (e.g. the thoracic region) meets a movable region (e.g. the cervical or lumbar). In the cervical region, the cord is enlarged and passes through a relatively narrow vertebral canal. Numerous neurones that supply the upper limbs arise from this section of the cord. This contributes to cervical injuries being the most common; accounting for approximately 50% of injuries in the USA since 2005 (National Spinal Cord Injury Statistical Center 2012), and 47% in the United Kingdom in 2009 (Spinal Injuries Association, 2009) and the remainder being spread between the thoracic, thoracolumbar and lumbosacral regions.

Two thirds of the blood supply to the cord is provided by the anterior artery. The posterior arteries and radicular arteries provide the final third, with input provided at different levels in the cervical and thoracic regions. Injury to the anterior artery can result in ischaemia of the cord and has a far greater impact on a larger area of tissue (two thirds of the anterior aspect of the cord). Traumatic or non-traumatic injury that results in a space-occupying lesion such as a haematoma or foreign body can cause compression to the cord and ischaemia that result in neurological damage.

In children, the vertebral facets have a shallow angulation and the vertebral bodies, particularly cervical, are more wedge-shaped. The structure is also more cartilaginous, providing much more ligamentous laxity. This can lead to false negative X-ray results. This is known as Spinal Cord Injury Without Radiologic Abnormality (SCIWORA) and is considered in more detail in Chapter 24. Children may be wrongly sent home with little or no intervention. Younger children are less able to participate in neurological examinations and may present several days or even weeks later with evidence of delayed onset neurological changes. It is recommended to always maintain a high index of suspicion in cases where there may be relatively minor trauma.

Older people may have concurrent conditions such as osteoporosis, ankylosing spondylitis and spinal stenosis, making them more vulnerable to spinal cord compression from minor trauma such as falls from standing or a low height. Forced hyperextension is a classic example that results in stretching of the cord and compression from subsequent oedema and haematoma often presenting as Spinal Cord Injury Without Radiographic Evidence of Trauma (SCIWORET).

Pathophysiology of the injury

There are several stages of injury within the cord itself (Sapru, 2002). Immediately following the primary injury (within minutes) there is disruption to cell bodies and axonal activity leading to haemorrhage and oedema in and around the site of injury, releasing inflammatory mediators. This results in a neurochemical cascade, leading to further injury and damage to the cord secondary to the primary injury (within hours). This can eventually result in a CSF-filled cyst in the centre of the cord (weeks to years) with the potential for elongating the damage caused from the initial injury that can result in neurological loss higher than that initially sustained. The resulting scar tissue in the cord prevents any growing nerve fibres from crossing and, with inhibitory substances and lack of nerve growth factors in the surrounding tissues, the adult spinal cord does not regenerate spontaneously after injury. Neuro-protection and neuro-regeneration are currently being researched but, at this time, spinal cord injury remains 'incurable.'

Emergency care and management

Principles of care at the site of trauma include the standards for Advanced Trauma Life Support (ATLS) as discussed in Chapter 16. As previously discussed, SCI should always be suspected in the unconscious trauma patient. It is important to maintain spinal alignment during care and management, but life threatening injuries take priority along with extraction from areas of danger for the patient, practitioner or others. If the patient is awake, assessing sensation and movement will provide information regarding voluntary movement and sensation, pain in the neck and/or back, pins and needles, burning and electric shock sensations should be noted as part of the assessment. For the conscious patient the practitioner should check hand-grip function and breath and voice sounds to give an early indication of where the injury may be. Diaphragmatic breathing (paradoxical, 'see-saw' breathing) can indicate a cervical or high thoracic neurological deficit along with weakness of hand-grasp or soft low volume voice.

If a high cervical injury is suspected the team should immediately instigate respiratory support as the effort to maintain respiratory function may very quickly not be sustained. Monitoring should be commenced and maintained throughout the emergency period for signs of hypotension (spinal/neurogenic shock – if there are no obvious signs of blood/fluid loss), bradycardia, diaphragmatic breathing, priapism (semi or full erection of the penis), floppy/flaccid limbs and warm peripheries with a low BP. These are all signs of neurological compromise. Priapism is a medical emergency and seeking medical advice and action should be taken to resolve it within six hours. The patient should be transported to the emergency department/trauma centre as quickly as possible under spinal immobilisation precautions using a hard collar, spinal board and head immobilisation (BOA 2006) with the spine in neutral alignment (normal curvature of spine, lying flat). Methylprednisolone is no longer recommended in acute SCI initial management (Bonner and Smith 2013).

As soon as it is safe to do so, the patient should be turned using a five-person log roll (see Figure 16.5 Chapter 16) to examine for tenderness and deformity and to insert a spinal board, hard collar and head blocks with strapping to completely immobilise the whole spine ready for transportation. In the emergency department the spinal board should be removed as soon as possible to avoid excessive pressure on the bony prominences and pre-hospital care practitioners should inform the receiving team how long the board has been in place so that they can make an informed plan to remove the board (BOA 2006) and check the pressure areas for skin trauma.

Spinal stability and management of the injury

Once the patient's condition has been stabilised, detailed clinical assessment and investigations will assist in the diagnosis of SCI. Plain X-rays of the whole spine will identify spinal fractures. The gold standard recommendation is to use whole spine MRI when a SCI is suspected. MRI imaging may be accompanied with CT to enable the team to more clearly understand the nature of the bony and soft tissue spine injury and ascertain whether this is 'stable' or 'unstable.' This will inform the management/treatment plan.

The term 'unstable' refers to the ability of the spinal column to withstand further stress without further deformity or neurological damage (Greaves *et al.*, 2009). Unstable fractures and soft tissue injury of the spine can result in further trauma to the spinal cord or damage where there was none previously. Care must be provided that prevents further insult to the cord which causes the level of neurological damage to worsen; for example, through inappropriate or poor manual handling, hypoxia or further hypotension. A medical assessment and decision about spinal stability will be based on an understanding of the cause of the injury and the forces placed on the structures and cord, the reviews of CT/X-ray and MRI and assessment of the patient. This must be documented by the medical team and the patient moved with all precautions requested to ensure no further damage to the spinal cord. If the injury has been deemed stable by the medical team, this must be documented in the notes before the patient is moved without any precautions. Senior medical practitioners may specify continued use of collars or braces or limitations on movement with or without such supports. Practitioners must ensure that this is clearly documented and fully explained as understanding the medical rationale for these decisions helps the team to be safe, clear and consistent in their management of the patient. If there are any doubts, the patient must be treated as having an unstable injury with full spinal precautions. The risks of being immobilised such as pressure ulcers must be weighed against the risks of being removed from immobilisation devices and care adapted accordingly. Hard collars should be removed routinely (during a head hold procedure, where the cervical spine is secure) and the patient's skin palpated or visualised for signs of pressure, particularly the occiput and clavicles. Guidelines for movement and handling of the patient with an unstable spinal/spinal cord injury are discussed in Box 19.1.

Box 19.1 Evidence digest: Moving and handling patients with actual or suspected spinal cord injuries

It is not possible to provide research based guidelines for all aspects of musculoskeletal care. One example of this is the manual handling of patients following spinal injury. In such instances expert practitioners often work together to provide guidelines that are based on expert clinical opinion. Although, as discussed in Chapter 2, expert opinion is not a higher level form of evidence, it is nevertheless an important way of ensuring that care is effective and based on the best possible practice. The Multidisciplinary Association of Spinal Cord Injury Professionals (MASCIP) is an example of a national organisation (UK) that endeavours to provide evidence-based guidelines representing current research and the consensus opinion of the best care of the patient with SCI. Guidelines are based on clinical and service user expertise and are created by inviting key representatives of specialist and national organisations and interest groups to form a working group. Core themes for the production of MASCIP guidelines are originated within the Annual MASCIP Scientific Meetings.

Existing guidelines at http://www.mascip.co.uk/guidelines.aspx include:

- Moving and handling patients with actual or suspected spinal cord injuries (SCI) (2009). These provide detailed pictorial guidance on recommended techniques for the movement and transfer of patients and should be referred to for further guidance. The guidelines include, for example, how to turn the patient with an unstable spinal injury.

Additional guidelines include:

- Guidelines for management of neurogenic bowel dysfunction in individuals with central neurological conditions (2012)
- Management of the older person with a new spinal injury (2010)
- Guidelines for the management of neuropathic pain in adults following spinal cord injury (2008)

Conservative or surgical management of the spinal column injury will vary depending on medical opinion and protocol in the unit in which care is being provided as there is currently no consensus as to whether surgical treatment or conservative management is ultimately better for patient outcomes. Conservative options involve the use of an orthosis, halo brace, plaster jacket or bed rest with or without traction. The availability of staff who can provide expert care such as in a dedicated spinal cord injury centre can be central in this decision as the complications of both the spinal cord injury and the immobilisation of conservative management make care complex. Cervical traction is often chosen as the immediate method of reduction and stabilisation of dislocated vertebrae. As the injured spinal cord is very vulnerable to distraction it is essential that the traction device is monitored closely during any intervention and neurological observations are carried out on a regular basis reporting any loss/change of neurology (BOA, 2006) (see below for neurological assessment).

Subsequent care and rehabilitation

Following surgery or initiation of conservative treatment, the next priority is for the injured person to be under the care of the best team of professionals to take them through a rehabilitation programme specifically designed with the SCI person's care needs in mind. In the UK, for example, the Spinal Injuries Association (SIA) have campaigned vigorously to ensure that all patients with SCI have access to a specialist SCI centre to ensure that their optimal rehabilitation potentials are achieved. Not all patients, however, can be moved to a specialist centre and one of the ways currently being used to address this is with spinal outreach services (SOS). Practitioners will visit, assess, support and train practitioners in other settings (such as the general hospital, trauma centre or regional intensive care unit) on how to care for the patient safely and effectively. The priority is for the patient to receive care that will allow them to rehabilitate without complications such as pressure ulcers and infections as well as respiratory problems that prolong stays in intensive/critical care units when there is a need for mechanical ventilation.

Documenting the neurological loss in the initial stage is essential on admission, at 72 hours following admission and prior to and after any surgery. This should include documentation of the neurological deficit, including the lowest sacral segments (deep anal pressure, sensation pin prick and light touch and voluntary anal contraction). This is known as the International Standard for Neurological Classification of SCI (ISNCSCI), however it is better known as the American Spinal Injuries Association Impairment Scale (AIS) (Box 19.2). The AIS assesses where the last 'normal' neurological motor and sensory levels are on both sides of the body in the last sacral segments, enabling diagnosis of 'complete' and 'incomplete' SCI as shown. This diagnosis allows for accurate information to be given to the clinical team on how to manage their patients until they can be admitted to a specialist spinal cord injury centre. The completion of the AIS chart requires specialist training to ensure accuracy of diagnosis.

Box 19.2 American Spinal Injuries Association Impairment Scale (ASIA) (2006). Reproduced with permission from American Spinal Injury Association

A Complete: No motor or sensory function is preserved in the sacral segments S4–S5

B Incomplete: Sensory but not motor function is preserved below the neurological level and includes the sacral segments S4–S5

C Incomplete: Motor function is preserved below the neurological level and more than half of key muscles below the neurological level have a muscle grade less than 3

D Incomplete: Motor function is preserved below the neurological level and at least half of key muscles below the neurological level have a muscle grade of 3 or more

E Normal: motor and sensory function are normal

The associated assessment chart can be downloaded and copied (permission provided on the chart at http://www.asia-spinalinjury.org/elearning/ISNCSCI_Exam_Sheet_r4.pdf

As the cord is an extension of the brain from the medulla oblongata, it has many characteristics that the brain has. Not only does it relay messages up the cord to the brain (sensory/ascending pathways) and relay messages back down the cord (motor/descending pathways), it also sends messages within the cord via interneurons. Following spinal cord injury this creates a reflex and allows electrical messages to move quickly within the cord without the brain controlling it. With injuries in the region of the conus medullaris (the base of the cord) there can be a mixed picture of some reflex activity and some flaccidity. This is often referred to as a conal injury. Injury above this level is referred to as a supraconal injury. If injury is sustained in the cauda equina region, there is no ability to create this connectivity between neurones, as the cord (as a single entity) no longer exists. There are only peripheral spinal nerves exiting the cord from approximately L1 bony level and thus no reflex activity can be seen in injuries that affect this level and below (generally below L1).

Understanding if the patient's cord injury is complete or incomplete and from which level provides predictive information for nursing care such as the patient's ability to breathe, swallow or feed themselves, VTE prevention and bladder and bowel management.

Neurogenic and spinal shock

These two terms are often used interchangeably. However, they present quite differently. After trauma to the spinal cord there is often a period of spinal 'shock' depending on the severity of the insult to the cord and the amount of cord damage. This can result in a 'shut down' of functions controlled by that area of the cord resulting in an absence of reflexes i.e. flaccid paralysis of all skeletal muscle and loss of all spinal reflexes below the level of injury. This is a temporary state and will resolve in hours or weeks from the injury. Spinal shock does not indicate the severity of paralysis in the long term and neurological recovery will vary as cord oedema subsides and spinal neurons regain excitability.

Neurogenic shock should be suspected if there is a cervical or high thoracic injury with hypotension and bradycardia with no signs of systemic fluid loss. With the initial flaccid paralysis and neurogenic shock it is common for there to be a low resting BP (e.g. 80/50 or 90/60). This is due to passive vasodilation of the blood vessels, lack of sympathetic tone and reflex activity below the level of injury. It may also lead to blood pooling in the extremities resulting in oedema in the hands and feet.

Neurogenic shock may require inotropic therapy to keep the cardiovascular system supported whilst it is in crisis. The autonomic reflexes that normally control BP can be unreliable in maintaining the body's equilibrium while in 'shock' and increasing fluid input may simply result in overloading a system that already has full circulating volume (providing no hypovolaemia has been diagnosed). Conservative use of crystalloids, principally normal saline, is often adequate and fluids should be given based on urine output (approximately 0.5 mg/kg/hr). Incomplete injuries may have less significant changes if any.

As well as close monitoring of the blood pressure and pulse, frequent monitoring of body temperature is also advisable. Passive vasodilation of the blood vessels and inability to moderate temperature below the level of injury through the usual mechanisms such as shivering may lead to poikilothermia (assuming the ambient temperature of the environment), resulting in hypo- or hyperthermia.

In higher level SCI usual signs and symptoms of VTE (venous thromboembolism) such as leg pain and chest pain may be absent due to loss of sensory pathways. VTE may present as persistent tachycardia with recurrent fevers in the absence of sepsis. Prophylaxis with LMWH (low molecular weight heparin) and use of usual VTE prevention regimes is mandatory along with other prophylactic measures such as passive and or active limb movements and deep breathing. Regular measurements of calf and thigh width in order to identify unilateral increase can give an early indicator of VTE (see Chapter 9 for further information).

During this time of flaccidity it is essential to use the correct handling of vulnerable limbs. It is most important for practitioners to understand that poor handling/mishandling may have detrimental future outcomes for hand and arm function and lower limb function. For example, a poorly placed hand on a pillow can lead to the patient losing the ability to grip that will be required later during rehabilitation for feeding and holding utensils. Unsupported feet can lead to foot drop.

Bradycardia

In cervical SCI, while in neurogenic shock, the unopposed activity of the parasympathetic vagus (10th cranial) nerve results in bradycardia and there is a risk of asystole secondary to stimulation such as with pharyngeal suction, attempted intubation, endotracheal suction, passing of nasogastric tubes or turning the patient during or following surgery. Exaggerated vagal responses, however, tend to be temporary and reduce over time.

Respiratory

Airway maintenance is a priority of care in the acute phase. The patient is often nursed on flat bed rest and this may have an effect on their respiratory function. It is suggested that all critical/intensive care patients should have the whole bed tilted to 30 degrees head up (reverse trendelenburg). However, SCI persons benefit from being nursed flat. The flat position has a beneficial effect on the patient's vital capacity by maintaining diaphragmatic curvature through use of abdominal content pressure. When sat up the pressure from the abdominal contents is reduced therefore increasing the effort of breathing (RISCI, 2012). SCI patients have increased respiratory secretion production due to the unopposed stimulation of the parasympathetic nervous system and management of this becomes a priority if the secretions become difficult for the patient to cope with, particularly while in neurogenic shock.

Knowing the neurological level of injury will give the practitioner information on the muscles that the patient can still control and the muscles that are affected by the SCI. The major breathing muscle is the diaphragm. This is innervated by the cervical 3/4/5 segmental nerve level. The usual breathing pattern for a high level tetraplegic is paradoxical due to the lack of intercostal muscle control and abdominal muscle control. The higher the level of injury, the more likely the patient is to need mechanical ventilation support in the early stages, especially while they are in spinal or neurogenic shock, as they will tire easily due to respiratory muscle weakness, increased secretions and retention of secretions. Abdominal guarding may also occur along with paralytic ileus. If any neurological symptoms are identified such as pins and needles in the limbs, increasing loss of sensation or uncontrolled pain in the patient who had previously maintained sensation, immediate medical attention should be sought. There may be nerve impingement, a developing haematoma or oedema around the cord, any of which require immediate action.

Baseline respiratory assessment and observations of breathing pattern including vital capacity must be recorded. The practitioner should also pay close attention to the possibility that swelling and oedema in the cord may make the neurological level rise and that this may have an impact on spontaneous breathing. If the patient presents as a cervical 4 AIS A level with swelling that ascends up the cord, the level may rise to C3 level, making spontaneous breathing silently laboured or impossible, leading to respiratory failure. If the patient has underlying respiratory problems (such as asthma or COPD) or if they are obese, particular attention must be paid to respiratory assessment. Care should consist of regular turning, monitoring of respiratory effort, rate and breath sounds and vital capacity, paradoxical breathing or asymmetry of the chest wall movements, regular physiotherapy, blood gas monitoring and SaO_2 should be maintained at 95% or above (Bonner and Smith, 2013).

It is important to observe for swallowing problems in patients with an acute cervical SCI as this will have an impact on their respiratory function and nutritional status. A range of factors increase the risk of dysphagia including the need for tracheostomy, ventilation, collar, nasogastric tube, type of surgery and any additional brain injury. There may also be problems with dry mouth and weak voice and patients may benefit from a swallowing assessment by a Speech and Language Therapist. Stress gastric ulceration from unopposed sympathetic activity means that risk of gastric ulceration and haemorrhage is possible. Use of proton pump inhibitors or H2 antagonist drugs can be helpful.

Skin care and avoiding pressure ulcers

Pressure ulcer prevention is a very significant aspect of care for patients with SCI. Significant weight loss due to metabolic and nutritional status and the loss of superficial tissues, subcutaneous fat and muscle to cushion the bony prominences, together with a lack of sensation, makes the SCI patient one of the most vulnerable groups. From the beginning of the SCI, immunity, skin integrity, vasomotor control and sensation will all be different to the pre-injury state and will make the SCI person more vulnerable to acquiring pressure ulcers. Risk assessment on admission along with an associated plan of care is essential. Both of these must be reviewed regularly and as the patient's condition changes, especially if there is any sign of sepsis or extreme weight loss or after spinal surgery. The principles of pressure ulcer prevention discussed in more detail in Chapter 12 also apply to the person with SCI.

Skin observation or signs of damage should begin immediately on admission. A base line observation should be recorded as soon as the skin can be visualised with the patient's clothing removed. There may be tissue damage from lacerations, bruising etc. and this should also be noted. As soon the skin state has been assessed a pressure ulcer prevention plan should be instigated. It is safe to position the patient in a side lying position as long as spinal alignment is maintained and pillows are used to support the position firmly. Maintaining spinal alignment makes the use of the 30-degree tilt discussed in Chapter 12 inappropriate in patients with SCI. A regular turning plan should be instigated along with use of pressure redistributing mattresses and cushions. Alternating pressure mattresses should not, however, be used if the spinal fracture is unstable. Many SCICs use specialist 'turning' beds when prolonged immobilisation of the unstable spine is likely. Such equipment can facilitate care in the general hospital, but should only be used if staff are trained to use them in a safe and effective manner. Regular care should consist of good nutrition, adequate hydration, skin inspection, keeping the skin clean and dry and action planning.

Initial bladder and bowel management

Immediately following SCI the bladder will be flaccid (without tone) while the spinal shock is present. Free drainage of the bladder should be maintained with an indwelling urinary catheter initially to avoid over-distension of the bladder, urinary incontinence and stagnation of urine leading to UTI (urinary tract infection). If priapism is present and has not resolved, urethral catheterisation should not be attempted and a suprapubic catheter inserted instead. Once spinal shock has resolved, an appropriate bladder regime can be commenced.

The gut suffers from neurogenic shock and paralytic ileus is possible during the first 48 hours. The patient should, therefore, be fasted ('nil by mouth') for at least this period or until bowel sounds return. Enteral nutrition is recommended if the patient is unable to take an oral diet after this as metabolic changes following severe injury can impact on the nutritional status for several weeks after injury. Within the first 48 hours baseline enteric neurological reflexes usually return. It is important to check bowel sounds daily, perform a daily rectal check and perform digital removal of faeces (DRF) to ensure that the rectum is clear of faeces as well as observe for abdominal distension. A free draining nasogastric tube is recommended with observation for bradycardia and vagal stimulation when it is being passed.

As the patient's condition improves and bowel sounds return, a bowel management regime should be established in light of the AIS to ensure that faeces is of the right consistency to enable DRF. There should be continued observation for signs of paralytic ileus which can return at any time. As reflexes return, autonomic dysreflexia can occur in response to rectal stimulation for those persons with SCI above T6.

Autonomic dysreflexia

This is a medical emergency. Autonomic dysreflexia (AD) is an exaggerated response of the sympathetic nervous system to any noxious or painful stimuli. This is most likely when the SCI is above T6. Noxious stimuli include bladder outflow obstruction, constipation, pressure ulceration or even restrictive clothing – anything that would cause pain or uncomfortable sensations in those who are able-bodied. The stimuli are picked up by the sympathetic nervous system and trigger reflex responses that cause vasoconstriction of the large blood vessels in the gut. This rapidly elevates the blood pressure, which then continues to rise. Above the level of the injury the body responds by trying to lower the BP by sweating and dilating the vessels of the skin of the face, head and shoulders (which appear flushed) and the blood vessels in the nose. There is usually an associated bradycardia as the parasympathetic nervous system (via the vagus nerve) may be stimulated. If the stimulus that triggered the AD is not removed the patient may have a myocardial infarction or stroke leading to death.

Once spinal shock has resolved and reflexes have returned AD can present at any time and must be considered whenever the BP is elevated. In a tetraplegic patient the resting BP may be as low as 80/50 mmHg due to passive vasodilation of peripheral blood vessels below the level of injury. The higher the level of injury the more there will be autonomic changes and altered observations. AD should be suspected with a rise of 15–20 mmHg in BP above usual for that patient. Initial management is to find the stimulus and remove it. Sitting the patient up (if the spine is stable) may help to reduce the BP while the cause is sought such as urinary outflow obstruction, constipation or pressure ulcer. Further stimulus to the bowel or bladder in performing evacuations to resolve the AD can actually trigger further stimulus and reflexes, potentially exacerbating the problem. Using local anaesthetic gel to perform the examination can help to reduce local stimuli in the rectum. If the stimulus cannot be found, removed or resolved a quick-acting hypertensive agent such as Nifedipine can be given sublingually (up to twice) to reduce the BP. It is important to be aware the BP will drop rapidly once the cause has been resolved. If the problem cannot be resolved, such as ingrowing toenails or pressure ulcer, advice and action from senior medical staff or the resuscitation team should be sought. Regular administration of anti-hypertensive agents may be required to keep the BP under control until the stimulus is treated or resolved.

Early rehabilitation

Following surgery, close attention should be paid to post-operative instructions for patient handling and turning, pain management and the use of collars and orthoses. Instructions may contain advice about the maximum angle to which patients can sit without a collar or brace (e.g. the patient can sit to 45 degrees without a collar but with a collar for all other activity, or no collar when flat but collar for all mobilising activity including bed mobility). The clearer the instructions the easier it is for practitioners to apply the correct techniques for moving and handling in and out of the bed and these should be followed carefully. Care should follow the standard pathways for all orthopaedic and spinal surgery with particular attention to neurovascular assessment so that any deterioration in sensation, for example, is identified quickly.

At this point the person with a new SCI will receive information about the care they will be receiving with a view to moving gradually towards self-care. This will include a discussion of the level of independence or otherwise they are likely to achieve so that they can begin to perceive this goal. Ensuring that patients are fully informed and start their rehabilitation is essential in giving people back control over the decisions that affect them and their lives. These conversations can be difficult and distressing for patients and need to be handled by experienced staff with appropriate sensitivity and honesty.

Pain

Pain after SCI is often misunderstood. Some people think that because the person is paralysed that they will not feel any pain. The reality is quite the opposite. Pain can fit into 2 categories; nociceptive (musculo skeletal and visceral) or neuropathic either at the level of injury, below the level of injury or above the level of injury. It is essential that assessment is carried out by the appropriate practitioners and that a plan for treatment is included. This will involve taking a full history and physical examination. Another misconception is that people with pain have incomplete spinal cord injuries, which is also not the case. Complete SCI people may have high levels of pain that are not fully treatable with medication and may require a support network that enables them to live with the pain. Pain management and assessment are considered in more detail in chapter 11.

Spasm

Spasm can occur once spinal and neurogenic shock have subsided. It is a velocity-dependent increase in the muscle stretch reflex usually stimulated by touching the SCI person's skin or movement during daily patient care. It can present in complete and incomplete injuries but is most prevalent in sensory incomplete lesions. If the patient is still considered as unstable or is being managed conservatively then maintaining alignment and staff safety during care provision can be an additional challenge. Spasticity should be expected and discussed with the patient and their family and information about the cause and physiology should be provided. It is not a sign of return of normal movement but is a reflex initiated response to a stimulus. Spasm can be useful in providing clues as to injury, pain or infection below the level of the lesion (e.g. full bladder or bowel) and can also be used for standing and transferring. Too much reflex activity and spasm can also be detrimental and need to be monitored and treated as appropriate. Correct positioning in bed, physiotherapy for stretching and exercising limbs and use of antispasmodic medication such as baclofen can be used initially until the rehabilitation team explore the benefits and use of spasm for the patient.

Starting mobilisation

The decision to begin mobilisation will be made by the senior medical practitioner in discussion with the multidisciplinary team. When spinal shock and neurogenic shock have resolved there should be no need for inotropic support of the BP. In the high level tetraplegic person there will be a common propensity for hypotension and when their position is altered the BP will often change up or down accordingly. For example, on sitting up the BP will drop and when elevating the legs above the heart the BP will rise. This 'orthostatic hypotension', when moving to an upright position, requires adequate preparation for initial mobilisation involving advanced planning for enough staff members to be available. An abdominal binder (large abdominal elasticated band) is often used to brace the abdominal contents in an effort to keep the pooled blood in the abdomen and avoid it escaping into the lower extremities when moving to upright. Eating before mobilising for the first time should be avoided as this often leads to vomiting on sitting up and increases the likelihood of hypotension.

A graduated sitting program in a 4-section profiling bed is the most effective approach to minimising risk to staff and patients. Gradual gentle inclines of 30 degrees, while monitoring BP, helps to ascertain if the person can progress without risk. This should begin with a 30-degree tilt for 5-10 minutes with full supervision and monitoring for nausea, vomiting, fainting and increased pain. Vasoconstrictor medication can be administered 30 minutes prior to sitting up if it is difficult to keep the systolic BP above 90 mmHg. It may take 2 or 3 sessions before the patient can achieve 30 minutes sitting up in bed. If the patient cannot tolerate sitting with the feet tilted down they are not ready to get out of bed. Once the patient is sitting upright in bed to roughly 90 degrees for 30 minutes, tilting the whole bed feet down (reverse Trendelenburg) will mimic more accurately what it will be like when they sit out in a wheelchair. The therapist should have measured the patient for a wheelchair that will accommodate the relevant level of injury with the right space and tilt. A pressure redistributing cushion will also be required from the outset. It is good, psychologically, to dress the patient for sitting up in bed in preparation for sitting out in the wheelchair. This helps to build up some skin tolerance to clothing with a view to building up from softer to more rigid clothing (such as jeans) over time. Shoes are needed to protect the feet from injury and pressure and should be a size bigger to accommodate any swelling in the legs, ankles and feet.

The first session sitting out in the wheelchair provides the opportunity to adapt the wheelchair to fit the patient more individually; for example, to adjust foot plates or alter lateral supports. Someone should stay with the patient for the whole time that they are up in the wheelchair as BP monitoring will still be required. This activity is extremely tiring for the patient and can be painful at the site of injury. Tetraplegic patients often complain of neck pain because it is now unsupported or only supported with a hard collar. Time sitting up in the chair should be increased slowly and gradually until longer periods can be tolerated with no BP drops or other symptoms.

Ongoing pressure ulcer prevention

Once the patient is up for an hour, a plan for pressure relief in the wheelchair should be instigated such as tilting laterally to each side for 2 minutes or bending forwards for 2 minutes in each hour. If the skin is reddened at all after sitting, especially over the bony prominences, a further check should be made within 30 minutes of return to bed. If the mark remains non-blanching the time in the wheelchair should not be increased but reduced to a time that does not produce a non-blanching skin reaction. This can then gradually progress to sitting up all day with pressure relieving position changes every hour for 2 minutes as long as there is no skin deterioration. Increasing skin tolerance to pressure needs to continue gradually to ensure that eventually the person can sleep overnight without requiring position changes. Education to ensure the SCI person develops the ability to manage or perform their own skin checks with a mirror or carer assistance is crucial. Once a pressure ulcer has been sustained there is a higher likelihood of sustaining more damage, particularly in same area. Living with the risk of pressure ulcers significantly impacts on home and work life, affecting the feasibility of holding down a job and maintaining life satisfaction.

Longer-term bowel management

The process of defecation and micturition is a complex and coordinated process in an able-bodied person. Voluntary control is mostly via the sacral nerves S2-4. Any SCI is, therefore, likely to cause disconnection between the brain the anorectal structures. The rectum is normally empty and when faeces arrive in the rectum a conscious urge to defecate is triggered which is usually controlled by the brain until a socially acceptable time for elimination. The internal anal sphincter is composed of smooth involuntary muscle and the external anal sphincter is composed of skeletal voluntary muscle (refer to the MASCIP bowel management guidelines 2012 for further information). As reflex activity returns and the patient commences mobilisation, a bowel management regime can be commenced based on the AIS with the aim of ensuring the person is able to empty their bowel fully within an acceptable timeframe on a regular basis. Consideration of past bowel patterns and medical/surgical history is crucial. Assistance will be required to ensure appropriate stool consistency and passage of stool through the gut as well as emptying of the rectum.

Depending on the level of neurological damage some enteric reflexes may exist and digestion, absorption and peristalsis will be slower, leading to an increased transit time of faeces. Stools can become hard due to reabsorption of fluid from the bowel and the risk of constipation is high. Appropriate fluids and diet are essential elements in counteracting this and use of the gastrocolic reflex (reflex contraction of the colon in response to ingestion of warm food or fluid 15–20 earlier) is also useful. Aperients may be commenced to ensure stools are the right consistency for evacuation and that the patient does not become constipated or impacted. Digital removal of faeces (DRF) is an appropriate and required procedure for the emptying of the neurologically damaged bowel

Box 19.3 Evidence digest: Neurologic bowel management

Krassioukov *et al.* (2010) carried out a systematic review of studies that assessed pharmacological and non-pharmacological intervention for the management of neurogenic bowel after SCI with the aim of reviewing the evidence for neurogenic bowel management. They considered 57 RCTs and prospective cohort, case-control and pre-post studies. The review found that multifaceted programmes tend to be the first approach to neurogenic bowel management, but that this is supported by lower levels of evidence. It was reported that transanal irrigation is a promising non-pharmacological intervention to reduce constipation and faecal incontinence. When conservative bowel management is not effective, the authors report that pharmacological interventions such as prokinetic agents have strong evidence of being effective for the management of chronic constipation. The quality of the evidence varies, but provides practitioners with some advice on which to base practice and suggests that more than one option is necessary in establishing a successful bowel management strategy for individuals.

(MASCIP 2012). Some of the evidence for bowel management is considered in Box 19.3.

Care should include a daily assisted bowel movement using Digital Removal of Faeces (DRF) until such time as sphincter reflexes appear in an upper motor neurone (UMN) reflex lesion (usually above T12). If the person has a complete SCI and has a reflexic sphincter (the sphincter contracts involuntarily when a PR check is done, and they have a strong positive bulbospongiosis reflex test) it can be assumed it is likely to be an UMN or reflex lesion. For this type of lesion the bowel will have reflex over-stimulation of the external anal sphincter, pelvic floor and the colon, meaning that there is less compliance or stretch and the sphincter is tightly contracted. Intervention is required to ensure the rectum is fully emptied on a regular basis as sphincter dyssynergia (lack of co-ordination between the contraction and relaxation of the sphincters) may result in stool retained in the rectum. The person may appear to be evacuating their bowel by themselves, but this may not mean it is emptying fully as it is being evacuated through a reflex contraction and not a coordinated contraction and expulsion. The bowel regime will consist of regular aperients or laxatives for stimulation and softening of faeces, massage of the abdomen, use of the gastrocolic reflex and suppositories. Anal stimulation for the UMN neurogenic bowel involves insertion of a lubricated, gloved finger into the rectum and gently circling the finger for 15–20 seconds or until the external anal sphincter can be felt to relax (through overstimulation of skeletal muscle) and the internal anal sphincter contracts. The finger is then removed as the faeces is expelled. The external anal sphincter will reflexly contract again and this process may be repeated several times until the rectum is empty or the reflexes tire and DRF can be used to ensure the rectum is empty. Failure to completely empty the rectum may result in an unplanned bowel evacuation later which is emotionally and physically distressing.

For those persons with a SCI that results in a flaccid presentation (LMN – generally below T12/L1), the external anal sphincter will appear soft and does not reflexly contract when a gloved lubricated finger is inserted and no bulbospongiosis reflex will be seen. The colon has increased compliance and there is little intrinsic peristalsis. The pelvic floor is relaxed as is the internal anal sphincter. This means there is a high risk of faecal incontinence as the external gateway mechanisms are impaired and any abdominal pressure can result in loss of faeces if the rectum is not emptied regularly. The bowel regime will consist of regular aperients or laxatives for stimulation and softening of faeces and massage of the abdomen. Use of the gastrocolic reflex may be of some help for enteric reflexes but suppositories will be of little help as no reflex emptying or stimulation of the rectum will be gained. DRF will be required to ensure emptying of the bowel.

The aim in all instances is to ensure that the faeces is in the rectum at the established time and of the right consistency to ensure complete emptying, so timing of the bowel evacuation and the ingestion of laxatives (8–12 hours prior) is important. A single digital check 5–10 mins after the last faeces has been expelled is important in ensuring faeces is not left in the rectum. Bowel management is mostly performed on the bed due to the risks involved for the carer in moving and handling and positioning for DRF. Use of gravity by using toilets or commodes, if appropriate, is also useful. Phosphate enemas should be used with caution as there is a risk of autonomic dysreflexia with a SCI above T6.

Quality of life for the SCI person is positively affected by having an effective bowel and bladder regime. It is crucial this is established as soon as possible and education and involvement of the person in this process is key. They may not wish or be able to provide their own care, but the options should be discussed and education be provided so that problem solving and decisions regarding their future choice of bowel management are in their control. Persons with SCI at C4 and above will have no or very limited ability to self-care for bowel evacuation, but they can direct carers to provide this assistance if educated to do so. Other options for bowel evacuation are available such as transanal irrigation, retrograde colonic irrigation, nerve stimulator or stoma, but these are not usually offered as the initial choice. Being aware of all options offers awareness, choice and discussion. The medical practitioner or specialist nurse can help with decision making as people living with SCI have can change their bowel evacuation methods and bladder evacuation methods over time depending on need and lifestyle.

Genitourinary management

Genitourinary function is both autonomic (involuntary) and somatic (voluntary). The level of SCI and diagnosis (complete and incomplete and UMN and LMN) as well as hand function and patient choice will define the treatment programme put in place. In the able-bodied person the bladder fills, the stretch receptors in the detrusor (bladder) muscle stretch and a conscious urge to void is triggered which is usually received and controlled by the brain until the person finds a socially acceptable time and place to void. Following SCI these processes are interrupted, voluntary control is impaired and autonomic control remains with either a reflex or flaccid presentation (UMN above T 12 or LMN usually below T12/L1).

Understanding the AIS will help to predict what type of input the healthcare professional will need to plan. For example, if the patient is an AIS "B" then the patient may have some degree of sensation but will not have voluntary control of the sacral nerves that control the urinary sphincter. They may report that they feel ready to void but will have no ability to relax the muscle in order to void. This may mean that they will ask when they need to void but that an intermittent catheter may be needed to assist with drainage of urine. The overall aim is to ensure complete emptying of the bladder in order to protect the kidneys, maintain continence and avoid complications such as UTI, bladder stones, kidney damage or trabeculated bladder (Bonner and Smith 2013).

The reflexic (UMN) cord injury will usually lead to the detrusor muscle contracting involuntarily and not being able to coordinate with the external sphincter (detrusor sphincter dyssynergia) and this will lead to a 'high pressure' system where damage can be caused to the kidneys by refluxed urine under pressure. Involuntary escape of urine under pressure in this type of bladder should not be perceived as complete voiding as it would in an able-bodied person. It usually leads to incomplete emptying.

Box 19.4 Case studies illustrating bladder management options

Case study 1

A C5 tetraplegic, day 1 post injury. AIS A – there is no voluntary anal contraction and no sensation preserved in the S4–S5 segments.

Day 1 post-injury will often lead to flaccid paralysis initially due to spinal shock and then over time this flaccid phase will resolve and the person will experience UMN symptoms. This patient will not have bladder filling sensation and will not have voluntary contraction of the bladder sphincter. An indwelling urethral catheter (IDUC) may start off as the desired management. When the flaccidity has resolved and reflexes have returned there may be wetness noted around the catheter even when the catheter is patent and draining. This is involuntary expulsion of urine usually under pressure and may not empty the bladder completely. This high pressure system can be dangerous and lead to renal reflux (backflow of urine to the kidneys). This pressure can be treated with the use of anticholinergics and a good emptying regime. As soon as possible the IDUC should be reviewed and another options discussed for the long term for example a suprapubic catheter.

Case study 2

L4 paraplegic, day 30 post-injury AIS C – there is voluntary anal contraction and sensation preserved in the S4–S5 segments

In this case the SCI is the LMN type (not a high pressure system), this patient will have some sensation of bladder filling and some 'urge' that they want to pass urine. There will probably be some ability to pass urine, but it is difficult to say how much urine they may pass voluntarily. It is imperative that investigations such as a post-residual intermittent catheter or a bladder scan highlight how much residual volume was left in the bladder after they tried to void. For example, when passing 300 ml of urine on urge, a bladder scan shows 30 ml of residual urine. If the residual is less than 20% of the total then this is enough to keep the patient voiding on urge. It is important to check more than once to ensure that they are consistently emptying.

Flaccid (LMN) cord injury will usually lead to a detrusor muscle that is prone to over stretching if not emptied regularly. Unlike the UMN bladder there is no involuntary muscle contraction, it continues to fill with urine and may overflow with increased abdominal pressure. This should also not be perceived as complete voiding as would be the case for an able-bodied person. It is usually incomplete emptying.

Both types of neurogenic bladder require a good working knowledge of SCI. AIS, possible options, investigations and patient choice are required to ensure a healthy genito-urinary (GU) system. In the long term urodynamics will be needed to fully assess the GU system. See Box 19.4 for two case studies illustrating bladder management in two different scenarios.

Planning for discharge and future life

To help the person to aim for and achieve a degree of wellness and quality of life following SCI, there is a need to determine what priorities or life domains are important to them. In the initial phase after injury, this may not be clear. It is essential to work continuously with the person and their family/significant others in determining goals that facilitate the rehabilitation process. The sooner this can be instigated, the sooner rehabilitation for discharge can commence. Preparing for the transition to community and "home" using open and clear communication between the patient, family, MDT and rehabilitation team is key. Goal planning and case conferences are the usual means to keep this communication and the ensuing rehabilitation process moving forwards. If the client is in a SCI centre, community liaison teams will usually facilitate this process, but for those without access to this, such advice can still be offered via telephone referral to spinal services and access to peer support organisations.

Key issues in planning for discharge and return to a lifestyle of choice include:

- Determining physical needs such as personal care, housing, adaptations and equipment, work and finances. Referrals to agencies such as social services and health services need to happen as soon as possible after admission once the SCI person is stabilised. Regular communication and referral to the correct agencies ensures that all are working towards the same goal in a timely fashion. The most common delays usually relate to suitable housing or adaptations and putting in place and funding of care packages.
- Benefits and income must be applied for as soon as is possible to ensure adequate resources are available in the short and long term. Referral to specialist solicitors for advice on compensation options is important in the early stages after admission. If there is a case for compensation it may be that interim payments can be obtained to speed up the process of discharge and enable purchase of equipment and adaptions to housing or temporary housing.
- Work is a crucial aspect of life, contributing to social wellbeing, offering structure and support, development of self and social networks and income. Loss of work through injury has a great impact and vocational rehabilitation is not well supported in many countries. For children, contact with their education provider is essential as soon as possible so that they can be involved in case conferences and planning and schooling can be incorporated into rehabilitation. For a smooth transition referral must be made with community teams as soon as possible after admission.
- Social support for people with SCI is central to successful rehabilitation (See evidence digest box 19.5). Spinal Cord Injury organisations in a given area or country can all be of support to the person with SCI and their families and significant others. They offer peer support, advice and information and education on living with a SCI and are invaluable in helping people learn to live with SCI long term. Peer support advisers can visit acute care centres such as district general hospitals or trauma centres. Online support and information and phone helplines are also available in many countries including information for healthcare professionals through publications and other educational opportunities.

Box 19.5 Evidence digest Social support and social skills following spinal cord injury

Muller *et al.* (2012) conducted a systematic review of the literature with a view to examining current knowledge about how social support and social skills are associated with aspects of health, functioning and quality of life for persons living with SCI. Examination of 58 studies showed that social support is positively related to physical and mental health and pain. The studies considered issues such as social problem solving, assertiveness, verbal communication and self-monitoring. All of these issues were related to better outcomes for the person with SCI although the area has not been studied in detail. A better understanding of these issues is advised but the existing literature illustrates the importance of the role of the practitioner in helping persons with SCI and their families to develop social support mechanisms.

Conclusion

Care and management of the patient following SCI is complex. However, a fundamental understanding of the pathophysiology of injury to the spinal cord can help the practitioner to make sense of the fundamentals of that care. Ideally, such care should be provided in a specialist SCI centre, but where this is not possible the practitioner working in the general hospital setting can seek advice and support from their nearest centre and from various organisations which specialise in this aspect of care.

Recommended further reading

As the scope of this chapter has been limited, recommended further reading should be accessed. The following are examples that may be supplemented by other, locality-specific sources in the reader's own country:

American Spinal Injury Association (ASIA) Learning Center. Available at: http://asia-spinalinjury.org/elearning/elearning.php (accessed 18 April 2014).

BASCIS (British Association for Spinal Cord Injury Specialists). Includes good practice guides. Available at: http://www.bascis.co.uk (accessed 18 April 2014).

BOA (British Orthopaedic Association) (2006) The Initial Care and Transfer of Patients with Spinal Cord Injuries. BOA, London. Available at: http://www.sbns.org.uk/index.php/download_file/view/19/112/

www.elearnsci.org A website for medical and paramedical professionals working the field of spinal cord injury containing elearning modules.

Harrison, P. (ed.) (2007) *Managing Spinal Cord Injury: The First 48 Hours*. Spinal Injuries Association, Milton Keynes.

MASCIP – Multidisciplinary Association of Spinal Cord Injury Professionals http://www.MASCIP.co.uk (accessed 18 April 2014).

Spinal Cord Injury Association (UK) http://www.spinal.co.uk/ (accessed 18 April 2014).

References

American College of Surgeons Committee on Trauma (ACS) (2008) *Advanced Trauma Live Support Manual for Physicians*, 8th edn. ACS, Chicago.

American Spinal Injury Association (ASIA) (2006) *Standard for neurological and functional classification of spinal cord injury*. Available at: http://asia-spinalinjury.org/elearning/ISNCSCI_Exam_Sheet_r4.pdf (accessed 14 June 2013).

Barr, F. (2009) *Preserving and Developing the National Spinal Cord Injury Service. Phase 2 – Seeking the Evidence*. Spinal Injuries Association. Available at: http://www.spinal.co.uk/userfiles/images/uploaded/pdf/234-242491.pdf (accessed 14 June 2013).

BASCIS (British Association of Spinal Cord Injury Specialists) (2006) *Good Practice Guide*. Available at: http://www.bascis.co.uk (accessed 14 June 2013).

BOA (British Orthopaedic Association) (2006) *The Initial Care and Transfer of Patients with Spinal Cord Injuries*. BOA, London. Available at: http://www.sbns.org.uk/index.php/download_file/view/19/112/ (accessed 14 June 2013).

Bonner, S. and Smith, C. (2013) Initial management of acute spinal cord injury. *Continuing Education in Anaesthesia, Critical Care & Pain*. Available at: http://ceaccp.oxfordjournals.org/content/early/2013/07/11/bjaceaccp.mkt021.short?rss=1 (accessed 22 April 2014).

Greaves, I., Porter, K. and Garner, J. (2009) *Trauma Care Manual* 2nd edn. Edward Arnold, London.

Harrison, P. (2007) (ed.) *Managing Spinal Cord Injury: The First 48 Hours*. Spinal Injuries Association, Milton Keynes.

Krassioukov, A., Eng, J.J., Claxton, G., Sakakibara, B.M. and Shum, D. (2010) Neurogenic bowel management after spinal cord injury: a systematic review of the evidence. *Spinal Cord*, **48**, 718–733.

MASCIP (2012) *Guidelines for Management of Neurogenic Bowel Dysfunction In Individuals With Central Neurological Conditions*. Coloplast Ltd., Peterborough.

Muller, R., Peter, C., Cieza, A. and Geyh, S. (2012) The role of social support and social skills in people with spinal cord injury – a systematic review of the literature. *Spinal Cord*, **50** (2), 94–106.

National Spinal Cord Injury Statistics Center (2012) *Annual Statistical Report*. Available at: https://www.nscisc.uab.edu/PublicDocuments/fact_figures_docs/Facts%202012%20Feb%20Final.pdf

Norton, L. (2009) *Spinal Cord Injury Australia 2007-08* Australian Institute of Health and Welfare. Available at: http://www.nisu.flinders.edu.au/pubs/reports/2010/injcat128.pdf (accessed 14 June 2013).

RISCI (Respiratory Information in SCI) (2012) *Weaning Guidelines*. Available at: http://www.risci.org.uk/NSCISB%20RISCI%20final.doc (accessed 22 April 2014).

Sapru, H. (2002) Spinal Cord Injury: Anatomy, physiology and pathophysiology, in *Spinal Cord* Medicine (eds S. Kirschblum *et al.*). Lippincott, Williams and Wilkins, Philadelphia.

Spinal Injuries Association (SCI) (2009) *Moving and Handling Patients with Actual or Suspected Spinal Cord Injuries*. Available at: http://www.spinal.co.uk/userfiles/images/uploaded/pdf/288-709666.pdf (accessed 14 June 2013).

CHAPTER 20

Soft tissue, peripheral nerve and brachial plexus injury

Beverley Wellington

New Victoria Hospital, Glasgow, UK

Introduction

The aim of this chapter is to provide evidence-based guidance for the assessment, investigation, surgical and conservative care, management and rehabilitation for patients who have sustained a soft tissue injury, peripheral nerve injury or injury to the brachial plexus. Each section will also provide a brief overview of the associated anatomy.

Soft tissue injuries

Soft tissue injuries have several mechanisms of injury but are often caused by either overuse of musculoskeletal soft tissue or a single specific injuring event. The impact on the patient of such injuries can be underestimated and it is important to make a full assessment and follow this with an effective plan of care. Evidence suggests that multiple risk factors, including a genetic predisposition, may be involved particularly in relation to the injuries to the Achilles tendon of the heel, rotator cuff tendons of the shoulder and cruciate ligaments of the knee. In the future, this may allow practitioners to consider genetic risk factors when assessing or treating individuals (Collins and Raleigh 2009).

Ligaments and tendons

Ligaments and tendons are fibrous tissues that have an important role in the musculoskeletal lever system. They are flexible bands of strong, dense connective tissue that connect the articular ends of bones or cartilages together, providing strength and mechanical stability to joints.

Tendons are inelastic fibrous connections between muscles and their points of insertion into bone, transmitting movement forces through joints. They are constructed of fibrous cords which are an extension of the fascia (the fibrous connective tissue found superficially beneath the skin and more deeply which forms a covering sheath for muscles and broad surfaces for muscle attachment). They have no elasticity and are of different lengths and thickness, making them very strong, but with few blood vessels and nerves. Tendons do not cope well with friction and are thus protected at areas of pressure or activity by bursae (sacs filled with a viscous fluid, cushioning movement of one bony part over another) (Hardy and Snaith 2011).

Sprains and strains

Soft tissue injuries are often treated in primary and secondary care settings. Strains and sprains are both soft tissue injures, but the tissue affected is different.

A ***sprain*** is an injury to a ligament supporting a joint. A twisting mechanism usually causes damage to fibres of the affected ligament and/or the joint capsule itself, resulting in decreased joint stability. Three grades of ligament injury/sprain are recognised (Altizer 2003):

- ***Grade I, Mild*** – stability is maintained, but can be decreased. The injury is often caused by a wrenching or twisting mechanism and commonly seen at the ankle. The site may be tender with bruising and mild oedema. The patient can usually walk, but with some discomfort.
- ***Grade II, Moderate*** – partial rupture or tear. Some fibres are torn, but some remain intact although with some loss of stability. More than one ligament may be

Orthopaedic and Trauma Nursing: An Evidence-based Approach to Musculoskeletal Care, First Edition. Edited by Sonya Clarke and Julie Santy-Tomlinson.

torn, increasing the severity of the injury and affecting the treatment regime that follows. The joint is tender, painful and difficult to move usually with some swelling and bruising.

- ***Grade III, Severe*** – complete rupture with loss of continuity of one or several ligaments. This causes loss of stability and a weakened, painful joint with significantly decreased range of movement. The patient is unable to actively move the joint or to weight bear, and the injury has a significant impact on mobility and activities of living.

A ***strain*** is an injury caused by overstretching of the muscle or tendon and may be severe enough to cause a partial or complete tear. These may also be mild, moderate or severe:

- ***Mild*** – pain and stiffness lasting a few days
- ***Moderate*** – partial tears causing more pain and swelling, with bruising with symptoms lasting for 1–3 weeks
- ***Severe*** – complete tears resulting in significant swelling, bruising and pain and often resulting in the need for surgical repair.

Management and care

There are some general principles of management for all soft tissue injuries:

Pain management

The most obvious symptom of soft tissue injury is pain, caused by the traumatic damage to tissue, cell hypoxia and release of chemicals such as histamine, bradykinin and prostaglandin as well as pressure on local nerve endings from swelling in the tissue. Pain relief is usually provided with simple analgesia and non-steroidal anti-inflammatory drugs (Chapter 11). Cryotherapy (the application of cold) has also been shown to have a positive effect on pain relief (Airaksinen *et al.*, 2003) as the cold reduces nerve conductivity.

Control of swelling

Swelling is due to the release of chemicals including prostaglandin, histamine and serotonin which increases the permeability of the cell membrane resulting in protein escaping into the interstitial space. This increases the osmotic pressure and causes increased oedema and associated pain and discomfort. The control of swelling is facilitated by rest, ice, compression and elevation.

Rest, ice, compression and elevation (mnemonic: RICE)

- ***Rest.*** It is important to maintain the normal correct anatomical alignment of the injured structures while immobilising the area until a full clinical examination and diagnosis is made. This will dictate the recovery time that can be expected and the subsequent plan of care. This may include a period of non-weight-bearing or supported weight-bearing with mobility aids, the application of a cast, brace, splint or supporting bandage and advice on when to return to physical activities.
- ***Ice.*** In an acute phase of injury, ice can help reduce pain and inflammation and muscle spasm. It decreases the inflammatory responses and cold-mediated vasoconstriction can help to decrease oedema. Protection of the injured area is important in avoiding ice burns. The ice is best applied frequently for moderate periods of time and for a minimum of three days (Airaksinen *et al.*, 2003).
- ***Compression***. This can be applied using elastic tubular bandage or equivalent with the aim of controlling the oedema at the injury site and to aid venous return. The evidence for this practice is, however, limited. Care is advised with the amount of compression applied to avoid other complications such as tourniquet effect and compartment syndrome. The aim is to assist with venous and lymphatic drainage and the dispersal of inflammatory fluid whilst preventing an accumulation of oedema.
- ***Elevation.*** This assists in lymphatic and venous drainage and reduces pain by reducing pressure on the capillaries and tissues. The injured part should be elevated above the level of the heart, but caution is advocated with any suspected compartment syndrome.

The goal of treatment, management and rehabilitation is to improve the condition of the injured area to allow a return of functional ability so that the patient can return to full daily activities. Depending on the level of mobility of the patient, significant nursing support may be needed along with assisted personal care.

Peripheral nerve injury

Peripheral nerve injuries are usually associated with another musculoskeletal injury such as a fracture and can have far-reaching effects for the patient. The practitioner needs an understanding of the peripheral

Table 20.1 The origins of the main peripheral nerves of the arm. Reproduced with permission from Crown copyright

Cord	Spinal nerve root	Nerve
Posterior	C5, C6	Axillary
Posterior	C5, C6, C7, C8	Radial
Lateral	C5, C6, C7	Musculocutaneous
Lateral and medial	C6, C7, C8, T1	Median
Medial	C8, T1	Ulnar

nerve supply in order to understand the impact of nerve injury on the patient. Table 20.1 provides a summary of the origins of the main peripheral nerves of the arm.

Radial nerve injury

The radial nerve is the most commonly injured nerve of the upper limb, often alongside fractures of the humerus. The nerve is derived from spinal nerve roots at level cervical 5 to 8 with contribution from thoracic 1 nerve root. The posterior cord of the brachial plexus is supplied from all 3 trunks of the plexus (upper, middle and lower) and terminates in both radial and axillary nerves. As the radial nerve travels into the arm its direction moves from medial to lateral and it enters near the spiral groove of the humerus running posterolaterally beneath the triceps. It then remains anterior to the humerus and passes anterior to the capitellum at the elbow before dividing at the level of the radial head. This position makes it prone to injury when the arm suffers trauma.

The radial nerve supplies the muscles on the posterior aspect of the arm and forearm. These include triceps brachii (the large muscle on the back of the arm principally responsible for extension of the elbow joint), brachioradialis (muscle of the forearm that acts to flex the forearm at the elbow and facilitates both pronation and supination) and the main muscles that control movements at the wrist as well as sensation to the posterior aspect of the arm and forearm, the radial side of the posterior hand and the dorsum of the fingers.

The causes of radial nerve injury are closely associated with its anatomical position:

- Radial nerve (and axillary nerve) injury may be caused by incorrectly administered intramuscular injection into the deltoid muscle.
- Radial nerve palsy can be caused by pressure damage from a spiral fracture of the distal shaft of humerus or from a cast applied too tightly around the mid humerus.
- Radial nerve neurapraxia can occur following dislocation of the radial head creating a traction-type injury.
- Radial nerve compression occurs when the arm is left hanging over the side or back of a chair, bed or trolley (often associated with alcohol intoxication and poor sleep posturing). It may also be compressed by the use of axillary/shoulder crutches.
- Radial nerve palsy can occur post-operatively due to prolonged use of or poor technique in the use of a tourniquet or blood pressure cuff.
- Other causes include compression by a limb cast, direct trauma to the nerve from an open wound, tumour and idiopathic neuritis.

Patients usually present with weakness in their hand grip and pinch and may also have sensory changes or loss over the dorsum of the thumb and first web space, although this may be minimal due to overlapping of the sensory innervations by other adjacent nerves. Any severe injury causing paralysis of the wrist extensor muscles results in wrist drop, inability to extend the wrist and fingers with a flexion of the hand at the wrist with flaccidity. Conservative management of the wrist drop is provided with a correctly fitting wrist drop support/splint and specific physiotherapy exercises.

Ulnar nerve injury

The ulnar nerve is derived from spinal nerve roots at level cervical 8 to thoracic 1. The medial cord of the brachial plexus is supplied from the lower trunk of the plexus and supplies the ulnar nerve and part of the median nerves. As the ulnar nerve travels into the arm it descends along the posteromedial aspect of the humerus. In the forearm, it enters the anterior (flexor) compartment through the two heads of flexor carpi ulnaris and runs alongside the ulna bone. The nerve also supplies the anteromedial muscles of the forearm and most of the muscles of the hand including the medial side of the hand, little finger and medial half of ring finger.

The causes of ulnar nerve injury are closely associated with its anatomical position and it can be:

- trapped or pinched as it passes through the cubital tunnel at the elbow
- damaged in association with fractures to the medial epicondyle of the humerus
- stretched or compressed when the forearm is extended and pronated.

Patients usually experience paraesthesia in the fourth and fifth digits. They may also be unable to spread the fingers apart, flex the metacarpophalangeal joints or extend the interphalangeal joints. Severe entrapment or complete severing of the ulnar nerve can present with a 'claw hand' and hypothenar wasting with an inability to flex the thumb. If cubital tunnel syndrome is diagnosed then surgical management with nerve decompression may be undertaken. Conservative management of ulnar clawing of the fingers is provided with splinting to maintain functional position and specific exercises to prevent further joint stiffness.

Median nerve injury

The median nerve is derived from spinal nerve roots at level cervical 5 to thoracic 1. The medial cord of the brachial plexus is supplied from the lower trunk of the plexus (C8 and T1) and the lateral cord is supplied from the upper and middle trunks of the plexus (C5 to C7). The nerve enters the arm from the axilla and then passes vertically down and alongside the brachial artery along the medial side of the arm between the biceps brachii and brachialis muscles. It moves from being lateral to the artery to lie anterior to the elbow joint and then crosses anteriorly to run medial to the artery in the distal arm and into the cubital fossa, travelling between the flexor muscles before entering the hand through the carpal tunnel. This nerve supplies most of the flexor muscles in the forearm which activate pronation and wrist and finger flexion. In the hand it supplies motor innervation to the first and second lumbrical muscles and also supplies the muscles of the thenar eminence which activate thumb opposition along with sensation to the skin of the lateral side of the palm side of the thumb, the index and middle finger and the lateral half of the ring finger.

The causes of median nerve injury are closely associated with its anatomical position and include:

- Above the elbow, an injury may result in loss of pronation and a reduction in flexion of the hand at the wrist.
- At the wrist, an injury by compression at the carpal tunnel causes carpal tunnel syndrome.
- Severing the median nerve causes median 'claw hand.'
- In the hand, the thenar muscles are paralysed and will atrophy over time causing a loss to thumb opposition and flexion.

Patients with carpal tunnel syndrome usually experience paraesthesia (pins and needles and tingling) in the thumb, the index finger, the middle finger and half of the ring finger. They may also present with dull aching and discomfort in the hand, forearm or upper arm. There may also be dry skin, swelling or changes in the skin colour of the hand and eventually weakness in the thumb when trying to bend it at a right angle away from the palm (abduction) with weakness and wasting of the muscles in the thumb.

If carpal tunnel syndrome is diagnosed then surgical management with a nerve decompression may be undertaken. Conservative management is provided with splinting to maintain functional position and specific physiotherapist-led exercises to prevent further joint stiffness. Corticosteroid injection into the joint may provide some temporary relief.

Sciatic nerve injury

The sciatic nerve arises from the sacral plexus from the roots of spinal nerves L4 and L5 and S1 to S3. It is actually two nerves (the tibial and common fibular) that are bound together with a sheath of connective tissue before dividing around the knee region. Injury can result from improperly performed injections into the buttock resulting in sensory loss. It is more commonly associated with pelvic injuries, specifically fractures of the acetabulum with posterior dislocation of the hip joint with displacement through the greater sciatic notch. It can also be damaged during hip arthroplasty surgery when surgical exposure can put the nerve at risk of being damaged or when the hip is dislocated and after the prosthesis is inserted the nerve may be stretched. More rarely the nerve may be damaged by the growth of a Schwannoma (a tumour – usually benign – of the tissue that covers nerves) on the nerve sheath. These tumours develop from a type of cell called a Schwann cell.

The symptoms of sciatic nerve damage include paraesthesia over the nerves' dermatomal distribution. They will have a loss of sensation below the knee (except in the medial border of the foot supplied by the saphenous nerve). The patient may also have severe weakness or paralysis of the hamstring muscles causing an inability to flex the knee with a weakness of ankle dorsiflexion resulting in plantar flexion (foot drop). Management of sciatic nerve injuries is usually conservative with the use of orthotics, splints, walking aids and lifestyle adaptation advice.

All peripheral nerve injuries require a complete patient history and thorough clinical examination (see also Chapter 7) to establish the level of the injury. The most commonly used tool to grade muscle power and

Table 20.2 MRC scale for assessment of muscle power (Medical Research Council 1981)

Motor function	
M 0	No muscle contraction is visible
M 1	Return of perceptible contraction in proximal muscles
M 2	Return of perceptible contraction in proximal and distal muscles
M 3	Return of proximal and distal muscle power to act against resistance
M 4	Return of function as stage 3 + independent movement possible
M 5	Complete recovery
Sensory function within the autonomous area	
S 0	Absence of sensibility
S 1	Return of deep cutaneous pain
S 2	Return of some degree of superficial cutaneous pain and touch
S 3	Return of some degree of superficial cutaneous pain and touch with disappearance of previous overreaction
S 3/4	As stage 3 with some recovery of 2-point discrimination
S 4/5	Complete recovery

Box 20.1 Evidence digest. Reproduced with permission from British Orthopaedic Association

Guide for Practice: Management of Nerve Injuries (BOA 2011)

This booklet is intended mainly for trauma and orthopaedic surgeons dealing with orthopaedic trauma and elective orthopaedic surgery where nerve injury may occur, but also has three purposes:

1 To provide advice and assistance
2 To assist towards the prevention of iatrogenous injuries
3 To emphasise the importance of rehabilitation.

The evidence base for the guide was taken from a large study of 3600 cases of compound nerve injury operated on during the years 1965 to 2007 at specified hospitals and from the many patients referred to the clinics at those hospitals. Many colleagues, from plastic surgery and neurosurgery as well as orthopaedics, in other British units provided important and extensive experience. Although there is no nursing focus in this booklet there is useful information to extend the nurse's knowledge in this field of practice and the guidance includes information about:

1 Urgent nerve injury management – presenting within 48 hours.
2 Delayed nerve injury management – presenting after 48 hours: general principles
3 The timing of surgery
4 Upper limb nerve injuries
5 Lower limb nerve injuries
6 Operation-related nerve injury
7 Compartment syndrome.

sensory function is the Medical Research Council (MRC) scale (Table 20.2). Best practice in the management of nerve injuries is discussed in Box 20.1

Brachial plexus injuries

The anatomy of the brachial plexus

A ***plexus*** is a network of nerves or blood vessels and *brachial* is an adjective relating to or affecting the arm. The ***brachial plexus*** is a network of nerves that is formed from the union of five spinal nerves: the anterior (ventral) rami of spinal nerves from the four lowest cervical roots (C5, C6, C7 and C8) and the first thoracic root (T1) (Figure 20.1). The spinal nerves result from a fusion of many smaller spinal rootlets that have all passed through cells in the spinal ganglion. The spinal nerves exit from the vertebral foramen and then undergo a complex joining and division of nerve fibres to form the brachial plexus. This network of nerves extends inferiorly and laterally on either side of the last four cervical and first thoracic vertebrae before passing above the first rib posterior to the clavicle and then entering the axilla. The brachial plexus descends into the posterior triangle of the neck between the scalenus anterior and medius muscles. The nerves form three trunks:

- upper (from C5 and 6)
- middle (C7)
- lower (C8 and T1).

Each trunk divides into two branches: anterior and posterior. The anterior branch forms the two anterior cords: lateral and medial. The musculocutaneous nerve and the lateral root of the median nerve stem from the lateral cord. The medial cord gives rise to the medial root of the median nerve, the ulnar nerve, the medial cutaneous nerve and the medial antebrachial cutaneous nerve. The lateral and medial roots of the median nerve unite to form the median nerve. The three posterior branches (divisions) unite to form the posterior cord which gives rise to the axillary and radial nerve (Tortora and Grabowski 2003).

The brachial plexus provides the entire nerve supply of the shoulders and upper limbs. Five important nerves arise from the brachial plexus (each nerve has sensory and motor components):

- ***axillary nerve*** – supplies the deltoid and teres minor muscles
- ***musculocutaneous nerve*** – supplies the flexor muscles of the arm

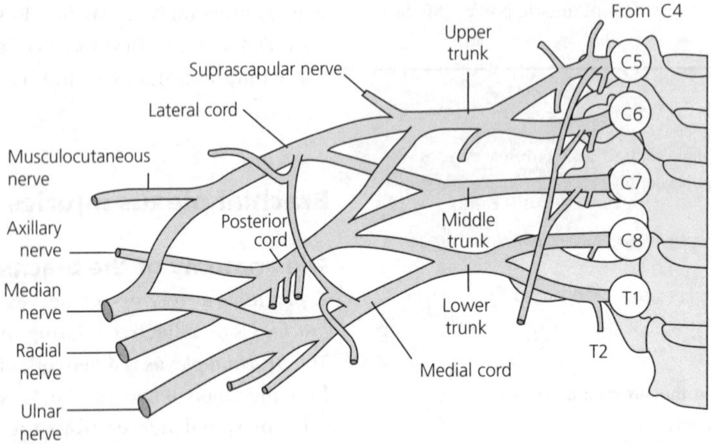

Figure 20.1 The brachial Plexus
(With permission: Scottish National Brachial Plexus Injury Service, Information for patients, Dec 2012. Medical Illustration Services, NHS Greater Glasgow and Clyde)

- ***radial nerve*** – supplies the muscles of the posterior aspect of the arm and forearm
- ***median nerve*** – supplies most of the muscles of the anterior forearm and some of the muscle of the hand
- ***ulnar nerve*** – supplies the anteromedial muscles of the forearm and most of the muscles of the hand.

Mechanisms of injury

Brachial plexus injuries are caused by damage to some or all of the nerves. Injuries can be classified in different ways and are often referred to as being open or closed injuries or high impact or low impact injuries:

- ***Open injuries*** occur as a result of a penetrating wound that can lacerate the nerves e.g. injury from an assault by a broken bottle, knife or falling through a glass door.
- ***Closed injuries*** occur as a result of either high impact injury or low impact injury.
- ***High impact injuries*** are often associated with motor vehicle collisions and cause a traction injury from a violent stretching or pulling force between the clavicle and the shoulder girdle. The plexus can also be compressed from injured and damaged tissues in the vicinity or from adjacent bony injury such as comminuted fractures of the clavicle, causing local haematoma formation (Krishnan *et al.*, 2008). There are also conditions in babies which are obstetric in origin causing brachial plexus palsies known as Erb's palsy or Klumpke's paralysis.
- ***Low impact injuries*** are usually the result of blunt trauma to the neck and upper limb causing crushing of the nerves. Rarely there may be radiation-induced damage to the plexus causing a brachial radiopathy from locally treated malignancies (e.g. breast, sarcoma) or a malignant infiltration into the area.

If the injury was sustained due to a high velocity accident e.g. a motorcycle collision, the likelihood of a more serious pathology is much greater than when the injury is sustained from a comparably low velocity fall. Patients involved in high velocity accidents are also more likely to sustain other injuries such as head injuries, spinal and upper limb fractures and vascular damage (see Chapters 16 and 19 for further information). These other injuries have to be considered when prioritising care for the newly injured patient.

Grades of injury

Patients who have sustained an injury or damage to the brachial plexus will present with motor and sensory loss in all or part of the upper limb depending on the extent of the injury. The damage to the brachial plexus nerves can be classified into four different grades (SNBPI Information for Patients 2012):

1. *Pre-ganglionic tear – Nerve root avulsion*. The nerves are torn away from their roots in the spinal cord. The nerve root cannot be rejoined to the cord. Some function of the arm will be permanently lost. Any possibility of surgery may mean that nerves may be transferred from other areas to improve function.
2. *Post-ganglionic tear – Neurotmesis*. The nerve has been stretched to breaking point and has been snapped or

torn (similar to an overstretched elastic band). Ruptures will not heal without surgery.

3 *Severe lesion in-continuity – Axonotmesis*. The nerve is stretched but remains intact, damaged but not torn apart. The nerves may recover to a variable degree on their own, but this may take some months. This type of injury may not require surgical treatment.
4 *Mild lesion in-continuity – Neurapraxia*. With this injury the nerve is minimally stretched or compressed with no structural damage. The sensitive nerve fibres temporarily stop working but will usually recover without surgery.

The number and combination of nerves injured are very variable. It should be noted that some patients can present with a combination of root avulsions, post-ganglionic tears and lesions in-continuity. Injuries can also be classified depending on the anatomical region of the plexus that is affected e.g. supraclavicular or infraclavicular.

Supraclavicular injuries

Supraclavicular injuries can be caused by a traction injury to the brachial plexus e.g. in a motorcycle accident where the head is flexed sideways and the shoulder girdle is depressed or through direct trauma e.g. a knife injury or gunshot wound. Common patterns of supraclavicular injury can be subdivided into three groups:

1 *Upper plexus* – from C5, C6 (+/– C7 and +/– C8). If C7 and C8 are involved the roots are sometimes avulsed. There is less likelihood that the roots of C5 and C6 will be avulsed.
2 *Total plexus* – there is damage to all nerve roots. C5, C6 may have post-ganglionic ruptures (neurotmesis) with the roots of C8 and T1 avulsed.
3 *Lower plexus* – the roots of C8 and TI are avulsed but C5 and C6 are working normally.

A high velocity accident is more likely to cause avulsion of the nerve roots from the spinal cord. Patients presenting with avulsion injuries usually complain of an instantaneous onset of pain. This is commonly described as a deep burning pain with frequent shocks of shooting pains throughout the day. The pain is caused by deafferentation of the dorsal horn of the spinal cord, which means that without input from the periphery, pain information passes from the dorsal horn to the brain unmodulated. Interestingly, these patients usually do not have problems with sleep disturbance due to pain.

There are a number of clinical factors that indicate a more serious lesion:

- high impact injury
- burning or shooting pains present since the time of injury
- possible Horner's sign.

Horner's sign (syndrome) – symptoms include a constricted pupil (miosis), drooping of the upper eyelid (ptosis) and absence of sweating of the face on the affected side (anhydrosis). These symptoms are due to a disorder of the sympathetic nerves.

Infraclavicular injuries

This type of injury can affect any one or all of the peripheral nerves. The most common presentations are:

- a complete lesion (neurotmesis)
- damage to the axillary nerve
- damage to the musculocutaneous nerve.

Injuries are usually caused by excessive traction of the brachial plexus e.g. following shoulder dislocation or in conjunction with a fracture of the humerus.

It is especially important to check with patients presenting following shoulder dislocation that the disruption of shoulder movement is not caused by a tear in the rotator cuff. Where there has been a severe infraclavicular injury affecting several peripheral nerves, the surgeon may choose to reconstruct only some of the peripheral nerves. This could be because the gap between the damaged nerve ends is too wide to successfully bridge. If a nerve is irreparable it is sometimes used to reconstruct another peripheral nerve.

There are some clinical factors that indicate a relatively mild lesion:

- low impact injury
- no pain
- Tinel's sign
- absent Horner's sign.

Tinel's sign is a method of checking the regeneration or activity of a nerve by direct tapping over the pathway of the nerve sheath to elicit a distal tingling sensation (axonal regeneration advances by approximately 1 mm per day) (Hems 2000).

Diagnosis and investigations

A thorough clinical examination is essential, noting all nerve actions and muscle power using the Medical Research Council (MRC) Scale for Muscle Strength (Table 20.2). This should be documented in detail according to muscle group. X-rays of the cervical spine, shoulder and clavicle may be taken to exclude any skeletal/bony injury. A MRI scan will often help to confirm the diagnosis. The location of any root avulsion can sometimes be seen on the scan image if there is a meningocele (sack filled with cerebrospinal fluid leaking from the spinal cord). Neurophysiology or electrical nerve conduction tests record the passage of electrical signals along nerves in the limbs using small electrical pulses on the skin. This may include a recording of the electrical activity of muscles using fine needles. These tests can be used to diagnose a variety of nerve or muscle problems.

Management of a patient with a brachial plexus injury

Surgical management

If there is a diagnosed nerve injury that is suitable for surgical intervention, there are a few options available. It is possible to repair damaged nerves. In order to have a chance of success this surgery must be performed within a few months of the injury. Exploratory surgery is advised to ascertain the anatomical state of the damaged nerve and then the most appropriate surgical procedure is performed. There are a number of factors that are collectively considered prior to surgery, including the level or grade of injury, the age and fitness of the patient and any other co-morbidities.

Surgical options include:

- ***Direct nerve suturing*** – if there is minor damage to the nerve and the ends are in approximation and can be directly micro-sutured/glued.
- ***Nerve graft*** – usually when the nerves are torn, the damaged segment of nerve either side of the injury must be removed and repaired using grafts from elsewhere. Common nerve donor sites are the cutaneous nerves in the forearm or the sural nerve in the lower leg. These are sensory nerves and will leave a feeling of paraesthesia or numbness over the nerve distribution area, but have little effect on function. The nerve graft acts as a guide through which new nerve fibres can grow and cross the gap caused by the injury. Growth is very slow, recovery time is lengthy and complete recovery may be impossible due to the way that each individual microscopic nerve fibre grows.
- ***Nerve Transfer*** – undamaged nerves in the area that are performing less valuable functions can be transferred to other parts of the brachial plexus to try and regain some function within the limb. As the nerves used in this transfer start to recover, the patient needs to work very hard at retraining these nerves to move the arm and initially they may have to engage different movements to make the arm function.

These primary surgical options are undertaken as soon as is reasonably possible after full investigations and preparation of the patient. Recovery following primary surgery varies according to the individual, the level of injury and the type of surgery performed. There may be a period of complete immobilisation of the arm in a sling or a plan for immediate physiotherapy. It is important to follow the postoperative care plan as advised by the surgeon and ensure the patient is fully informed at every stage. The need for later or secondary surgical procedures is entirely dependent on the individual's recovery from injury or primary surgery. The main aim of any surgery is to improve functional ability and secondary surgery is often not considered until two years after injury or primary surgery. This is a recognised time scale for ultimate recovery potential to be reached, although it is known that some nerve regeneration can continue for a longer period of time.

Secondary surgical procedures fall into three categories:

- bony/joint fusion (arthrodesis) – commonly wrist or shoulder
- tendon transfer
- muscle transfer.

Arthrodesis

The joints most commonly fused are the wrist and the shoulder. Bony fusions will only be considered when there is no chance of further useful recovery. This is one of the most common secondary operations undertaken. It is performed at the shoulder because the patient has poor shoulder control but has gained other functional return in the hand and elbow. The main aim of this surgery is to stabilise the shoulder to optimise elbow and hand function but allow some active movement of the upper limb through the scapulothoracic joint (Sousa *et al.*, 2011). The patient must have good thoracoscapular muscle power (e.g. upper trapezius, serratus anterior) to be suitable for this type of surgery. Fusion of the joint may also be helpful in relieving pain.

Following shoulder arthrodesis the joint is immobilised in an abduction brace for at least six weeks. Patients are given advice about the position, function and appearance of the brace. Once the brace is removed they can start passive and active movements. The increase in range of movement usually progresses quite quickly, with the expectation that they will be able to achieve between 60 and 90 degrees of elevation and abduction. The patient is warned that they will have loss of medial rotation and putting their 'hand behind back' and that the arm will hang in a slightly abducted position. It is vital to manage the patient's expectations carefully and ensure they are thoroughly informed about expected improvements and expected limitations.

Arthrodesis is performed at the wrist to correct the effects of muscle dysfunction. The fusion of the wrist joint can assist in maximising finger function by stabilising the wrist in a neutral position. It can provide the possibility of synchronising movements and enable easier tasks such as lifting and holding objects using the hand (Terzis and Barmpitsioti 2009).

Tendon transfer

Tendon transfer surgery is most commonly performed in the hand and is necessary when the function of a specific muscle is lost because of nerve injury. If a nerve is injured and cannot be repaired, the nerve no longer sends signals to particular muscles. Those muscles are paralysed and their function is lost. Tendon transfer surgery can be used to attempt to replace that function by leaving the origin of the muscle in place and moving the tendon insertion (attachment) to a different position. It can be sutured into a different bone or a different tendon. When the muscle fires after the insertion point has been moved it will produce a different action to previously, depending on where it has been inserted. Patients who present only with avulsion of the lower trunk (C8–T1) nerve roots may eventually be considered for tendon transfer. In order for this to be successful it is important to teach the patient how to maintain range of joint movement and to maximise the strength in the muscle groups that are still functional.

Tendons used for transfer must be of good quality (Grade 4 or better). It is important that tendon transfers in the hand are planned so that pinch and grip will be improved. Rehabilitation involves the re-education of function, occasionally with trick movements or with the co-ordination of other movements e.g. wrist extension with finger flexion.

Muscle transfer

A variety of muscles may be used as free transfers or transplantations and this surgery is often performed by a plastic surgeon. The aim is often to restore elbow flexion or wrist extension. The muscles used include latissimus dorsi and gracilis.

Non-surgical management

Some patients will have suffered temporary damage to the conduction of the nerve e.g. a neurapraxia or an axonotmesis or those who have had a virus causing a brachial neuritis. These injuries/pathologies can take from several months to over a year to recover and it is essential that the patient understands this and the importance of maintaining range of joint movement while waiting for recovery. It may be necessary to provide some form of splinting to aid function and/or to maintain hand position. Early signs of recovery are sometimes difficult to detect and this highlights the importance of accurate record keeping. Once a flicker of muscle contraction can be detected the patient should then commence prescribed exercises to maximise this improvement. This can include muscle stimulation and gravity-assisted exercises. Muscle stimulation is an option that can be helpful at this stage. When the muscles that have not been working start to show signs of working, it will often be a very small flicker. In the early recovery phase this may not be enough to move the joints involved so it can be difficult for the individual to exercise. Muscle stimulation works by using a device that electrically stimulates the muscles with pads placed on the skin over the muscle that is to work. It stimulates the muscles to contract and can help to give the feeling of moving them again, but it does not replace an exercise programme.

Rehabilitation and ongoing care and support

Many patients will experience pain of a neuropathic nature which can be difficult to treat and requires specific neuro-analgesics. Some of these drugs have another mode of use as antidepressants or antiepileptics. The use of other techniques in addition to drug therapy can be useful to help the patient 'live with' the pain. These may include psychological exercises such as relaxation, visualisation of pain and guided imagery, cognitive behavioural therapy and specific directed counselling. General pain management issues are considered in more detail in Chapter 11.

Acceptance of the effects of the injury and changes to body image should be addressed with counselling support. The purpose of therapy is to focus on the effects of pain on behaviour, mood, function and activity.

Intervention involves setting goals such as being more active, returning to previous activities and how to use the pain relief achieved to reach these goals. The aim is to improve the individual's ability to function and enhance their ability to cope with the pain. The use of a TENS device may also be useful. This is a small portable electrical device which is designed to help relieve pain. It works by sending a harmless electrical current through pads that are placed on the skin. This is felt as pins and needles and these sensations can help to block pain messages. It can be used on various parts of the body but only on skin that has normal feeling.

Current developments in relieving deafferentation pain following brachial plexus injury are starting to filter into clinical practice. The dorsal root entry zone (DREZ) procedure is performed as a last resort for resolution of intractable pain associated with some neuropathic pain syndromes. This invasive procedure is performed via a myelotomy or laminectomy. Thermo-coagulation (the use of heat generated by an electric current to destroy tissue) is selectively applied and destroys the posterolateral aspect of the spinal cord corresponding to the area through which dorsal (sensory) root fibres enter the cord itself. When used in appropriately selected patients, particularly in those with post-traumatic avulsion of the brachial plexus, the DREZ procedure may produce lasting pain relief (in a majority of patients), but carries some significant potential side effects including loss of feeling and temperature sensitivity (the pathway is blocked at the spinal cord and messages no longer cross over), weakness and a loss of proprioception (Blaauw *et al.*, 2008).

Physical activity of any type is advantageous for a number of reasons:

- It is known to release endorphins into the bloodstream which can act as natural analgesics and help to improve the patient's mood.
- It is good for the body to stay in good physical condition to help with the healing process.
- If an individual enjoyed sports or other physical activities before their injury it is very helpful to return to them as soon as possible to fulfil their enjoyment.

There are many ways of adapting activities to allow a return to them even with an injured or non-functioning upper limb. Participation in sport has well known benefits to health, wellbeing and self-esteem. The majority of activities can be adapted to allow participation. Patients have been reported as being able to return to a variety of sport, leisure and hobby activities using adaptations including fishing, playing guitar, running, cycling, playing snooker and gardening. Quality of life issues for patients with brachial plexus injury are considered in Box 20.2.

Box 20.2 Evidence digest. Reproduced with permission from Elsevier

Quality of life for patients following a traumatic brachial plexus injury (Wellington 2009 and 2010)

Wellington (2009 and 2010) undertook research into the quality of life for patients following a traumatic brachial plexus injury and published the findings in a series of two papers. The first paper (Wellington 2009) discusses a literature review which aimed to gather evidence regarding the extent of quality of life issues for adult patients following traumatic brachial plexus injuries so that this could provide the clinical team with additional knowledge from the patient's perspective of their subjective experiences in order to enhance their provision of care. The second paper (Wellington 2010) describes a qualitative research study and concludes with recommendations for future research. Participants were selected using purposive sampling from those who were on the database of the Scottish National Brachial Plexus Injury Service. Five patients were finally selected and data collected using semi-structured audio taped interviews and field notes. Themes were identified from the experiences described by the patients including employment, pain, body image and sexuality/emotions. These two papers demonstrate the importance of addressing quality of life issues for patients with traumatic brachial plexus injuries. Further research in this area would be beneficial to test various quality of life assessment tools for applicability and usefulness with this group of patients.

There may be a need for an orthosis to be fitted to aid in supporting a flail or paralysed arm that is not functional. Specialised orthoses that work using biomechanical principles may be provided on an individual basis according to the level of injury and functional ability.

The aims of orthoses are to:

- Reduce shoulder pain (as subluxation from poorly controlled shoulder musculature can be problematic).
- Allow improved positioning of the hand for functional activities (the ability to 'crank' the orthosis from a position of elbow extension to flexion is possible).
- Improve cosmetic appearance of the upper limb (which may 'sit' in a more neutral position).

The patient may also require adaptations or modifications to a vehicle so that they may safely drive it. These may include steering wheel 'rotators', change to automatic transmission, positioning of indicator switches etc.

Even though brachial plexus injury is uncommon, practitioners working in the trauma setting are likely to care for patients in the early stages of their recovery. The complexity of brachial plexus injuries can provide a challenge to the healthcare professional. A holistic approach to the assessment, treatment, care and support of the patient and their family is best provided by an interdisciplinary team with specialist knowledge and expertise. Team members will include consultant medical staff, nurse specialists and therapy practitioners as well as other professionals such as psychologists, pain specialists and orthotists. In the UK, for example, such care is currently provided in only three specialist brachial plexus injuries units who receive referrals from around the country.

Suggested further reading

Anscomb, S.J. (2007) Managing sprains and strains. *Practice Nurse*, **33**(5), 44, 46, 48–49.

Bailey, R., Kaskutas, V., Fox, I., Baum, C.M. and Mackinnon, S.E. (2009) Effect of upper extremity nerve damage on activity participation, pain, depression and quality of life. *Journal of Hand Surgery*, **34**(a), 1682–1688.

Elton, S.G. and Rizzo, M. (2008) Management of radial nerve injury associated with humeral shaft fractures: an evidence-based approach. *Journal of Reconstructive Microsurgery*, **24**(8), 569–573.

Norris, B.L. and Kellam, J.F. (1997) Soft tissue injuries associated with high-energy extremity trauma: principles of management. *Journal of the American Academy of Orthopaedic Surgeons*, **5**(1), 37–46.

Wardrope, J., Barron, D., Draycott, S. and Sloan, J. (2008) Soft tissue injuries: principles of biomechanics, physiotherapy and imaging. *Emergency Medicine Journal*, **25**, 158–162.

References

Airaksinen, O.V., Kyrklund, N., Latvala, K. *et al.* (2003) Efficacy of cold gel for soft tissue injuries. *American Journal of Sports Medicine*, **31**(5), 680–684.

Altizer, L. (2003) Strains and sprains. *Orthopaedic Nursing*, **22** (6), 404–409.

Blaauw, G., Muhlig, R.S., and Vredeveld, J.W. (2008) Management of brachial plexus injuries. *Advances and Technical Standards in Neurosurgery*, **33**, 201–231.

British Orthopaedic Association (BOA) (2011) the Management of Nerve Injuries: A Guide to Good Practice. BOA, London. Available at: http://www.boa.ac.uk/Publications/Documents/The%20Management%20of%20Nerve%20Injuries.pdf (accessed 7 April 2014).

Collins, M. and Raleigh, S.M. (2009) Genetic risk factors for musculoskeletal soft tissue injuries. *Medicine and Sport Science* **54**: 136–149.

Hardy, M. and Snaith, B. (2011) *Musculoskeletal Trauma*. Churchill Livingstone, Edinburgh.

Hems, T.E.J. (2000) Nerves, in *Bailey and Love's Short Practice of Surgery*, 23rd edn (eds R.C.G. Russell, N.S. Williams and C.J.K. Bulstrode), Arnold, London, pp. 530–568.

Krishnan, K.G., Mucha, D., Gupta, R., and Schackert, G. (2008) Brachial plexus compression caused by recurrent clavicular non-union and space-occupying pseudoarthrosis: definitive reconstruction using free vascularised bone flap – a series of eight cases. *Neurosurgery*, **62**(5 Suppl 2), 461–469; discussion 469–470.

Medical Research Council (1981) *Aids to the Examination of the Peripheral Nervous System*. Memorandum 45. Her Majesty's Stationery Office, London.

Scottish National Brachial Plexus Injury Service (SNBPI) (2012) *Information for Patients*. Available at: www.brachialplexus.scot.nhs.uk (accessed 7 April 2014).

Sousa, R., Pereira, A., Massada, M. *et al.* (2011) Shoulder arthrodesis in adult brachial plexus injury: what is the optimal position? *Journal of Hand Surgery (European Volume)*, **36**(7), 541–547.

Terzis, J.K., and Barmpitsioti, A. (2009). Wrist fusion in post-traumatic brachial plexus palsy. *Plastic and Reconstructive Surgery*, **124**(6), 2027.

Tortora, G.J. and Grabowski, S.R. (2003) *Principles of Anatomy and Physiology*. John Wiley and Sons Inc., New York

Wellington, B. (2009) Quality of life issues for patients following traumatic brachial plexus injury – Part 1. *Journal of Orthopaedic Nursing*, **13**(4), 194–200.

Wellington, B. (2010) Quality of life issues for patients following traumatic brachial plexus injury – Part 2. *International Journal of Orthopaedic and Trauma Nursing*, **14**(1), 5–11.

PART V
Children and young people

CHAPTER 21

Key issues in caring for the child and young person with an orthopaedic or musculoskeletal trauma condition

Sonya Clarke[1] and Lorna Liggett[2]

[1] *Queen's University Belfast, Belfast, UK*

[2] *Queen's University Belfast, Belfast, UK (Retired)*

Introduction

This chapter, although dedicated to 'children', continues to build upon the transferable knowledge and skills discussed in earlier sections of this book. The terms 'child' and 'children' will be used collectively to refer to the neonate, infant, child and young person. The common concepts of informed consent, pain assessment/management and safeguarding are included. Assessment and planning of care alongside educational and psychological issues considered pertinent to this client group will provide a foundation for this. Subsequent chapters will then build upon this within the context of 'children's nursing' for the child presenting with a common orthopaedic condition or injury. Additional team members who help to create a positive child and family experience are further introduced within this chapter. Chapter 22 further reflects fundamental aspects of care pertinent to orthopaedics and trauma, but from a child perspective e.g. caring for the child in spica cast (Figure 21.1).

The United Nations Convention on the Rights of the Child (1989) recognises that children are a vulnerable group who need special consideration in all respects, including healthcare. Children's nurses are, therefore, committed to safeguarding vulnerable children and improving standards of care. A significant review of the UK National Health Service (NHS) (Kennedy 2010) in respect of meeting the needs of children and young people in light of widespread concerns expressed about a particular case (Laming 2009) found many services needing improvement with only a minority deemed excellent. The report also found that general practitioners had little or no experience of paediatrics as part of their professional training. Safeguarding was also considered an ongoing challenge alongside transition into adult services, with parents who were frustrated due to poor sharing of information by health professionals. The report stated that children were a low priority in health care and that they needed a 'champion' within such complex care organisations. The Kennedy report (2010) was positive about the value of 'benchmarking' to develop a range of standards. A benchmark is a process of comparison between the performance characteristics of separate, often competing, organisations intended to enable each participant to improve its own performance. An example relating to children's musculoskeletal wellbeing is examined in Box 21.1.

Age definitions

Variations exist, but a general consensus suggests that key phases in respect of age are:

- *Neonate* – a newborn infant less than four weeks old
- *Infant* – less than one year but more than four weeks old
- *Child* – over one year old but before puberty
- *Young person/adolescent* – between puberty and adulthood (up to 18 years old).

Psychosocial and educational issues that relate to the infant, child and young person are central to their wellbeing and the outcomes of the care they receive. The

Orthopaedic and Trauma Nursing: An Evidence-based Approach to Musculoskeletal Care, First Edition. Edited by Sonya Clarke and Julie Santy-Tomlinson.

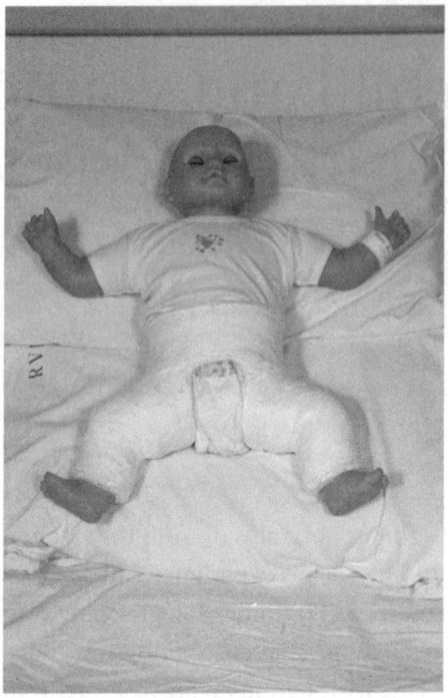

Figure 21.1 Spica cast/hip spica in human position

term 'psychosocial' refers to the child's ability to, consciously or unconsciously, adjust and relate themselves to their social environment. The term 'educational' refers to the provision of knowledge or instruction required as part of the child's development that must be incorporated into the care process.

The overarching family dynamics, culture, language and age of a child affect their physical and cognitive development and the achievement of expected milestones. Age is central, as the needs of an infant are very different from that of a young person. For example, a young person may experience anxiety and fear related to insults to dignity and altered body image and need acceptance within their peer group. They have a right to have a voice, to be heard and to have their vulnerability acknowledged regardless of their presenting condition and treatment. At the opposite end of the age continuum, the infant has increased vulnerability and dependence and their growth and development must be central to individualised and holistic nursing care. The child's experience of health professionals, hospital admission and pain are an important consideration in planning care and a full and effective assessment is needed, even for day surgery, as it must identify associated risk and promote a positive child experience of the care episode.

Assessment of the child on admission to hospital must include involvement of the parent and child when possible. History taking can be confounded by the child and parents failing to remember old or previous conditions and incidents but which remain pertinent to anaesthetic, surgery and planning of care. Honesty should be maintained whenever possible as children do not often forgive or forget if an untruth is revealed,

Box 21.1 Evidence digest. Reproduced with permission from RCN

Benchmarks for children's orthopaedic care: RCN guidance (2007)

This publication offers a portfolio of succinct evidence on the key elements required to effectively care for the infant, child and young person requiring orthopaedic and fracture trauma-related nursing care. The indicators of best practice are identified as factors (F) for each of the nine benchmarks. The RCN guidance document was developed by an expert group of paediatric nurses experienced in orthopaedic related nursing care.

The benchmarks:

1 *Pre-op assessment* – F1 screening and assessment; F2 practitioner competence; F3 informing child/young person and carers; F4 implementation of an individualised plan.
2 *Cast care* – F1 education and training; F2 patient care; F3 upper body cast; F4 lower body cast; F5 discharge planning.
3 *Neurovascular assessment* – F1 education and competence; F2 recording and documentation; F3 communication and information; F4 clinical action; F5 discharge planning.
4 Traction – F1 education and application of traction; F2 education, management of traction and nursing care; F3 communication and information
5 Pin site care – F1 screening and assessment; F2 education; F3 evidence, knowledge and competence; F4 clinical care; F5 discharge planning.
6 Kirchner wire removal – F1 competence and knowledge; F2 preparation of chid/ young person and carers.
7 *Bone or joint infection* – F1 admission; F2 assessment and screening; F3 treatment; F4 discharge planning.
8 *Spinal injury* – F1 assessment of injury; F2 stabilisation; F3 acute care and rehabilitation programme; F4 psychological impact of a spinal cord injury; F5 discharge planning.
9 *Spinal surgery* – F1 pre-operative assessment; F2 nursing care plan; F3 pain management; F4 post-surgical mobility.

The nine benchmarks reflect pertinent areas relating to this client group and the speciality of orthopaedics and fracture trauma. The publication has also been reported upon by Shields and Clarke (2011) who described it as limiting, when used to guide clinical practice within a children's ED setting. This book builds upon the RCN publication as each benchmarked area of practice is further explored here.

Box 21.2 The importance of telling the truth to children

> One example of a difficult admission involved a six-year old child carrying a suitcase who appeared somewhat confused on arrival. The assessment process uncovered parents who thought their child unable to cope with the truth so told her she was going on holiday. The lack of parental truth-telling had a direct impact on the child's hospital experience, but proactive inclusion of 'clown doctors' and a play specialist helped the child's experience to be salvaged, resulting in a positive outcome.

affecting the nurse/child relationship leading to an anxious or non-compliant child and an angry parent (Box 21.2). Resources, culture, language, social services, school, peer group, age, body image and discharge planning can present barriers to parent and child education and communication. Benchmarks (RCN 2007) identify a number of areas that relate to this (Box 21.1).

Assessment of children and young people

The needs of the infant, child and young person have been charted across the decades by a variety of government reports (Platt Report 1959, Laming 2003, Children Act 2004). Even with the differences and similarities of children and adult patients acknowledged and continually debated, there is a widely accepted recognition that the 'children's nurse' is best placed to care for this client group (Clarke 2007). It must be noted, nonetheless, that not all children will have a children's nurse caring for them in all health care settings. Pre-qualifying children's nursing programmes have evolved with increasing degrees of academic demand. Registered nurses are often 'dual' qualified, having a professional and academic award in both children's and adult/general nursing. Depending on individual need, children requiring continued care in the community are ideally placed under the care of the Children's Community Nurse (CCN) or Public Health Nurse. Many adult registered nurses and other fields of nursing may be able to care for this client group effectively but often not in a child-friendly environment. Clarke (2007) advocates that the children's nurse should have equal opportunity to complete recognised continuing education in caring for the child with orthopaedic conditions and fracture trauma – adult orthopaedic and trauma nurses currently have better access to such continuing professional development.

Hydration and nutrition are key components of child health and wellbeing. The child's immature and developing skeletal system can result in an extreme metabolic response to injury, surgery and fasting, resulting in a high risk of poor outcomes if diet and hydration are not carefully considered. The practitioner needs to be aware of the importance of a balanced diet in maintaining normal childhood development and expected milestones. Dietary assessment history is essential in identifying the child's likes and dislikes for food texture and presentation. While BMI (body mass index) charts are used in adult patients, standard practice with children is to plot the child's weight and height on centile charts which provide better indicators of child growth and development. Hydration is equally as important as diet, but assessing fluid balance can be problematic in the child. For example, assessing urinary output can be difficult due to the use of nappies and obtaining a midstream specimen of urine (MSSU) can be problematic due to lack of understanding and anxiety associated with using a 'bedpan' for the younger child. Diet and hydration are explored in greater detail in Chapter 10.

Children receiving orthopaedic or trauma care come from a variety of diverse patient groups, ages and cultures. Challenges often exist in communicating with the child and family in respect to cultural and language barriers and difficulties, for example, the use of touch in some cultures. Family dynamics, especially where there is obvious dysfunction, can also have an impact on the care process.

The infant, child and young person can struggle to have a say in their care and the practitioner caring for children is best placed to advocate for the patient (NMC 2008). The management of disclosure of sensitive information needs to be carefully handled. The child who presents with a fracture and has a learning disability may present specific challenges to the assessment and delivery of care particularly in the acute environment, which may not be well organised to address their specific needs. The 'complex' or 'special needs' child reinforces the need for a multidisciplinary team (MDT) approach with the children's nurse as the 'key worker' within the team. This group of children requires additional knowledge and skill in providing safe and effective care. Chapter 22 further explores these issues.

Assessment of risk is fundamental to wellbeing and positive outcomes in all parts of the journey of care and in all settings (Corkin *et al.*, 2012). All children undergoing surgery, for example, require care that gives a high priority to their ASA level (the American Society of Anaesthesiologists grade given to each patient using a scale in relation to their fitness for undergoing an anaesthetic), as this predicts the need for 24-hour Paediatric Intensive Care Unit support (see Chapter 14 for further detail).

The care environment

Children are cared for in a wide range of settings with an emphasis on home care with the intention of reducing hospital acquired infections and keeping the child within the family home and normal routine. Even so, the child is often cared for within acute hospital settings, day procedure units, outpatient clinics, hospices and residential units which are not dissimilar to adult care settings. Because of concerns about child safety, however, children should be cared for in units that have specific security measures in place including closed circuit television surveillance and locked doors to promote safety. The ideal environment should meet the specific needs of children; it should be light, spacious and colourful with appropriate decoration, pictures and toys for young children and a dedicated area for young people. Bathroom and toilet facilities need to meet the needs of the child and specifically the child with mobility problems. Sensory rooms can provide a relaxing atmosphere for those with special needs.

Livesley and Long (2013) contemporarily explored the views of hospitalised children using an ethnographic design and two-stage research method that valued children throughout the whole research process. A theme of 'different worlds' was identified which relates well to the philosophical assumptions of qualitative research, as 'one ward' was noted as two worlds, even when the children and nurses were actually within the same environment, they lived there differently with each having different goals and realities. Challenges around the child's voice and competence were also uncovered as the nurse held power around lighting, TV and access to the playroom etc. The parent was also undervalued and often viewed as incompetent like the child, by the nurse. Children had to accept the change of routine which often differed from home. This recent empirical study, although small, is important for policy makers, nurse educators and for the professional who cares for children.

The team

A wealth of health professionals and lay persons participate in the care of the child, from the specialist/advanced nurse to the allied health professional working within a multidisciplinary team, CCN, parent and beyond. Chapter 5 provides an overview of the team approach and nursing roles within orthopaedics and fracture trauma with some principles that can be transferred to the care of the child. Additional roles have been developed to promote effective care of children. The fundamental role of play in child wellbeing and development must be considered in providing the right care environment for children, again with a specific focus on the child who has difficulty mobilising. Playing is a familiar activity for most children and is central to relieving stress and boredom. Dissimilar to adult care but highly valued within children's nursing the parent, play specialist/therapist and arts-based 'clown doctors' are all utilised to generate a more positive hospital experience for the child.

- ***Play specialists*** work with children of all ages regardless of their health problem. They plan and supervise activities that help the child to express their feelings through play and encourage development of creative skills to provide an outlet for the child's thoughts and worries and offering ways to adapt to the new environment. This involves managing pre-admission 'clubs' and using play to welcome children to hospital and preparing them to cope with surgery or other procedures. This enables the child to express and manage their fears about separation from parents and encourages the child to maintain their usual interests whilst using specific play techniques to minimise stressful events by acting them out in advance.
- ***Clown doctors*** are professional performers who are specially trained to work in hospitals with the aim of creating fun, laughter, play, communication and creativity in clinical environments. They visit children who are chronically and acutely ill and who are hospitalised, children who are in hospice care, children and young people with severe or profound disabilities and those with life-limiting conditions. Further information can be found at the http://www.artscare.co.uk/clowndoctors/ website. It is important to note, however, that not all children like clowns.
- ***The parent or guardian*** has parental responsibility for a child. Simons *et al.* (2001) suggest that children benefit from their parents' presence during a hospital

admission and this is a key principle commonly adopted by children's units. Parental involvement can also be challenging for the attending nurse due to child-focused anxiety. It is also recognised that a child's siblings and other family members such as grandparents can play an important part in the child's wellbeing and in maintaining social links in hospital.

Planning care

Effective care planning through all care phases and health care settings is pivotal in achieving positive outcomes for the child and family. The complexity of modern families, however, makes this challenging, especially when the child's long-term care transfers to adult services as they become older. Transition is often not seamless and can be problematic for both the service provider and family, as developed relationships within the child's service are family-centred and built on trust and respect. A variety of frameworks, models and approaches to care planning are available (Corkin *et al.*, 2012) and a joint approach is commonly adopted when planning care for children i.e. Casey's partnership model (Casey 1988) and the Roper Logan Tierney (2000) model of care; one is family-centred and the latter encompassing the 12 activities of living with the aim of care to move from dependence to independence.

An essential aspect of care planning is assessment. Chapter 22 discusses the commonly applied **look, feel, and move** approach with 'ears' that listen to the child and parent, underpinned by a holistic and family-centred approach. Family-centred care (FCC) recognises that the parent is a valued part of the child's care team but should not to be taken for granted. Some parents adopt an 'expert' role when their child has complex needs. Examples of FCC include:

- Parental facilities: kitchen, shower and overnight facilities or purpose build parent accommodation.
- One parent is routinely expected and welcomed in the anaesthetic and recovery room, the parent needs to be educated and supported by the nurse as an anaesthetised or recovering child can be upsetting for the parent.
- One parent should be present during routine, painful and stressful procedures e.g. wound dressings, cast removal, venepuncture. The older child is given the choice. The rights of the child and consent are complex and challenging within all health care settings.

Consent and capacity

Adults

At 18 years of age mentally competent adults are considered able to make all decisions in relation to their medical care providing they have the capacity to do so. This right does not diminish with age and all mentally competent adults have the right to refuse treatment even when it will clearly benefit them. The Mental Health Capacity Act (2005) introduced in England and Wales in 2007 permits courts to appoint a proxy decision maker who has power to grant consent to medical treatment if the patient becomes incapacitated.

For consent to be valid the person must have **capacity**, the consent must be **voluntary** and not be given under **duress**. Furthermore, the person must have received **sufficient information** upon which to base their decision. The person must also be able to communicate their decision. No adult is able to give consent for another adult. Here, 'surgical, medical or dental treatment' includes any procedure undertaken for the purposes of diagnosis and this section applies to any procedure (including, in particular, the administration of an anesthetic) which is ancillary to any treatment as it applies to that treatment.

Young person: 16–17 years of age

In many localities 16–17 yr olds are legally entitled to consent to their own medical treatment (without parental involvement). However, in certain circumstances they may not be permitted to refuse therapeutic care where they are at risk of suffering harm as a result of their decision.

Young person: under 16 years of age

A high profile test case of child consent (*Gillick v West Norfolk and Wisbech Area Health Authority 1985)* saw Victoria Gillick attempting to set a legal precedent in England and Wales which would have meant that medical practitioners could not give young people under the age of 16 treatment or contraceptive services without parental permission. After Initial success, the House of Lords ruled that under-16 s who are fully able to understand what is proposed, and its implications, are competent to consent to medical treatment regardless of age. This test case leads to 'Gillick competence', which states:

(As a matter of law the parental right to determine whether or not their minor child below the age of 16 will have medical treatment terminates if and when the child achieves sufficient understanding and intelligence to enable him to understand fully what is proposed.)

This also establishes that a child who is competent to consent to a course of treatment is entitled to the same obligation of confidentiality. Disclosures, however, need be considered against:

- the young person's right to privacy
- the degree of current harm or likely harm
- what any such disclosure is likely to achieve
- what the potential benefits are to the young person's wellbeing and, of course, the criminal law in this regard.

Those under 16 years may be able to consent if they are 'Gillick competent', meaning they have **sufficient understanding and intelligence** to make relevant decisions. In under 16s, parental involvement is desirable but not always essential (e.g. contraception) except where it is in the child's best interests (e.g. sexual abuse). If a person with parental responsibility (PR) consents, they are subject to the same tests for capacity, duress and information as all adults. It is routine practice to gain consent from only one person with PR i.e. parent or guardian.

Pain

Childhood may require hospital admission and surgical intervention as a result of developmental disorders, disease or injury. The 'total pain' concept which considers the **physical, psychological, spiritual** and **social** aspects should be valued with the last three being met only after pain and related symptoms (e.g. anxiety) are controlled. Anxiety and fear are often overlooked or cause confusion for those caring for the child in pain. Chapter 11 concentrates on the fundamentals and exploration of orthopaedic and musculoskeletal trauma conditions. There is a need, however, to consider specific issues for the child in pain.

Pain is commonly experienced following surgery, but research highlights that pain is not always well controlled (Twycross 2007). It is well established that pain is an individual and subjective phenomenon, with three approaches commonly used in isolation or in combination to assess child pain i.e. self-report (what the child says); behavioural (how the child behaves) and physiological indicators (how the child's body reacts). Self-report of pain intensity is a valuable source of information although there are many sources of bias and error (von Baeyer 2006). Children younger than five years of age can point to where they hurt but may be unable to accurately offer a reliable description of pain intensity due to age-related development (Twycross *et al.*, 2009). Consequently, behavioural and physiological approaches are also commonly used. A one-dimensional approach is limited whereas multidimensional approaches promote optimal pain management. The child's ability to describe pain increases with age and experience and changes throughout their development.

Pain assessment is central to successful management of pain. Commonly adopted child-specific assessment tools include the Wong and Baker (1988) six-point cartoon face rating scale (see Chapter 11 for further discussion of pain assessment tools). FLACC (Merkel *et al.*, 1997) is an observer-rated pain scale for the non-verbal child. The abbreviation FLACC stands for face, legs, activity, crying and consolability. The FLACC pain scale was designed for children between the ages of two and seven years with McKay and Clarke (2012) recently reporting it suitable for children with a learning disability within the orthopaedic and trauma setting.

Pain management for children following orthopaedic trauma and surgery is further complicated by it commonly being difficult to obtain self-report of the pain experience of the child (Clarke 2003a). Such complexity has historically led to nurse-reporting of pain. Parents commonly adopt a central or supportive role when their child is too young to self-report their pain. However, parents' and nurses' judgements of facial expression or 'how the patient looks' mean that children's pain is frequently underestimated (Goubet *et al.*, 2009). Twycross *et al.* (2009) demonstrate that practices can be suboptimal when children are asked to report on how well their pain is managed. This problem may relate to nurses' continuing belief in misconceptions about children's pain; for example that a sleeping child cannot be in pain. There is evidence to suggest, however, that a sleeping child may, in fact, be exhausted because of persistent pain. If pain management is dependent solely on nurse-assessment then the outcome may be suboptimum. The role of the parent within the domain of family-centred care is deemed paramount (Corkin *et al.*, 2012), with seminal and contemporary literature openly debating the value of the parent to score pain equal to the child post-surgery. The subjective nature of reporting pain severity and a reliance on the use of nurse and parent report when communication and cognition is absent, questions how effectively and consistently the documenting nurse and parent assess a child's pain. Caution is advised due to the impact of fear and anxiety and not actual pain, alongside a need to identify pain location as the child could be reporting pain associated with, for example, their cannula. Children communicate their pain in many different ways; for example a child may 'hide' under their duvet, stop talking or become vocal, aggressive or 'lash out'.

Misconceptions around children's pain continue to impact upon practice, pain outcomes and wellbeing; these include:

- neonates do not feel pain
- children experience pain differently to/less than adults
- children cannot express their pain
- children do not remember pain
- it is not safe to give children opiates due to the risk of respiratory depression.

Pain assessment is commonly considered the 'fifth vital sign' and undertaken as part of pre-existing clinical observations, blood pressure, pulse, respiration and temperature (von Baeyer 2006). (See Box 21.3 for examples of evidence related to pain assessment in children following orthopaedic surgery).

Harrop (2007) suggests there is widespread inadequate prevention and relief of pain, supporting findings documented by the National Service Framework for Children in 2004. Conversely, Clarke and Richardson (2007) report on evolving practice that includes the recognition and deeper understanding of the child's individual pain experience and the benefits of using an age-appropriate pain assessment tool that demonstrates validity and reliability and is taught preoperatively to the child (if possible) with parental involvement. Others include recent pharmacological advances such as intravenous (IV) paracetamol, continuous epidural infusions, caudal blocks and recognising the benefits of non-pharmacological interventions. Non-pharmacological options include behavioural and supportive methods such as information, empathy, belief and choices. Psychological treatment should be an integral part of orthopaedic and fracture trauma pain management with cognitive methods such as imagery and hypnosis potential options. Deep breathing and progressive

Box 21.3 Evidence digest

Childrens', parents' and nurses' reports of pain following orthopaedic surgery

An unpublished prospective exploratory study drew upon three convenience sample groups; the child, parent and attending nurse within an acute UK orthopaedic unit (Clarke 2003). Children were included ($n=32$) aged five to fifteen years old who were scheduled for an overnight admission following orthopaedic surgery. The sequence of data collection was nurse, child and parent. Each participating/attending nurse collected the pain scores on day one post-surgery between 10 and 11 am, with both scores blinded to parent and child. All three groups used the same modified 'FACE' rating pain assessment tool. Non-parametric testing found no statistical significance between the small sample groups of child, parent and nurse report of pain.

Statistically significant differences were, however, reported more recently by Rajasagaram *et al.* (2009) using a larger ($n=86$) sample of child, parent and nurse groups. Findings should be viewed with caution due to inappropriate testing i.e. a Mann Whitney U-test was used to test for difference in three groups instead of the recognised two (Connolly 2007). The small exploratory study undertaken by Clarke (2003) showed a statistically significant difference between boys and girls self-reporting of pain, with girls reporting a higher level of pain. A positive correlation was also found between parent- and nurse-report of child pain which would suggest parent/nurse agreement but not with the child. Interestingly Belville and Seupaul (2005) report a tradition of asking adults for information about the health status of children.

More recently, Twycross *et al.* (2007) completed a qualitative observational study of post-operative pain management practices in England. Thirteen registered nurses working in a surgical ward were observed continuously for a period of five hours per shift for two to four shifts. Data were collected for 36 shifts in total (185 hours). The study involved children aged 0–16 years. The nurses were observed administering pain relief when the child self-reported pain. They did not, however, routinely assess a child's pain, nor use non-drug methods of pain relief on a regular basis. Reasons offered included a deficit in the nurses' knowledge of pain and a lack of priority given to pain management. Parents were also not consistently encouraged to be involved in their child's pain and on five occasions children's behavioural cues were used as an indicator that a child was in pain, rather than appropriately assessing the child.

relaxation should not be used in isolation for intense pain. Parents sometimes need to be given permission to touch and stroke their child.

Fear and anxiety management play key roles in children's pain management and the nurse needs to take into account the stage of child development, cognitive abilities, gaining child and family trust and ensuring pain intensity is being measured and not the anxiety or fear. Influences on the pain experience for any child include past experiences, socialisation (how they see pain managed at home), personal values, cultural patterns and differences in assessment and intervention of pain (e.g. phobia of needles due to previous analgesic injections). Developments and innovative practice should be managed by a dedicated integrated multidisciplinary 'pain team' (Clarke 2003a) with the contribution of a children's nurse educated in orthopaedics and fracture trauma. Pain management continues to challenge practitioners caring for children but particularly within orthopaedics and trauma as surgical intervention often produces pain of medium to severe intensity.

Safeguarding children

This section of the chapter aims to provide an overview of safeguarding plus the signs of child abuse and neglect. It will also identify the key government policies and guidelines which have been produced for all health professionals. The focus will be upon physical abuse as it is aligned to the field of orthopaedics and trauma with an emphasis on fractures in young children who present to emergency departments and surgical wards.

The case of Victoria Climbie has had a significant impact on children's services in the UK over the last decade. Victoria suffered maltreatment at the hands of her great aunt and partner (Laming 2003). A wide range of agencies were involved and they missed opportunities to protect Victoria. Laming (2003) made multiple recommendations regarding assessment and observation, documentation and communication between all agencies and clearly stated that this was a lesson to be learned and never to happen again. But it did happen again; in August 2007 a 17-month old boy, 'Baby P', died having suffered fatal injuries at the hands of his mother and her boyfriend (Laming 2009). Baby P was visited 60 times by health and social care professionals and had been on the child protection register for nine months. There was a public outcry and a national review of child protection. The message was clear, it must not happen again.

During the period 2007–2012 a further 100 children have died in similar circumstances in the UK alone (www. nspcc.org.uk). These statistics show that the publishing of further guidelines to help health professionals to recognise, assess and protect children who may be at risk of significant harm appears, so far, to have had inadequate effect.

Recognition of child abuse

The categories of child abuse fall into the following areas:

- physical abuse
- sexual abuse
- emotional abuse
- neglect.

All staff involved need to be alert to signs of child abuse and act accordingly, following the guidelines set out by government and professional bodies.

Physical abuse

This type of abuse may involve hitting, slapping, throwing, burning or scalding, poisoning or suffocating the child resulting in injury or death of the infant or child. Signs and symptoms include:

- bruising
- broken bones
- bites, scratches
- burns, scalds
- black eyes.

Additional mediating factors include (Corkin *et al.*, 2012):

- where there is delay in seeking medical attention
- where there is conflicting history as to what has happened
- where a pattern appears linked to recurrent injuries
- where there is poor parental anxiety shown.

NICE (2009) guidance suggests a focus on the concepts of 'alerting features', 'consider' or 'suspect':

- ***Alerting features*** are symptoms, signs and patterns of injury or behaviour, which may indicate child abuse.
- ***Consider*** means that abuse is one possible explanation for an alerting feature (but there are other possible diagnoses).
- ***Suspect*** means there is a serious level of concern about abuse, but not proof. It may trigger a child

protection investigation. This may lead to child protection procedures being put in place, offering the family more support or may lead to alternative explanations being found.

Fractures are a common manifestation of child abuse that may be found incidentally on X-rays ordered for another reason. A majority of non-accidental fractures occur in children under 18 months old. There are few genuine accidental fractures in this age group as fracture requires significant force in a child with normal bone development and does not occur during normal child care. Nurses are often one of the first to assess a child with an injury or fracture so they require a good level of knowledge of bone and child development.

When a child has a fracture, concerns are raised by the following issues:

- age/developmental level – fractures in non-ambulatory children are unusual
- location – metaphyseal, post-ribs, scapula, vertebrae and sternum fractures are highly suggestive of non-accidental injury
- pattern – e.g. multiple fractures, complex skull fractures may suggest non-accidental injury
- age of injury – delay in seeking medical attention, fractures of different ages.

Eighty-five percent of fractures from non-accidental injury (NAI) occur in children under the age of three and 69% under the age of one year. Fractures under the age of one are highly associated with non-accidental trauma, as the infant would not have the ability to exert the force required to cause a fracture (Wade Shrader *et al.*, 2011). Long bone fractures can be suggestive of NAI. Long bone fracture may present initially with a cry/scream, then the child may be irritable with decreased movement/use of limb and crying on movement of the affected area (i.e. changing, bathing) along with swelling. Fractures usually occur as a result of a twisting fall with foot planted – i.e. less force than expected. Fractures that occur due to traction/torsional forces can sometimes be attributed to forceful yanking, tugging which twisting which rarely occur accidentally and can suggest non-accidental injury.

Spiral humeral fractures and metaphyseal fractures of the distal femur and tibia are thought to be more likely to be caused by non-accidental injury (NAI). If an infant is pulled sharply, the corner of the metaphyseal region of the bone can be torn; this is referred to as 'bucket handle' fracture. Finding spiral fractures in a bone shaft is indicative of a twisting injury. Violent squeezing of the rib cage can result in anterior and posterior rib fractures which are difficult to acquire as children's ribs are quite flexible. Additionally skull fractures such as linear fractures in the parietal bone are uncommon in a child under eighteen months and result from a direct force to the skull (refer to Chapter 24 for an evidence digest that highlights the incidence of non-accidental fractures in infants).

Assessment for non-accidental injury

The assessments of children, following local and national guidance, are a fundamental part of recognising non-accidental injury. Assessment frameworks set out to improve the quality of assessment and to assist in communicating the needs of children across all agencies involved. They also aim to avoid the escalation of a 'child in need' in relation to child protection through early identification and effective intervention. Guidance provides information to practitioners on how and when to refer a child to the dedicated child protection agency/team. A detailed documented assessment can lead to action that ensures child protection is maintained. Throughout the process the child is the main focus and the child's views must be listened to throughout. The family's circumstances must also be considered; including their strengths, needs and potential risks, in order to make robust plans that can lead to improving the outcomes for the child. All practitioners must be aware of the assessment tool in use and be responsible for ensuring that the assessment process and subsequent action are carried out effectively and in a timely manner to ensure the safety of the child.

Role and responsibilities of practitioners

All practitioners must be aware they have a role to play in recognising abuse or neglect in infants and children. They must work closely with other disciplines and act accordingly. They must place the interests of the child at the centre of their work and act on the child's behalf if they have concerns (DES 2006). UK nurses, for example, must adhere to the Nursing and Midwifery Code of Conduct (2008) which states that

Box 21.4 Nurse responsibility: safeguarding

- Refer to hospital policies and procedures
- Inform line manager
  - consultant
  - hospital social worker
  - child protection nurse specialist.
  - follow up with a written referral; include: names of child and carer, DoB, address, GP, Health Visitor, school, language spoken
- State concerns/issues/reason for referral
- All referrals must be followed up in writing within 24 hours
- Observe and document anything that may be of significance
- Never confront a suspected abuser
- Do let parents know you are concerned
- Document
- Note outcome.

(all nurses have duty and personal responsibility to act in the best interest of the child or young person, and to alert and to inform appropriate personnel if they suspect a child is at risk or has been abused.)

As well as having the skills of recognition and communication, all staff must have good record keeping and report writing skills. These must be clear, comprehensive, accurate, accessible, dated and signed in a chronological order (RCN 2007). The nurse's responsibility around safe guarding children is summarised in Box 21.4.

Summary

The first chapter in this section highlights the needs of the child and family presenting with either an orthopaedic condition or fracture to be, ideally, cared for by a children's nurse who has received post-qualifying education in orthopaedics and trauma. Key issues within this client group include challenges around assessment and planning care, informed consent, safeguarding, separation from parents, change of environment, anxiety and fear and the effective assessment and management of pain. Although similar to that of the adult, the team of health and non-health care professionals differs in placing family-centred care as an approach fundamental to good care outcomes for the child. In order to fully appreciate the wider context of caring for children within orthopaedic and fracture trauma the reader should review Chapters 22, 23 and 24 while taking into account the principles covered in this introductory chapter.

Recommended further reading

Corkin, D., Clarke, S. and Liggett, L (eds) (2012) *Care Planning in Children and Young People's Nursing*. Wiley Blackwell, Oxford.

Glasper, A. and Richardson, J. (2011) *A Textbook of Children and Young Persons Nursing*, 2nd edn. Elsevier Press, London.

Liverley, J. and Long, T. (2013) Children's experiences as hospital in-patients: voice, competence and work. Messages for nursing from a critical ethnographic study. *International journal of Nursing Studies*. DOI: dx.doi.org/10.1016.

Royal College of Anaesthetists (2013) *Guidance on the Provision of Anaesthesia Services for Acute Pain Management*. RCA, London. Available at: http://www.rcoa.ac.uk/document-store/guidance-the-provision-of-anaesthesia-services-acute-pain-management-2013 (accessed 22 April 2014).

References

Casey, A. (1988) A partnership with child and family. *Senior Nurse*, **8**(4), 8–9.

Clarke, S.E. (2003a) Postoperative pain in children: A retrospective audit of continuous epidural analgesia in a paediatric orthopaedic ward. *Journal of Orthopaedic Nursing*, **7**(1), 4–9.

Clarke, S.E. (2003b) Orthopaedic paediatric practice: an impression pain assessment. *Journal of Orthopaedic Nursing*, **7**(3), 132–136.

Clarke, S. (2007) Changing paediatric orthopaedic education and certification for the RN in Northern Ireland? *Orthopaedic Nursing*, **26**(2), 126–129.

Clarke, S.E. and Richardson, O. (2007) Using intravenous paracetamol in children following surgery: a literature review. *Journal of Children's and Young People's Nursing*, **1**(6), 273–280.

Connolly, P. (2007) *Quantitative Data Analysis in Education: A Critical Introduction Using SPSS*. Routledge, London.

Corkin, D., Clarke, S. and Liggett, L. (eds) (2012) *Care Planning in Children and Young People's Nursing*. Wiley Blackwell, Oxford.

Department for Education and Skills (DES) (2006) *What to do if You Are Worried a Child is Being Abused*. DES, London.

Department of Health (2004) *National Service Framework for Children*. DoH, London.

Department of Health and Social Services and Public Health (2004) *Understanding the Needs of Children in Northern Ireland (UNOCINI)*. DHSS, Belfast.

Department of Health (2000) *Framework for the Assessment of Children in Need and their Families*. DoH, London.

Gillick v West Norfolk & Wisbech Area Health Authority (1985) UKHL 7 British and Irish Legal Information Institute (BAILII). Available at: http://www.nspcc.org.uk/Inform/research/briefings/gillick_wda101615.html#How_is_Gillick_competency_assessed? (accessed 7 April 2014).

Goubet, L., Vervoort, T., Cano, A. and Crombez, G. (2009) Catastrophizing about their children's pain is related to higher parent-child congruency in pain ratings: an experimental investigation. *European Journal of Pain*, **13**(2), 196–201.

Harrop, J.E. (2007) Management of pain in childhood. *Archives of Disease in Childhood*, **92**: 101–108.

HMSO (2004) *The Children Act*, Chapter 31. HMSO, London.

Kennedy, I. (2010) *Getting it Right for Children and Young People: Overcoming Cultural Barriers in the NHS so as to Meet Their Needs*. Department of Health, London.

Laming Report (2003) *The Victoria Climbie Inquiry: Report of an Inquiry by Lord Laming*. The Stationery Office (TSO), Norwich.

Laming Report (2009) *The Protection of Children in England. A Progress Report*. The Stationary Office, London.

Livesley, J. and Long, T. (2013) Children's experiences as hospital in-patients: voice, competence and work. Messages for nursing form a critical ethnographic study. *International Journal of Nursing Studies*. DOI: dx.doi.org/10.1016.

McGrath, P., Rosmus, C., Canfield, C., Campbell, M.A. and Hennigar, A. (1998) Behaviours caregivers use to determine pain in nonverbal, cognitively impaired individuals. *Developmental Medicine and Child Neurology*, **40**(5), 340–343.

McKay, M. Clarke, S (2012) Pain assessment tools for the child with severe learning disability: a review and application to orthopaedic practice. *Nursing Children and Young People*, **24** (2), 14–19.

Mental Health Capacity Act (2005) London, The Stationery Office.

Merkel, S.I., Voepel-Lewis, T., Shayevitz, J.R. and Malviya, S. (1997) The FLACC: a behavioral scale for scoring post-operative pain in young children. *Pediatric Nursing*, **23**(3), 293–297.

Murat, I., Baujard, C., Foussat, C. *et al.* (2005) Tolerance and analgesic efficacy of a new IV paracetamol solution in children with inguinal hernia repair. *Pediatric Anaesthesia*, **15**, 663–670.

National Institute for Health and Clinical Excellence (NICE) (2009) *When to Suspect Maltreatment: Clinical Guideline CG89*. NICE, London.NSPCC www.nspcc.org.uk (accessed September 2012).

Nursing and Midwifery Council (NMC) (2008) *The Code – Standards of Conduct, Performance and Ethics for Nurses And Midwives*. NMC, London.

Platt report (1959) *The Report of the Committee on the Welfare of Children in Hospital*. Ministry of Health, London.

Roper, N., Logan, W. and Tierney, A.J. (2000) *The Roper-Logan-Tierney Model of Nursing: Based on Activities of Living*. Elsevier Health Sciences, Edinburgh.

Royal College of Nursing (RCN) (2007) *Safeguarding Children and Young People – Every Nurse's Responsibility*. RCN, London.

Royal College of Nursing (RCN) (2007) *Benchmarks for Children's Orthopaedic Nursing Care – RCN guidance*. Available at: www.rcn.org.uk/__data/assets/pdf_file/0007/115486/003209.pdf (accessed 15 April 2013).

Shrader, W.M., Nicholas, M.D., Bernat, B.A., Lee, S. and Segal, M.D. (2011) Suspected non accidental trauma and femoral shaft fractures in children. *Orthopaedics*, **34**, 5.

Simons, J., Frank, L. and Robertson, E. (2001) Parent involvement in children's pain care: views of parents and nurses. *Journal of Advanced Nursing*, **36**(4), 591–599.

Twycross, A. (2007) Children's nurses' postoperative pain management practices: an observational study. *International Journal of Nursing Studies*, **44**, 869–881.

Twycross, A., Dowden, S.J. and Bruce E. (2009) *Managing Pain in Children: A Clinical Guide*. Wiley Blackwell, London.

UNICEF (1989) *A New Charter for Children 3/88*. UNICEF/UK Information Sheet No. 8. UNICEF, London.

van Aken, H., Veekman, L. and Buerkle, H. (2004) Assessing analgesia in single and repeated administrations of propacetamol for postoperative pain: comparison with morphine after dental surgery. *Anaesthesia Analgesia*, **98**: 159–195.

von Baeyer, C.L. (2006) Children's self-reports of pain intensity: Scale selection, limitations, and interpretation. *Pain Research and Management*, **11**(3), 157–162.

Wong D. and Baker, C. (1988) Pain in children: comparison of pain assessment scales. *Paediatric Nursing*, **14**(1), 9–17.

CHAPTER 22

Common childhood orthopaedic conditions, their care and management

Julia Judd

University Hospital Southampton, Southampton, UK

Introduction

The purpose of this chapter is to review current knowledge and management of paediatric orthopaedic conditions and discuss some of the health issues which affect bone development of children. This will serve as a source of information for nurses caring for children with a musculoskeletal condition in hospital, in the outpatient setting and in primary care. The selected topics, description of the subject matter and the child's pathway of care are of value to the practitioner in the advancement of their knowledge. The evidence base for this is represented through current literature in the subspecialty of paediatric orthopaedics, although in some areas the evidence may be old or lacking.

Musculoskeletal assessment

In the assessment of children it is important to use your ears, eyes and hands along with listening to the history given by the family and the child. It is vital to obtain a clear history about the presenting problem. The term 'OLD CART' is a useful tool for clinical examination (Dawson *et al.*, 2012). Each 'letter' aims to prompt the recall of a series of statements which encourages the practitioner to ask the child and family about the **O**nset of the problem; **L**ocation of problems; **D**uration and **C**haracteristics of symptoms; **A**ssociated factors that contribute to the problem; **R**elieving factors that make the problem better and **T**reatment so far.

Throughout the assessment the practitioner must take into account the family dynamics and involve the child, however young they are, listening to their description of the problem, using language that is age appropriate and using toys or favourite items to help the child to understand what is being asked. Information needs to be accessible in a variety of forms including written, visual and through play (Dawson *et al.*, 2012). The environment should be friendly and welcoming to alleviate any fear that the child may have in coming into the hospital.

Try and build a rapport with the child before examining them. If they are very young it may be more appropriate to examine them on the parents lap. One format for examination is to use the *look, feel, move* approach to assess the presenting problem. This involves looking at the problem area, feeling and moving where the problem is and assessing associated joints whilst observing the child's facial expressions and noticing pain or discomfort.

The orthopaedic practitioner should have sound domain-specific knowledge to be able to clinically assess the child and reach conclusions (Judd 2005). This means knowing what the normal musculoskeletal development for different age groups is and being able to interpret X-rays dependent on the child's age and the bone or joint that is being assessed. Collectively the history and clinical examination should lead the practitioner to a plan for investigations and diagnosis.

A systematic approach is helpful when assessing a child. Look at the overall appearance, taking note of the child's colour (pale or healthy), their stature and posture. How does the child stand? Look at the leg alignment. Is there evidence of asymmetry, such as genu varum/valgum (Figure 22.1), an abnormal rotational profile or leg length

Orthopaedic and Trauma Nursing: An Evidence-based Approach to Musculoskeletal Care, First Edition. Edited by Sonya Clarke and Julie Santy-Tomlinson.

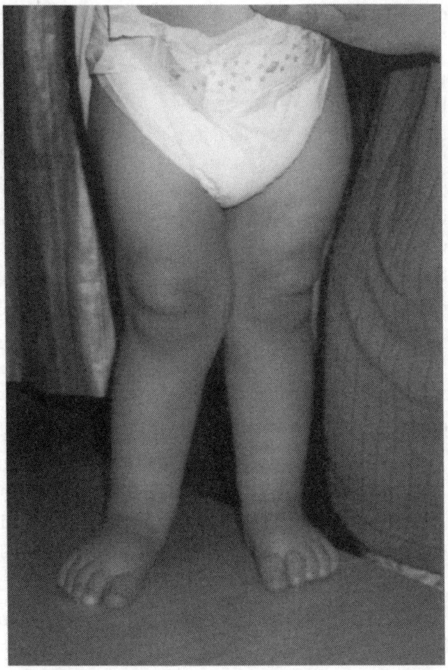

Figure 22.1 Genu Valgum

difference? Is there evidence of dysfunction? For example, tripping up, a limp, reduced range of motion in a joint or disability.

Normal variants

Many referrals from general practitioners to orthopaedic services relate to concerns regarding deviation from what parents believe to be the norm. Moloney *et al.*, (2006) determined that half of child referrals (53%) to the hospital present with normal variants, predominated by in-toeing gait and flexible flat feet. In-toeing may be caused by femoral anteversion, tibial torsion or metatarsus adductus (forefoot adduction). An out-toeing gait may be due to femoral retroversion, external tibial torsion or flat feet. All of these are normal variants and are expected to resolve naturally with growth.

Developmental dysplasia of the hip, a neuromuscular problem, clubfoot or a slipped capital femoral epiphysis, however, contribute to in-toeing or out-toeing torsional abnormalities and will require orthopaedic intervention. Flat feet are commonly referred as a result of concern raised by a shoe shop. If the foot is flexible with the arch restored on tip toe standing, then parents can be reassured. The normal age for arch development is by age six although, if the child has ligamentous laxity, they may always have normal flexible flat feet. Orthotics are not required to restore an arch in a normal foot and are used only for the symptomatic foot.

Genu varum (bow legs) and genu valgum (knock knees) deformities can be physiological or pathological and diagnosis is made based on the age of the child, X-ray appearances and progression versus resolution. At birth, a baby's legs are naturally bowed and this can look progressively worse, especially if the child walks at a young age. By the age of two years the legs will straighten, followed by valgus deformity between the ages of three to four years and gradual correction to normal by age six. It is important to exclude pathology such as rickets, Blounts disease or a metaphyseal dysplasia and to be aware that a unilateral deformity is probably pathological in origin.

Common conditions presenting in the neonate, infant, child and young person

Congenital muscular torticollis

Congenital muscular torticollis is a benign condition that is usually detected in early infancy. The baby tilts their head towards the affected side and turns their face in the opposite direction. This is caused by a fibrous tissue mass within the sternocleidomastoid muscle (SCM). The reason for this is unclear, but may be due to in-utero crowding or a decrease in the blood supply to the muscle. On palpation a firm tumour can be felt in the neck and there may be accompanying plagiocephaly (Luther 2002). Hollier *et al.* (2000) report a high incidence of 1 per 250 live births, associating difficult births as a causative factor. Resolution is usually within four to six months with stretching exercises if the condition is without other association. The incidence of developmental dysplasia of the hip in an infant with torticollis varies between 2–29% and should be excluded with a hip scan at six weeks of age (von Heideken *et al.*, 2006). Physiotherapy is the mainstay of treatment and parents are taught stretching exercises to continue at home. For those who do not respond favourably by twelve months, a surgical release of the SCM is performed.

Developmental dysplasia of the hip

Developmental dysplasia of the hip (DDH) is the term used to describe a spectrum of disorders affecting the infant hip. Previously known as congenital dislocation of the hip (CDH), the term was changed to DDH to reflect that the condition is dynamic, can change and is not always detectable at birth. The hip joint may be dysplastic with a shallow acetabulum (acetabular dysplasia) that is unstable and subluxing or completely dislocated. Early recognition and appropriate treatment by skilled practitioners, predetermines a good outcome. Clinical guidelines (NIPE 2010) promote a uniform approach to infant screening and detecting abnormality promptly. Treatment decisions are determined by abnormal clinical and sonographic examination (Clarke and Castaneda 2012) and are reliant on the competence of the practitioner (RCN 2012). The primary aim of DDH treatment is to achieve a concentric and stable hip joint and ultimately normal development of the acetabulum and proximal femur with minimal possibility for subsequent reconstructive surgical intervention (Bolland *et al.*, 2010). Early osteoarthritis, chronic pain and a reduction in activity levels are all possible sequelae of DDH and the earlier the intervention the more likely a successful outcome.

Aetiology and epidemiology

DDH is the most common congenital newborn defect (75%). The cause is unknown, although there are multifactorial traits; gender, hormonal influence, race, hyperlaxity, uterine malposition, geographic and environmental influences. Box 22.1 outlines some of the associated risk factors. The incidence of true DDH is difficult to determine accurately as the definition lends itself to a broad spectrum of the condition, giving variance to the accurate incidence. Over the years, authors have strived to clarifiy the terminology and there have been improved methods of detection and diagnosis. The introduction of screening of neonates at risk and sonography has improved diagnostic technique (Kokavec and Bialik 2007). Reported incidence of hip instability is as high as 20 per 1000 live births and varies depending on geographic location. Many of these, which are due to ligamentous laxity, stabilise within the first couple of weeks. The incidence of true hip dislocation in the United Kingdom (UK) is reported as one to two per 1000 live births (Clarke and Taylor 2012).

DDH is more common in females, with increased prevalence in first born infants. The latter is believed to be due to the tight structure of the uterus and subsequent reduced capacity for foetal movement. The risk of late DDH was found to be 29% in breech presentation at four to six month follow-up (Imrie *et al.*, 2010), despite normal ultrasound at six weeks. Research studies to assess prophylactic hip abduction splints for this category of patient are ongoing (Clarke and Judd 2012).

Box 22.1 Associated risk factors for DDH

- Oligohydramnios
- Firstborn child
- Large baby for gestational age
- Packaging disorders e.g. torticollis, positional/structural club foot
- Caesarean section delivery
- Cerebral palsy
- Breech presentation

The infant hip is at risk of DDH if the baby is subject to the recognised risk factors. Early appropriate intervention will result in normal hip development in the majority of babies.

Diagnosis

A routine part of the neonate's postpartum check is hip examination. The practitioner assesses for equal leg length and looks for asymmetry of the gluteal and thigh folds. More importantly, reduced hip abduction and instability are indicative of DDH. In the UK the NHS Newborn and Physical Examination Programme (NIPE) recommend examiners be trained and are competent in the Ortolani and Barlow tests (NIPE 2010). The Barlow test demonstrates hip instability as the hip displaces posteriorly out of the actebulum and the Ortolani test produces an audible clunk as the dislocated hip is relocated back into the acetabulum. Babies with a positive clinical examination and those that meet the screening criteria are referred to a specialist clinic for hip ultrasound (see Box 22.2 and Figure 22.2).

As an adjunct to clinical assessment, ultrasound clarifies clinical findings. It is not feasible, however, to scan all babies' hips due to the inordinate expense and requirement for resources (American Academy of Pediatrics 2000). Guidelines ensure practitioners make the appropriate referrals at the correct time (Box 22.2).

It is important to obtain a good family and birth history (Judd 2012a) prior to a clinical and sonographic

Box 22.2 Infant hip screening criteria (NIPE 2010)

Babies with a positive clinical examination

Abnormal/unstable hips

⇩

Refer for expert paediatric orthopaedic consultation and hip ultrasound by three weeks of age

Positive risk factors

Family history of DDH

Breech presentation

In utero postural deformities (torticollis, club foot)

Multiple births

⇩

Refer for ultrasound by four to six weeks of age

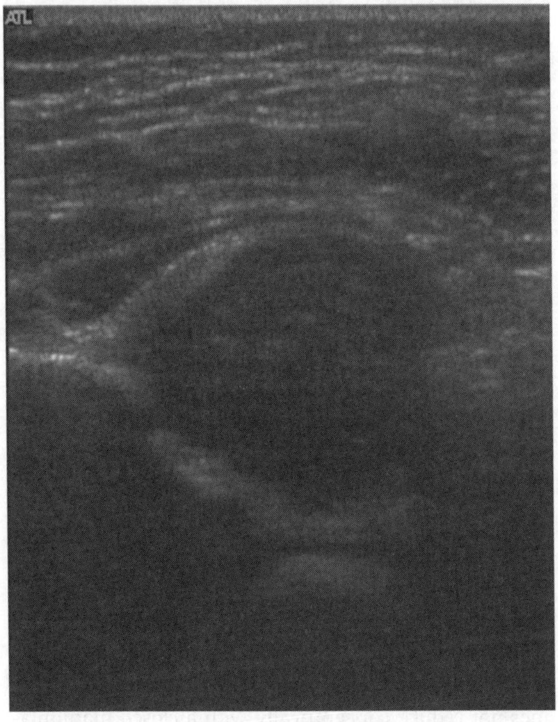

Figure 22.2 Hip ultrasound showing a dysplastic hip

examination. The ossific nucleus (secondary ossification centre) is normally present in the infant's hip at the approximate age of four months but later in an infant with DDH. An X-ray therefore is not helpful in determining the hip structure and ultrasound is the gold standard to show true hip dislocation or dysplasia. A static coronal view can be measured using the Graf method to assess for dyplasia (Eastwood and de Gheldere 2010). A further dynamic stress test in the transverse plane will assess for instability. Combined, the two images detect the degree of abnormal hip morphology.

Late diagnosis of DDH is commonly detected by the parent who notices their child has a short leg or a limp when there is a unilateral presentation. A child with bilateral dislocated hips will present with a waddling gait. Confirmation is made by X-ray (see Figure 22.4) and clinical examination. Hip abduction is markedly reduced and if unilateral, the affected side shows a shortened limb. The later the diagnosis, the more interventional the treatment and potential for the development of degenerative joint disease. Because DDH is often neglected or treated inappropriately it has become the most common cause of secondary osteoarthritis of the hip.

Guidelines (NIPE 2010) advise the practitioner on when to refer to a specialist paediatric orthopaedic doctor and tested algorithms of treatment are available in the literature (Clarke and Taylor 2012). Multi-centred research studies aim to amalgamate findings to improve knowledge of DDH management and to test new theories. The Institute of Infant Hip Dysplasia (IHDI) strives to create a gold standard for referral and treatment, looking at timing of intervention, method of treatment, failure and complication rates.

Treatment

Treatment of DDH is dependent on the age of the child at presentation (Clarke and Taylor 2012):

Newborn to four months

The Pavlik harness is the most common hip abduction orthosis for the treatment of DDH. Reported as having a 95% success rate, it is effective for dysplastic and unstable hips. It should be abandoned early if a fixed irreducible hip fails to respond to treatment in the first week as there is an increased risk of subsequent avascular necrosis (AVN). It is also contraindicated in neurological hip dislocation (Clarke and Taylor 2012). The harness consists of shoulder and leg straps secured to a chest band (Figure 22.3).

The optimum position for treatment and prevention of complications, such as femoral nerve palsy and AVN, is 90 degrees of hip flexion and 60 degrees of hip abduction. Weekly ultrasound scans confirm successful treatment and allows the practitioner to check and adjust the harness position and ensure compliance. The infant wears the harness for six weeks full time, following which they

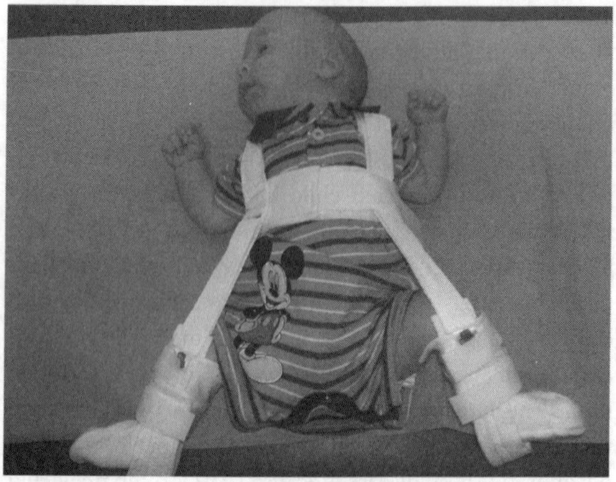

Figure 22.3 Pavlik harness. Reproduced with permission from Wiley.

are gradually weaned out of it. Follow-up is recommended with serial X-rays until the age of five years to exclude residual dysplasia and late onset complications.

Parents are often upset by the diagnosis and the visual appearance of their baby in the harness. Close observation of the infant and reassurance and support of the parents are required to ensure successful treatment (Atalar *et al.*, 2007). The consequence of not treating the infant's hip is extremely detrimental and will condemn the child to significant surgical intervention later. It is important to give parents written information on how to care for their baby (Box 22.3 shows an abbreviated sample information leaflet) and advice on appropriate and useful websites (for further information of the care of a baby in a harness, see: www.steps-charity.org.uk).

Early years treatment

Between the ages of 4–12 months, surgical correction is necessary to reduce the hip. For these infants either the Pavlik harness failed and was abandoned early or the diagnosis was not detected on initial clinical examination. Surgical correction is usually deferred until the ossific nucleus is evident on scan, to prevent potential for subsequent AVN (Luedtke *et al.*, 2000).

There is some consensus that a week of pre-operative gallows traction to stretch the vascular supply to the femoral head reduces the risk of post-operative AVN although this is not proven (Luedtke *et al.*, 2000). Gallows traction is not a pre-requisite and does not affect whether the hip reduces by closed manipulation or by open surgery. An arthrogram and adductor tenotomy is

Box 22.3 Parent's information – Care of your baby in a Pavlik harness (NIPE 2010). Reproduced with permission from Crown copyright

The harness does not hurt your baby. It is designed to gently position your baby's hips normally.
Cuddle and feed them as you would normally do.
Do not remove the harness or adjust it.
The harness will be checked and adjusted weekly when you come to clinic.
Your baby will have an ultrasound scan to check the hip position each week.

Clothing

- It is recommended that a vest is worn underneath to prevent skin chafing.
- To change the vest: first loosen the chest band. Undo one shoulder strap. Take the vest up the body and off one arm. Do up this shoulder strap.
- Undo the second shoulder strap and remove the vest.
- Check your baby's skin and wash with a cloth or cotton wool and water.
- The new vest can be put on in the same way as when taking it off.
- Replace the chest band to its marked position.
- Each day remove the legs one at a time from its straps to wash and replace socks.

General care

- The best position for your baby's health and hips is to place them on their back.
- If the harness is soiled, clean with detergent and a nail brush. Dry with hairdryer on a cool setting, taking care not to harm your baby's skin.
- All clothes on top of the harness need to be loose around the legs to maintain the correct position.
- Do not swaddle your baby's legs tightly as this prevents normal hip development.
- Contact the team at the hospital if you have any questions or concerns.

performed as part of the surgical procedure and if the hip does not reduce concentrically with a closed manipulation, the hip joint is opened to remove obstructing soft tissue such as the labrum. The hip position may be confirmed post-operatively by CT scan to confirm concentric reduction. A hip spica in the human position maintains the femoral head in the acetabulum for six weeks if an open reduction or 12 weeks for a closed reduction (Chapter 21). Sequential broomstick casts (six weeks) and night splint casting (six weeks) may be used to complete the surgical programme (Table 22.1) or as

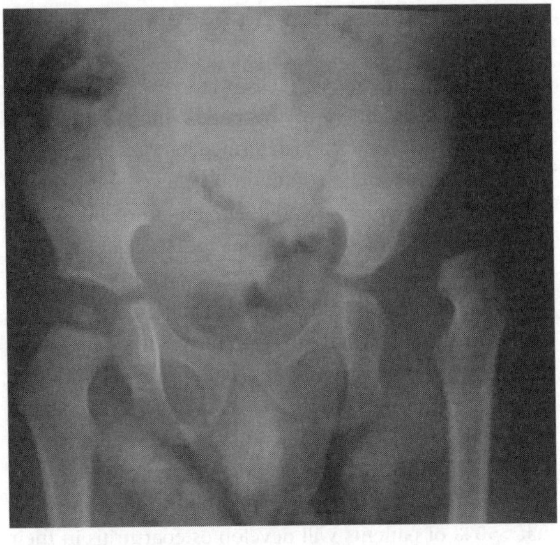

Figure 22.4 X-ray showing a dislocated left hip: the ossific nucleus is absent

Table 22.1 An example Surgical programme

Gallows raction		
Closed reduction	**Open reduction**	
Six weeks hip spica	Six weeks hip spica	
Six weeks hip spica		Changed under GA
Six weeks Broomstick plasters	Six weeks Broomstick plasters	Changed under GA
Six weeks night splints	Six weeks night splints	Changed under GA

an alternative ring splints or a hip abduction orthosis. For the older child who presents late (aged >18 months) a femoral shortening is required in addition to the open hip reduction to reduce the tension on the hip and protect from AVN. The 18-month-old child is too heavy for Gallows traction as they would be heavier than the upper weight limit of 16 kg (Davis and Barr 1999).

Further surgical procedures

Children who have undergone a closed or open hip reduction for either late presentation or failed Pavlik harness may subsequently need further surgery to improve acetabular cover. Residual hip dysplasia following treatment for DDH has a reported incidence of 2–17% (Cashman *et al.*, 2002). Of those children requiring pelvic osteotomy 60% previously underwent a closed reduction of the hip and 20% open reduction. This is usually by the age of three to four years to prevent progressive dysplasia, instability and eventual early osteoarthritis. The most important predictive factor for further surgery was found to be the initial achievement of a stable concentric reduction at closed or open reduction (Bolland *et al.*, 2010).

A pelvic osteotomy aims to realign the bony structure of the hip joint and therefore the weight bearing forces. A triangular shaped bone graft taken from the iliac crest is inserted into the osteotomy site above the acetabulum. This is fixed with two pins which are removed at six weeks under general anaesthetic (Figure 22.5). Post-operatively the child is nursed in a one and half hip spica cast to immobilse the hip joint until the bone graft has fused. The optimum timing is before school age, giving the femoral head and acetabulum opportunity to remodel with growth.

Specific nursing considerations

The child in a hip spica requires considerable care. It is a stressful time for the parents who require support emotionally and practically as well as needing written information on caring for their child (Clarke and McKay 2006).

An epidural is effective pain management for the first 48 hours if the child has had an open hip reduction after which Paracetamol is usually sufficient. This modality can provide excellent pain relief but can also be problematic. The line can migrate (comes out of

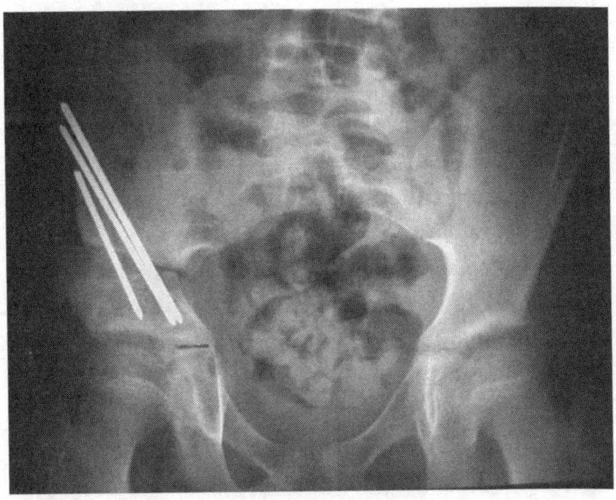

Figure 22.5 X-ray showing a pelvic osteotomy - the graft is secured with pins

epidural space), the child requires close observation and monitoring and the epidural site cannot not be visualised due to being covered by the spica.

The spica needs to dry naturally and the child is nursed on pillows alternating from front to back for the first 24 hours. A fibreglass covering is applied on day one post-operatively and waterproof tape is secured around the edges of the spica cast for protection (Sparks *et al.*, 2004). The parents are taught 'nappy care' and instructed on the frequency of checking the nappy for dampness and changing promptly to prevent the spica from becoming soiled. The parents should check their child's skin daily for signs of friction or rash. They can use a cloth to wash their child taking care not to get the cast wet. Hair washing is possible with the child resting on the legs of an adult who sits beside the bath. Holding the child's head over the edge of the bath, another adult can use the shower attachment to wash the hair.

The child in a spica cast is both heavy and awkward to lift; refer to Chapter 21 to view a picture of a hip spica in the human position. The occupational therapist (OT) can teach the parents handling techniques and how to turn their child safely. An assessment of the home will highlight issues early. A hoist may be required in the home. If the child cannot be securely and safely transported in the car, it may be necessary to arrange ambulance transfer home.

There are a number of ways to clothe a child in a spica. Trousers can be split and Velcro added to secure seams. Dresses are the easiest clothing for girls. Online companies advertise specific clothing made especially for children in spica casts.

Intervention for the young person

As the child gets older, a hip with residual dysplasia will give intrusive pain. A total hip arthroplasty for young and active patients, however, is not the best option. There is a risk of loosening and the revision rates are high. Alternative non-arthroplasty choices for the young patient include proximal femoral and periacetabular osteotomies to re-align the femoral head or re-position the acetabulum to delay the onset of arthritis. Surgical management of the problematic hip in adolescent and young adult patients can be challenging and technically difficult to do. As well as hip pain the patients may also have associated chronic instability. The optimum time for operative intervention is before there is too much wear on the cartilage and before arthritis sets in.

Legg Calvé Perthes disease

Legg Calvé Perthes disease (LCPD) (also known as Perthes disease) is a condition of the child's hip of unknown aetiology which results in a deformed femoral head due to avascular necrosis. The condition is believed to be due to ischemia of the femoral head due to an interruption of its blood supply. Studies suggest that the articular cartilage, the bony femoral epiphysis, the growing physis and the metaphysis are all affected (Catterall *et al.*, 1982). The aim of treatment, whether conservative or surgical, is to manage the child's symptoms and preserve hip joint congruency throughout the approximate two year disease process (Herring, 1998). Outcomes of Perthes disease are largely dependent on age at diagnosis as well as on treatment modalities (Daly *et al.*, 1999). Studies suggest that >50% of patients will develop osteoarthritis in their 60s (Perry *et al.*, 2012) and require early total hip replacements. Recent research has investigated the effect of bisphosphonates on animals with induced Perthes. Early results of ongoing research have shown effectiveness on increasing bone density, bone mineral content and strength (Little and Kim 2011).

Aetiology and epidemiology

The cause of Perthes is unknown. A study by Glueck *et al.* (1996), however, found 75% of participants had abnormal coagulation properties. Thrombophilia as a cause, however, has not been proven and debate regarding the reason for the temporary deficient blood supply of the femoral head continues (Kim 2010). Studies of epidemiology indicate a varied incidence of between 6–15.6 per 100000. A higher incidence is reported in lower socioeconomic and urban areas and a lower incidence in rural areas. Ethnicity may be a factor as Caucasians are affected more than other races with fewer numbers affected in the African and Chinese populations. It is also more common in the Japanese and in some parts of central Europe (Nochimson 2011). The condition predominantly affects boys from four to eight years and children who are small for their age and have a low BMI (body mass index) (Judd and Wright 2005). The condition is bilateral in 10% of cases.

Diagnosis

The child usually presents to the general practitioner with a history of limp and complaints of pain in either their hip or knee. Clinical examination frequently

Box 22.4 Herring classification for grading stage of Perthes disease (Herring et al., 2004)

Group A: Lateral pillar of femoral head not involved. No loss in femoral head height. No changes in bone density.
Group B: Lateral pillar of femoral head shows lucency and a loss of height of up to 50%.
Group C: Lateral pillar of femoral head has increased lucency and collapse of over 50%.

reveals reduced hip abduction with pain at the extreme of movement on the affected side. An initial radiograph may show evidence of the disease, but often it is the subsequent X-rays or an MRI which demonstrates changes in the appearance of the femoral head and confirms the diagnosis (Dillman and Hernandez 2009) (see Figure 22.6). There is a number of classification systems used to grade the stage of the disease and used in the further monitoring of the disease status (Box 22.4). A bone age (left hand X-ray) is also useful in determining the child's actual skeletal and chronological ages which assists with treatment planning strategies. MRI can also be used.

The disease process covers an approximate two year period from when the femoral head starts to collapse to the remodeling phase; eventually with the blood supply re-innervated (Figure 22.3). The duration of the disease and its course is variable and treatment outcomes are therefore difficult to predict (Maxwell *et al.*, 2004). During the early stages, when the femoral head is collapsing and softening, there is a risk of extrusion beyond the outer rim of the acetabulum. Left untreated the enlarged femoral head can impinge and become deformed. The best treatment for Perthes disease is debated. The aim of treatment is to prevent femoral head deformity, containing it within the acetabulum to allow for optimal re-modelling and resulting in a better long term outcome (Bowen *et al.*, 2011). However, the expected result is worse if the child is over the age of eight years at diagnosis.

Treatment

The treatment of Perthes disease is dependent on the age of the child, the stage of the disease, the X-ray appearance and the child's symptoms and clinical evaluation. The aim is to maintain femoral head containment through the disease process either non-operatively or operatively. Conservative management includes

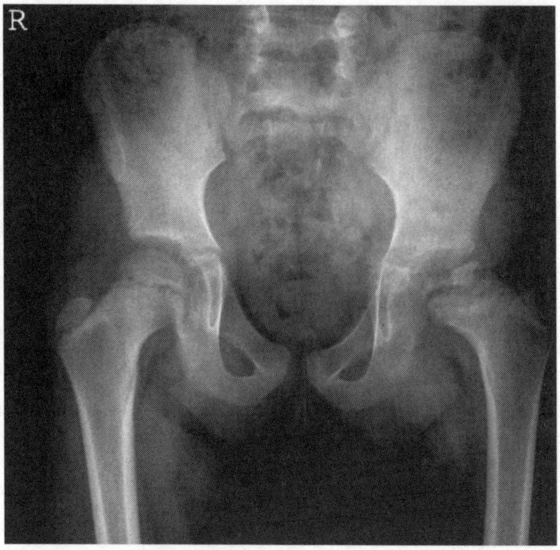

Figure 22.6 X-ray showing Perthes disease of the left hip – note the collapsing femoral head. Reproduced with permission from The Journal of Bone and Joint Surgery, Inc.

Box 22.5 Four stages of Perthes disease

Stage 1: Necrosis: Increased radiodensity of the femoral head. The joint space is wider.
Stage 2: Fragmentation: subchondral fracture of the femoral head. Metaphyseal cysts. Bone resorption
Stage 3: Reossification: Healing phase
Stage 4: Remodelling: Residual deformity with new femoral head shape – dependent on hip joint congruency

non-steroidal therapy such as Ibuprofen to minimise inflammation of the hip joint synovium, 'slings and springs' traction to maintain hip joint movement, non-adhesive traction and physiotherapy with hydrotherapy. Hip abduction orthoses are used in some centres to protect the femoral head.

Under five years – treatment is usually non-operative with 3–6 monthly X-rays monitoring the hip's progression with symptoms managed with simple analgesics and a change in lifestyle. The child needs to refrain from impact sports and activities which are likely to cause pain such as jumping from a height. Swimming is recommended to prevent stiffness in the hip and maintain the joint's range of movement. If symptoms become severe and unmanageable at home, the child may be admitted to hospital. A period of bed rest and hydrotherapy (with or without simple skin traction) is normally sufficient to settle pain and muscle spasm (Judd and Wright, 2005). The child may need to use crutches or a Zimmer frame to assist mobility and offload the affected hip when symptomatic. Occasionally, if symptoms are relentless, the hip can be protected by applying broomstick plasters (Petrie cast) for 4–6 weeks. This is a temporary measure which, in many units, has been replaced with a surgical shelf acetabuloplasty.

Over five years – there are a variety of surgical options to treat Perthes ranging from femoral or pelvic procedures to improve both hip containment and articular congruence.

Shelf acetabuloplasty – the aim is to provide additional cover for the extruding femoral head (Figure 22.7) and facilitate maintenance of a free range of hip movement. In turn the femoral head will remodel in the revascularisation phase of the disease to the shape of the new hip socket. A hip arthrogram is performed to show the cartilaginous component of the femoral head and the degree of subluxation. The shelf is a corticocancellous graft taken from the ilium. It is inserted into a previously made notch on the outer edge of the acetabulum and secured in position by reattaching the reflected head of the rectus femoris muscle (van der Geest *et al.*, 2001). Post-operatively the child may be nursed on simple skin traction for 48 hours to allow muscle spasm to settle, prior to application of a single hip spica to immobilise the hip joint and reduce post-operative pain.

Varus derotation femoral osteotomy – reserved for the older child with residual deformity at the end of treatment. The proximal femur is realigned, tilting the femoral head into the acetabulum to achieve improved containment and facilitate femoral remodelling ability. This prevents subluxation and redirects the force through the hip when weight bearing.

Arthrodiastasis – designed to protect the femoral head and preserve its height during the early fragmentation stage of the disease. The hip joint is distracted using an external monolateral fixator for two to six months. The distraction causes the hip joint to open, thereby increasing the space, reducing the weight bearing forces and encouraging restoration of the synovial circulation. Although good results have been achieved, this significant interventional procedure is not without complications; including pin site infection and residual stiffness in the hip and knee joint (Chapter 8). Studies are of small numbers and long-term follow up to skeletal maturity are required to assess whether arthrodiastasis results in a better outcome (Maxwell *et al.*, 2004). From the child's point of view the fixator is unsightly and cumbersome and psychological support from the outset is recommended.

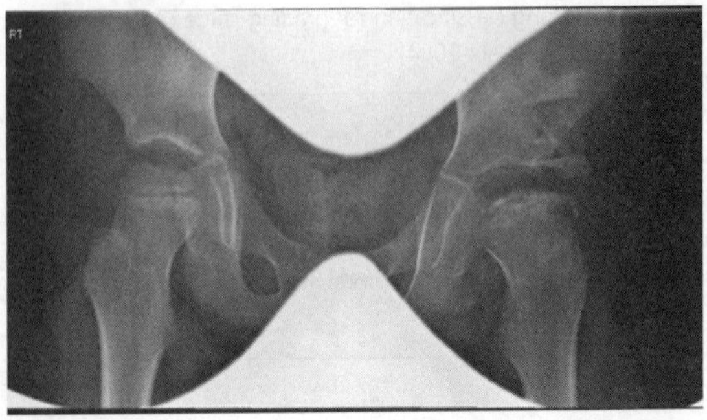

Figure 22.7 X-ray showing Shelf acetabuloplasty of the left hip

Slipped capital femoral epiphysis

A slipped capital femoral epiphysis (SCFE) is a condition where the head of the femur slips off the physis. The neck or the metaphysis of the femur is the section that moves, normally migrating anteriorly and superiorly (Sun *et al.*, 2011), while the femoral head maintains its normal position in the acetabulum. The slip occurs through the widened hypertrophic zone of the growth plate and may be acute (sustained after a traumatic episode) or chronic (occurring slowly over a period of time). 25% of cases are bilateral, half of which present sequentially.

Aetiology and epidemiology

The incidence of SCFE is two to three per 100 000 and is more common in male adolescents. Although the cause is unknown, risk factors and associated traits include: obesity, delayed skeletal maturity, hypothyroidism, endocrine abnormalities, puberty and vitamin D deficiency (Clarke and Page 2012). It is suggested that the growth plate plays a part in the cause. The perichondral fibrocartilaginous ring which surrounds the physis contributes to its strength. It is at its strongest during infancy, diminishing as the child gets older. In addition, the physis is widened and therefore potentially weakened during the adolescent growth spurt which is the most common time for a slip to occur. The condition is more common in boys with a ratio of 2.4 per female and more prevalent in the 10–16 year age group in boys (average 13.4 years) and 10–14 year age group in girls (average 11.5 years). Children presenting outside these age perimeters should be investigated for causative factors such as endocrine or systemic disorders.

Diagnosis

A child who presents with pain and a limp over the age of eight years should be investigated for SCFE with an anteroposterior (AP) and frog lateral X-ray views. The AP view is not always helpful and will be normal in 14% of cases (Benson *et al.*, 2002). For a suspected SCFE, which is not evident on X-ray an MRI is useful in detecting a pre-slip (Lalaji *et al.*, 2002) in a child who presents with symptoms.

Slipped Capital Femoral Epiphysis can be classified as (Southwick, 1967):

- acute – symptoms <2 weeks
- chronic – symptoms >2 weeks
- acute-on-chronic – long term pain with a sudden episode of acute pain.

The X-ray findings are described according to the degree of displacement:

- mild (grade 1, 0°–30° of displacement),
- moderate (grade 2, 30° to 60°)
- severe (grade 3, 60° to 90°+).

On presentation with an acute slip the child will complain of pain of less than three weeks' duration in their groin, thigh or knee. They will limp and have an out-toeing gait. With a chronic slip their symptoms will have been more insidious in nature (Uglow and Clarke 2004). They may be able to weight bear, indicating that the slip is stable. If there is an unstable slip the child is unable to bear weight due to pain. In a severe unstable slip the examination will show a shortened leg lying in external rotation with markedly restricted range of movement. X-ray findings may be subtle or obvious. The AP view will show widening of the physis and a loss of epipyhseal height. There is increased density in the femoral neck (Blanch sign) and Klein's line drawn up the superior aspect of the femoral neck does not cross the femoral head (see Figure 22.8).

Treatment

The prognosis of SCFE is linked to the prompt recognition of the condition and the severity of the slip. The aim of treatment is to reduce the complication rate of AVN and chondrolysis (Uglow and Clarke 2004). Early intervention within 24 hours of diagnosis reduces the rate of AVN to 7% with surgery; after this time increasing the rate of AVN to 87.5% (Walter *et al.*, 2011). It is important to determine whether the slip is stable or unstable. The latter has a poorer prognosis with increased probability of avascular necrosis whilst a stable slip may deteriorate and become unstable if not treated. Attempting to realign the femoral head will damage the blood supply and risk AVN. Stabilisation of the slip with single screw fixation (see Figure 22.9) is advocated for mild to moderate slips to prevent further slipping and maintain position until physeal fusion (Judd and Wright 2005).

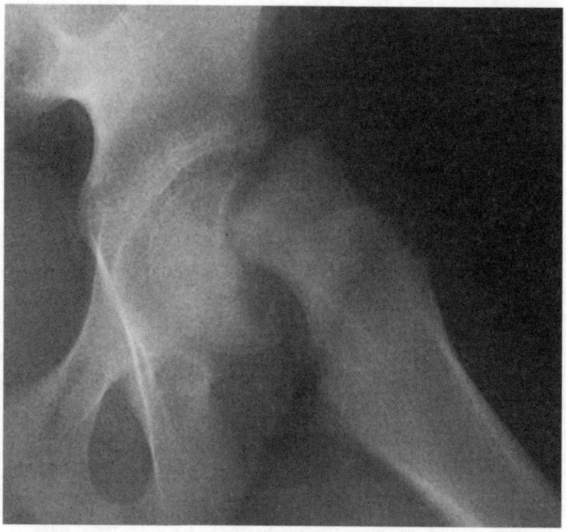

Figure 22.8 X-ray showing slipped left femoral capital epiphysis where Klein's line does not intersect the epiphysis

Moderate and severe slips are difficult to manage. Gentle intra–operative reduction of the hip, taking care not to damage the blood supply, is advocated by some surgeons prior to screw fixation. Osteotomies of the femoral neck can be performed to realign the femoral neck in a severe slip but subsequent AVN, chondrolysis and reduced range of hip movement are all significant complications (Lawane *et al.*, 2009). There is some debate whether the contralateral hip of a child with a unilateral slip should be fixed at initial presentation. A study by Riad *et al.* (2007) demonstrated that the younger the patient, the greater the probability of increased development of a contralateral slip.

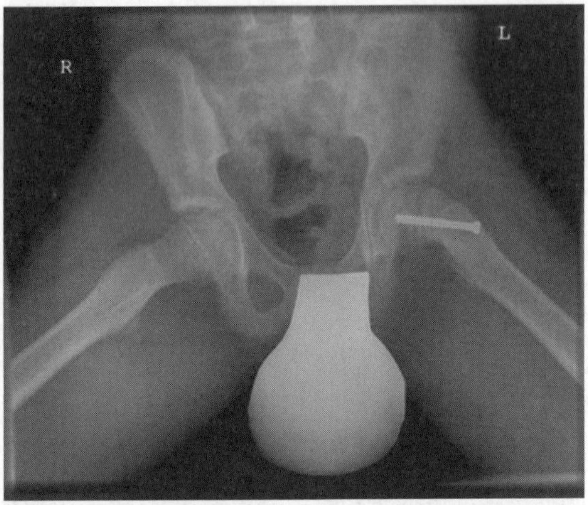

Figure 22.9 X-ray showing slipped left femoral capital epiphysis, fixed with a left screw

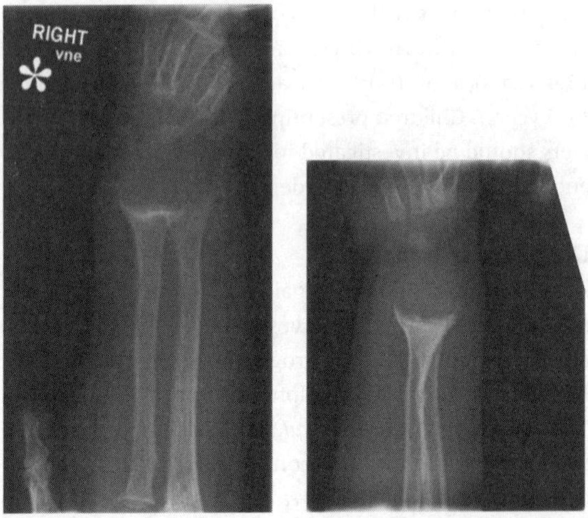

Figure 22.10 Wrist X-ray showing widened and cupped physis

Post-operatively the child mobilises non-weight bearing with crutches for the first six weeks, progressing to partial weight bearing for another six weeks. X-rays are taken at each stage to assess position of screw fixation and possible AVN. Patients are followed up radiographically until the physis has fused, negating the possibility of further slippage.

Vitamin D deficiency

Vitamin D deficiency is associated with rickets, fractures and musculoskeletal symptoms (Judd 2011). Previously thought of as a condition of the past, it is no longer a rarity and is linked to a number of health issues. Studies suggest a concerning association with deformity and generalised bone and muscle pain. In the UK the increase in vitamin D deficiency is attributed to the varied ethnic population, poor diet and lifestyle choices made by families.

Accepted sufficient blood serum levels of vitamin D have been agreed as >75 nmols/L (Pearce and Cheetham 2010) with some variance according to population and environmental factors. Below 20 nmols/L is considered deficient. 80–90% of vitamin D is made through synthesis in the skin and the remaining 10–20% is acquired through diet. In efforts to protect children from sun exposure parents use high factor sun protection creams and cover children's skin with clothing. A reduction in time spent outdoors due to a preference for indoor activities also contributes to lack of sunlight exposure as do cultural dress codes (Judd and Wright 2011). The best source of vitamin D is exposure to sunlight with 20–30 minutes a day recommended without application of sunscreen (Judd and Wright 2011). Dark skinned children do not synthesise vitamin D well due to increased melanin and are therefore prone to deficiency. In addition to reduced synthesis in the skin, hypovitaminosis D is the primary cause of rickets as it results in poor absorption of calcium and phosphorus minerals from foods. Circulating blood levels of vitamin D are low, resulting in bone softening, non-specific musculoskeletal symptoms and deformity.

Vitamin D deficiency is a global problem and is not restricted to culture, race or demographics. Low vitamin D levels have been associated with musculoskeletal problems such as SCFE, cerebral palsy, fractures and poor bone healing (Clarke and Page 2012). Guidance (DoH 2012) advises practitioners to be aware of at-risk groups within the population and recommends that older people, pregnant women, infants and young children receive vitamin D supplementation.

An X-ray of a child with rickets will show evidence of widened growth plates which have a cupped and splayed appearance (see Figure 22.10). Due to loading on the leg's long bones, genu varum and valgum is noticeable with abnormality depicted on leg alignment radiographs (see Figure 22.11). Clinical findings are of bowed legs (tibia vara) or knock knees (genu valgum). Skeletal deformity may be symmetric or asymmetric. The wrists and ankles are swollen and enlarged due to reduced mineralisation of the physis. The incidence of fracture and re-fracture rates are increased. There may be permanent skeletal deformities such as rachitic rosary (ends of the ribs are enlarged) and scoliosis. Children may present due to a delay in walking, have poor muscle development and tone and complain of muscle pain.

Management

Vitamin D deficiency is an ever-increasing problem with new evidence linking it to a number of health issues. Shared care of the child and family is important with both orthopaedic and endocrinology teams contributing to the overall management. Where levels are simply insufficient (20–75 nmols/L) supplementation of 400 iu per day is recommended. At risk population groups (pregnant women, infants, young children and older people) should receive supplements routinely (Gillie 2006). Deficient levels of vitamin D require a treatment dose of 6000 iu of cholecalciferol daily for three months with calcium supplements for two weeks. Dosages are adjusted according to the results of repeated blood tests at the end of three months (Judd 2012b). Supplementation should be supported by maintaining a dietary intake of vitamin D rich foods (Chapter 10) and adequate exposure to the sun.

Poor diet, whether an excess of the 'wrong' foods or a reduced intake of the 'right' foods, can contribute to both vitamin D deficiency and future osteoporosis. Obese children tend to have low vitamin D; vitamin D is a fat soluble vitamin and obesity may prevent the storage of the vitamin (Elizondo-Montemayor *et al.*, 2010). An excess consumption of carbonated drinks affects the body's ability to absorb calcium due to the presence of phosphoric acid (Wyshak 2000). This results in poor bone density and an increased risk of fracture as well as poor fracture healing (Tucker *et al.*, 2006). Eating disorders can result in a reduced intake of calcium and vitamin D; if there is concern review by a dietician, who can advise parents and monitor the child, should be requested.

Uncorrected deformity following treatment with 25 hydroxyvitamin D may need surgical intervention. A classical picture of rickets is deformed leg alignment. Genu varum or valgum can be simply corrected through a minimally invasive procedure using guided growth plates. These slow down the physeal growth on one side whilst the other continues to grow. They are removed when the limbs are clinically straight (Ballal *et al.*, 2010). More invasive procedures are reserved for residual tibia vara, requiring proximal tibial and/or femoral osteotomies (Zaki and Rae 2009). An alternative is to correct the deformity using an external fixator following the osteotomy. The literature reports non-union of the osteotomy, the possibility of fracture through the regenerate and the recurrence of the deformity (Petje *et al.*, 2008, Fucentese *et al.*, 2008, Choi *et al.*, 2002).

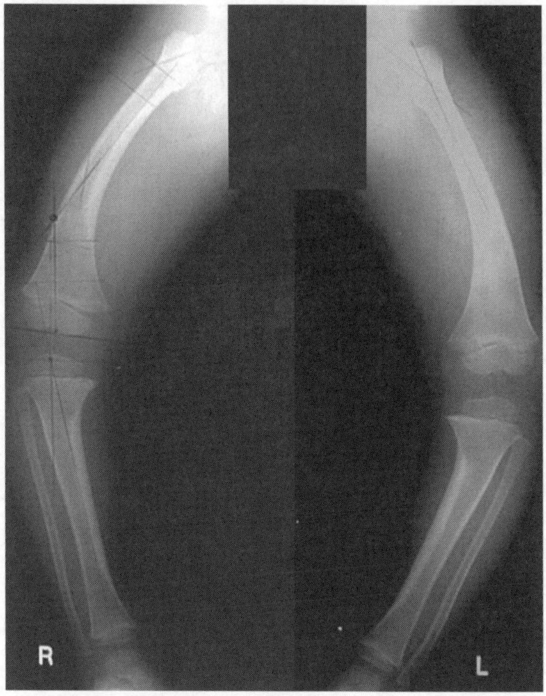

Figure 22.11 X-ray showing rickets

Congenital talipes equino varus

Congenital talipes equino varus (CTEV), or 'club foot', is the most common structural deformity of the lower limb present at birth (see Figure 22.12).

The name comes from:

- Congenital – at birth
- Talipes (talus = ankle bone)
- Pes (pes = Foot)
- Equino – characteristic of a horse; the term describes the position of the heel
- Varus – inward turning

The condition involves abnormal alignment of the foot bones and contractures of the joint capsules, ligaments and tendons:

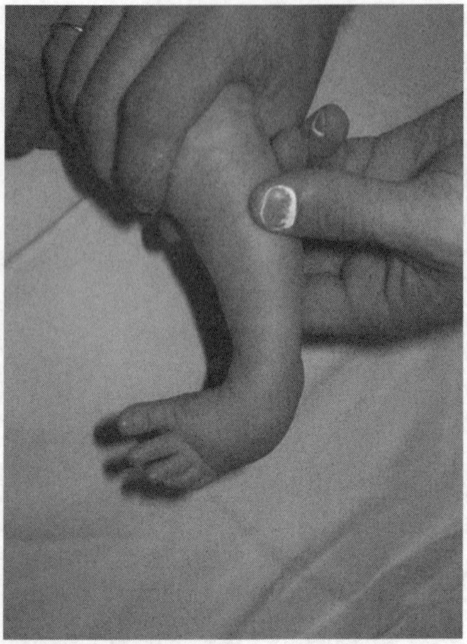

Figure 22.12 Club foot (CTEV)

- The deformity is seen at the hindfoot and forefoot
- The heel is in equinus (high) and in varus (turned inward)
- The forefoot is supinated (rotated) and adducted (turned inwards).

The core problem of the foot deformity is the abnormal positioning of the talus and subsequent malaligned relationship with the calcaneus and navicular bones. Muscle, tissue and vascular structure are all abnormal (Cummings *et al.*, 2002). The deformity may be detected antenatally on the mother's 20-week ultrasound scan or noted at birth. Pre-natal counselling has proven to be valuable for the expectant parents; giving an explanation of the proposed treatment and reassurance of the excellent functional outcomes (Bar-on *et al.*, 2005). They should be made aware that as the child grows they will notice the affected foot to be shorter by 1–2 sizes and the calf muscle to be thinner.

Aetiology

The cause of club foot (CTEV) is unknown. It occurs in one per 1000 births in Caucasians but varies in different races, with an incidence in Polynesians of 6.8 per 1000 for example. It is bilateral in 50% of cases and more common in males. Strong genetic links are reported in the literature; a sibling has a 30% chance of having club foot deformity and a reported 24% of children with CTEV will have a positive family medical history.

Treatment

Treatment for idiopathic club foot is primarily non-operative, although this may be dependent on place of birth and treatment availability (Judd and Wright, 2005). The overall aim of treatment is to give the child a pain-free, functional 'foot-shaped' foot, so they are able to wear normal shoes and perform normal daily activities (Ponseti, 1992). At birth the foot will have varying degrees of stiffness in the hind-foot and forefoot. For the best results, early intervention before the age of one month is advocated since much of the skeleton is cartilaginous, allowing the ligaments, tendons and muscles to be readily stretched (Hart *et al.*, 2005, Ponseti and Smoley 2009).

Prior to initial orthopaedic assessment parents can be taught simple stretching exercises and massage to maintain suppleness in the foot. They are usually extremely keen for their baby to be reviewed by a paediatric orthopaedic specialist and to commence treatment. Information available via the Internet has meant parents have enhanced knowledge and choice regarding their baby's treatment (Judd 2004).

The management of the foot begins with an assessment of its severity using a grading system. Different assessment tools exist to classify the foot deformity and are useful in the evaluation of patient outcomes (Judd 2004). The **Pirani scoring system** is a recognised and universally accepted simple tool to use (Dyer and Davis 2006). Divided into sections to give a score for the hind-foot and for the forefoot, it gives an assessment of the flexibility in the foot as a whole (Figure 22.13). An audit of outcomes using the Pirani score as an assessment tool demonstrated that higher total scores and a high hind-foot score predicted a potential relapse of deformity (Goriainov *et al.*, 2010).

The **Ponseti method** is a conservative technique for the treatment of club foot which has gained popularity over the last ten years. Commenced ideally before one month of age, weekly gentle manipulation and application of above knee moulded serial casts, will gradually correct each component of the foot deformity (Figure 22.14). The average number of casts is six, with more or less required dependent on the severity of the foot deformity. Parents can remove the casts in the bath on the morning of the clinic. If done earlier, the foot may relapse from its new position. Parents should be reassured

Right Total	Right 0	Right 0.5	Right 1		Left 0	Left 0.5	Left 1	Left Total
				Posterior crease				
				Empty Heel				
				Ankle DF				
				Medial crease				
				Lateral Head Talus				
				Lateral Border				

Figure 22.13 Pirani score

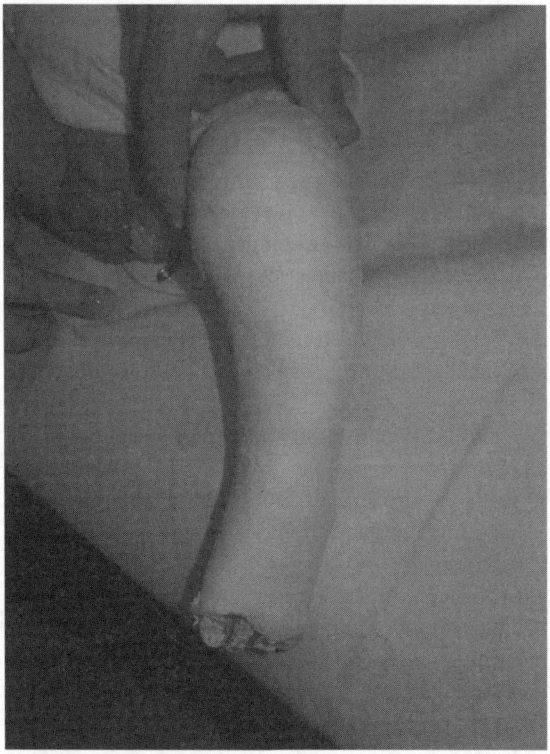

Figure 22.14 Ponseti cast

that the treatment is not painful, but their baby will dislike having their leg held still. Feeding at the same time as the procedure is calming (Faulks and Luther 2005).

Approximately 70% of babies will require a percutaneous Achilles tenotomy to correct the heel equinus (Ponseti, 1992, Goriainov *et al.*, 2010). This is commonly performed using a topical anaesthetic cream, following which a final cast is applied for three weeks, holding the ankle in a dorsi-flexed position while the tendon heals in its new position. The final stage of the correction is maintained by the infant wearing 'boots on a bar' in the overcorrected position of 70 degrees of abduction (Figure 22.15). These are worn for three months for twenty three hours per day and then at night time only until the age of four.

The child is reviewed in the clinic at three to four monthly intervals to review the progress of the foot as it grows. Compliance with the boots and bar can sometimes be problematic and it is vital to ensure they fit correctly, with the heel positioned snuggly down in the boot. Poor outcomes of club foot correction using the Ponseti method have been attributed to lack of compliance with the boot and bar for the four-year duration (Ponseti 1992).

Approximately 20–40% of children will require a tibialis anterior tendon transfer to correct dynamic forefoot supination. Considered to be part of the Ponseti technique, the problem is usually detected in the early years when the child is up and running around. The tendon is transferred into the lateral cuneiform adjusting the muscle pull to bring the forefoot around. Postoperatively a cast is required for six to eight weeks.

Assessment of the atypical club foot

The atypical club foot commonly co-exists with other diagnoses, such as arthrogryposis. It is important to examine the baby by fully assessing the upper and lower limbs and spine and hips, looking for associated anomalies. Assessment of the foot demonstrates a deep posterior heel crease and a deep plantar crease that extends across the entire sole of the foot, creating tightness in the plantar aspect. This type of foot tends not to respond well to conservative management alone and may require minimal surgical intervention (Faulks and Luther 2005).

Surgical correction

Surgical correction is reserved for the recalcitrant club foot, when there is little or no progression in correction with manipulation. The procedure may be minimal, with a soft tissue release, or more interventional

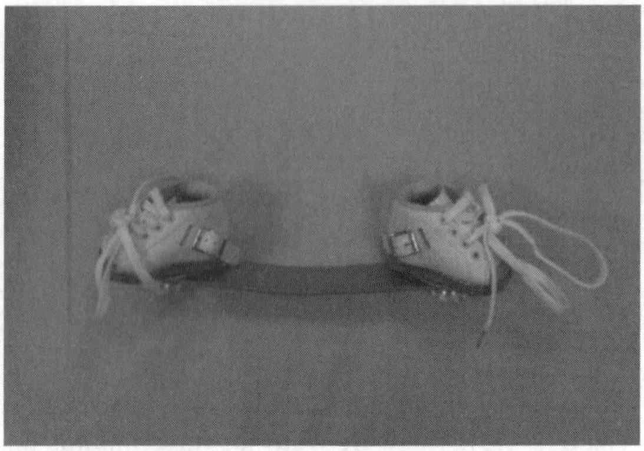

Figure 22.15 Boot on a bar

addressing all the components of the deformity and requiring a posteromedial plantar lateral release (Cummings *et al.*, 2002). Surgery may be performed in either one or two stages, the latter proven to reduce the incidence of wound infection (Uglow and Clarke 2000). The corrected position is held with casts for three months (Judd and Wright 2005).

Relapsed club foot

Bradish and Noor (2000) report a 20% recurrence rate of clubfoot deformity. Severely stiff feet have a greater tendency to relapse. The child needs regular follow-up throughout growth to detect deformity recurrence, which commonly occurs in the hind foot with reduced ankle dorsiflexion and heel varus. With walking on the lateral border of the foot, forefoot supination may also feature (Ponseti 2002). Surgery may involve capsular releases, tendon transfers or osteotomies. Plaster casts hold the corrected foot for 6–12 weeks depending on the surgery. Routine plaster care and neurovascular observations should be carried out. Pain is controlled with a nerve block and Oramorph initially, with subsequent simple analgesics. If the child has had bony surgery an epidural for 48 hours is optimal (Judd and Wright 2005).

Amplified musculoskeletal pain syndrome

Amplified musculoskeletal pain syndrome (AMPS) is also known as:

- Chronic regional pain syndrome
- Reflex sympathetic dystrophy
- Fibromyalgia.

There is no assumed cause and the pain is increased to a point that the child can no longer manage. Commonly AMPS in children is initiated by minor insignificant trauma, psychological stress or an illness. The trauma maybe a simple fracture or a soft tissue injury and, although the injury itself heals, the pain does not resolve within the expected time frame. The pain pathway is dysfunctional. There is an abnormal short circuit within the spinal cord so that the transmission of pain to the brain is also transmitted to the neurovascular nerves. The signal causes the blood vessels to constrict, resulting in a reduced blood flow and deprivation of oxygen to the bones, muscles and skin. The result is a buildup of acid waste products such as lactic acid with the subsequent production of pain. The new pain signal transmits across the abnormal circuit, further reducing the blood flow and consequently produces more pain (Sherry 2008). How pain is perceived and how individuals cope with pain is influenced by a number of external factors (Chapter 11). The child with AMPS is noted to experience higher levels of stress. The pain, however, not only affects the individual but also has a psychological and social impact on the immediate family.

Signs and symptoms of AMPS may include some or all of the following (Miller, 2003):

- allodynia – pain that comes from a stimulus that is not normally painful e.g. wearing a sock or gentle light touch
- hyperalgesia (increased sensitivity to a pain) – pain that is disproportionate to the injury
- burning sensation
- muscle cramps
- X-rays may reveal some osteoporosis as a result of disuse
- intermittent colour changes of the skin
- shiny appearance or mottling of the skin
- clammy skin or increased sweating
- diffuse swelling
- coolness or warmth of the affected limb
- reduced mobility.

Epidemiology

The majority of children who present with AMPS are female and are from higher socioeconomic backgrounds. It is more common in the adolescent population with a mean age of onset at 12 to 13 years. In a study by Perquin *et al.* (2000) of 6636 Dutch children, 25% reported recurrent or continuous pain for >3 months. Similarly Roth-Isiqkeit *et al.'s* (2005) study of 749 children in Germany gave a result of 30.8% reporting symptoms for >6 months. The prevalence is significantly higher in females and is increased with age. The site of symptoms is frequently the lower limb and overall AMPS is the commonest reason for school non-attendance. Predisposing factors to AMPS have been reported as:

- hypermobility
- significant previous pain experiences
- family members response to pain and their coping strategies
- emotional personality – high achievers, pleasers, high anxiety levels.

Management

The patient pathway begins immediately on diagnosis. Early recognition of the problem and prompt action is key to success in treatment (Taylor 2002, Littlejohn 2004). Once all investigations such as bloods, radiographs and scans have proven that there is no organic cause for the pain, medical intervention should be stopped with emphasis placed on rehabilitation (Clinch and Ecclestone, 2009). Management of children with AMPS involves the whole family. A clear discussion with the child and family supported with written information regarding the diagnosis and requirement for involvement with the rehabilitation programme is vital to a successful outcome. It is important to get the child and family on-board (Clinch and Ecclestone 2009) and help them to understand the necessity of physiotherapy and continued compliance. Early intervention for mild symptoms that are suggestive of impending AMPS will abate further deterioration with a reassuring prognosis.

Background history may reveal a role model within the family who has chronic pain (Littlejohn 2004), a major life event as a trigger to symptoms, such as parental marital problems, a house or school move, sporting stressors and high parental expectations. All of these can affect the child's response to their pain and their involvement and progression with rehabilitation. Family interactions can be intense with enmeshment between the child and mother or sometimes the father.

A major part of the rehabilitation programme is the emphasis on ownership. The child needs to acknowledge that to get better they have to participate at all levels and work with practitioners and therapists to improve. The perception from the child and family may be an expectation that the health professionals will solve the problem. A usual course of action would be to identify the problem, to review what the child can or cannot do and discuss treatment that has failed. This problem-focused approach is negative whereas the aim is for positivity.

Solution-focused approach

The solution-focused approach encourages ownership of the problem, involving the child in their rehabilitation. The focus is to get to the problem via the solution, utilising positive discussion which always focuses on strengths and achievements (Iveson 2002, Sherry *et al.*, 1999). The child is encouraged to think forward to the future and where they would like to be in terms of wellness and activity. 'Scaling' is used where the child allocates a score to where they are currently and where they are aiming to get to in their rehabilitation. The aim of the practitioner is to empower the child and encourage them to aim high. A successful tool is to use a scenario where the child endeavors to climb a mountain on which they have placed goals to reach at each stage of improvement. It is crucial that the team have a unified approach, with the nurses and therapists working with the child and family to build a rapport, aiming to help them to reach their goals. Early psychological support may also be useful especially if progress is slow. Guided imagery, externalising the pain, distraction techniques, and teaching the child relaxation methods can all be employed with the assistance of the play specialist. It is important for the team to stress their understanding of the symptoms and not to ignore the fact that the pain exists. However, the pain that the child feels is not harmful or protective of the body. Pain medication is gauged and is dependent on symptoms and progress. It varies from simple analgesics to antidepressants (Amitriptyline) and anticonvulsants (Gabapentin). The latter two are used for neuropathic pain (nerve damage) (Sherry 2008).

Recommended further reading

Glasper, E.A., McEwing, G. and Richardson, J. (eds) (2007) *Oxford Handbook of Children's and Young People's Nursing*. Oxford University Press, Oxford.

Kelsey, J. and McEwing, G. (eds) (2008) *Clinical Skills in Child Health Practice*. Churchill Livingstone Elsevier, Edinburgh.

References

American Academy of Pediatrics, Committee on Quality Improvement, Subcommittee on Developmental Dysplasia of the Hip (2000) Clinical Practice Guideline: Early Detection of Developmental Dysplasia of the Hip. *Pediatrics*, **105**(4), 896–905.

Atalar, H., Sayli, U., Yavuz, O.Y., Uras, I. and Dogruel, H. (2007) Indicators of successful use of the Pavlik harness in infants with developmental dysplasia of the hip. *International Orthopaedics*, **31**(2), 145–150.

Ballal, M.S., Bruce, C.E. and Nayagam, S. (2010) Correcting genu varum and genu valgum in children by guided growth: temporary hemiepiphysiodesis using tension band plates. *Journal of Bone Joint Surgery (Britain)*, **92**(2), 273–276.

Bar-On, E. Mashiach, R. Inbar, O. Weigl, D. Katz, K. and Meizner, I. (2005) Prenatal ultrasound diagnosis of club foot. *Outcome and recommendations for counselling and follow up. Journal of Bone and Joint Surgery*, **87-B**(7), 990–993.

Benson, M.K.D., Fixsen, J.A., Macnicol, M.F. and Parsch, K. (2002) *Children's Orthopaedics and Fractures*. 2nd edn. Churchill Livingstone, London.

Bolland, B.J., Wahed, A., Al-Hallao, S., Culliford, D.J. and Clarke, N.M.P. (2010) Late reduction in congenital dislocation of the hip and the need for secondary surgery: radiologic predictors and confounding variables. *Journal of Pediatric Orthopaedics*, **30**(7), 676–682.

Bowen, J.R., Guille, J.T., Jeong, C. *et al.* (2011) Labral support shelf arthroplasty for containment in early stages of Legg-Calve-Perthes disease. *Journal of Pediatric Orthopaedics*, **31**(2 Suppl), S206–S211.

Bradish, C.F. and Noor, S. (2000) The Ilizarov method in the management of relapsed clubfeet. *Journal of Bone Joint Surgery (British)*, **82B**, 387–391.

Cashman, J.P., Round, J., Taylor, G. and Clarke, N.M. (2002) The natural history of developmental dysplasia of the hip after early supervised treatment in the Pavlik harness: a prospective, longitudinal follow-up. *Journal of Bone Joint Surgery (British)*, **4-B**, 418–412.

Catterall, A., Pringle, J., Byers, P.D. *et al.* (1982) A review of the morphology of Perthes' disease. *Journal of Bone and Joint Surgery (Britain)*, **64**(3), 269–275.

Choi, I.H., Kim, J.K., Chung, C.Y. *et al.* (2002) Deformity correction of the knee and leg lengthening by Ilizarov method in hypophosphataemic rickets: outcomes and significance of serum phosphate level. *Journal of Pediatric Orthopaedics*, **22**, 626–631.

Clarke, N.M.P. and Castaneda, P. (2012) Strategies to improve non-operative childhood management. *Orthopaedic Clinics of North America*, **43**, 481–489.

Clarke, N.M.P. and Judd, J. (2013) La cadera neonatal limítrofe: observación versus Pavlik. *Revista Mexicana de Ortopedia Pediátrica*, **15**(1), 14–18. www.medigraphic.org.mx

Clarke, N.M.P. and Page, J.E. (2012) Vitamin D deficiency: a paediatric orthopedic perspective. *Current Opinion in Pediatrics*, **24**(1), 46–49.

Clarke, S. and McKay, M. (2006) An audit of spica cast guidelines for parents and professionals caring for children with developmental dysplasia of the hip. *Journal of Orthopaedic Nursing*, **10**(3), 128–137.

Clarke, N.M.P. and Taylor, C.C. (2012) Diagnosis and management of developmental hip dysplasia. *Paediatrics and Child Health*, **22**(6), 235–238.

Clinch, J. and Ecclestone, C. (2009) Chronic musculoskeletal pain in children: assessment and management. *Rheumatology*, **48**(5), 466–474.

Cummings, R.J., Davidson, R.S., Armstrong, P.F. and Lehman, W.B. (2002) Congenital clubfoot. An instructional course lecture, American Academy of Orthopaedic Surgeons. *Journal of Bone and Joint Surgery*, **84A**(2), 290–308.

Daly, K., Bruce, C. and Catterall, A. (1999) Lateral shelf acetabuloplasty in Perthes'disease. A review at the end of growth. *Journal of Bone and Joint Surgery (Britain)* **81**, 380–384.

Davis, P. and Barr, L. (1999) Principles of traction. *Journal of Orthopaedic Nursing*, **3**(4), 222–227.

Dawson, P., Cook, L., Holliday. LJ. and Reddy, H. (2012) *Oxford Handbook of Clinical Skills for Children's and Young People's Nursing*. Oxford University Press, Oxford.

Department of Health (DoH) (2012) *Vitamin D: Advice On Supplements For At Risk Groups*. Available at: http://www.dh.gov.uk/en/Publicationsandstatistics/Lettersandcirculars/Dearcolleagueletters/DH_132509 (accessed 3 March 2012).

Dillman, J.R. and Hernandez, R.J. (2009) MRI of Legg-Calvé-Perthes Disease. *The American Journal of Roentgenology*, **193** (5), 1394–1407.

Dyer, P.J. and Davis, N. (2006) The role of the Pirani scoring system in the management of club foot by the Ponseti method. *Journal of Bone Joint Surgery (Britain)* **88-B**(8), 1082–1084.

Eastwood, D.M. and de Gheldere, A. (2010) Clinical examination for developmental dysplasia of the hip in neonates: how to stay out of trouble. *British Medical Journal*, **340**, c1965.

Elizondo-Montemayor, L., Ugalde-Casas, P.A., Serrano-González, M., Cuello-García, C.A. and Borbolla-Escoboza, J.R. (2010) Serum 25-hydroxyvitamin d concentration, life factors and obesity in Mexican children. *Obesity (Silver Spring)*, **18**(9), 1805–1811.

Faulks, S. Luther, B. (2005) Changing Paradigm for the Treatment of Clubfeet. *Orthopaedic Nursing*, **24**(1), 25–30.

Fucentese, S.F. Neuhaus, T.J. Ramseier, L.E. Ulrich Exner, G. (2008) Metabolic and orthopedic management of X-linked vitamin D-resistant hypophosphatemic rickets. *Journal of Children's Orthopaedics*, **2**(4), 285–291.

Gillie, O. (2006) A new health policy for sunlight and vitamin D, in *Health Research Forum Occasional Reports: No 2*. Available at:

http://www.healthresearchforum.org.uk/reports/sunbook.pdf (accessed 13 April 2013).

Glueck, C.J., Crawford, A., Roy, D. *et al.* (1996) Association of antithrombotic deficiencies and hypofibrinolysis with Legg-Calve Perthes' Disease. *Journal of Bone and Joint Surgery (British)*, **78A**: 3–13.

Goriainov, V., Judd, J. and Uglow, M. (2010) Does the Pirani score predict relapse in clubfoot? *Journal of Childrens Orthopaedics*, **4**(5), 439–444.

Hart, E.S., Grottkau, B.E., Rebello, G.N. and Allbright, M.B. (2005) The newborn foot. Diagnosis and management of common conditions. *Orthopaedic Nursing*, **24**(5), 313–321.

von Heideken, J., Green, D.W., Burke, S.W. *et al.* (2006) The relationship between developmental dysplasia of the hip and congenital muscular torticollis. *Journal of Pediatric Orthopaedics*, **26**, 805–808.

Herring, J.A. (1998) Legg-Calve Perthes Disease, in *Pediatric Orthopaedic Secrets* (ed. L.T. Staheli). Hanley and Belfus, Philadelphia.

Herring, J.A., Kim, H.T. and Browne, R. (2004) Legg-Calve-Perthes disease. Part I: Classification of radiographs with use of the modified lateral pillar and Stulberg classifications. *Journal of Bone and Joint Surgery (America)*, **86-A**(10), 2103–2120.

Hollier, L., Jeong, K., Grayson, B. and McCarthy, J. 2000 Congenital muscular torticollis and associated craniofacial changes. *Plastic and Reconstructive Surgery*, **105**(3), 827–834.

Imrie, M., Scott, V., Stearns, P., Bastrom, T. and Mubarak, S.J. (2010) Is ultrasound screening for DDH in babies born breech sufficient? *Journal of Children's Orthopaedics*, **4**(1), 3–8.Institute of Infant Hip Dysplasia (IHDI). www.hipdysplasia.org

International Association for the Study of Pain (IASP). http://www.iasp-pain.org/Content/NavigationMenu/GeneralResourceLinks/PainDefinitions/default.htm

Iveson, C. (2002) Solution-focused brief therapy. *Advances in Psychiatric Treatment*, **8**: 149–156. Available at: http://apt.rcpsych.org/content/8/2/149.full (accessed 3 March 2012).

Judd, J. (2004) Congenital talipes equino varus – evidence for using the Ponseti method of treatment. *Journal of Orthopaedic Nursing*, **8**(3), 160–163.

Judd, J. (2005) Strategies used by nurses for decision-making in the paediatric orthopaedic setting. *Journal of Orthopaedic Nursing*, **9**(3), 166–171.

Judd, J. (2011) Rickets: a 21st-century disease? *Nursing in Practice* (March/April). Available at: www.nursinginpractice.com (accessed 3 March 2012).

Judd, J. (2012a) History taking, in *Oxford Handbook of Clinical Skills for Children's and Young People's Nursing* (eds P. Dawson, L. Cook, L. Holliday and H. Reddy), Oxford University Press, Oxford.

Judd, J. (2012b) Rickets in the 21st century: A review of the consequences of low vitamin D and its management. *International Journal of Orthopaedic and Trauma Nursing*, **17**, 199–208.

Judd, J. and Wright, E. (2005) Joint and Limb Problems in Children. In: Kneale, J. and Davis, P. (Eds) *Orthopaedic and Trauma Nursing*, 2nd edn. Churchill Livingston, Edinburgh.

Judd, J. and Wright, E. (2011) *Vitamin D deficiency in the paediatric orthopaedic patient: the epidemiology and evidence of sunlight exposure – a follow-up audit on the sun habits of families.* Poster presentation, Pediatric Orthopedic Society of North America Conference, 11–14 May 2011.

Kim, H. (2010) Legg-Calvé-Perthes Disease. *A review article. Journal of American Academy of Orthopaedic Surgeons*, **18**, 676–686.

Kokavec, M. and Bialik, V. (2007) Developmental dysplasia of the hip. Prevention and real incidence. *Bratislavske lekarske listy* **108**(6), 251–254. Available at: http://www.bmj.sk/2007/10806-03.pdf (accessed 16th September 2012).

Lalaji, A., Umans, H. and Schneider, R. (2002) MRI features of confirmed 'pre-slip' capital femoral epiphysis: a report of two cases. *Skeletal Radiology*, **31**, 362–365.

Lawane, M., Belouadah, M. and Lefort, G. (2009) Severe slipped capital femoral epiphysis: The Dunn's operation. *Orthopaedics Traumatology and Surgery Research*, **95**(8), 588–591.

Little, D.G. and Kim, H.K. (2011) Potential for bisphosphonate treatment in Legg-Calve-Perthes disease. *Journal of Pediatric Orthopaedics*, **31**(2), S182–S188.

Littlejohn, G.O. (2004) Reflex sympathetic dystrophy in adolescents: lessons for adults. *Arthritis and Rheumatism (Arthritis Care and Research)*, **51**(2), 151–153.

Luedtke, L.M., Flynn, J.M. and Pill, S.G. (2000) Review of avascular necrosis in developmental dysplasia of the hip and contemporary efforts at prevention. *The University of Pennsylvania Orthopaedic Journal*, **13**, 22–28.

Luther, B.L. (2002) Congenital muscular torticollis. *Orthopaedic Nursing*, **21**(3), 21–28.

Maxwell, S.L., Lappin, K.J., Kealey, W.D., McDowell, B.C. and Cosgrove, A.P. (2004) Arthrodiastasis in Perthes' disease. Preliminary results.The *Journal of Bone and Joint Surgery (Britain)*, **86**(2), 244–250.

Miller, R.L.S. (2003) Reflex sympathetic dystrophy. *Orthopaedic Nursing*, **22**(2), 91–99.

Moloney, D., Heffernan, G., Dodds, M. and McCormack, D. (2006) Normal variants in the paediatric orthopaedic population. *Irish Medical Journal*, **99**(1), 13–14.

NHS Newborn and Infant Physical Examination Programme (NIPE) (2010) *Ultrasound Examination of the Hips in Screening for Developmental Dysplasia of the Hips (DDH)* Available at: http://newbornphysical.screening.nhs.uk/standards#fileid10855 (accessed 3 March 2012).

Nochimson, G. (2011) *Legg-Calve-Perthes Disease in Emergency Medicine*. Available at: http://emedicine.medscape.com/article/826935 (accessed 16 September 2012).

Pearce, S.H.S. and Cheetham, T.D. (2010) Diagnosis and management of vitamin D deficiency. *British Medical Journal*, **340**, b5664.

Perquin, C.W., Hazebroek-Kampschreur, A.A.J.M., Hunfeld, J.A.M. *et al.* (2000) Pain in children and adolescents: a common experience. *Pain*, **87**(1), 51–58.

Perry, D.C., Green, D.J., Bruce, C.E. *et al.* (2012) Abnormalities of vascular structure and function in children with Perthes disease. *Pediatrics*, **130**(1), 126–131.

Petje, G., Meizer, R., Radler, C., Aigner, N. and Grill, F. (2008) Deformity correction in children with hereditary hypophosphatemic rickets. *Clinical Orthopaedics and Related Research*, **466** (12), 3078–3085.

Ponseti, I.V. (1992) Treatment of Congenital Clubfoot. *Journal of Bone and Joint Surgery (American)*, **74A**(3), 448–454.

Ponseti, I.V. and Smoley, E.N. (2009) The classic congenital club foot: the results of treatment. *Clinical Orthopaedics and Related Research*, **467**(5), 1133–1145.

Riad, J., Bajelidze, G. and Gabos, P.G. (2007) Bilateral slipped capital femoral epiphysis: predictive factors for contralateral slip. *Journal of Pediatric Orthopedics*, **27**(4), 411–414.

Roth-Isigkeit, A., Thyen, U., Stöven, H., Schwarzenberger, J. and Schmucker, P. (2005) Pain among children and adolescents: restrictions in daily living and triggering factors. *Pediatrics*, **115**(2), e152–e162.

Royal College of Nursing (RCN) (2012) *A Competence Framework for Orthopaedic and Trauma Practitioners*. RCN, London.

Sherry, D., Wallace, C., Kelley, C., Kiddler, M. and Sapp, L. (1999) Short and long-term outcomes of children with complex regional pain syndrome type I treated with exercise therapy. *The Clinical Journal of Pain*, **15**, 218–223.

Sherry, D. (2008) Amplified musculoskeletal pain: treatment approach and outcomes. *Journal of Pediatric Gastroenterology and Nutrition*, **47**(5), 693–694.

Southwick, W.O. (1967) Osteotomy through the lesser trochanter for slipped capital femoral epiphysis. *Journal of Bone and Joint Surgery*, **49-A**, 807–835.

Sparks, L., Rush Ortman, M. and Aubuchon, P. (2004) Care of the child in a body cast. *Journal of Orthopaedic Nursing*, **8**(4), 231–235.

Sun, W., Li, Z., Shi, Z. *et al.* (2011) Early and middle term results after surgical treatment for slipped capital femoral epiphysis. *Orthopaedic Surgery*, **3**(1), 22–27.

Taylor, G.R. and Clarke, N.M.P. (1997) Monitoring the treatment of developmental dysplasia of the hip with the Pavlik harness. *Journal of Bone and Joint Surgery (Britain)*, **79-B**, 719–723.

Taylor, L.M. (2002) Complex regional pain syndrome: comparing adults and adolescents. *Topics in Advanced Practice Nursing eJournal* **2**(2). Available at: http://www.medscape.com/viewarticle/430537_1 (accessed 3 March 2012).

Tucker, K.L., Morita, K., Qiao, N. *et al.* (2006) Colas, but not other carbonated beverages, are associated with low bone mineral density in older women: The Framingham Osteoporosis Study. *American Journal of Clinical Nutrition*, **84**(4), 936–942.

Uglow, M.G. and Clarke, N.M.P. (2000) Relapse in staged surgery for congenital talipes equinovarus. *Journal of Bone and Joint Surgery (Britain)*, **82B**(5), 739–743.

Uglow, M.G. and Clarke, N.M.P. (2004) The management of slipped capital femoral epiphysis. *Journal of Bone and Joint Surgery (British)*, **86-B**(5), 631–635.

Walter, K.D., Lin, D.Y. and Schwartz, E. *Slipped Capital Femoral Epiphysis*. Available at: http://emedicine.medscape.com/article/91596-overview (accessed 16 September 2011).

Wyshak, G. (2000) Teenaged girls' carbonated beverage consumption and bone fractures. *Archives of Pediatric and Adolescent Medicine*, **154**(6), 610–613.

Zaki, S.H. and Rae, P.J. (2009) High tibial valgus osteotomy using the Tomofix plate – Medium-term results in young patients. *Acta Orthopædica Belgica*, **75**, 360–367.

CHAPTER 23

Fracture management in the infant, child and young person

Elizabeth Wright
University Hospital Southampton, Southampton, UK

Introduction

Children are not small adults but *'different'* due to their state of development and growth, resulting in physiological differences between the child and adult skeleton. The growing skeleton has an enormous capacity for more rapid healing and remodelling. Injuries that involve skeletal growth plates can potentially cause permanent growth irregularities. Children sustain more fractures than healthy adults (Jones *et al.*, 2002) and Schalamon *et al.* (2011) estimated that 10% to 25% of all children's injuries worldwide will be fractures. In a study of 3421 children's fractures 34.7% were sport related, 17.6% occurred at home and 16.7% happened outdoors. The incidence of childhood fractures varies across the age spectrum. This is influenced by a child's physical mobility, language development, their comprehension of danger, ability to identify risk in their immediate environment and more adventurous behaviour with age. The principles of fracture management are considered in Chapter 17 while this chapter, along with Chapter 24, focusses specifically on fractures in the infant, child and young person.

The pre-ambulant child

The pre-ambulant child, newborn to around 13 months of age, is dependent and vulnerable with crying the only means of communication. This can sometimes seem relentless and frustrating for carers. This age group has minimal capacity to place themselves in danger; therefore, for any child from this age group presenting with a fracture, there should be a high index of suspicion for non-accidental injury (Clarke *et al.*, 2012). Skellern *et al.* (2000) report 24% of fractures in children under one year of age to be due to non-accidental injury. It is essential that practitioners working with this age group always obtain a full medical history and seek continuity between the mechanism of injury and the actual injury (Clarke *et al.*, 2012) (see Chapter 21 for further discussion). Accidents that do happen are often attributed to unexpected mobility by the child, for example the first time a baby independently rolls over and falls from a surface or unexpectedly crawling and falling down stairs. Other accidents are inadvertently caused by the child's carer; for example dropping the child while carrying them or placing a child seat on a high surface from which it can fall. It is known that pre-school age children are most likely to sustain fractures in the home environment (Majori *et al.*, 2009) and there is a role here for parental/carer education in accident prevention.

The pre-school child

Pre-school children, aged 13 months to five years of age, are gradually becoming independently mobile. They are inquisitive about their environment and need to interact with things in order to learn. It is in their nature to be impetuous, excitable, trusting, naïve and quick. However, they have little knowledge of what can potentially harm them. Language skills are developing but they may not fully comprehend instructions. For those three to five years of age the most likely reason for emergency department attendance for 1 to 2 year olds is accidental poisoning followed by musculoskeletal injury (Orton *et al.*, 2012). Valerio *et al.* (2010) researched paediatric fracture patterns in 382 subjects and found that 19.9% of pre-school children sustained a fracture, 83%

Orthopaedic and Trauma Nursing: An Evidence-based Approach to Musculoskeletal Care, First Edition. Edited by Sonya Clarke and Julie Santy-Tomlinson.

of these injuries were to the upper limb, there was no gender difference and 68% of the fractures occurred in the home environment.

The school aged child

School age children, aged five to twelve years, continue to interact with the environment and gradually form some independence. It is at this age they start to play outside away from direct supervision. Their understanding of risk is developing but is still limited. They form friendships and may start to engage in risk taking behaviours to impress their friends. Language comprehension has developed and instructions can be followed unless the child chooses to be disobedient. This is reflected in the injury patterns for this age group. Most injuries still occur in the home (46%) but 28% of fractures are sustained at playgrounds and 18% at sports facilities (Valerio *et al.*, 2010). Children are seen with injuries that relate to trends in their play activities such as skating (Ruth *et al.*, 2009), trampolining and skateboards (Lustenberger *et al.*, 2010). It is important to look at these trends and consider health and safety initiatives to help reduce the number of fractures that children sustain such as the type of surfaces in playgrounds (Howard *et al.*, 2009). Such initiatives have health benefits but are also important because school attendance is reduced when a child has a limb immobilised in a cast (Hymen 2011) and this may impact on their education. Young children often don't pay attention and are at particular risk of injury from road traffic accidents (Doong and Lai, 2012; Dunbar 2012). Children at the younger end of this age group are short in stature and have small body mass, rendering them more vulnerable to significant injury if involved in a road traffic accident. Often the child is a pedestrian, possibly playing in the street or on a bike, and because of their smaller size they are harder to see, the main trunk of their body comes into contact with the vehicle and they can be thrown further. Even at slow speeds the child involved in a road traffic accident is likely to sustain more significant injuries.

The young person/adolescent

Adolescents are known for being adventurous and engaging in risk-taking behaviours. Many are thrill seeking, attention seeking, respond to peer pressure and confidently believe that they are indestructible. Most adolescents have adult appearance but it is important to remember that they have not fully reached skeletal maturity. Wang *et al.* (2010) suggest the higher fracture incidence in this age group is related to the very rapid pubertal growth spurt that weakens the bone cortex. Mathison and Agrawal (2010) attribute the recent increase in the number of paediatric fractures to the emergence of more adventurous sporting activities that appeal to this age group. Most adolescent fractures are sustained when participating in contact sports such as rugby and football or more adventurous activities like skiing and mountain biking (Aleman and Meyers 2010).

Key stages of musculoskeletal development of bone and fracture healing

Childhood skeletal growth

Skeletal formation commences in the embryo and continues until skeletal growth is complete at around 21 years of age. Before eight weeks gestation the foetal skeleton is formed entirely of fibrous membranes and hyaline cartilage. Two types of bone tissue development occur: intramembranous ossification when bone develops from a fibrous membrane and is called membranous bone and endochondral ossification when bone develops from hyaline cartilage and is called cartilage or endochondral bone. Interstitial growth at the epiphyseal plates or physes lengthens bone and appositional growth widens bones. During bone lengthening the epiphyseal plate cartilage that abuts the diaphysis produces new cartilaginous cells that transit towards the diaphysis and then form new bone. Appositional growth occurs along the periosteum. Osteoblasts form new bone on the inner side of the periosteum whilst osteoclasts erase bone along the outer edge of the endosteum. Osteoblast formation is more prolific than osteoclast activity. The end result is a thicker and stronger bone shaft and a widening medullary canal in proportion to the bone diameter. Bone growth is said to be complete when the epiphyseal plates fuse. Growth of the young child's femoral head demonstrates this. Figure 23.1 shows a series of radiographic images of the hip illustrating development from birth to skeletal maturity.

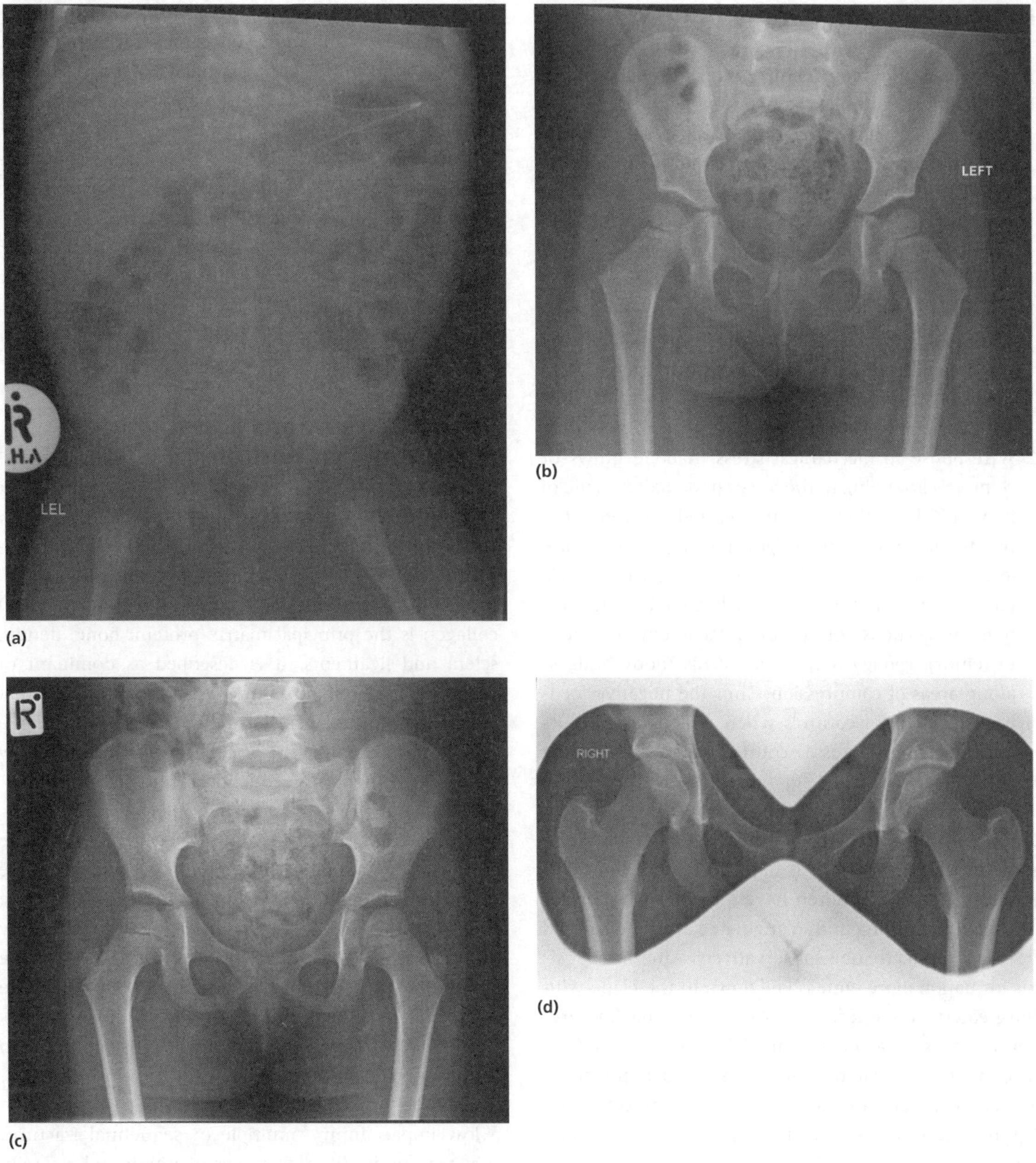

(a) (b) (c) (d)

Figure 23.1 Series of child hip X-rays from birth to skeletal maturity

At birth the femoral head is a cartilaginous template that is not evident on X-ray. By eight months of age the ossific nuclei of the femoral head (secondary centre of ossification) is evident. At around eight years of age the femoral heads are fully formed, with the epiphyseal plate (physis) clearly evident. At skeletal maturity the physis of the proximal femur is fused.

Bone repair and remodelling

Bone repair and remodelling occurs throughout life. Remodelling is controlled in two ways:

1 A hormonal negative feedback mechanism in which parathyroid hormone and calcitonin control the blood calcium concentration. When blood calcium concentration falls, parathyroid hormone stimulates osteoblasts to release calcium from the skeleton. When blood calcium levels rise the thyroid gland releases calcitonin that stimulates the calcium to be deposited into bone. Calcium is essential for many physiological processes and this mechanism exists to maintain the blood calcium level rather than assist with skeletal wellbeing.
2 A response to mechanical stress. A bone grows or remodels according to the forces or demands made of it (Wolff's law). Bones are thicker and stronger at the points of maximum weight bearing and muscle attachment/pull. Long bones are thickest mid shaft, curved bones are thickest at the bend point and form bony projections for muscle attachment (i.e. neck of femur), spongy bone forms struts (bony bridges) along areas of compression. Thus the negative feedback mechanism controls when remodelling occurs and mechanical stresses control where remodelling occurs (see Chapter 4 for musculoskeletal structure and development).

Fracture healing in the child fundamentally follows the same process as in adults (Chapter 17) with some differences. Younger children have a greater capacity for fracture remodelling and so angulated and/or displaced fractures can be treated conservatively. After initial callus formation more bone is laid down in the plane with the greatest mechanical stress. As a general rule fractures within the sagittal plane remodel well whereas fractures with axial rotation are unlikely to remodel. In adults similar injuries would require surgical correction. Figure 23.2 provides a pictorial overview of the healing process.

Children have a growing skeleton; consequently fracture healing is faster in children than adults. It is estimated that a two-year old will heal a long bone fracture in three weeks whereas a ten-year old will take three months and children have a greater capacity for fracture remodelling. When managing children's fractures it is acceptable for the fracture fragments not to be in true alignment and/or have some degree of angulation. It is important to know the age of the child and the injury. The younger the child the faster the healing capacity and the greater the remodelling capacity.

Vitamin D is essential for calcium homeostasis and thus affects bone development and remodelling. This is considered in more detail in Chapter 22. The practitioner should consider assessing the vitamin D level of children that present with repeat fractures and when considering the possibility of non-accidental injury.

Specific conditions and fractures presenting in children

Osteogenesis imperfecta

Osteogenesis imperfecta (OI) is a genetic skeletal dysplasia in which the skeleton is osteoporotic (Cole 2002). It is clinically manifested in tissues in which type I collagen is the principal matrix protein: bone, dentin, sclera and ligaments. It is described as dominant or recessive. In dominant OI there is a protein defect that affects type I collagen formation. Either there is a reduction in the amount of collagen manufactured by the body or there is a reduction in the amount of collagen mixed with some defective collagen (Cole 2002). In recessive OI genetic mutations cause deficiency in the collagen components. Both dominant and recessive forms result in reduced bone mass and strength, making the bone fragile and susceptible to fracture, deformity and growth deficiency (Forlino *et al.*, 2011). The condition is rare, affecting around six per 100 000 of the population (van Dijk *et al.*, 2011). Its clinical presentation ranges from silent forms with osteoporosis to intrauterine death.

Children with OI usually present with a fracture from a low impact injury, multiple or sequential fractures that may be in different stages of union and a family history of 'easy' fractures and/or bone disease. Fractures often heal with abundant callus. Abnormal reparative bone may give rise to malunion or pseudarthrosis. Children with more severe forms of OI tend to present earlier and with more numerous fractures. Fracture incidence decreases after puberty. Other main musculoskeletal features are short stature, pectus excavatum,

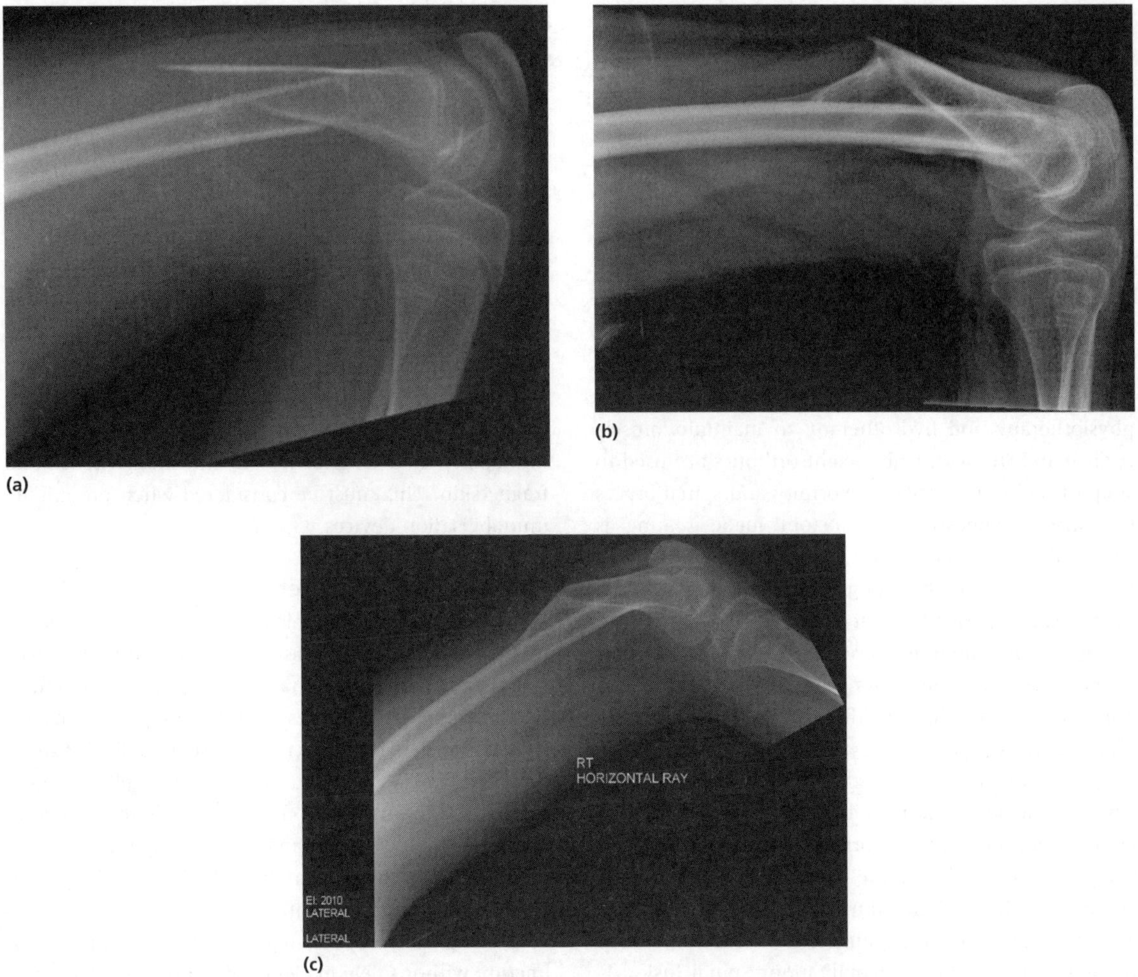

Figure 23.2 Series of X-rays to show fracture remodelling in a femur. 23.2a new injury; 23.2b two months post-injury; 23.2c eight months post-injury

kyphoscoliosis and Wormian bone. Kyphoscoliosis occurs in 40–60% of cases and may be progressive after maturity. In Wormian bone small independent areas of primary ossification are seen within membranous bone on X-ray, most often seen on a skull X-ray. Alteration of the tissues containing type I collagen also causes dentinogenesis imperfecta, blue sclera and ligamentous laxity.

OI is classified in to four types:

- The mildest form is type 1, these patients have blue sclera, bone fragility varies from mild to severe; dentinogenesis imperfecta may be present.
- Type 2 is the severest form of OI. It is incompatible with life and usually results in intrauterine death. Babies rarely survive the neonatal period and there is extreme bone fragility with crumpled long bones.
- In type 3 bone fragility is variable, being more severe in infancy; skeletal deformity is progressive with blue sclera.
- In type 4 OI there is bone fragility, normal sclera with variable skeletal deformity and dentin abnormality.

OI is difficult to diagnose; 20.5% of children with OI are initially diagnosed as non-accidental injury (Pandya *et al.*, 2011).

Children with OI should be managed by the multidisciplinary team. Systemic management aims to improve skeletal strength. A group of drugs called bisphosphonates may be prescribed. These decrease osteoclast activity to improve the mineral content of bone (van Dijk *et al.*, 2011) with the intention of decreasing fracture risk. Calcium, vitamins C and D, fluoride and calcitonin are used to try and strengthen the bone with growth hormone used in an attempt to correct short stature.

Management aims to maximise independent mobility by minimising disability that can result from fractures and skeletal deformity. OI is a chronic condition and requires long-term routine therapy. This consists of physiotherapy and hydrotherapy to maintain muscle control and strength. Lightweight orthotics are used to support limbs and prevent deformity and spinal braces to control kyphoscoliosis. Custom made seating is provided for non-ambulators. Parents and carers need to be taught proper handling and positioning to avoid fractures. It is preferable that fractures are treated conservatively and are immobilised in lightweight casts for short durations to allow for early motion. Prolonged immobilisation results in further osteoporosis leading to repeat fractures.

Surgery can be used to stabilise skeletal deformity. Options include intramedullary nailing of the long bones, with or without correctional osteotomies, or using telescopic rods that are fixed in the epiphysis and elongate with the bone during growth. Stabilisation aims to improve bone alignment, decrease the risk of refracture and improve rehabilitation. Spinal fusion is recommended for curves over 35 degrees but surgical fixation is complicated by the poor bone quality and the lack of autogenous bone graft. It is important to remember that patients with OI have the tendency to bleed excessively.

Fractures in children with special needs

Children with special needs are at increased risk of pathological fractures because of low bone mineral density. Many have a decreased weight bearing status that contributes to osteoporosis (Marreiros *et al.*, 2010), require parenteral nutrition because of poor gastrointestinal absorption that affects their nutritional status, may have epilepsy and need anti-convulsant drugs that have been shown to lower bone mineral density (Gniatkowska-Nowakowska 2010) and/or underlying pathology such as osteomyelitis that affects skeletal strength (Belthur *et al.*, 2012) or neurofibromatosis. Some syndromes (e.g. Turner's syndrome) have a known association with increased fracture risk but the physiology is not yet fully understood (Holroyd *et al.*, 2010).

There is a tri-partite approach to caring for the disabled child with a fracture. The main principles of fracture management apply, pain control and limb immobilisation, conservative or surgical treatment appropriate for the underlying pathology and the child's ability to manage the suggested treatment. Traction may be a preferable treatment. Early mobilisation is preferable, splints and braces may be more appropriate than casts and all need to be lightweight. Many children with special needs are at greater risk of pressure ulcers due immobility, neurological deficit, nutritional issues and fragile skin. This must be considered when prescribing immobilisation devices.

Pathological fractures

Some fractures are pathological in origin. This means that there is underlying disease or alteration of the biochemistry of the bone that predisposes it to fracture. There can be many causes; malnutrition, neurophysiological disorders that affect the musculoskeletal system, osteomyelitis, skeletal syndromes and dysplasias, bone cysts and tumours. Bone chemistry is altered and bone density is reduced. Pharmacological regimes used to treat other conditions can affect the bone density, (e.g. epilepsy drugs and chemotherapy).

To complicate matters, when a child presents with a fracture without clear evidence of injury the practitioner must consider non-accidental injury (NAI) but must also be mindful of pathological causes. Each hospital must have sound child protection procedures/safeguarding in place and designated child protection specialists. The practitioner needs to know and follow the local child protection guidelines if there is any concern about the mechanism of the injury. Sadly, this is especially significant as reported child maltreatment continues to rise (Gilbert *et al.*, 2012). The consequences of not identifying child abuse are severe with 50% presenting with further injury and 10% dying from abuse. See Chapter 21 for further discussion of safeguarding children.

The first priority when managing a child with a pathological fracture is to diagnose the cause (Saraph and Linhart 2005). Attempting to treat the fracture without understanding the pathological cause is largely futile. If a child has osteomyelitis, then the fracture will not heal until the infection has been appropriately treated. Expediency is also key. A pathological fracture from a bone lesion diagnosed on X-ray, may have resulted from a simple bone cyst or an osteosarcoma of which the latter is life threatening. Initial principles of fracture management apply, pain control and limb immobilisation but further management is dependent on the underlying diagnosis (Chapter 15).

Fracture diagnosis, classification and management in childhood

The principles of diagnosis, classification and management of fractures in the adult are considered in a previous chapter. For the sake of completeness in this chapter an overview of fracture care in children are also considered here with some overlap but the reader may also wish to refer to Chapter 17.

Diagnosis

A fracture is described as a disruption of bone continuity and is most often the result of accidental trauma. On initial presentation the child experiences pain, swelling and loss of function of the affected limb, although in stable undisplaced fractures not all these criteria may be present. It is important to obtain a full medical history, complete a clinical examination and obtain an X-ray to assist with diagnosis. Not all fractures are clearly evident on X-ray and it may be necessary to use other forms of imaging to clarify the injury, such as MRI (magnetic resonance image) or CT (computerised tomography).

The medical history should identify how the injury happened, the age of the child and the age of the injury. Information about the mechanism of injury will allow for any concerns regarding non-accidental injury to be considered and, hopefully, ruled out. Information about the velocity and impact of injury can give vital information. If a fracture that is normally associated with a high impact injury, for example fractured femur, occurred as a result of low impact then the clinician should be suspicious of a pathological fracture and further investigations are needed. If the child has been involved in major trauma (i.e. road traffic accident) then the clinician must consider the possibility of other injuries (Chapter 16).

Fractures can be diagnosed clinically. The main indices are pain, swelling and loss of function. Palpation over the suspected site of injury will be uncomfortable if there is an underlying fracture. Assessment of the limb must include assessment for neurovascular deficit/compartment syndrome (Wright 2007b). Radiological imaging is used to confirm the diagnosis of a fracture. Initially an X-ray is obtained. It is important to obtain two views – anterior-posterior and lateral. The body is three dimensional and thus one X-ray view may not show evidence of fracture. If an X-ray does not illustrate a fracture but there is a high index of clinical suspicion, then other imaging such as an oblique X-ray view, MRI or CT may be requested. MRIs show the soft tissues and CTs provide better definition of bones. Also if the injury is complex, for example a triplane fracture of ankle – which as the name suggests is a three dimensional injury, then further imaging is requested so that the surgeon can have a full understanding of the injury.

Fracture classification

Fractures are generally classified as closed or open injuries, by the anatomical location, the direction of fracture line, the level of the fracture within the bone, as a description of the fracture pattern and, if the injury involves the growth plate, using the growth plate classification called Salter Harris. There is a detailed and, complex fracture classification system for long bones called the AO system of long bone fracture classification (Müller at al., 1990); a further version was created for paediatric long bone fractures by Slongo and Audigé (2007).

In closed fractures the skin surrounding the fracture is intact. If a fracture is described as open then the skin has been punctured and the skin integrity has been compromised. In this instance there is a high risk of infection especially as debris from the scene of the incident may be embedded inside the bone and surrounding tissues. This is also known as a compound fracture and the bone may be protruding from the skin. Haemorrhage is likely with an open fracture.

Primary fracture description involves identifying the fractured bone, for example fractured left tibia or fractured right metacarpal of index finger. The anatomical reference points are used to describe the level of the fracture i.e. diaphysis, epiphysis. The Salter Harris classification system is used to describe fractures that involve the physis (Chapter 24). The fracture is then further described by the direction of the fracture line: transverse, linear, oblique or spiral as demonstrated in

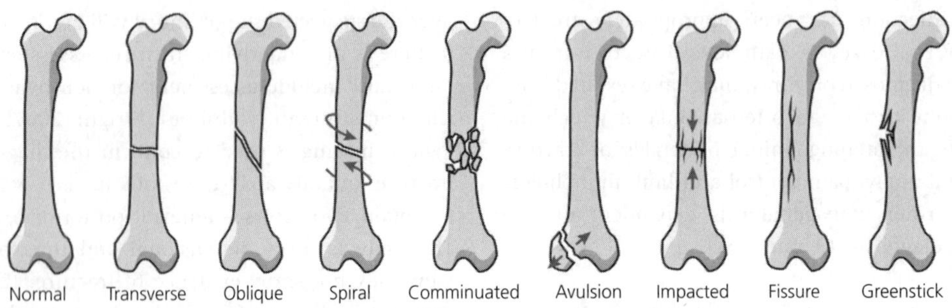

Figure 23.3 Types of fracture. Roproduced with permission from ASU Ask A Biologist.

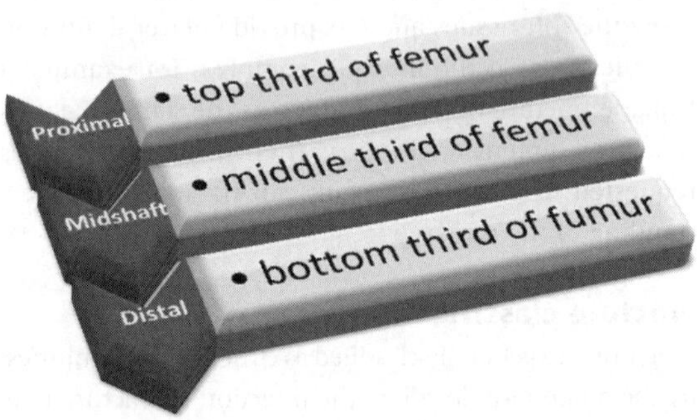

Figure 23.4 Bone descriptors applied to the femur

Figure 23.3. In a transverse fracture the fracture line crosses the shaft of the bone at a right angle to the bone's long axis. In a linear fracture the fracture line is parallel along the bone's long axis. In an oblique fracture the fracture line is diagonal and in a spiral fracture the fracture line twists around the long axis of the bone. Other terms used to describe fractures are impacted, comminuted and avulsed. Impacted fractures occur when the bone fragments are driven into each other. In comminuted or multi-fragment fractures the bone has broken into a number of fragments. With an avulsion fracture the muscle that attaches to the bone via a tendon has been pulled away by sudden contraction of the muscle. The sudden and forceful muscle contraction results in a fragment of bone being pulled off from the bone. The levels of the fracture site are also used in fracture description: proximal, mid shaft and distal, Figure 23.4 applies these terms to the femur.

It is also described as the proximal third, middle third or distal third. Terms that describe the fracture pattern are also used. A hairline fracture is a thin, fine fracture where there is no clear evidence of fracture on X-ray but clinical indices are high. Depressed fractures are inwardly displaced, often caused by a direct blow. Intra-articular fractures involve part of the joint surface. Pathological fracture occurs when the bone is weakened by disease and fractures with minimal force.

Fractures unique to childhood

Buckle fractures and greenstick fractures are unique to children. The juvenile skeleton has thicker periosteum and this partially protects the bone from injury when a high impact force is sustained, reducing the severity of the fracture. The result is an incomplete 'buckle' or 'greenstick' fracture. The term buckle refers to the buckling of the bone without disturbing the whole bone. This is also known as a torus fracture, from the Latin word *'tori'* meaning swelling or protuberance. Buckle fractures most commonly occur in the distal radius, typically when a child falls on an outstretched hand. These fractures can be successfully treated using a temporary removable wrist splint (Wright 2011). The term greenstick fracture describes a fracture in which one cortex of the bone is broken and the other cortex is intact. These fractures are treated conservatively, by immobilising in a cast because angulation can occur at the fracture site due to the asymmetry of the fracture (Chapter 24).

Growth plate injuries

Fractures that include the epiphyseal plate are classified using the Salter Harris (SH) classification. This classification describes the physeal injury and appoints a number to each type. The gradient is from one to five; a Salter Harris 5 injury is the severest injury and poses the greatest likelihood of an angulatory deformity or bone length discrepancy. Salter Harris classification and management is further explored in Chapter 24.

Potential diagnostic pitfalls

The altered physiology of the child's skeleton complicates diagnosing children's fractures. The cartilaginous component of the child's skeleton does not show on X-ray and may result in the true extent of the injury not being appreciated. This is particularly true of SH1 and fractures of the lateral condyle of the humerus. A Salter Harris 1 fracture of long bone presents with the fracture line traversing the physis; a child's physis is cartilage and will therefore not be evident on radiological imaging (Gaston *et al.*, 2012). Similarly, the physis of the lateral condyle of the humerus is the last growth plate in the elbow to fuse – at around 13 years of age – making radiological diagnosis difficult. This is particularly significant because there is a high incidence of non-union (Storm *et al.*, 2006). These injuries are usually treated conservatively (Marcheix *et al.*, 2011) but, due to the risk of non-union, some surgeons prefer to treat them surgically with fracture reduction and K wire fixation. Either way, children with these injuries should be followed up in the outpatient clinic until fracture healing has been confirmed radiologically.

Hairline or stress fractures are not always evident radiologically. These injuries are usually the result of minor trauma or repeated stress (e.g. when participating in sports). Mostly they are stable fractures that will heal well, but the scaphoid is an exception. Scaphoid fractures usually occur in the adolescent (Bhatti *et al.*, 2012) and have a high incidence of painful non-union (Eastley *et al.*, 2012). If there is clinical suspicion of a scaphoid fracture, the limb should be immobilised in a cast. Further imaging by MRI is recommended to aid diagnosis (Yin *et al.*, 2012). Once the cast is removed the child is reviewed in clinic until there is radiological evidence of fracture healing and the patient is symptom free.

Overlooking these injuries can result in deformity and disability. If there is a clinical suspicion of a fracture, even if the injury is not confirmed on X-ray, the limb should be immobilised and further imaging requested to confirm or refute the diagnosis. Furthermore, children's ligaments are stronger than bone which makes it rare for a child to sustain a 'strain' or 'sprain'. When a child presents, for example, with ankle pain and a history of trauma with no evidence of fracture on X-ray, the practitioner should suspect SH type 1 fracture and take appropriate action.

Joint dislocations

Joint dislocations occur with high impact events, usually sport related. The two bones that constitute a joint are completely displaced from one another. There is no articulation and the joint cannot function. Subluxation is a variance of this where the two bones are partially dislocated but some contact is maintained. Dislocation of joints most commonly occur in the shoulder and the patella. Treatment involves manipulating the bones back into the correct position followed by a period of immobilisation then gradual rehabilitation with physiotherapy to strengthen the musculature that supports the joints.

Fracture dislocations

Fracture dislocations are a complex group of injuries where a joint is dislocated alongside a fracture. These injuries usually require surgical reduction but can be difficult to reduce and may be unstable. Children with these injuries require close supervision as joint stiffness and avascular necrosis are common complications. An uncommon but unique fracture dislocation in children is the Monteggia fracture. This is a fracture dislocation in which a fracture of the proximal ulna is coupled with dislocation of the radial head (Beutal 2012). While the ulna fracture is usually identified, the radial head dislocation is sometimes initially overlooked (Babb and Carlson 2005). This can cause a valgus deformity of the elbow, restriction of forearm rotation and pain with activity (Bhaskar 2009). With all ulna fractures the position of the radial head should be confirmed. Surgical reduction of a displaced ulna fracture is needed with which the radial head spontaneously reduces (Ring *et al.*, 1998).

Articular fractures

If the fracture extends into a joint surface it is classified as an articular fracture. Two descriptions are used; 'complete' and 'partial'. In a complete articular fracture the joint line is completely separated. These injuries can also be considered fracture dislocations. In partial articular fractures, also described as intra-articular, part of the joint is separated. The significance of these injuries is that there is usually residual joint stiffness and they can predispose to early osteoarthritis.

Main principles of fracture treatment

The priorities of initial fracture management are to ensure that the neurovascular status of the limb is healthy and that there are no indications of compartment syndrome (Wright 2008a), relieve pain and support the injured limb. The aim of secondary management is to ensure the bone ends are in continuity so that healing can occur without residual deformity and the limb is restored to full normal function. Fractures can be treated conservatively using casts, splintage or traction. If the fracture is displaced then surgical correction is required; this ranges from manipulation under anaesthetic to open reduction with either internal or external fixation (refer to Chapters 8 and 17).

Casting

Casts made of plaster of Paris (POP) or resin can be used to support and align fractured limbs. Plaster of Paris casts are easier to mould by the clinician but are heavier and take longer to dry. Resin casts dry within 30 minutes, are available in different colours and are lightweight. The purpose of casting is:

- to maintain bone alignment for fracture healing
- to maintain surgical correction until healed
- to promote pain relief by resting the affected limb or joint
- to correct deformities by wedging or serial casting.

Casts should always be applied by a suitably qualified practitioner. There are three layers:

- stockinette to protect the skin
- wool to add padding and further protection
- the casting material.

Each layer should be applied smoothly, to avoid creasing that may cause pressure sore, and snugly, to support and mould the cast to the limb (Wright 2008b).

After application the plaster will feel warm due to chemical reaction. The wet cast should be handled by the palm of the hand to avoid cast denting that may cause pressure. The cast should be allowed to dry naturally. Casts can conduct heat and resting a casted limb on a radiator or using a hair drier may cause a burn. The affected limb should be elevated to reduce swelling so the limb should be rested/elevated on pillows covered with a towel to absorb the moisture from the cast. Children in large body casts should be turned two hourly to facilitate drying of the cast. The practitioner should observe the cast for dents, cracks or skin rubbing and assess the patient for complaints of pain or discomfort. If any of these are noted then medical staff should be informed. It may be necessary to modify or remove the cast (Wright 2008). See Chapter 8 for further information.

When discharged the child and family should be advised to keep the cast dry. It should not be covered with plastic for showering or bathing as steam condenses on the inside of plastic bags and will make the cast wet. The best advice is to cover the cast with a towel to absorb water splashes. Nothing should be put down the cast because of the risk of developing pressure ulcers and nothing should be used to scratch under the cast as the skin may be lacerated and there is a risk of subsequent infection. The family should be advised to avoid beaches and sandpits to prevent sand getting inside the cast that can rub the skin and cause excoriation (Wright 2007a).

The patient should be advised to observe for the following and to seek medical assistance should any of the following signs and symptoms occur. (Lucus and Davis 2005):

- the toes or fingers become blue, swollen and painful to move
- the limb becomes more painful
- pins and needles or numbness are felt in the digits
- if the cast feels uncomfortable or is rubbing
- if an unpleasant smell is noticed from the cast and/or a discharge is seen on the cast.

Orthotic splints

Orthotic splints are used in the management of fractures to immobilise and rest a limb. They are particularly useful when a child has underlying pathology and traditional treatment such as casting may do more harm than good. Orthotic splints are either dynamic or fixed. A fixed splint is rigid and will support and control the limb and/or correct deformity (Wright 2012); for example, removable wrist splints used in the management of buckle fractures (Wright 2011). Dynamic splints support the limb but allow for a controlled range of movement that can help soft tissue development and healing (Wright 2012). The IROM brace is an example of a dynamic splint; following patellar dislocation it is used to allow controlled knee flexion.

Traction

Traction is a pulling force that is applied to an injured limb using weights and pulleys. This is considered in more detail in Chapter 8 but is considered briefly here for the sake of completeness of this chapter. Traction is applied superficially to the limb with the force being indirectly exerted on the underlying structures:

- In fixed traction the traction force is exerted against a fixed point (e.g. Thomas splint traction).
- In balanced traction the traction pull is exerted against an opposing force usually provided by the weight of the body when the foot of the bed is raised.

There are three types of traction; skin, skeletal and manual.

- In skin traction the traction apparatus is applied directly to the patient's skin.
- In skeletal traction the traction pull is exerted via pins, screws, wires or tongs that have been surgically applied to the skeleton (e.g. Steinman pin through the tibia).
- Manual traction is applied by a person pulling on the affected limb, used during traction application and fracture manipulation.

Traction is used in fracture treatment to restore and maintain fracture alignment and to assist with pain relief by controlling muscle spasm. Different types of traction are used according the injury (Table 23.1) and is described in more detail in chapter 8.

Surgical management

Surgical management falls into four categories:

- closed reduction
- closed reduction with surgical pinning
- open reduction with or without internal fixation
- external fixation.

Closed reduction is achieved by manipulating the fracture while the patient is anaesthetised. With general anaesthetic the muscles are relaxed and the patient is unaware of pain allowing the surgeon to manipulate the fracture ends back to anatomical position. This is used when the fracture is minimally displaced. First manual traction is applied, pulling the limb distally. This corrects limb shortening and often, because the muscles are relaxed from the general anaesthetic, this may be enough to correct the bone alignment. The next step is to push or angulate the bone ends until reduction is achieved. Alignment is radiologically confirmed in theatre and a cast is applied. If the fracture position slips, percutaneous Kirschner wires (K wires) are inserted across the fracture site. After confirmation of alignment by X-ray a back slab cast is applied. The K wires loosen in the bone over the next few weeks and are normally removed four to six weeks after insertion. There is a best practice debate about whether the K wires should be removed in the outpatient clinic or as a day case procedure under general anaesthesia. Removing the K wires in a clinic takes a few seconds and is slightly uncomfortable, although the sight of the pliers used to remove the wires can be frightening. To have the wires removed in theatre means having to fast the child and it carries the risks of general anaesthesia. The practitioner should discuss this with the child and family. As a general rule, if the child is under eight years of age the K wires should be removed under general anaesthesia and in the clinic if older.

Table 23.1 Traction type and injury

Traction type	Injury
Bucks or Pughs	Hip injury or infection
Gallows	Fractured femur under two years of age Pre hip surgery
Halter neck	Torticollis
Dunlop	Supracondylar fracture of humerus (rarely used now)
Thomas splint	Fractured femur over two years of age
Tibial (Denham or Steinmann pin)	Fractured femur – adolescent (rarely used now)
Skull/halo	Spinal injuries and deformities (rarely used now)

Open reduction and internal fixation

Open reduction is used if satisfactory fracture reduction has not been achieved with closed reduction or the best way to achieve fracture alignment is to expose the fracture to allow reduction under direct vision with or without internal fixation. If the injury is an open fracture then the site is already exposed and further surgical opening may be needed to fully debride the wound and apply the necessary internal fixation. With open fractures there is added complication of poor skin integrity. It may not be possible to surgically close the wound and plastic surgery may be needed. Internal fixation secures the anatomical alignment and is beneficial for complex injuries such as intra-articular or fracture dislocation.

A variety of devices can be used for internal fixation, screws, plates, wires, nails and tension sutures. Internal fixation may be beneficial in major trauma, stabilising the limb injuries and allowing focus on more life threatening aspects of the patient's care. It also allows for early mobilisation. This may be particularly beneficial to a child with special needs. To internally fix a fracture the surgery is more invasive with the possibility of infection and the child will be under general anaesthesia for longer.

External fixation

External fixation is particularly useful when managing open and/or comminuted fractures. Pins are inserted percutaneously into the bone above and below the fracture site. The pins are then attached to a rigid external frame and the fracture ends can then be brought into alignment by manipulation of the frame. When there is severe soft tissue damage, the external fixator allows the fracture to be stabilised whilst the skin can be accessed for wound management. External circular frames such as the Ilizarov and Taylor spatial frame use wires that are thinner than pins and can be placed in individual bone fragments for comminuted fractures. External fixators are visible, there is a risk of pin site infection and the patient needs to be involved in pin site care (see Chapter 8 for further detail).

Factors complicating healing

Infection can delay fracture healing. The more interventional the management strategy employed to stabilise the fracture the greater the risk of infection. Sometimes there is delayed healing that proceeds to non-union. Non-union in otherwise healthy children is rare but can happen if fibrous tissue is within the fracture. Smoking and poor diet can contribute to delayed or non-union. It is known that certain fractures, of the scaphoid for instance, are at risk of non-union due to poor vasculature of the scaphoid bone. Mal-union occurs when the fracture ends have united in a suboptimal anatomical position. It is unusual in children and the management depends on the presenting clinical deformity and effect on function.

Recommended further reading

Benson, M.K.D. (2010) *Children's Orthopaedics and Fractures,* 3rd edn. Churchill Livingstone, London.

Rang, M., Pring, M. and Wenger, D (2005) *Rang's Children's Fractures,* 3rd edn. Lippincott Williams and Wilkins, Philadelphia.

Valerio, G., Gallè, F., Mancusi, C. *et al.* (2010) Pattern of fractures across pediatric age groups: analysis of individual and lifestyle factors. *BioMedCentral Public Health,* **10**, 656. Available at: http://www.biomedcentral.com/1471-2458/10/656 (accessed 20 March 2013).

References

Aleman, K.B. and Meyers, M.C. (2010) Mountain biking injuries in children and adolescents. *Sports Medicine,* **40**(1), 77–90.

Babb, A. and Carlson, W.O. (2005) Monteggia fractures: beware! *South Dakota Journal of Medicine,* **58**(7), 283–285.

Belthur, M.V., Birchansky, S.B., Verdugo, A.A. *et al.* (2012) Pathologic fractures in children with acute staphylococcus aureus osteomyelitis. *Journal of Bone and Joint Surgery America,* **94**(1), 34–42.

Beutel, B.G. (2012) Monteggia fractures in pediatric and adult populations. *Orthopedics,* **35**(2), 138–144. DOI:10.3928/01477447-20120123-32.

Bhaskar, A. (2009). Missed Monteggia fracture in children: is annular ligament reconstruction always required? *Indian Journal of Orthopaedics,* **43**(4), 389–395.

Bhatti, A.N., Griffin, S.J. and Wenham, S.J. (2012) Deceptive appearance of a normal variant of scaphoid bone in a teenage patient: a diagnostic challenge. *Orthopedic Reviews (Pavia),* **4**(1), e6. Epub 2012 Feb 2.

Boyce, A. and Gafni, R. (2011) Approach to the child with fractures. *Journal of Clinical Endocrinology and Metabolism,* **96**(7), 1943–1952. DOI:10.1210/jc.2010-2546 PMCID: PMC3135196.

Clarke, N.M., Shelton, F.R., Taylor, C.C., Khan, T. and Needhirajan, S. (2012) The incidence of fractures in children under the age of 24 months in relation to non-accidental injury. *Injury,* **43**(6), 762–765. Epub 2011 Sep. 19.

Cole, W. (2002) Bone, cartilage and fibrous tissue disorders, in *Children's Orthopaedics and Fractures* 2nd edn (eds M. Benson., J. Fixen., M. Macnicol, and K. Parsch), Churchill Livingstone, London, pp. 67–92.

van Dijk, F.S., Cobben, J.M., Kariminejad, A. *et al.* (2011) Osteogenesis imperfecta: a review with clinical examples. *Molecular Syndromology,* **1**: 1–20. Epub 2011 Oct. 12.

Doong, J.L. and Lai, C.H. (2012) Risk factors for child and adolescent occupants, bicyclists, and pedestrians in motorized vehicle collisions. *Traffic Injury Prevention,* **13**(3), 249–257.

Dunbar, G. (2012) The relative risk of nearside accidents is high for the youngest and oldest pedestrians. *Accident Analysis and Prevention,* **5**, 517–521. Epub 2011 Sep. 25.

Eastley. N., Singh, H., Dias, J.J. and Taub, N. (2012) Union rates after proximal scaphoid fractures; meta-analyses and review of available evidence. *Journal of Hand Surgery (European Volume)* Epub 2012 Jun. 26.

Forlino, A., Cabral, W.A., Barnes, A.M. and Marini, J.C. (2011) New perspectives on osteogenesis imperfecta. *Nature Reviews Endocrinology* **9**, 540–557. DOI:10.1038/nrendo.2011.81.

Gaston, M.S., Irwin, G.J. and Huntley, J.S. (2012) Lateral condyle fracture of a child's humerus: the radiographic features may be subtle. *Scottish Medical Journal* **57**(3), 182.

Gilbert, R., Fluke, J., O'Donnell, M. *et al.* (2012) Child maltreatment: variation in trends and policies in six developed countries. *Lancet,* **379**(9817), 758–772. Epub 2011 Dec. 9.

Gniatkowska-Nowakowska, A. (2010) Fractures in epilepsy children. *Seizure,* **19**(6), 324–325. Epub 2010 May 20.

Holroyd, C.R., Davies, J.H., Taylor, P. *et al.* (2010) Reduced cortical bone density with normal trabecular bone density in girls with Turner syndrome. *Osteoporosis International* **21**(12), 2093–2099. Epub 2010 Feb. 5.

Howard, A.W., Macarthur, C., Rothman, L., Willan, A. and Macpherson, A.K. (2009) School playground surfacing and arm fractures in children: a cluster randomized trial comparing sand to wood chip surfaces. *PLoS Medicine* **6**(12), e1000195. Epub 2009 Dec. 15.

Hyman, J.E., Gaffney, J.T., Epps, H.R. and Matsumoto, H. (2011) Impact of fractures on school attendance. *Journal of Pediatric Orthopaedics,* **31**(2), 113–116.

Jacobsen, S.T., Hull, C.K. and Crawford, A.H. (1986) Nutritional rickets. *Journal of Pediatric Orthopaedics* **6**(6), 713–716.

Jones, I.E., Williams, S.M., Dow, N. and Goelding, A. (2002) How many children remain fracture free during growth? A longitundinal study of children and adolescents participating in the Dunedin Multidisciplinary Health and Development Study. *Osteoporosis International,* **13**, 990–995.

Kraus, R. and Wessel, L. (2010) The treatment of upper limb fractures in children and adolescents. *Deutsches Arzteblatt International,* **107**(51–52). 903–910. DOI:10.3238/arztebl.2010.0903

Lucus, B. and Davis, P. (2005) Why restricting movement is important, in *Orthopaedic and Trauma Nursing* (eds J. Kneale and P. Davis) Churchill Livingstone, London, pp.105–139.

Lustenberger, T., Talving, P., Barmparas, G. *et al.* (2010) Skateboard-related injuries: not to be taken lightly. *A National Trauma Databank analysis. Journal of Traumatic Stress,* **69**(4), 924–927.

Majori, S., Ricci, G., Capretta, F. *et al.* (2009) Epidemiology of domestic injuries. *A survey in an emergency department in North-East Italy. Journal of Preventative Medicine and Hygiene,* **50**(3), 164–169.

Marcheix, P.S., Vacquerie, V., Longis, B. *et al.* (2011) Distal humerus lateral condyle fracture in children: when is the conservative treatment a valid option? *Orthopaedics & Traumatology: Surgery & Research* **97**(3), 304–307. Epub 2011 Apr. 7.

Marreiros, H., Monteiro, L., Loff, C. and Calado, E. (2010) Fractures in children and adolescents with spina bifida: the experience of a Portuguese tertiary-care hospital. *Developmental Medicine and Child Neurology* **52**(8), 754–759. Epub 2010 Mar 19.

Mathison, D.J. and Agrawal, D. (2010) An update on the epidemiology of pediatric fractures. *Pediatric Emergency Care* **26**(8), 594–603; quiz 604–606.

Müller, M.E., Nazarian, S. and Koch, P. (1990) *The Comprehensive Classification of Fractures of Long Bones,* 1st edn. Springer-Verlag, Berlin.

Orton, E., Kendrick, D., West, J. and Tata, L.J. (2012) Independent risk factors for injury in pre-school children: three population-based nested case-control studies using routine primary care data. *PLoS One* **7**(4): e35193. Epub 2012 Apr 5. Available at: http://injuryprevention.bmj.com/content/18/Suppl_1/A231.3.abstract (accessed 8 April 2014).

Pandya, N.K., Baldwin, K., Kamath, A.F., Wenger, D.R. and Hosalkar, H.S. (2011) Unexplained fractures: child abuse or bone disease? A systematic review. *Clinical Orthopaedics and Related Research* **469**(3), 805–812.

Ring, D., Jupiter, JB. and Waters PM. (1998). Monteggia fractures in children and adults. *Journal of the American Academy of Orthopaedic Surgery,* **6**(4), 215–224.

Ruth, E., Shah, B. and Fales, W. (2009) Evaluating the injury incidence from skate shoes in the United States. *Pediatric Emergency Care,* **25**(5), 321–324.

Saraph, V. and Linhart, W.E. (2005) Modern treatment of pathological fractures in children. *Injury* **36** Suppl 1: A64–74.

Schalamon, J., Dampf, S., Singer, G., *et al.* (2011) Evaluation of fractures in children and adolescents in a Level I Trauma Center in Austria. *Journal of Trauma,* **71**(2), E19–E25.

Slongo, T.F. and Audigé, L. (2007) AO Pediatric Classification Group. Fracture and dislocation classification compendium for children: the AO pediatric comprehensive classification of long bone fractures (PCCF). *Journal of Orthopaedic Trauma,* **21** (10 Suppl), S135–S160.

Skellern, C.Y., Wood, D.O., Murphy, A. and Crawfordm M. (2000) Non-accidental fractures in infants: risk of further abuse. *Journal of Paediatric Child Health,* **36**(6), 590–592.

Storm, S.W., Williams, D.P., Khoury, J. and Lubahn, J.D. (2006) Elbow deformities after fracture. *Hand Clinics,* **22**(1), 121–129.

Valerio, G., Gallè, F., Mancusi, C. *et al.* (2010) Pattern of fractures across pediatric age groups: analysis of individual and lifestyle factors. *BioMedCentral Public Health* **10**, 656. Available at: http://www.biomedcentral.com/1471-2458/10/656 (accessed 20 March 2013).

Wang, Q., Wang, X.F., Iuliano-Burns, S. *et al.* (2010) Rapid growth produces transient cortical weakness: a risk factor for metaphyseal fractures during puberty. *Journal of Bone and Mineral Research,* **25**(7), 1521–1526.

Wood, A.M., Robertson, G.A., Rennie, L., Caesar, B.C. and Court-Brown, CM. The epidemiology of sports-related fractures in adolescents. *Injury* **41**(8), 834–838. Epub 2010 May 23.

Wright, E. (2007a) Care of Child in a Plaster, in *Oxford Handbook of Children's and Young People's Nursing* (eds E.A. Glasper, G. McEwing and J. Richards), Oxford University Press, Oxford, p. 510.

Wright, E. (2007b) Evaluating a Paediatric Assessment Tool. *Journal of Orthopaedic Nursing,* **11**, 20–29.

Wright, E. (2008a) Neurovascular impairment and compartment syndrome: a literature review. *Journal of Children's and Young Peoples Nursing*, **2**(3), 126–130.

Wright, E. (2008b) Application of plaster and observation for neurovascular deficit. In: J. Kelsey and G. McEwing (Eds) *Clinical Skills in Child Health Practice*. Edinburgh: Churchill Livingstone Elsevier, pp. 374–378.

Wright, E. (2011) Treating children's buckle fractures with removable splints. *Nursing Children and Young People*, **23**(10), 14–17.

Wright, E. (2012) Musculoskeletal system – splints, in *Oxford Handbook of Clinical Skills for Children's and Young People's Nursing* (eds P. Dawson, L. Cook, L.J. Holliday and H. Reddy), Oxford University Press, Oxford, pp.486–489.

Yin, Z.G., Zhang, J.B., Kan, S.L. and Wang, X.G. (2012) Diagnostic accuracy of imaging modalities for suspected scaphoid fractures: Meta-analysis combined with latent class analysis. *Journal of Bone Joint Surgery (Britain)*, **94**(8), 1077–1085.

CHAPTER 24

Key fractures relating to infant, child and young person

Thelma Begley[1] and Sonya Clarke[2]
[1] *Trinity College Dublin, Dublin, Ireland*
[2] *Queen's University Belfast, Belfast, UK*

Introduction

Up to 25% of all childhood injuries are fractures (Rennie *et al.*, 2007). The aim of this chapter is to provide evidence-based guidance for the most common fractures in children and adolescents, the mechanism of injury and the typical management and treatment. As a child grows they become more involved in sport, have further freedom and the incidence of fracture increases (Hooton and Scott 2006). A child's musculoskeletal system and the biomechanical composition of children's bones are different to adults. These differences affect how children's fractures occur and are managed. Differences reduce as a child grows, especially as they reach adolescence (Hart *et al.*, 2006a). Fractures in children tend to heal much more rapidly than in adults as their growth plates/physis are open. This results in shorter periods of immobility and less stiffness. Mal-union and non-union occur rarely with children also having great potential for remodelling and reshaping of bone after a fracture heals (Berg 2005).

The factors that need to be considered when assessing children with fractures include:

- age of the child
- mechanism of injury
- location of fracture
- any potential complications
- possibility of physeal injury
- continuing bone growth
- the possibility of non-accidental injury.

The inclusion of the family in the child's care and awareness of family circumstances also need to be considered.

Physeal injuries

Children are at risk of physeal (growth plate) injuries until bone growth is complete. In boys this is age 18 years approximately and girls two years after the beginning of puberty (Lipp 1998). These injuries are common during periods of active growth and more common in boys due to their sporting activities. Injury to the upper limb is more common with the distal radius most affected (Lipp 1998). See Figures 24.1 and 24.2 for examples of growth plate injuries.

The signs of physeal injury are similar to those of a fracture; predominantly with pain and swelling specifically located at the ends of bones (Lipp 1998). Diagnosis of the injury is usually by X-ray. Any child presenting with signs and symptoms should be thoroughly assessed as an initial displacement of the epiphysis may occur before returning to a normal position and result in a shearing injury (Lipp 1998). Any injury that involves the physis should be referred to a specialist orthopaedic surgeon for definitive treatment and follow up. The history of how the injury happened (mechanism) is an essential element of the diagnosis. Injuries are commonly classified using Salter Harris (Salter and Harris 1963) classification (Box 24.1).

Management of the injury and length of immobilisation will depend on the location and extent of injury:

- Salter Harris Type I and II are managed by closed reduction and application of a cast.
- Salter Harris Type III and IV may require open reduction and internal fixation and application of a cast.

A return to mobilisation with full range of motion is the priority following removal of the cast, and may take up

Orthopaedic and Trauma Nursing: An Evidence-based Approach to Musculoskeletal Care, First Edition. Edited by Sonya Clarke and Julie Santy-Tomlinson.

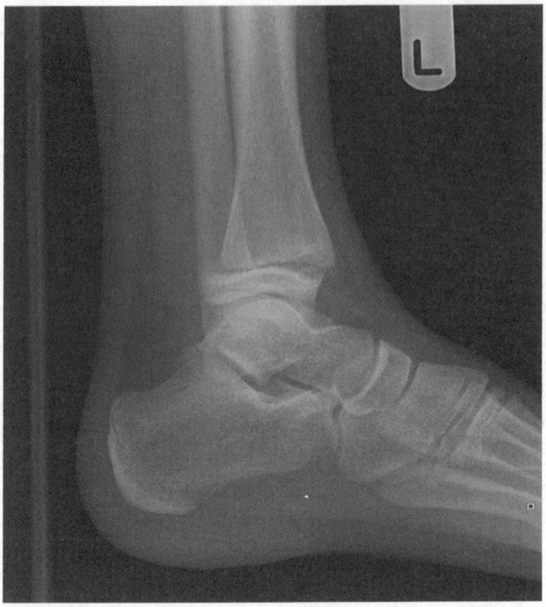

Figure 24.1 Salter Harris Type 1 displaced fracture through the inferior tibial growth plate in a ten-year-old girl

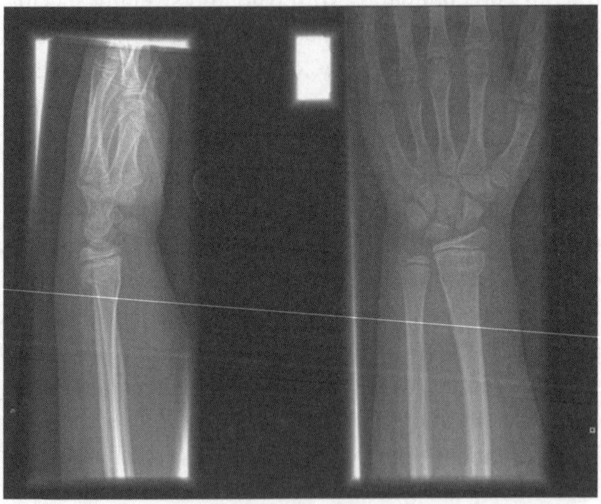

Figure 24.2 Fracture of distal radius-Salter Harris type II with slight displacement

to four weeks. Disturbance of growth may be associated with this injury but is dependent on the bones involved, the extent of the injury and the age at which injury occurs along with the amount of expected remaining growth (Lipp 1998). Complications are uncommon if injuries are managed effectively (Pring and Wenger 2005).

Box 24.1 Salter Harris classification of physeal Injuries

Salter Harris I – the fracture is across the physis and through the weak zones of growth cartilage.
Salter Harris II – fractures extend from the physis into the metaphysis.
Salter Harris III- fracture involves the physis and extends into the epiphysis.
Salter Harris IV- fractures include the physis and extend into both the epiphysis and metaphysis. There is a great potential for growth disruption with this injury.
Salter Harris V – fracture represents a crush to the growth plate and death of the reserve zone cells. It is difficult to identify on X-ray as the physis may appear normal or slightly narrowed so there is risk of delayed diagnosis and potential risk for growth disturbance or deformity.

Upper limb injuries

Clavicle fractures

Clavicle (collar bone) fractures are common in children (see Figure 24.3), often occurring due to a fall or trauma directly to the bone with an incidence of 198 per 100 000 in the 0–14 age group (Nordqvist and Petersson, 1994). Most fractures (80–90%) occur in the middle third of the bone (Hart *et al.*, 2006b) with some fractures incomplete due to the strong periosteum of the clavicle (Shannon *et al.*, 2009).

Signs of a clavicle fracture are:

- tenderness directly over the fracture site
- bruising
- swelling
- crepitus that is easy to palpate as the bone is near the skin surface
- restriction of movement
- holding the arm close to the body and supporting it with the opposite hand.

Neonatal fractures are usually caused by birth trauma especially in infants with a birth weight greater than 4kg and following a difficult delivery (Pring and Wenger 2005). Neonatal fractures may be associated with brachial plexus palsy and will require further evaluation (Dunham 2003; Pring and Wenger 2005) as infants may present with a lack of spontaneous movement. Neonatal clavicle fractures usually heal spontaneously and successfully with the infant starting to move the arm in two to three weeks.

With this fracture, neurovascular observation should be performed on the distal extremities to include pulses, motor function, sensation and reflexes (Shannon *et al.*

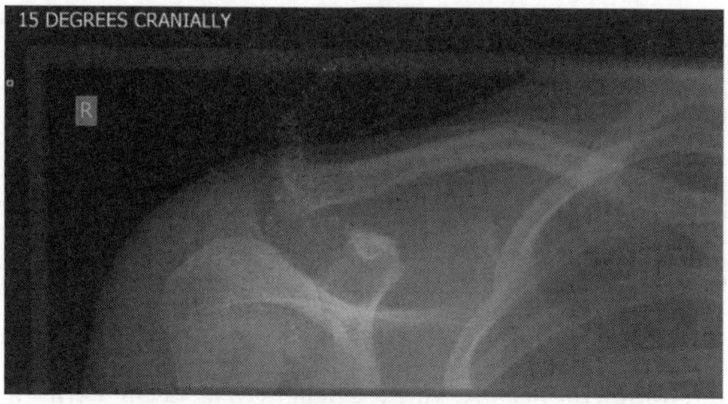

Figure 24.3 Fracture of the mid clavicle with slight angulation in a two-year-old. The shoulder joint is normal

2009). A simple sling is advocated for two to three weeks until the child is comfortable. Pinning the sleeve to the body or wrapping the arm to the body with bandage may be useful for infants (Pring and Wenger 2005) as it may be difficult to restrict movement in this age group. While the majority of fractures heal uneventfully with the use of a simple sling, some angulation and deformity may occur. Fractures may heal with a visible and palpable bump obvious at the fracture site due to increased callus formation. The child will require follow-up X-rays in four to six weeks and contact sports should be avoided for another two to three weeks after that (Hart *et al.*, 2006b).

Surgery is rarely indicated but considered if the fracture is open, the skin is broken, the fracture is complicated or comminuted and where there is neurovascular injury (Moonot and Ashwood 2009). Complications from clavicle fractures in children are rare.

Elbow fractures

Elbow fractures are common in children usually following a fall on an outstretched hand (FOOSH). Care needs to be taken when interpreting X-rays of the elbow and using X-ray as a diagnostic tool; recognition is difficult as the bones of the elbow are poorly developed in childhood and ossify at different rates (Hart *et al.*, 2006b). The location of nerves and vascular structures around the elbow plus the limited ability of the elbow to remodel post fracture mean that elbow fractures are commonly subject to open or closed reduction.

The most common fracture in the elbow region in children is a supracondylar fracture of the humerus (Babel *et al.*, 2010) with peak incidence at ages four to seven years (Hart *et al.*, 2011). It has the highest rate of complications of any fracture in children with a neurological injury or deficit occurring in 20% of cases (Robertson *et al.*, 2012).

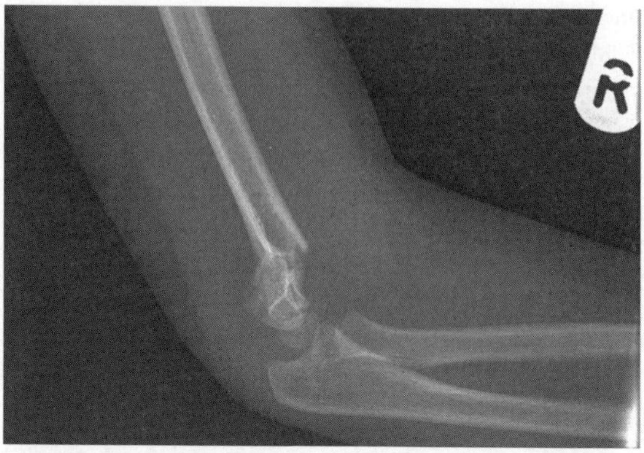

Figure 24.4 Supracondylar fracture of the distal right humerus with significant dorsal angulation of the distal humerus in an eight-year-old

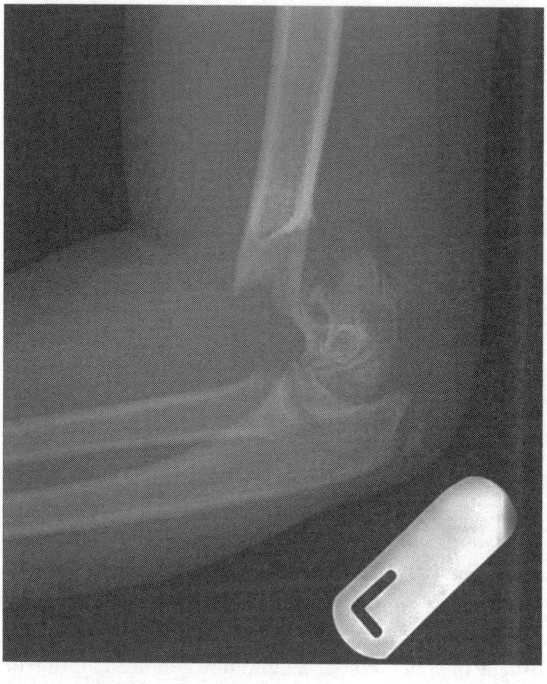

Figure 24.5 Supracondylar fracture of the distal left humerus with gross deformity, displacement and swelling in a nine-year-old

The most common mechanism of injury is a FOOSH. During the fall the child's arm hyperextends and causes a fracture with the distal fragment normally being displaced posteriorly (Hart *et al.*, 2006b) which may affect both the vessels and nerves posterior to the fracture (Figures 24.4 and 24.5). Neurovascular assessment of the

Box 24.2 Evidence digest. Reproduced with permission from BioMed Central Ltd

Neurological status in paediatric upper limb injuries in the emergency department – current practice (Robertson *et al.*, 2012)

Robertson *et al.* (2012) retrospectively reviewed the case notes of all children admitted to an emergency department (ED) with upper limb injuries over a three month period. Inclusion criteria were that the child had an upper limb injury that required admission and intervention from the orthopaedic team under general anaesthetic. 121 patients were identified, 61 males and 60 females and another six who were referred from an ED at another hospital. The age range was from 1–12 years. The commonest injury was a fractured radius and ulna (39.8%) with a fall the most common mechanism of injury (42.1%). Neurological status was documented in 107 cases (88.4%) using the terms 'NVI', 'CSM', 'sensation' and 'moving.' There was no mention of particular nerves being examined in 114 cases with the anterior interosseous nerve never mentioned.

In the three months ten patients had neurological deficits (8.2%) with supracondylar fracture involved in 40% of these. None of these deficits were identified on initial examination in the ED. The authors acknowledge that while some of these may have occurred after ED assessment, this is unclear due to the lack of documentation.

Discussion: Over 90% of patients had no documentation of neurological examination. There were no records of which nerves were assessed or what tests had been performed to assess neurovascular status. This included those who had confirmed neurological injury. The authors concluded that this area of practice was deficient and that there should be documentary evidence that the radial, median, ulnar nerve and anterior interosseous nerve had all been assessed in the ED. Neurovascular assessment of all limb injuries should be standard practice.

arm should involve a thorough evaluation of motor, sensory and vascular structures (Box 24.2). The brachial or radial pulse needs to be assessed to ensure that there is no vascular injury. A white or cool hand or absence of pulse usually indicates arterial compromise and need for urgent reduction. Owing to extensive swelling the arm also needs to be assessed for compartment syndrome (Chapter 9) so neurovascular assessment must be performed regularly and documented accurately. The fractured bone may also cause puckering of the skin (Platt 2004) with an urgent need for reduction so as to prevent the overlying skin becoming ischaemic and necrotic. Neurovascular assessment can be difficult as there will be significant swelling and pain with the child experiencing considerable fear and anxiety. Gaining their cooperation is essential but often difficult because of the challenges associated with a child's level of understanding and compliance (Robertson *et al.*, 2012). Neurovascular observations are also necessary pre- and post-surgery/treatment alongside elevation of the arm with fingers above the elbow recommended. The anatomy of this region is complex leading to high complication rates. Damage to the brachial artery, median nerve and/or ulnar nerve may be possible. A complication associated with the fracture is Volkman's ischaemic contracture; a permanent flexion contracture.

Box 24.3 Gartland's classification (1959)

- Type 1 – undisplaced
- Type 2 – minimally displaced with some bony contact (Figure 24.4)
- Type 3 – completely displaced (no contact between fracture fragments) (Figure 24.5)

Classification is most commonly based on displacement using Gartland's classification (Gartland 1959) (Box 24.3). Treatment will depend on the grade of fracture. Type 1 is usually placed in an above elbow cast or sling for three to four weeks with the elbow held in 90 degrees of flexion unless swelling impedes this (Hart *et al.*, 2006b). Type 2–3 fractures may require surgical intervention with closed or open reduction with pins or Kirschner (K) wires to hold the position after reduction. Three weeks after surgery K wires are removed and the child should be allowed to resume most activities. Children will continue to be monitored for another two to three months. If reduction cannot be achieved with closed reduction open reduction is necessary.

Forearm fractures

Radial fractures (Figures 24.6 and 24.7) are common at any age (Schneider *et al.*, 2007) and this is an expected fracture in older children with the usual mechanism of injury a FOOSH. Increased engagement in sporting activities has increased the incidence of radial fractures (Khosla *et al.*, 2003) and de Putter *et al.* (2011) report that fractures in the five to nine age group are mainly caused by accidents in the home. Those older than nine years primarily fracture their forearm during sporting activity. Radial fractures can be classified as 'plastic deformation' (bowing), 'buckle' (torus) (Figure 24.7), greenstick, transverse, comminuted or physeal (Hart *et al.*, 2006b). Confirmation of fracture is made by antero-posterior (AP)

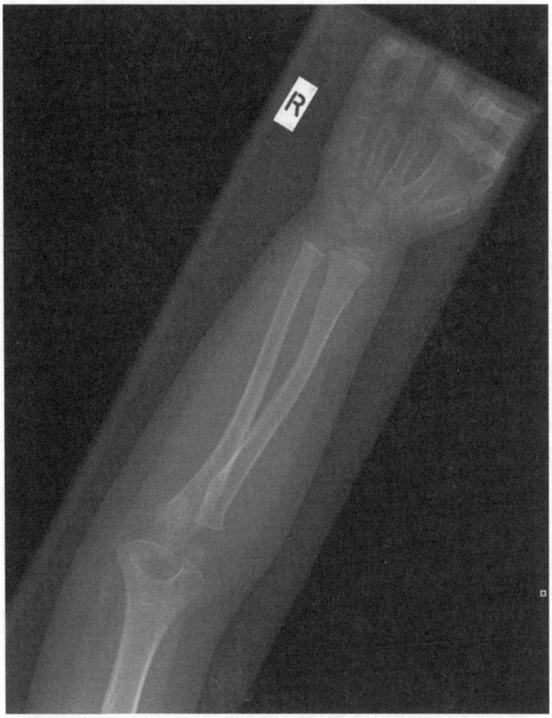

Figure 24.6 Deformity through the proximal radial metaphysis with gross displacement. Displaced and angulated fracture of the proximal ulna shaft

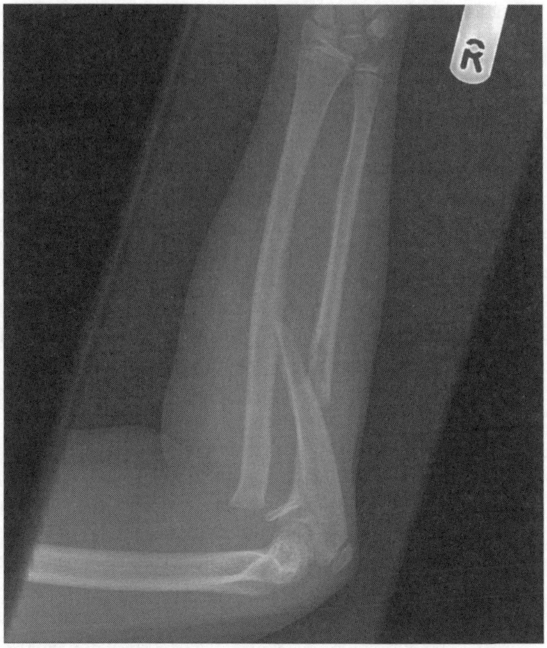

Figure 24.7 Distal radius and ulna buckle fracture without significant deformity and displacement

and lateral X-rays which will also confirm the type of fracture and the bones involved. It is essential in a mid-forearm fracture that both the wrist and elbow are X-rayed to assess for displacement at the joints above and below.

The management of the fracture will depend on the type and location. Closed reduction and immobilisation remains the main treatment option in children (Schneider *et al.*, 2007). Simple stable fractures such as the 'buckle' are managed in a short arm cast for three to four weeks mainly for pain control. After the cast is removed normal activities can resume without restrictions and no review appointment. A splint is an alternative immobilisation option but keeping the splint in place in children can be difficult. This has been the subject of a Cochrane systematic review (Box 24.4).

A thorough examination of the arm must be carried out to identify if ulnar fractures are present as the management changes i.e. application of a long arm cast and possibly a longer period of immobilisation. The arm must also be assessed for other fractures caused by a FOOSH such as a scaphoid or supracondylar fracture (Hart *et al.*, 2006b). Injuries to the radial, median or ulnar nerve can also occur with this fracture. Increased swelling is also a feature especially if the fracture is displaced and compartment syndrome can be a complication. The fracture may heal with some displacement but there is no consensus in the literature on how much displacement is acceptable and can be left to normal remodelling (Schneider *et al.*, 2007).

Hand and finger fractures

Hand fractures (Figure 24.8) are common in children and young people with the fifth metacarpal and phalanges the most common bones affected. Treatment is by closed reduction with casting/splinting. It can be difficult to keep a splint on a young child with hand and finger fractures but they usually heal quite quickly with casts in place for 3–6 weeks depending on the injury (Hart *et al.*, 2006b).

Different casts are applied depending on the area of the hand involved. Thumb fractures are treated by immobilisation in a 'thumb spica'. Fractures of the index finger are often treated in a radial 'gutter' short-arm cast and those of long, ring and little fingers with an ulnar gutter short-arm cast (Hart *et al.*, 2006b). Finger fractures must also be assessed for physeal injuries.

Box 24.4 Evidence digest. Reproduced with permission from Cochrane

Cochrane review: casting v splinting in forearm fractures (Abraham *et al.*, 2008)

This systematic review evaluated removable splintage versus plaster casts for undisplaced 'buckle' forearm fractures. Cast length, position and surgical fixation for displaced wrist fractures in children were considered. Ten trials involving 827 children concluded that minor buckle fractures could be treated by a removable splint. Fractures that have the potential to displace should be placed in below elbow casts. While surgery helped to avoid re-displacement of some types of fractures the long-term benefits were unconfirmed. Two of three search authors evaluated the quality of the studies and extracted data. Searches between 1966 to 2007 were performed of the Cochrane Bone, Joint and Muscle Trauma Group Specialised Register (2007) and Central Register of Controlled Trials, Medline, Embase, Cinahl and their reference lists. Randomised and quasi-randomised controlled trials comparing types and position of casts plus surgical fixation were considered.

Findings: four trials compared removable splints versus traditional below-elbow casts in children with buckle fractures. No short term deformity was noted in the four trials with one having no re-fracture in six months. The 'Futura' splint was shown to be cheaper, less restrictive and preferred by child and parent. Children were able to bathe and be active with less restriction. A soft bandage was more comfortable, convenient and less painful. Home removal plaster casts by parents did not produce less favourable outcomes and were preferred. Two trials evaluated below-elbow and above-elbow casts – cast type did not affect re-displacement of reduced fractures or cast-related complications. One trial considered the effect of arm position in above-elbow casts and found no effect on deformity. Three trials found percutaneous wiring significantly reduced re-displacement and re-manipulation – one found no advantage in function at three months after injury.

Summary: Limited evidence supports the use of removable splintage for buckle fractures instead of above-elbow casts in fractures of the forearm after reduction. Percutaneous wiring prevents re-displacement but the effects on long-term arm function are unclear. Further research is required to establish the optimum approach to splints and above-elbow casts after reduction of displaced fractures. Minor buckle fractures can be treated by a splint that is removable at home. Fractures that have the potential to re-displace could be put in below-elbow casts. Surgery helps to avoid re-displacement in some types of fractures, but long-term benefit is unconfirmed.

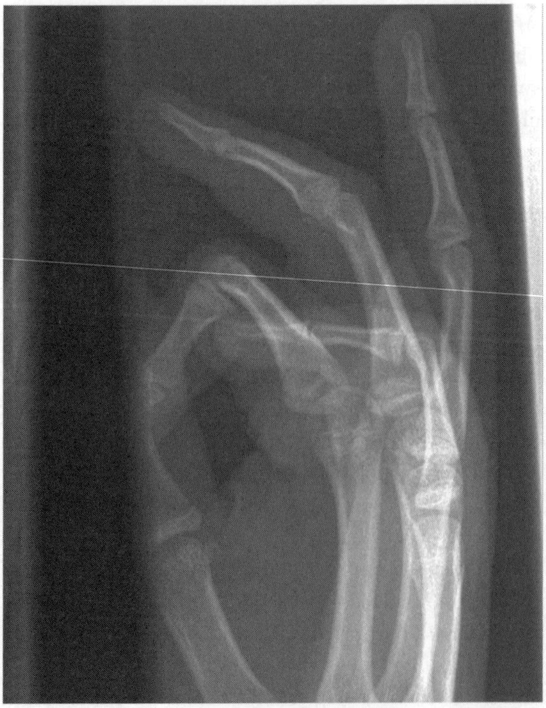

Figure 24.8 Fractures of the palmar aspects of the proximal ends of middle phalanges of the 3rd and 4th fingers

Fractures of the scaphoid bone are common in young people, presenting in isolation or with other injuries of the hand (see Figure 24.9). Diagnosis is made on the basis of patient history, examination and clinical signs plus tenderness of the 'anatomical snuff box' and X-ray. There is a risk of non-union and osteonecrosis with this fracture type and if displaced internal fixation may be necessary to maintain blood supply to fragments (Gillon 2001).

Lower extremity fractures

Femoral shaft fractures

While fractures of the femoral shaft are less common in children than adults (see Figure 24.10) it is the most typical fracture requiring hospitalisation as it is associated with high impact trauma usually resulting from road traffic accidents. Bener *et al.* (2007) conducted a retrospective review of femoral fracture incidence in Qatar between January 1992–December 2004. There were 256 femoral fractures in young people aged 1–16 in that timeframe in 82% boys and 18% girls. The frequent sites of presenting femoral fractures included 16 of the neck (6.3%), 33 upper third (12.9%), 147 middle (57.4%), 38 lower (14.8%) and 22 condyle

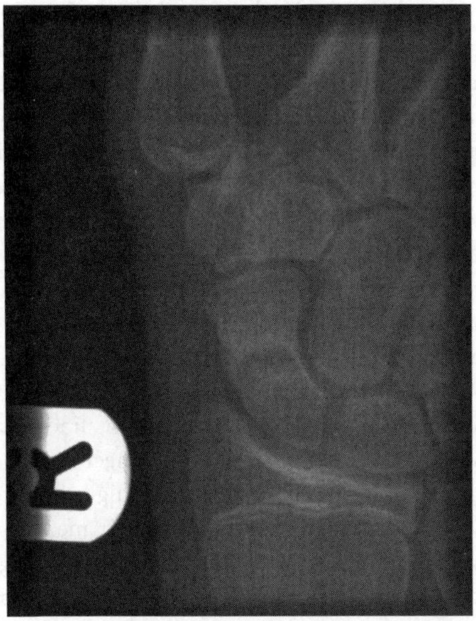

Figure 24.9 An ununited fracture of the mid scaphoid with no evidence of avascular necrosis following an injury six months earlier

(8.6%). The most common mechanism of injury was pedestrian motor vehicle accident (43.4%).

Treatment of femoral shaft fractures depend on the site and extent of fracture, the age of the child and if open or closed reduction is required. Standard treatment is for infants to be immobilised in a Pavlik harness (Chapter 22) younger children in traction (Chapter 8), Thomas splint (Chapter 8) or spica cast (Chapter 22) and adolescents treated with internal fixation with an intramedullary nail. The length of hospitalisation may vary greatly depending on the method of treatment (Table 24.1).

While age-based algorithms are useful in suggesting treatment methods there are other factors to be considered. The ability to care for a child at home is an important consideration. Traction still remains a viable option where other treatment options are not suitable. Anglen and Choi (2005) advocate that spica casting in children over 100 pounds (approximately 45 kg) may not be effective or safe and size, weight, activity level and family circumstances will also need to be considered.

Surgical treatment may be considered superior in older or larger children and adolescents. This is especially the case following multiple trauma and with soft tissue injury, obesity or head injury. Box 24.5 discusses evidence that highlights the increased risk of complications in children who are obese. Adolescents who have

Table 24.1 Options for treatment of femoral shaft fractures depending on age (Pring *et al.*, 2005). Reproduced with permission from LWW

Age of child	Standard treatment	Complex/ open fractures
Under two	Pavlik harness, single leg spica	Skin traction with delayed casting
Two to six years	Early spica cast	Skin or skeletal traction, plate fixation or external fixator
6–14 years	Traction followed by application of spica cast, external fixation or flexible intramedullary nails	Skeletal traction, plate fixation, external fixator
Over 14 years	Interlocking rigid intramedullary nails	Skeletal traction, plate fixation, external fixator

Box 24.5 Evidence digest

Obesity and surgery for fractured shaft of femur

Leet *et al.* (2005) undertook a retrospective review of the charts of children who were admitted with femoral shaft fractures between the ages of 6–14 and had surgery. 104 children were identified with 59 having external fixation and 45 an intramedullary rod inserted. Six children were considered obese and four were overweight at the time of surgery and of those ten, four (40%) had complications post-surgery that required admission to hospital. These complications were infections that required IV antibiotics or wound dehiscence. Twelve percent of the remaining children had a complication.

The authors concluded that obese children have an increased risk of postoperative complications compared with children who are not obese and that parents of children who are obese should be warned about this increased risk.

reached an acceptable size may be considered for rigid nailing and in younger children flexible nailing may be used (Anglen and Choi 2005). Flexible nailing is well suited to fractures of the central 2/3 of the diaphysis. However, surgery is not without complications. Leet *et al.*'s (2005) limitations highlighted a lack of consistency in the measurement of obesity.

Fractures of the femur in children under five years usually have further investigation as non-accidental injury may be suspected (Anglen and Choi 2005, Pring *et al.*, 2005). However, it must also be noted that this is not the cause in the majority of cases, with a fractured femur also occurring from minimal trauma during play in the young child (Pring *et al.*, 2005). Therefore, this fracture type needs to be managed by experienced professionals in a non-judgmental manner (Chapter 21). Complications associated with fractures of the femur depend on the site of the fracture and the method of treatment. Attention is required in the management to ensure leg length is maintained (Pring *et al.*, 2005) especially as the age of the child increases as there is less time for remodelling.

Tibial fracture

Tibia fracture is also a common injury in children with 50% of all tibial fractures occurring in the distal third (Setter and Palomino 2006). The mechanism of injury is usually direct or indirect force. Indirect force is mainly sports, motor vehicle accidents and falls (Mubarak *et al.*, 2009) with football, skiing and rugby all associated with this type of fracture (Rennie *et al.*, 2007). Fractures are usually oblique or spiral (see Figure 24.11) with the younger child requiring less force than in those who are older. Typically a child with a tibial fracture will present with a history of a traumatic event (either witnessed or unwitnessed), pain, an inability to weight bear, swelling, bruising and deformity (Setter and Palomino, 2006). Younger children, especially toddlers, may not have swelling and deformity. In 30% of tibial fractures, a fracture of the fibula will also be present (Hart *et al.*, 2006c). AP and lateral X-ray views that include the knee and ankle are required to confirm the diagnosis.

Simple closed tibial fractures in children can be managed with closed reduction and immobilisation without a need for surgery (Hart *et al.*, 2006c). Surgery may be required if the fracture is open, comminuted and/or irreducible or if casting has been unsuccessful. As always, understanding the mechanism of injury may help in the reduction of the fracture (Mubarak *et al.*, 2009). The length of time in a cast following reduction will depend on type and location of fracture, the treatment and age of the child. The younger the child the less time they spend immobilised, ranging from three to four weeks for a toddler to three to four months for a young person/adolescent. A full or half (short) leg cast will be applied depending on the fracture location. Mubarak *et al.* (2009) recommends a long leg cast to be applied for four to six weeks for both non-displaced metaphyseal and physeal fractures. However, a displaced metaphyseal fracture requires a closed or open reduction under general anaesthetic plus a cast for six to eight weeks. For a displaced physeal fracture suggested treatment is open reduction with internal fixation which may

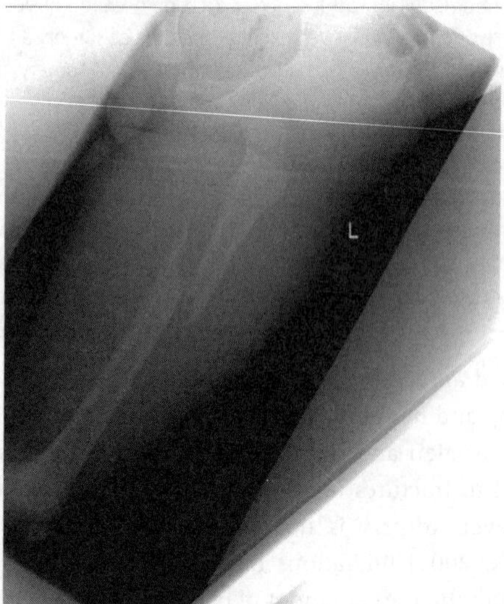

Figure 24.10 Oblique femoral mid-shaft fracture

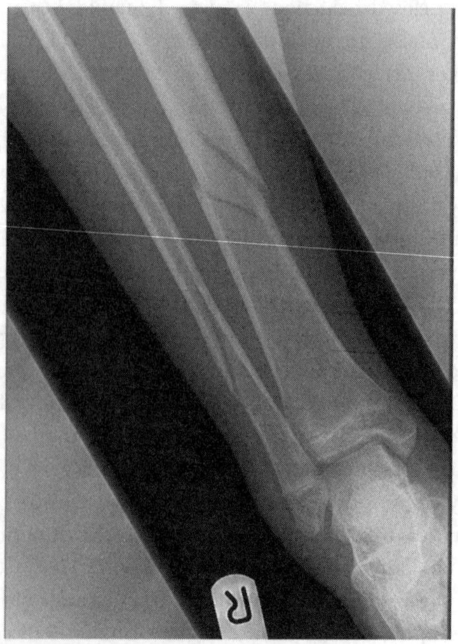

Figure 24.11 An oblique/spiral distal tibial and fibula fracture with minimal deformity

need CT (computerised tomography) to help plan for surgery and a long leg cast for four to six weeks. Finally, extra articular fractures (through a joint) involving the physis will require either a closed or open reduction with internal fixation and long leg cast.

Acute compartment syndrome (ACS) is also a complication of this fracture type. Careful observation of neurovascular status is required regardless of the method of treatment and immobilisation. An acceleration of pain is the predominant symptom of ACS with presence especially on passive movement which will require splitting of a cast or padding (Hart *et al.*, 2006c) and a thorough evaluation of the leg including possible measurement of incompartmental pressure (Chapter 9). Early recognition of compartment syndrome generally leads to a favourable outcome for the child and the importance of regular neurovascular observations performed accurately cannot be over-emphasised. In fractures with physeal involvement long-term follow-up for evaluation of physeal closure should be advocated (Mubarak *et al.*, 2009).

A 'toddler' fracture is an undisplaced tibial fracture in a child under three years of age (Shravat *et al.*, 1996). The child will present with guarding of the limb, a limp or an inability to weight bear (Hart *et al.*, 2006c). Swelling and deformity may not be presenting symptoms. The mechanism of injury varies and occasionally the history is vague with the injury not noticed until the child is limping. X-rays may be inconclusive with no fracture visible and follow-up not necessary. It will also be necessary to rule out other causes of a limp such as irritable hip or Perthes disease. Usual management is application of a cast for comfort with the child allowed to walk and the site of the fracture determining what kind of cast is applied.

A Cozen's fracture is a fracture of the proximal metaphyseal tibia in children mainly between ages three to six years. A typical mechanism of injury is trampoline jumping where often one child gets injured because there are several jumping (Mubarak *et al.*, 2009). Treatment of a non-displaced fracture is with a long leg cast for six weeks with the knee flexed to ten degrees and a varus mould (Setter and Palamino 2006). A displaced fracture will require reduction under general anaesthetic and a long leg cast applied for six to eight weeks. It is a Palomino, an uncommon fracture but clinically important as development of post-fracture progressive valgus deformity can occur. It is reported that this valgus deformity occurs in approximately 50% of fractures in this area (Setter and Palomino 2006). Treatment of valgus deformity in younger children is primarily conservative, monitoring the leg until after puberty as it is possible that some remodelling may take place. The importance of regular follow-up must be stressed to the family. Surgery may be considered if no significant improvement has taken place and the child has reached puberty.

Ankle fractures

Ankle fractures are also common in children and most fractures happen in the distal third of the tibia and fibula (medial and lateral malleolus) as a result of twisting, falls and direct trauma between the ages of 10–15. The clinical signs are pain, swelling, deformity and difficulty/inability to weight bear. Initial treatment of ankle fractures is known by the anagram 'PRICE' – *protection, rest, ice, compression* and *elevation* (Nicholas and Cooper 2009). Diagnosis is on the basis of both AP and lateral plain X-rays. It is also important to be aware that distal tibial fractures can involve the physis and this is the second most common site of Salter Harris injuries after the radius (Hart *et al.*, 2006c). The grading of injury will affect how the child is managed; closed reduction to grades I and II and open reduction and stabilisation to grades III and IV. All fractures will require casting for six to eight weeks (Figure 24.12). The majority of fractures in this area have

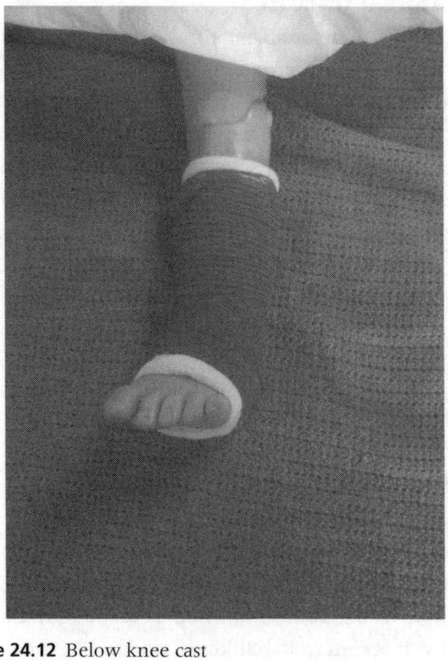

Figure 24.12 Below knee cast

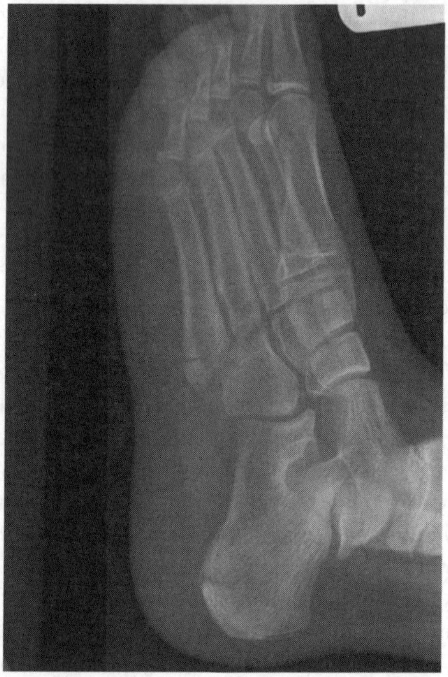

Figure 24.13 Fracture through the base of the fifth metatarsal

a good prognosis but this depends on the severity of the injury, the skeletal age of the young person, fracture type and the reduction achieved (Hart *et al.*, 2006c).

Metatarsal fractures

Fractures of the metatarsal are the most common fracture of the foot in children. See Figure 24.13 for an example. The first and fifth metatarsals are the usual sites. Mechanisms of injury include falling from a low height such as a bed or something heavy falling onto a foot. Physical examination reveals swelling, inability to weight-bear, bruising or limp. Diagnosis is determined using anterolateral and oblique X-rays (Hart *et al.*, 2006) with conservative treatment with application of a short leg walking cast for three to four weeks. Open, displaced or comminuted fractures will require further operative treatment.

Spinal cord injury (SCI)

Chapter 19 of this book is dedicated to spinal cord injury. SCI in children is uncommon (Vogel *et al.*, 2004; Johnston *et al.*, 2005; Mathison *et al.*, 2008) but the severity is greater. In children under five years the incidence of injury in males and females is equal. However, as they grow older the incidence in males far exceeds that in females. Worldwide, sports such as diving, soccer, rugby, horseback riding, skiing, wrestling, trampoline and bicycle accidents are common causes for spinal injuries. Motor vehicles are the greatest cause and result in more serious injury. It is hoped that the implementation of the correct use of car seats for children can result in a reduction of SCI (Vogel *et al.*, 2004). Violence is reported as a common cause in adolescents especially due to street violence (Mathison *et al.*, 2008). Johnston *et al.* (2005) retrospectively reviewed the records from 1986 to 2003 of 190 children who had suffered spinal cord injury in Pennsylvania and found the most common causes were vehicular (n=105), sports (n=25), gunshot wound (n=26), medical (n=16) and other (n=18). Other reasons included falls, direct trauma to the spine, roller coaster and birth injury.

The diagnosis of spinal cord injury in children is comparatively difficult as it is not always obvious on X-rays (Mathison *et al.*, 2008) and many children present with spinal cord injury without radiographic abnormality (SCIWORA). The advent of MRI has advanced the diagnosis of SCIWORA and it is estimated that 30–40% of children with traumatic spinal injury have such a condition (Li *et al.*, 2011). Laxity of ligaments in children means that the vertebral column can stretch without disruption but the spinal cord can only stretch minimally and so becomes damaged. As children grow this laxity decreases so SCIWORA is most common in children under eight years of age. Damage to the spinal cord can be complete or incomplete with the younger child more at risk of complete injury (Mathison *et al.*, 2008).

Assessment of the child with a spinal injury consists of history, physical examination, X-rays, CT and MRI. Treatment options are limited with immobilisation in an age-appropriate orthosis or surgical stabilisation recommended (Mathison *et al.*, 2008; Li *et al.*, 2011). Musculoskeletal complications in children with SCI are scoliosis and hip dysplasia with a large proportion of those who suffer SCI before puberty developing both and requiring corrective surgery (Vogel *et al.*, 2004). This reduces significantly in those injured after puberty.

The effect of the injury on the child and family is enormous with changes evident within family dynamics and the team focus to ensure both child and family adjust to the injury. The provision of coordinated care by a multidisciplinary team is essential. The goal for all is to maintain active participation at home, school and other activities so to ensure they continue to develop socially. The focus is on promoting independence, rehabilitation and transition from hospital to home (Vogel *et al.*, 2004). The reader should refer to Chapter 19 for further discussion of care following spinal cord injury.

Non-accidental injury

In frequent or multiple fractures in children the most likely cause is non-accidental injury (NAI) (Jenny 2006). Carty (1993) identified metaphyseal, rib, scapular, vertebral or subluxations plus fracture of the outer end of the clavicle. In addition finger injuries in non-ambulant children, bilateral and complex skull fractures plus fractures at different stages of healing were identified as the most common sites for NAI fractures.

Children under two and those who are pre-verbal are most at risk (Jenny 2006). Issues for practitioners to consider are:

- fractures are often found in cases of fatal abuse
- fractures of normal bones (non-pathological) require considerable force
- fractures that are sudden and painful – the child does not play normally afterwards
- pain is immediately worse after the fracture
- in late presentation loss of function may be the only symptom
- lack of associated bruising does not exclude NAI
- most abusive fractures are in children under three years
- most non-abusive fractures occur in children over five years (Selby 2011).

Practitioners also need to remember that several medical conditions may cause multiple fractures in children. These are osteogenesis imperfecta, preterm birth, rickets, osteomyelitis, copper deficiency or bones that are demineralised secondary to paralysis. Many parents whose child has such disorders report they were initially accused of abusing their child. Hence, children need a careful assessment if NAI is suspected including a full history, skeletal survey, bloods for metabolic or bone disease and eye examination (Jenny 2006). Most units have protocols for this and children less than two years of age will be reviewed by a paediatrician before discharge to ensure that children who may be at risk of future injury are not discharged until review is completed. The reader should review Chapter 21 for further detail regarding NAI.

Summary

This chapter updates the reader on how best to care for the infant, child and young person presenting with common fractures.

Recommended further reading

Pandya, N., Baldwin, K., Kamath, A., Wenger, D. and Hosalkar, H. (2011) Unexplained fractures: child abuse or bone disease – a systematic review. *Clinical Orthopaedic Related Research*, **469**, 805–812.

Rang, M., Pring, M. and Wenger, D (2005) *Rang's Children's Fractures*, 3rd edn. Lippincott Williams and Wilkins, Philadelphia.

References

Abraham, A., Handoll, H.H.G. and Khan, T. (2008) Interventions for treating wrist fractures in children (review). *Cochrane Database of Systematic Reviews* **2**(Art No: CD004576). DOI:10.1002/14651858.CD004576.pub2.

Anglen, J. and Choi, L. (2005) Treatment options in pediatric femoral shaft fractures. *Journal of Orthopaedic Trauma*, **19** (10), 724–733.

Babel, J.C., Mehlman, C.T. and Klein, G. (2010) Nerve injuries associated with pediatric supracondylar humeral fractures: a meta- analysis. *Journal of Pediatric Orthopaedics*, **30**(3), 253–263.

Bener, A., Justham, D., Azhar, A., Rysavy, M. and Al-Mulla, F. (2007) Femoral fractures in children related to motor vehicle injuries. *Journal of Orthopaedic Nursing*, **11**, 146–150.

Berg, E.E. (2005) Pediatric distal double bone formation fracture remodeling. *Orthopaedic Nursing*, **24**(1), 55–59.

Carty, H. (1993) Fractures caused by child abuse. *Journal of Bone and Joint Surgery (British)*, **75-B**, 849–857.

de Putter, C.E., van Beeck, E.F., Looman, W. *et al.* (2011) Trends in wrist fractures in children and adolescents, 1997–2009. *Journal of Hand Surgery*, **236A**, 1810–1815.

Dunham, E.A. (2003) Obstetrical brachial plexus palsy. *Orthopaedic Nursing*, **22**(2), 106–116.

Gartland, J.J. (1959) Management of supracondylar fractures of the humerus in children. *Surgery, Gynaecology and Obstetrics*, **109**(2), 145–154.

Gillon, H. (2001) Scaphoid injuries in children. *Accident and Emergency Nursing*, **9**, 249–256.

Hart, E.S., Albright, M., Gleeson, N.R. and Grottkau, B.E. (2006a) Common pediatric fractures – Part I. *Orthopaedic Nursing*, **25**(4), 251–256.

Hart, E.S., Grottkau, B.E., Rebello, G.N. and Albright, M.B. (2006b) Broken bones: common pediatric upper extremity fractures – Part II. *Orthopaedic Nursing*, **25**(5), 311–325.

Hart, E.S., Luther, B. and Grottkau, B.E. (2006c) Broken bones: common lower extremity fractures – Part III. *Orthopaedic Nursing*, **25**(6), 390–409.

Hart, E.S., Turner, A., Albright, M. and Grottkau, B. (2011) Common pediatric elbow fractures. *Orthopaedic Nursing*, **30**(1), 11–16.

Hooton, S. and Scott, D. (2006) Health needs of middle childhood, in: *A Textbook of Children's and Young People's Nursing*, 1st edn (eds A. Glasper and J. Richardson), Churchill Livingstone Elseiver, Edinburgh, pp. 686–699.

Hoskote, A., Martin, K., Hormbrey, P. and Burns, E.C. (2003) Fractures in infants: one in four is non-accidental. *Child Abuse Review*, **12**, 384–391.

Jenny, C. (2006) Evaluating infants and young children with multiple fractures. *Pediatrics*, **118**(3), 1299–1303.

Johnston, T.E., Greco, M.N., Gaughan, J.P., Smith, B.T. and Betz, R.R. (2005) Patterns of lower extremity innervation in pediatric spinal cord injury. *Spinal Cord*, **43**, 476–482.

Khosla, S., Melton, L., Dekutoski, M. *et al.* (2003) Incidence of childhood distal forearm fractures over 30 years. *Journal of the American Medical Association*, **290**, 1479–1485.

Leet, A., Pichard, C and Ain, M. (2005) Surgical treatment of femoral fractures in obese children: does excessive body weight increase the rate of complications? *Journal of Bone and Joint Surgery (American)*, **87-A**(12), 2609–2613.

Li, Y., Glotzbecker, M., Hedequist, D. and Mahan, S. (2011) Pediatric spinal trauma. *Trauma*, **14**(1), 82–96.

Lipp, E.J. (1998) Athletic physeal injury in children and adolescents. *Orthopaedic Nursing*, **17**(2), 17–22.

Mathison, D., Kadom, N. and Krug, S. (2008) Spinal cord injury in the pediatric patient. *Clinical Pediatric Emergency Medicine*, **9**, 106–123.

Moonot, P. and Ashwood, N. (2009) Clavicle fractures. *Trauma*, **11**, 123–132.

Mubarak, S., Ryul Kim, J., Edmonds, E., Pring, M. and Bastrom, T. (2009) Classification of proximal tibial fractures in children. *Journal of Children's Orthopaedics*, **3**, 191–197.

Nicholas, M. and Cooper, L. (2009) Assessment of ankle injuries. *The Journal of School Nursing*, **25**(1), 34–39.

Nordqvist, A. and Petersson, C. (1994) The incidence of fractures of the clavicle. *Clinical Orthopaedic Related Research*, **300**, 127–132.

Platt, B (2004) Supracondylar fracture of the humerus. *Emergency Nurse*, **12**(2), 22–30.

Pring, M. and Wenger, D. (2005) Clavicle, in *Rang's Children's Fractures*, 3rd edn (eds M. Rang, M. Pring and Wenger, D.), Lippincott Williams and Wilkins, Philadelphia, pp. 76–83.

Pring, M., Newton, P. and Rang, M. (2005) Femoral shaft, in *Rang's Children's Fractures*, 3rd edn (eds M. Rang, M. Pring and Wenger, D.), Lippincott Williams and Wilkins, Philadelphia, pp. 182–200.

Rennie, L., Court-Brown, C., Mok, J. and Beattie, T. (2007) The epidemiology of fractures in children. *Injury*, **38**, 913–922.

Robertson, J., Marsh, A. and Huntley, J. (2012) Neurological status in paediatric upper limb injuries in the emergency department – current practice. *BioMed Central Research Notes* **5**, 324. DOI: 10.1186/1756-0500-5-324.

Salter, R.B. and Harris, W.R. (1963) Injuries involving the epiphyseal plate. *Journal of Bone and Joint Surgery (American)*, **45-A**, 587–623.

Schneider, J., Staubli, G., Kubat, S. and Altermatt, S. (2007) Treating displaced distal forearm fractures in children. *European Journal of Trauma and Emergency Surgery*, **33**, 619–625.

Selby, M. (2011) Child protection and safeguarding. *Practice Nurse*, **41**(4), 32–39.

Setter, K.J. and Palomino, K.E. (2006) Pediatric tibia fractures: current concepts. *Current Opinion in Pediatrics*, **18**, 30–35.

Shannon, E., Hart, E. and Grottkau, B. (2009) Clavicle fractures in children: the essentials. *Orthopaedic Nursing*, **28**(5), 210–216.

Shravat, B.P., Harrop, S.N. and Kane, T.P. (1996) Toddler's fracture. *Journal of Accident and Emergency Medicine*, **13**, 59–61.

Vogel, L., Hickey, K., Klass, S. and Anderson, C. (2004) Unique issues in pediatric spinal cord injury. *Orthopaedic Nursing*, **23** (5), 300–310.

Index

Note: Page numbers in *italics* refer to Figures; those in **bold** to Tables.

Orthopaedic and Trauma Nursing: An Evidence-based Approach to Musculoskeletal Care, First Edition. Edited by Sonya Clarke and Julie Santy-Tomlinson.